CURRENT THERAPY IN PLASTIC AND RECONSTRUCTIVE SURGERY

Trunk and Extremities

Surgical Titles in the Current Therapy Series

Callaham:
Current Therapy in Emergency Medicine
Cameron:
Current Surgical Therapy
Charles, Glover:
Current Therapy in Obstetrics
Ernst, Stanley:
Current Therapy in Vascular Surgery
Fazio:
Current Therapy in Colon and Rectal Surgery
Foley, Payne:
Current Therapy of Pain
Garcia, Mastroianni, Amelar, Dubin:
Current Therapy of Infertility
Garcia, Mikuta, Rosenblum:
Current Therapy in Surgical Gynecology
Gates:
Current Therapy in Otolaryngology—Head and Neck Surgery
Grillo, Austen, Wilkins, Mathisen, Vlahakes:
Current Therapy in Cardiothoracic Surgery
Jay:
Current Therapy in Podiatric Surgery
Long:
Current Therapy in Neurological Surgery
Marsh:
Current Therapy in Plastic and Reconstructive Surgery
Parrillo:
Current Therapy in Critical Care Medicine
Resnick, Kursh:
Current Therapy in Genitourinary Surgery
Rogers:
Current Practice in Anesthesiology
Spaeth, Katz:
Current Therapy in Ophthalmic Surgery
Trunkey, Lewis:
Current Therapy of Trauma
Torg, Welsh, Shephard:
Current Therapy in Sports Medicine

CURRENT THERAPY IN PLASTIC AND RECONSTRUCTIVE SURGERY

Trunk and Extremities

JEFFREY L. MARSH, M.D.

Professor of Surgery
Plastic and Reconstructive
Washington University School of Medicine
Medical Director
Cleft Palate and Craniofacial Deformities Institute
Children's Hospital
St. Louis, Missouri

1989

B.C. Decker Inc • Toronto • Philadelphia

Publisher

B.C. Decker Inc
3228 South Service Road
Burlington, Ontario L7N 3H8

B.C. Decker Inc
320 Walnut Street
Suite 400
Philadelphia, Pennsylvania 19106

Sales and Distribution

United States and Puerto Rico
The C.V. Mosby Company
11830 Westline Industrial Drive
Saint Louis, Missouri 63146

Canada
McAinsh & Co. Ltd.
2760 Old Leslie Street
Willowdale, Ontario M2K 2X5

Australia
McGraw-Hill Book Company Australia Pty. Ltd.
4 Barcoo Street
Roseville East 2069
New South Wales, Australia

Brazil
Editora McGraw-Hill do Brasil, Ltda.
rua Tabapua, 1.105, Itaim-Bibi
Sao Paulo, S.P. Brasil

Colombia
Interamericana/McGraw-Hill de Colombia, S.A.
Apartado Aereo 81078
Bogota, D.E. Colombia

Europe
McGraw-Hill Book Company GmbH
Lademannbogen 136
D-2000 Hamburg 63
West Germany

France
MEDSI/McGraw-Hill
6, avenue Daniel Lesueur
75007 Paris, France

Hong Kong and China
McGraw-Hill Book Company
Suite 618, Ocean Centre
5 Canton Road
Tsimshatsui, Kowloon
Hong Kong

India
Tata McGraw-Hill Publishing Company, Ltd.
12/4 Asaf Ali Road, 3rd Floor
New Delhi 110002, India

Indonesia
P.O. Box 122/JAT
Jakarta, 1300 Indonesia

Italy
McGraw-Hill Libri Italia, s.r.l.
Piazza Emilia, 5
I-20129 Milano MI
Italy

Japan
Igaku-Shoin Ltd.
Tokyo International P.O. Box 5063
1-28-36 Hongo, Bunkyo-ku,
Tokyo 113, Japan

Korea
C.P.O. Box 10583
Seoul, Korea

Malaysia
No. 8 Jalan SS 7/6B
Kelana Jaya
47301 Petaling Jaya
Selangor, Malaysia

Mexico
Interamericana/McGraw-Hill de Mexico, S.A. de C.V.
Cedro 512, Colonia Atlampa
(Apartado Postal 26370)
06450 Mexico, D.F., Mexico

New Zealand
McGraw-Hill Book Co. New Zealand Ltd.
5 Joval Place, Wiri
Manukau City, New Zealand

Panama
Editorial McGraw-Hill Latinoamericana, S.A.
Apartado Postal 2036
Zona Libre de Colon
Colon, Republica de Panama

Portugal
Editora McGraw-Hill de Portugal, Ltda.
Rua Rosa Damasceno 11A–B
1900 Lisboa, Portugal

South Africa
Libriger Book Distributors
Warehouse Number 8
"Die Ou Looiery"
Tannery Road
Hamilton, Bloemfontein 9300

Southeast Asia
McGraw-Hill Book Co.
348 Jalan Boon Lay
Jurong, Singapore 2261

Spain
McGraw-Hill/Interamericana de Espana, S.A.
Manuel Ferrero, 13
28020 Madrid, Spain

Taiwan
P.O. Box 87–601
Taipei, Taiwan

Thailand
632/5 Phaholyothin Road
Sapan Kwai
Bangkok 10400
Thailand

United Kingdom, Middle East and Africa
McGraw-Hill Book Company (U.K.) Ltd.
Shoppenhangers Road
Maidenhead, Berkshire
SL6 2QL England

Venezuela
McGraw-Hill/Interamericana, C.A.
2da. calle Bello Monte
(entre avenida Casanova y Sabana Grande)
Apartado Aereo 50785
Caracas 1050, Venezuela

NOTICE

The authors and publisher have made every effort to ensure that the patient care recommended herein, including choice of drugs and drug dosages, is in accord with the accepted standards and practice at the time of publication. However, since research and regulation constantly change clinical standards, the reader is urged to check the product information sheet included in the package of each drug, which includes recommended doses, warnings, and contraindications. This is particularly important with new or infrequently used drugs.

Current Therapy in Plastic and Reconstructive Surgery–Trunk and Extremities ISBN 1–55664–101–X

Library of Congress catalog card number: 88–72309

10 9 8 7 6 5 4 3 2 1

CONTRIBUTORS
Volume 2

JAMES L. BAKER Jr., M.D., F.A.C.S.

Adjunct Professor of Surgery, College of Health, University of Central Florida, Orlando, Florida; Active Staff, Orlando Regional Medical Center, and Courtesy Staff, Winter Park Memorial Hospital, and Florida Hospital of Orlando, Florida
Augmentation Mammoplasty: A Personal Approach

ROBERT W. BERNARD, M.D.

Chief (Emeritus), Plastic Surgery, White Plains Hospital, White Plains, Chief, Plastic Surgery, Northern Westchester Hospital, Mount Kisco, and Chief, Plastic Surgery, United Hospital, Port Chester, New York
Reduction Mammoplasty

PATRICIA E. BURROWS, M.D., F.R.C.P.(C)

Assistant Professor, Radiology, University of Toronto Faculty of Medicine; Staff Physician, Department of Radiology, The Hospital for Sick Children, Toronto, Ontario, Canada
Vascular Problems in the Hand

H. HOLLIS CAFFEE, M.D., F.A.C.S.

Associate Professor, University of Florida College of Medicine, Gainesville; Chief, Plastic Surgery Service, Gainesville Veterans Administration Hospital, Gainesville, Florida
Augmentation Mammoplasty: Biology of Capsule Contracture

RICHARD W. CLEMENT, M.D.

Assistant Professor of Surgery, Plastic and Reconstructive, Washington University School of Medicine, St. Louis, Missouri
Gynecomastia

BENJAMIN E. COHEN, M.D., F.A.C.S.

Assistant Clinical Professor, Division of Plastic Surgery, Baylor College of Medicine; Academic Chief and Director, Plastic Surgery Residency Program, St. Joseph Hospital, Houston, Texas
Surgical Options and Aesthetic Considerations

I. KELMAN COHEN, M.D.

Professor of Surgery and Chairman, Plastic and Reconstructive Surgery, Medical College of Virginia, Virginia Commonwealth University, Richmond, Virginia
Immediate Breast Reconstruction

LAWRENCE B. COLEN, M.D.

Assistant Professor of Surgery (Plastic), Dartmouth Medical School; Staff Surgeon, Dartmouth-Hitchcock Medical Center, Hanover, New Hampshire
Diabetic Foot

R. EVAN CRANDALL, M.D.

Private Practice, St. Louis, Missouri
Implants in the Hand and Wrist

A. LEE DELLON, M.D.

Associate Professor, Plastic Surgery and Neurological Surgery, The Johns Hopkins University School of Medicine; Attending Hand Surgeon, Curtis Hand Center, Union Memorial Hospital, Baltimore, Maryland
Interruption of Nerve Function

BARRY FERNANDO, M.D.

Resident, Department of Plastic Surgery, Washington University Medical Center, and Barnes Hospital, St. Louis, Missouri; Private Practice, Paradise Valley, Arizona
Chest Reconstruction
Implants in the Hand and Wrist
Painful Hand Syndrome

JACK C. FISHER, M.D., F.A.C.S.

Professor of Surgery, University of California, San Diego School of Medicine, Head, Division of Plastic Surgery, UCSD Medical Center, and Chief, Section of Plastic and Reconstructive Surgery, Veterans Administration Medical Center, La Jolla, California
Who Can Benefit from Prophylactic Mastectomy?

ALAN E. FREELAND, M.D.

Professor of Orthopaedic Surgery, University of Mississippi Medical Center, Jackson, Mississippi
Internal Fixation of Metacarpal and Phalangeal Fractures

LOUIS A. GILULA, M.D.

Professor of Radiology, Washington University School of Medicine; Co-Director, Musculoskeletal Section, Edward Mallinckrodt Institute of Radiology, St. Louis, Missouri
Radiologic Examination

BURT M. GREENBERG, M.D.

Attending Plastic Surgeon, Northshore Hospital and Long Island Jewish Hospital, New York, New York
Chronic Traumatic Lower Extremity Wounds: Free Muscle Transfer and Skin Graft

DAVID C. HARDY, M.D.

Assistant Professor of Radiology, Edward Mallinckrodt Institute of Radiology, Washington University School of Medicine, St. Louis, Missouri
Radiologic Examination

CARL R. HARTRAMPF Jr., M.D.

Clinical Professor, Emory University School of Medicine; Private Practice, Atlanta Plastic Surgery, P.A. Atlanta, Georgia
TRAM Flap

VINCENT R. HENTZ, M.D.

Associate Professor of Surgery, Stanford University School of Medicine; Chief, Division of Hand and Upper Limb Surgery, Stanford University Hospital, Stanford, California
Phalloplasty

T. RODERICK HESTER Jr., M.D.

Associate Professor of Surgery, Plastic and Reconstructive, Emory University School of Medicine, Emory University Affiliate Hospitals, Atlanta, Georgia
Augmentation Mammoplasty: Polyurethane-Covered Mammary Implant

CHARLES E. HORTON, M.D., F.A.C.S.

Professor, Medical College of Hampton Roads, Norfolk, Virginia
Hypospadias

DENNIS J. HURWITZ, M.D.

Clinical Associate Professor of Surgery (Plastic), University of Pittsburgh School of Medicine; Attending Staff Surgeon, Montefiore Hospital, Children's Hospital of Pittsburgh, Eye and Ear Hospital of Pittsburgh, and Presbyterian-University Hospital, Pittsburgh, Pennsylvania
Perineal Defects

MICHAEL E. JABALEY, M.D.

Clinical Professor of Surgery (Plastic), University of Mississippi School of Medicine, Jackson, Mississippi
Internal Fixation of Metacarpal and Phalangeal Fractures

JOHN R. JARRETT, M.D., F.A.C.S.

Clinical Instructor in Plastic Surgery, University of Oregon Health Science Center, Portland; Department of Surgery, Sacred Heart Medical Center, Eugene, Oregon
Prophylactic Mastectomy

MORTON L. KASDAN, M.D., F.A.C.S.

Assistant Clinical Professor, University of Louisville School of Medicine, Louisville, Kentucky
Occupational Hand Dysfunction

JOHN G. KENNEY, M.D., F.A.C.S.

Associate Professor of Plastic and Maxillofacial Surgery, University of Virginia Medical Center, Charlottesville, Virginia
Gender Dysphoria

NEIL E. KLEIN, B.A., M.D.

Assistant Professor of Surgery, University of Southern California School of Medicine, Los Angeles, California; Chief, Division of Plastic Surgery, Rancho Los Amigos Medical Center, Downey, California
Pressure Sores

KENNETH E. KORBER, M.H.S.

Research Assistant Experimental Instructor, Microsurgery Laboratory, Division of Plastic Surgery, Washington University School of Medicine, St. Louis, Missouri
Use of Leeches in Plastic Surgery

BRUCE A. KRAEMER, M.D.

Assistant Professor of Plastic and Reconstructive Surgery Washington University School of Medicine, St. Louis; Staff Plastic Surgeon, Barnes Hospital and St. Louis Children's Hospital, Chief of Plastic Surgery, St. Louis Regional Medical Center, St. Louis, Missouri
Use of Leeches in Plastic Surgery

DONALD R. LAUB, M.D., F.A.C.S.

Associate Clinical Professor of Plastic Surgery, Stanford University School of Medicine, Stanford, California
Phalloplasty

DONALD R. LAUB Jr., M.S.

Medical Student, Medical College of Wisconsin, Milwaukee, Wisconsin
Phalloplasty

JOHN R. LEWIS Jr., M.D.

Clinical Professor of Surgery (Plastic), University of Kentucky College of Medicine, Lexington, Kentucky, Associate Clinical Professor of Surgery (Plastic), Emory University School of Medicine, Atlanta; Director, Institute of Aesthetic Plastic Surgery, Member of Hospital Staff, Metropolitan Hospital, West Paces Ferry Hospital, Crawford W. Long Memorial Hospital of Emory University, Piedmont Hospital, and Grady Memorial Hospital of Emory University, Atlanta, Georgia

Abdominoplasty

JOHN WILLIAM LITTLE III, M.D.

Professor and Director, Division of Plastic Surgery, Georgetown University Medical Center, Washington, D.C.; Consultant, National Cancer Institute, National Institutes of Health, Bethesda, Maryland

Nipple-Areola Reconstruction

SUSAN E. MACKINNON, M.D., F.R.C.S.(C), F.A.C.S.

Associate Professor, Department of Surgery, University of Toronto; Staff Plastic Surgeon, Chief, Hand Service, Sunnybrook Medical Centre, Toronto, Ontario, Canada

Nerve Compression Syndromes

RALPH T. MANKTELOW, M.D., F.R.C.S.(C)

Professor, Department of Surgery, and Chairman, Division of Plastic Surgery, University of Toronto Faculty of Medicine; Head, Division of Plastic Surgery, Toronto General Hospital, Toronto, Ontario, Canada

Microsurgical Muscle Transfer for Upper Extremity Motors

HALLENE MARAGH, M.D.

Assistant Professor of Plastic Surgery, Eastern Virginia Medical School; Full Attending Physician, J.K.T., M.D., Ltd., Norfolk, Virginia

Brachial Plexus Injuries

MARTHA S. MATTHEWS, M.D.

Assistant Instructor, Medical College of Hamptom Roads, Norfolk, Virginia

Hypospadias

G. PATRICK MAXWELL, M.D.

Assistant Clinical Professor, Department of Plastic Surgery, Vanderbilt University School of Medicine; Associate Professor, Department of Surgery, Meharry Medical College School of Medicine and Director of Research, HCA Center for Research and Education, Nashville, Tennessee

Latissimus Dorsi

JAMES W. MAY Jr., M.D.

Associate Clinical Professor, Harvard Medical School; Chief of Plastic and Reconstructive Surgery and Hand Surgery Service, Department of General Surgery, Massachusetts General Hospital, Boston, Massachusetts

Chronic Traumatic Lower Extremity Wounds: Free Muscle Transfer and Skin Graft

ROBERT M. MCFARLANE, M.D., M.Sc., F.R.C.S.(C), F.A.C.S.

Professor and Chief, Division of Plastic Surgery, University of Western Ontario Faculty of Medicine; Head, Division of Plastic Surgery, Victoria Hospital Corporation, London, Ontario, Canada

Dupuytren's Disease

TIMOTHY A. MILLER, M.D., F.A.C.S.

Professor of Surgery, UCLA School of Medicine; Chief of Plastic Surgery, Wadsworth VA Hospital, Los Angeles, California

Lymphedema

WILLIAM D. MORAIN, M.D.

Professor of Surgery (Plastic), Dartmouth Medical School; Staff Surgeon, Dartmouth-Hitchcock Medical Center, Hanover, New Hampshire

Diabetic Foot

FOAD NAHAI, M.D., F.A.C.S.

Associate Professor of Surgery, Emory University School of Medicine; Associate Professor of Surgery, Department of Plastic and Reconstructive Surgery, Emory Clinic, and Crawford W. Long Memorial Hospital of Emory University, Atlanta, Georgia

Infected Vascular Prostheses

HENRY W. NEALE, M.D., F.A.C.S.

Professor of Surgery, University of Cincinnati College of Medicine; Director, Division of Plastic, Reconstructive and Hand Surgery, University of Cincinnati Medical Center and Director, Burn Reconstructive and Plastic Surgery, Shriners Burn Institute, Cincinnati, Ohio

Reconstruction of Burns of the Trunk and Breast

MICHAEL G. ORGEL, M.D., F.A.C.S.

Associate Professor of Surgery (Plastic), University of Massachusetts Medical School; Attending Plastic Surgeon, Berkshire Medical Center, Pittsfield, Massachusetts

Rectal Sphincter Reconstruction

CALVIN R. PETERS, M.D.

Associate Clinical Professor of Surgery (Plastic), University of Florida College of Medicine, Gainesville, and University of South Florida College of Medicine, Tampa, Florida
Exstrophy

PAUL G. PIN, M.D.

Instructor of Surgery (Plastic and Reconstructive), Washington University School of Medicine, St. Louis, Missouri
Role of Physical Therapy
Extensor and Flexor Tendon Injuries

WILLIAM E. POWERS Jr., M.D.

Attending Plastic Surgeon, Kaiser Foundation Hospital, Sacramento, California
Replantation Surgery

RICHARD P. RAND, M.D.

Resident, Department of Plastic and Reconstructive Surgery, Emory University School of Medicine, Atlanta, Georgia
Infected Vascular Prostheses

ROGER E. SALISBURY, M.D., F.A.C.S.

Professor of Surgery and Chief, Plastic and Reconstructive Surgery, New York Medical College; Chief, Plastic and Reconstructive Surgery and Director, The Burn Center, Westchester County Medical Center, Valhalla, New York
The Burned Upper Extremity

ROBERT R. SCHENCK, M.D.

Director, Section of Hand Surgery and Associate Professor, Departments of Plastic and Orthopedic Surgery, Rush-Presbyterian-St. Luke's Medical Center, Chicago, Illinois; Senior Attending Staff, Rush-Presbyterian-St. Luke's Medical Center, Chicago, Illinois
Fingertip Injuries

PAUL L. SCHNUR, M.D., F.A.C.S.

Clinical Lecturer in Surgery, University of Arizona College of Medicine; Instructor, Tucson Hospital, Medical Education Program, Tucson, Arizona
Augmentation Mammoplasty: Ancillary Measures

WILLIAM W. SHAW, M.D., F.A.C.S.

Associate Professor of Surgery (Plastic), New York University School of Medicine; Chief of Plastic Surgery, Bellevue Hospital, New York, New York
Microvascular Free Flaps
Replantation Surgery

DAVID J. SMITH Jr., M.D.

Associate Professor of Surgery, Section Head, Plastic Surgery, University of Michigan Medical School, Ann Arbor, Michigan
Ganglions and Other Benign Tumors of the Hand

SCOTT L. SPEAR, M.D., F.A.C.S.

Associate Professor and Deputy Director, Department of Plastic Surgery, Georgetown University School of Medicine, Washington, D.C.
Intradermal Tattooing

THOMAS R. STEVENSON, M.D., F.A.C.S.

Assistant Professor of Surgery, Section of Plastic Surgery, University of Michigan Medical School, Ann Arbor, Michigan
Restoration of Stable Soft Tissue Coverage in Wounds of the Foot

BAHMAN TEIMOURIAN, M.D.

Associate Clinical Professor, Georgetown University School of Medicine, and Faculty Member, George Washington University, Washington, D.C.; Chairman, Department of Surgery, Suburban Hospital, Bethesda, Maryland, and Chairman, Department of Plastic Surgery, Southern Maryland Hospital, Clinton, Maryland
Suction Lipectomy: Body Contouring—Suction Versus Scalpel

JULIA K. TERZIS, M.D., Ph.D., F.R.C.S.(C)

Associate Professor of Plastic Surgery, Eastern Virginia Medical School; Director, Microsurgical Research Center, Eastern Virginia Medical School, and Staff, J.K.T., M.D., Ltd., Norfolk, Virginia
Brachial Plexus Injuries

GORDON R. TOBIN, M.D.

Professor of Surgery, University of Louisville School of Medicine, Louisville, Kentucky
Vaginal Reconstruction

JOSEPH UPTON, M.D.

Assistant Professor of Surgery, Department of Surgery, Harvard Medical School, Boston, Massachusetts
Pollicization for the Aplastic Thumb

PAUL M. WEEKS, M.D.

Professor of Surgery (Plastic and Reconstructive), Chief, Division of Plastic and Reconstructive Surgery, Washington University School of Medicine, St. Louis, Missouri
Role of Physical Therapy
Extensor and Flexor Tendon Injuries

MICHAEL J. YAREMCHUK, M.D.

Assistant Professor of Plastic Surgery, Harvard Medical School, Boston; Plastic Surgeon, Massachusetts General Hospital, Boston, Massachusetts, Former Assistant Director of Plastic and Maxillofacial Surgery, Maryland Institute for Emergency Medical Services Systems (MIEMSS), Baltimore, Maryland

Acute Flap Coverage of Open Fractures of the Lower Extremity

VERNON L. YOUNG, M.D.

Associate Professor, Washington University School of Medicine, St. Louis, Missouri

Chest Reconstruction
Implants in the Hand and Wrist
Painful Hand Syndrome

ELVIN G. ZOOK, M.D.

Professor of Surgery and Chairman of Plastic and Reconstructive Surgery, Southern Illinois University School of Medicine, Springfield, Illinois

Nailbed Injuries

RONALD M. ZUKER, M.D., F.R.C.S.(C), F.A.C.S.

Associate Professor of Surgery, Department of Surgery, University of Toronto Faculty of Medicine; Head, Division of Plastic Surgery, The Hospital for Sick Children and Staff Plastic Surgeon, Toronto General Hospital, Toronto, Ontario, Canada

Vascular Problems in the Hand

PREFACE

One may ask, as I did upon being invited to edit these volumes: is there a need for yet another book on plastic and reconstructive surgery?

Plastic surgeons are distinguished by their originality in conception and finesse in execution. They are a restless breed, preferring untrod paths to worn byways. Being unrestricted by anatomic region or system, their explorations often have yielded insights and techniques readily adopted by sister surgical specialties. This fluidity, which is plastic surgery's strength, makes creation of a contemporaneous text difficult, given the usual lag time between manuscript preparation and publication. In addition, the familiar encyclopedic text, which is cumbersome to produce, may bury creativity beneath historical review and therapeutic ecumenism.

The opportunity, therefore, to invite a large number of active contributors in the field of plastic and reconstructive surgery to write personalized submissions for prompt publication was intriguing. These contributors were chosen for their expertise, as demonstrated by recent presentations, study courses, or articles. They were instructed to submit succinct statements of personal preferences for solutions to problems confronted by practicing plastic surgeons. At publication, the first chapter received will be twenty months old and the last five months old. Publication of subsequent volumes every three years should maintain the currency of the contents and express the diversity of management opinions.

The successful production of this book was made possible by the promptness of the authors, the cooperation of my editor, Mary Mansor, the efficiency of my publisher, Brian C. Decker, the attention of my secretary, Karen Lask-McDonagh, and the tolerance of my wife, Rebecca, and my daughter, Kohli. I thank them all for participating in this project.

Following the invitation to edit, I did conclude that the uniqueness of this book, with respect to the currency and individualization of contents, did make the effort worthwhile. I hope that you, the reader, concur.

Jeffrey L. Marsh, M.D.
St. Louis, Missouri

CONTENTS

VOLUME 1

General Principles

Head and Neck

Trauma

VOLUME II

BREAST

POSTMASTECTOMY RECONSTRUCTION

THE TRUNK

GENITOURINARY STRUCTURES

BREAST

AUGMENTATION MAMMOPLASTY: A PERSONAL APPROACH

JAMES L. BAKER Jr., M.D., F.A.C.S.

Augmentation mammoplasty has been one of the most sought after cosmetic operations of the past decade. It has been estimated that 100,000 to 125,000 procedures are carried out annually in the United States and approximately 2,000,000 women now have silicone prostheses beneath their breast tissue.

For surgeon and patient alike, it is one of the most gratifying operations we have the privilege of performing. It yields instant alteration of body image for the woman, with rapid development of positive psychological feelings. Very few cosmetic operations can produce the high degree of patient satisfaction that augmentation mammoplasty repeatedly produces. In the past, patient surveys have shown that 96 to 98 percent of women who have undergone this operation, despite any number of postoperative complications, have stated that they are glad they underwent the procedure and would recommend it.

For the plastic surgeon to repeatedly produce an esthetic surgical result as well as a happy, satisfied patient, he should have a full understanding of the motivation of women seeking this procedure.

The breast is a symbol of femininity and the United States is an extremely breast oriented culture. In the psychological study of the patient who undergoes this operation, which I published in 1975, I found that the size and shape of a woman's breast are extremely important in her concept of self-image and how she interacts with her environment. Women compare their breast size and development to that of their peer groups, beginning in early puberty when breast development begins. It is during this formulative psychosexual development phase that deep rooted feelings of inferiority and low self-csteem can develop in those girls who have retarded breast development. The feelings of inadequacy become deeply rooted and play an important role in their interpersonal relationship with other women, as well as with men. They dislike padded bras, feeling that they are a deceptive device. For artificial devices to be effective in producing body image alteration, it is imperative that they be implanted beneath the skin and hence become incorporated into the patient's body image. In the early postoperative period, the augmentation patient spends a great deal of time viewing herself in the mirror and examining her new breasts. This mechanism encourages early incorporation of the implant into the body image, which then becomes "her own breast," and is no longer thought of as a breast implant. Early mobilization by massage helps deter capsular contracture, is important in the incorporation process, and should be encouraged.

Most commonly at the first dressing change, the patient's fears of having been made too large should be dealt with by the surgeon and his staff to reassure that patient that as the implants settle and the breast tissue attains its natural contour, she will become used to seeing this new projection from her body. In all probability, she will wish she were larger at the 3 month visit. This should be viewed as a positive finding by the surgeon and a compliment to his goal in producing a balanced esthetic result that looks natural. At this point the patient's preoperative photographs are given to her; they are usually viewed in amazement with the accompanying statement of "Gee, was I that flat?" The patient now becomes very pleased with the result you have produced and will be satisfied. The accompanying psychological alterations noted at this time will be a marked increase in self-esteem, adequacy, and self-confidence. Usually the quality and quantity of their sexual relations increase, due to the release of sexual inhibitions, which were caused by feelings of inadequacy due to small breast size prior to surgery.

PATIENT EVALUATION

Besides obtaining a complete medical history, including specific family history of breast pathology, the following three key questions will be excellent prognosticators regarding the patient's acceptance of operative change.

1. Why would you like your breast enlarged?
2. What size bra do you now wear and what size would you like to be?
3. If you have had a pregnancy, what were your feelings regarding breast enlargement during this time?

Motivation should be selfish. Thc patient should want the breast enlargement for herself so that she can look better in her clothing or discontinue wearing a padded bra. There is also a group of patients who have had adequate breast tissue prior to pregnancy. Following pregnancy they noted diminution in the volume and quality of their breast tissue. This group of patients desire to be returned to their "prepregnancy state." No woman who is basically satisfied with her self-image should undergo a surgical procedure for the selfish reason of a friend or marital partner. When a patient responds to my question regarding what they think of their present breast size with the answer "Well, I am happy with them, but my husband or boyfriend wants them to be bigger," my advice to them is to send that person in and we will augment him. When breast size is not a problem to the patient, then she is psychologically stable and would not harbor the feelings of inadequacy and low self-worth and esteem, and the operation would not produce an additional positive reinforcing effect on the patient. The interpersonal relationship between two people should be based on more than just the physical attributes, so long as the woman feels adequate about herself.

The patient must be realistic about what breast size can be obtained. The increase in size should be esthetically pleasing to body proportion. When asked the question "what size would you like to be," and a triple A cup size patient responds, "I want a quadruple D," she is not only being unrealistic about what can be safely accomplished through surgery, but also has no concept of what is esthetically pleasing for her. It is the responsibility of the surgeon to produce an esthetic result that is in balance and proportion to the general body build. Why create a massive bosom that would not only be nonesthetic, but grotesque and disfiguring? When expectations are beyond reality, the patient should be referred for psychological evaluation prior to surgery.

Since breast enlargement during pregnancy simulates, temporarily, breast augmentation, the patient's response to this enlargement is important. A woman who was not pleased with *this* breast enlargement, probably would not be pleased with the result of surgical augmentation. Contrariwise, most women state that they would gladly remain pregnant throughout their adult life, despite the nausea and vomiting frequently accompanying the pregnancy, just to maintain the larger breast size. These patients are excellent candidates for the procedure.

PHYSICAL EXAMINATION

The nurse prepares the patient for examination and should remain present at all times during the physician's examination and photograph taking. Proper consent regarding the photograph taking should be obtained prior to the examination. The photograph is taken from neck to waist level and only clothing to the waist need be removed. Your nurse should give the patient an examination gown for cover until you begin your examination. You should make every effort to make the patient feel comfortable and at ease.

After greeting the patient and introducing myself, I look on the patient information sheet to find out where the patient lives, what type of work she does, or some other general bit of information with which I can open conversation. Do not begin talking about her small breasts. These few moments of casual conversation prior to your asking her to disrobe "breaks the ice" and puts her more at ease.

Examination is begun on the patient's back to evaluate spinal alignment. It is rare that a patient does not have some degree of scoliosis. Any alteration in spinal alignment will create alterations on the anterior thoracic wall as well as shoulder and hip position. I utilize a body diagram and draw her anatomical variations on it as I proceed with the examination. After the patient turns and is facing me, I then evaluate the shoulder height. One shoulder will usually be slightly higher than the other, which usually produces an alteration in nipple alignment. One side of the thorax is usually rotated anterior and appears more prominent. Not infrequently, the midline between the breast is shifted to the right or left side depending on which side the thoracic wall rotates toward. The side which is more convex will produce more projection of that breast. When this rotation is prominent, despite the patient having equal volumes of breast tissue, it is best to increase the volume of the implant slightly on the nonrotated side to produce a better visual illusion of symmetry. Nipple position is measured from the sternal notch. The sternal width between the breast is noted as well as any lateralization of the thoracic wall, which produces lateralization of the projection of the breast. Once the external examination has been performed, palpation of the breast and axillae is carried out. Any areas of breast pathology are carefully evaluated and mammography is performed when indicated.

After the physical evaluation, the patient's height, bone structure, and general body configuration are taken into account, and the implant size is determined. I use a different volume on the two sides in approximately 75 percent of patients undergoing augmentation mammoplasty. This difference is most commonly due to alteration in bone structure as opposed to actual breast volume. A 15 to 30 cc difference in implant volume can create improved symmetry on the side in which the thoracic wall is slightly more posterior or where the ribs are lateralizing.

The patient then stands in front of a full length mirror while I point out the anatomical variations pertinent to her body configuration. I demonstrate any scoliosis, alteration in shoulder alignment, rotation of her thoracic wall, as well as the amount of cleavage that will be attainable and any lateralization of the ribs. She is reminded that the breasts lie on the thoracic wall just as a building lies on its foundation and the foundation cannot be altered by this procedure. The limitations of her anatomy will dictate her final result. I feel it is more important to warn the patient of the limitations (i.e., what you cannot change, more than what you can change). If the patient is aware preoperatively of these limitations, she will either accept or reject the procedure, and you will have a happy postoperative patient. If you fail to discuss these physical findings, which will influence her surgical result, she may have a preconceived mental image of what she will look like postoperatively (an image that you will not be able to create), and hence you will have an unhappy postoperative patient to deal with.

The degree of ptosis present is critical in your preoperative discussion. In general, augmentation mammoplasty can be successfully carried out on those patients whose nipples are at the inframammary crease or slightly below it. With the nipple at or slightly above the crease, the patient can expect a very pleasing esthetic result. Women who have low lying breasts, are warned that the breasts will not be elevated up on the chest wall, but that they will remain in their anatomical position. Nonetheless, a slight degree of upward migration of the nipple can be expected due to the volume filling in the diminished breast tissue below it. When the nipple is slightly below the inframammary crease, the woman is warned that the nipple will not appreciably rise and that she may have a slight downward deflection of the nipple areolar complex postoperatively. At this point, the operation of combined mastopexy with augmentation or mastopexy alone, can be discussed with the patient. Most commonly, once patients are made aware of the amount of scars which these procedures produce, they opt for augmentation alone and accept the compromised results.

When the nipple is more than 1 cm below the inframammary crease, augmentation usually produces a marked downward deflection of the nipple areolar complex. These patients are usually advised against augmentation mammoplasty.

INFORMED CONSENT

The possible routine complications of the operation are discussed in detail with the patient. (A two-page consent with NCR paper in which the patient receives a copy after she has signed it is shown in [Fig. 1]. Page 1 is the general consent utilized for all operations and page 2 is the specific consent related to the cosmetic operation performed.)

Any physical anomalies observed during the physical examination are rediscussed with the patient, and she is warned of those that will later have an effect on her final result. The average percentages of postoperative bleeding, infection, unattractive scars, which may require secondary revision, as well as the process of capsular contracture, which may require secondary surgery for correction, are explained in detail. If postoperative hematoma occurs, she is warned that this will require surgical evacuation, and with infection, normally the implant must be removed from 1 to 3 months on the affected side.

The possibility of loss of nipple sensation is specifically discussed in detail. The patient is asked the question "How important is nipple stimulation to your sex life?" They are then asked to grade it on a scale of 1 to 10 with 10 being the ultimate in sexual pleasure for the patient. The most common answer received is between 4 and 5. When the answer is 8 or higher or the patient can have orgasm purely from nipple stimulation without any genital play, I recommend that the patient be advised of the possibility of permanent alteration of sensation in the nipple areolar complex. Since this phenomenon is found in an extremely low percentage of women, it is a unique phenomenon, and the patient must consider the operation carefully. The national statistic for permanent loss of nipple sensation is approximately 15 percent and can involve both sides. I recommend that such a patient does not schedule the operation at this interview but goes home to discuss this with her partner and considers the operation very carefully; the gratification phenomenon of nipple stimulation may exceed the pleasure they would obtain from breast enlargement surgery. The woman is warned that although the operation of augmentation mammoplasty can be reversible, (the prostheses can be removed at a later date, thereby returning the patient to essentially her preoperative state), we cannot return nipple stimulation when it is permanently lost. Care should be taken to document carefully the importance of nipple stimulation, and to explain the consequences of possible loss of sensation from the procedure.

PREOPERATIVE PREPARATION

The patient should receive preoperative instructions regarding her preoperative preparation. This includes a systemic antibiotic beginning 2 days preoperatively and continued for 1 week postoperatively. The skin of the chest wall, breast, and axillae are to be washed with Betadine skin cleanser daily for 5 days prior to surgery. This reduces skin bacteria and gets the patient used to handling her breasts, which aids in psychological acceptance of the early massage exercises begun on the third postoperative day. All patients are warned against any aspirin ingestion for 2 weeks pre- and postoperatively due to its potent anticoagulant effect. Preoperative laboratory studies are obtained within 10 days of surgery and include a complete blood count, bleeding time, SMAC 23, the HIV AIDS antibody test, and urinalysis.

Patients are instructed to wear garments that are easy to slip on after their procedure, as well as a low-heeled slip-on shoe, since many patients experience some equilibrium disturbances due to pre- and postoperative medications. They must have someone accompany them to and from the office and to remain with them for the first 48 hours postoperatively.

Depending on the patient's preference, the procedure is carried out under general anesthesia or local anesthesia with sedation in the office surgical facility as an outpatient. Following the operation, the responsible party is given written instructions that cover the first 48 hours (Fig. 2).

OPERATIVE PROCEDURE

Almost all augmentation mammoplasties are performed under general anesthetic administered by a board-certified M.D. anesthesiologist, utilizing inhalation anesthetic technique. When local anesthetic is utilized, an intravenous catheter is inserted in an antecubital vein and connected to a solution of 5 percent dextrose and water, which is allowed to drip slowly throughout the procedure.

INFORMED CONSENT TO OPERATION

PATIENT: ____

DATE: ______________________ TIME: ______________________

I hereby authorize Dr. James L. Baker, Jr., and/or associates to perform the following procedures on myself:

____

____

____

1. I recognize that, during the course of the operation, unforeseen conditions may necessitate additional or different procedures than those set forth above. I therefore further authorize and request that the above-named surgeon, his assistants, or his designees perform such procedures as are, in his professional judgement, necessary and desirable, including, but not limited to, procedures involving pathology and radiology. The authority granted under this paragraph shall extend to remedying conditions that are not known to the above doctors at the time the operation is commenced.

2. I consent to the administration of local anesthesia to be applied by or under the direction and supervision of the above doctors, with the exception of

____

(None or a particular one)

3. I recognize that when general anesthesia is used it presents additional risks over which the above doctors have no control and I agree to discuss the risks of general anesthesia with the anesthesiologist before surgery is performed.

4. I am aware that the practice of medicine and surgery is not an exact science, and I acknowledge that no guarantees have been made to me as to the results of the operation or procedure.

5. I consent to be photographed before, during and after the treatment; that these photographs shall be the property of the above doctors and may be published in scientific journals and/or shown for scientific reasons.

6. I agree to keep the above doctors informed of any change of address so that they can notify me of any late findings, and I agree to cooperate with the above doctors in my care after surgery until completely discharged.

7. I am not known to be allergic to anything except: (List) ______________________

____

____

Figure 1 Informed consent to surgery.

AUGMENTATION MAMMOPLASTY: *(An operation for increasing the size of the breasts)*

8. This procedure has been personally explained to me by the above doctors, and I completely understand the nature and consequences of the procedure. The following points, among others, have been specifically made clear:

   a. The operation has been done for several years, but the end results are not, and cannot be determined for a number of years yet to come.

   b. Research indicates that the material implanted in the body does not cause malignancy in human subjects.

   c. There is a possibility that my body may not tolerate these implants, making it necessary to remove the implants. This occurs in a small percentage of cases.

   d. A cyst may form in the area adjacent to the implants, causing fluid accumulation which may require drainage by needle or removal of the implants.

   e. The breasts can become firm (capsule formation and contraction). This condition can be permanent and can cause pain and discomfort.

   f. No guarantee has been given as to size and shape of the breasts. Good results are expected but not guaranteed.

   g. In some patients the margin of the implants can be felt.

   h. The incision will heal with a scar which will be permanent.

   i. Postoperative bleeding may occur around the implant requiring a second operation for its removal.

   j. After being exposed to cold temperatures (i.e., swimming in cold water), the breasts may feel cooler than surrounding body tissues.

   k. Pregnancy is not recommended for at least six (6) months after the surgery.

   l. Numbness or hypersensitivity of the nipple may be experienced following surgery.

   m. The procedure is subject to the same postoperative complications as other surgical procedures.

   n. The implant shell theoretically could be broken at some point in the life of the implant or during the duration it is implanted. The gel contained within is medical grade and the same as the shell design and would in all probability be confined to the space behind the breast where the implant was implanted. This should not cause any serious side-effect.

I have read the above consent and received a copy of it. I fully understand the contents of the consent and authorize and request the above doctors to perform this surgical procedure on me.

______________________________________ ______________________________________

Witness Date Patient or Legal Guardian

BREAST AUGMENTATION—POSTOPERATIVE INSTRUCTIONS

1. After leaving the office, upon arrival at your destination, go to bed, preferably with two pillows under your back. Take 1 of your pain pills, even though you may not be experiencing any discomfort at this point. Then take the pain pills only as necessary for discomfort as directed. For the first 5 days you must sleep on your back, so no pressure is on the breast.

   DO NOT USE YOUR ARMS FOR THE NEXT 48 HOURS. This means pushing yourself up from a chair, opening doors, lifting heavy objects, etc.

   YOU MAY brush your teeth, comb your hair and feed yourself. (The first 48 hours are critical in an attempt to avoid any bleeding, thus the less the arms are used the better). Care should also be taken in getting dressed and undressed with excess arm movements.

2. Take your antibiotics as directed.

3. DO NOT WORRY if your brassiere does not fit you at this point. This brassiere is intended only as a dressing and is not meant to always have the cup filled out by the new breast. It may take several weeks to months before the breasts settle and contour. Consequently do not be alarmed if the point of the brassiere is not filled by the breast.

4. Leave the brassiere and padding exactly as it is until you are seen in the office. Do not attempt to take a bath or shower until seen in the office. Sponge bathing at the sink is allowed.

5. If there are any questions or doubts, please feel free to call this office.

6. Return to this office ______________________________

Figure 2 Breast augmentation—postoperative instructions.

The intravenous sedation of the surgeon's preference is administered slowly while the patient is constantly monitored with electrocardiography (ECG) and a pulse oximeter. Infiltration anesthesia is then accomplished utilizing 0.5 percent Xylocaine with Adrenalin 1:200,000 utilizing an 18-gauge spinal needle connected to a Pitkin syringe. The 18-gauge needle is preferred due to its rigidity that does not allow it to bend or deflect and enter the thoracic cavity if a rib is encountered during infiltration. Inadvertent thoracic entry is much more likely to occur when flexible, smaller gauges, such as 23- or 25-gauge spinal needles, are utilized. It is important to keep the needle at a right angle to the rib to avoid entering the intercostal space producing iatrogenic pneumothorax.

No skin preparation is utilized since the patient has diminished surface bacteria of the skin by washing with Betadine daily prior to the surgical procedure. Disposable paper drapes are utilized. Gloves are washed with alcohol to remove any powder residue and are rinsed with saline. Presterilized implants are left in the container and are not opened until the prostheses are ready for insertion to avoid any contamination. The surgeon alone handles the prostheses.

I utilize only the inframammary approach for breast augmentation as it affords easiest re-entry into the pocket in case of postoperative complications or bad scarring, which will be less obvious than the periareolar or transaxillary scar. A 4-cm curvilinear incision is drawn approximately 1 cm above the inframammary crease to avoid having a scar within the inframammary crease itself. The breast then falls over the crease hiding the incision on the inferior breast side of the inframammary crease. A subcutaneous flap approximately 1.5 cm in length is developed from this incision to the bottom of the inframammary crease, then dissection turns cephalad and a pocket is developed over the pectoralis muscle. I utilize the suprapectoral implantation on all patients as I feel it gives a more natural appearance and is certainly less painful in the postoperative recuperative period. Bleeders are coagulated and the pocket irrigated with copious amounts of saline. After a final check for hemostasis, the table is turned in a slight Trendelenberg position and 500 mg of Velosef in 3 cc of diluent and 40 mg of triamcinolone in 3 cc of diluent are instilled into the cavity and dispersed. Having the head in a slight downward position retains the fluids in the top of the pocket and avoids pooling of the steroid solution near the lower limits of dissection which could later cause some atrophy of the subcutaneous flap and ptosis of the implant. The prosthesis is then taken from the sterile container and inserted into the pocket. No drains are utilized. The subcutaneous flap is reapproximated with a running 3–0 nonabsorbable suture, and the skin is closed with several subcuticular inverted polyglactin sutures. A 4–0 Prolene intracuticular pullout suture is then utilized with Steri-Strip reinforcement. A new all elastic brassiere, one cup size larger than the patient wore preoperatively is then applied as final dressing. The patient is then observed for several hours in the recovery facility and, after final examination, is discharged home with the instruction sheet and returns on the second or third postoperative day.

POSTOPERATIVE CARE

Upper arm motion is limited in the first 48 hours. This diminishes movement of the pectoralis major muscle, which is the most common site of origin of postoperative hematoma. Bed rest and very limited activities are encouraged during this time as well.

The patient is seen between the second and third postoperative day at which time the brassiere is removed and the breasts are examined. She may begin showering daily and begin routine activity, such as driving an automobile, between the third and fifth postoperative day so long as she is not taking any pain medication. In essence, the old adage "if it does not hurt, do it," is employed to guide the patient's activities. A new printed instruction sheet is given to the patient at this time (Fig. 3). She is warned against sun exposure for a minimum of 4 to 6 weeks as well as any strenuous activity, such as exercise programs, which may be begun at that time as well. Routine walking or lower abdominal exercises may be reinstituted at the end of 2 weeks. The patient returns on the tenth postoperative day for removal of the pullout suture and a Steri-Strip is reapplied, which she removes in 5 days. She then returns to the office for routine follow-up at 3 months, at which time the postoperative photos are taken and given to the patient. She is then seen in 9 months and annually thereafter for routine examinations. She is encouraged to return to the office at any time should questions arise.

CAPSULAR CONTRACTURE

Capsular contracture following breast augmentation is most commonly seen approximately 6 months after surgery. Its relative occurrence appears as a bell-shaped curve, which tapers between 6 and 12 months. Although the exact etiology of capsular contracture remains obscure, in essence it occurs as a basic wound healing phenomenon common to all wounding. It appears, at least in part, to be host-related as opposed to implant-related. While multiple etiologic factors may be contributory, it has been shown that the myofibroblast plays an important role in the process of wound contracture. The mechanism controlling activation of this cell, however, remains obscure. Since myofibroblast cell population is present in greatest number during the early phases of wound contracture, the drug papaverine, 150 mg twice daily, can in some instances, cause a relaxation of contracture and an abatement of the process, although this may only prove a temporary situation. I am continuing research with this drug and do not have enough facts available for definitive time schedules of dosages.

Prophylaxis of Contracture

If capsular contracture can be prevented, this is more desirable than treatment for both surgeon and patient alike.

THIRD POSTOPERATIVE DAY

BREAST AUGMENTATION INSTRUCTIONS:

1. You may remove and discard padding and shower beginning ______________________

2. Beginning after you shower, each day, gently massage the breasts until the soreness is gone and then massage more vigorously. Do this at least twice a day, and do at least for the first year and preferably for all time. Hopefully, this will keep the breasts very soft.

3. You may sleep without a brassiere beginning ______________________, but wear one for the next week, during the day. After that, wear only if you desire, keeping in mind that a large breast has the forces of gravity pulling on it and continuously going braless for anyone will only accentuate later ptosis (sagging of the breasts).

4. The tapes may get wet, but pat them dry after coming out of the shower.

5. You may sleep on your abdomen beginning ______________________, if the breasts are not too sore.

6. Return to the office for suture removal ______________________

Figure 3 Third postoperative day—postoperative instructions.

CLOSED CAPSULOTOMY CONSENT

PATIENT: ______________________________

DATE: ______________________________

TIME: ______________________________

1. I hereby authorize ______________________ and/or his associates to perform a procedure to attempt to rupture the scar capsules surrounding my breast implants by squeezing the breasts, known as closed capsulotomy on:

____

(Name of patient or "myself")

2. The procedure listed in Paragraph 1 has been explained to me by the doctor and/or his nurse and I completely understand the nature and consequences of the procedure. The following points have been made specifically clear:

   a. There is a possibility that a blood clot may form in the area adjacent to the implants which might require surgical correction which may have to be performed in the hospital under general anesthesia.
   b. The procedure is not always successful and/or bizarre shape of the breast can occur which could necessitate surgery for correction.
   c. Recurrence of the contracture (hard breast) can occur even if capsulotomy is successful.
   d. Breakage of the implant can occur which would necessitate surgical correction.
   e. Thinning of an area of the tissue over the prosthesis may occur which could necessitate surgical correction or removal of the prosthesis.
   f. If surgery is necessary following the capsulotomy it may be necessary to make an incision in an area other than where the previous scar is located.
   g. No guarantee has been given as to the expected result.

3. I consent to the administration of drugs and/or anesthesia to be applied by or under the direction of the doctor, or such anesthesiologists as he shall select, and to the use of such drugs and/or anesthetics as they may deem advisable with the exception of:

____

(None or a particular one)

4. I am aware that the practice of medicine and surgery is not an exact science, and I acknowledge that no guarantees have been made to me as to the results of the operation or the procedure.

5. I agree to keep the doctor informed of any change of address so he can notify me of any late findings, and I agree to co-operate with the doctor in my care after surgery until completely discharged.

6. I have read the above consent and fully understand same and do authorize the doctor to perform this procedure on me.

7. I am not known to be allergic to anything except: (List) ______________________________

____

Witness: ______________________________

Witness: ______________________ ______________________

(Patient)

Figure 4 Closed capsulotomy consent.

Meticulous surgical technique should be employed to diminish the amount of tissue trauma. Microscopic foreign bodies in the pockets, such as glove powders, sponge lint, and so forth should be avoided. Triamcinolone instilled into the pocket in a dosage schedule, which will not create excessive tissue atrophy that could be symptomatic, can be employed to diminish the initial inflammatory response to wound healing. I do not advocate instilling any drugs into the implant since there is no way to predict the drug activity or release from the implant through the membrane and intraluminal administration can create more problems than it is intended to cure. Also one must be aware that breast implants come under the Device Legislation Act of 1977 and once a drug is instilled into an implant, a new drug has been created and should fall under FDA control and regulation. It is best to follow only the manufacturer's recommendations regarding instillation of saline into the prosthesis. Antibiotics are utilized to diminish the possibility of bacterial invasion and propogation.

Alpha-tocopherol (vitamin E) is effective in decreasing inflammatory response. Its effect is similar to that of the corticosteroids and weakens collagen strength. Its anti-inflammatory effect has been well known for many years and has been used successfully in the treatment of Peyronie's and Dupuytren's contractures. For this effect, synthetic vitamin E, 1,000 U is given twice daily, begun immediately after surgery and continued indefinitely. Vitamin E decreases the incidence of fibrocystic breast disease and usually improves the condition once it has occurred. Natural occurring vitamin E is very rich in oil and will usually stimulate sebaceous glands, which can activate old standing acne or skin conditions and should be avoided. Vitamin C in pill form, should be avoided due to its effects on increased strength of collagen, which can create increased tensile strength in the capsule. Since this is a water soluble vitamin, the high doses many people take are excreted by the urine in any case. Patients are instructed to drink orange juice, to eat salad, vegetables, and fruits rich in vitamin C to obtain more than an adequate daily supply of this vitamin. To be effective, vitamin E must be taken on a daily basis to maintain a constant blood level.

Breast massage is begun on the second or third postoperative day and the patients are encouraged to gently move and massage the breast tissue frequently throughout the day forever. In theory, the implant moving in the pocket has an effect similar to any bursal cavity in allowing the capsule to form at the outermost periphery of the wounded area. After capsule formation, the frequent motion of the prosthesis against the walls of the capsule will help keep the collagen fibers stretched and diminish contracture rate and activity.

Treatment of Capsular Contracture

The nonsurgical squeeze closed capsulotomy technique is performed after the possible complications have been discussed with the patient and a consent signed (Fig. 4). Antibiotics are given for 2 to 3 days postoperatively to diminish the possibility of mastitis developing due to potential release of any intraductal bacteria from the compression of breast tissue. No sedation is given and if the procedure is too painful for the patient it should be discontinued and attempted at another date.

Surgical capsulotomy is reserved for those few cases that are completely resistant to closed capsulotomy or have an extremely high and rapid recurrence rate following this nonsurgical treatment. Surgical capsulotomy is recommended to those patients in whom irretractible contracture is present. Many women however, will choose to live with firmer than natural breasts and this should be the patient's decision.

Augmentation mammoplasty can be one of the most gratifying operations to surgeon and patient alike, so long as patient selection has been carefully considered. An understanding of the woman's psychology regarding her breasts is of maximum importance in obtaining the desired result.

SUGGESTED READING

Baker JL Jr. The effectiveness of alpha-tocopherol (vitamin E) in reducing the incidence of spherical contracture around breast implants. Plast Reconstr Surg 1981; 68(5):696–698.

Baker JL Jr, Chandler ML, LeVier RR. Occurrence and activity of myofibroblasts in human capsular tissue surrounding mammary implants. Plast Reconstr Surg 1981; 68(6):905–912.

Baker JL Jr, Kolin IS, Bartlett ES. Psychosexual dynamics of patients undergoing mammary augmentation. Plast Reconstr Surg 1974; 53(6):652–659.

AUGMENTATION MAMMOPLASTY: ANCILLARY MEASURES

PAUL L. SCHNUR, M.D., F.A.C.S.

The purpose of augmentation mammoplasty is to enlarge the breasts and create a natural result. The breast should be soft and symmetrical, the scars should not be visible, the implant should not be palpable, and the sensation should be normal. The results should last the life of the patient. Although the perfect result is not always achieved, every attempt should be made to give the patient the best result possible.

In 1964, Cronin and Gerow reported the use of silicone breast prostheses for augmentation mammoplasty. Since then, many procedures, implants, and ancillary measures have been proposed to achieve the perfect augmented breast. No single procedure, implant, or ancillary measure has proved to be the best, and controversy still exists as to the proper methods of breast augmentation.

Many different breast implants are on the market today, and each manufacturer claims his implants to be the best for achievement of the desired results. There are three types of implants based upon contents of the implant: silicone gel-filled, saline-filled (inflatable), and a combination of the two (double lumen). Implant surfaces may be Silastic or polyurethane. All types of implants come in a variety of sizes and shapes. Dacron fixation patches, have, for the most part, been abandoned because of the high incidence of capsular contraction.

Location of the incision is important. At least three different positions have been advocated to achieve a favorable scar: inframammary, periareolar, and axillary. The location of the implant, with respect to the skin, breast tissue and chest wall musculature, is felt to affect the result. While the implant can be placed in the subcutaneous, subglandular or submuscular plane, placement in the subcutaneous plane has no role in augmentation mammoplasty. Ancillary measures such as immobilization, compression exercise, antibiotics, and vitamins have been proposed to achieve the perfect result.

PATIENT SELECTION AND CONSULTATION

Selection of patients for augmentation mammoplasty is not difficult; in fact, most patients select themselves. By the time the patient comes to the plastic surgeon, she usually has already decided to have the procedure performed, and is really in the process of selecting a surgeon. Seldom does a woman with large breasts request augmentation mammoplasty. The indication for the procedure is mammary hypoplasia. Some patients who want surgery may have breasts that the surgeon thinks are large enough. In this case, the surgeon can refuse to do the procedure, but, often, the patient will consult another surgeon who will do as she requests. This operation is performed to satisfy the patient; not the doctor.

The patient should have proper motivation and expectations. It is not wise to operate on a patient who wishes to have breast enlargement solely for someone else. If she says that she is doing it only to please her husband or boyfriend, I would not operate on her, since, in most cases, she will not be happy with the result. If she expects to salvage a marriage or an unhappy relationship, she is not a good candidate for the procedure.

The surgeon must rule out any contraindications and carefully evaluate any serious medical problems. Mitral valve prolapse, a common problem in young women, is not a contraindication. During an operation on a woman with mitral valve prolapse, one must use subacute bacterial endocarditis prophylaxis, a cardiac monitor, and have intravenous xylocaine ready for possible arrhythmia. Serious medical conditions, such as heart disease, bleeding disorders, collagen disease, or lung disease may be contraindications. In each case, the decision to operate should be made in consultation with the patient's internist.

Augmentation mammoplasty cannot correct extensive ptosis of the breast. These patients need a mastopexy with, or instead of, augmentation mammoplasty. Other physical contraindications, such as marked asymmetry, burn scars, or chest wall deformities are rare and require more extensive surgery for correction than augmentation mammoplasty alone.

Age is a relative factor. The youngest patient I have operated on was 17. Two factors are significant in the young patient. First, she must have a mature breast size—most women have developed maximum breast size by age 17. Second, she must be mature enough to recognize her needs and understand what effect the new breasts will have on her self-image and on her interpersonal relationships. If she has not yet reached majority, the decision for surgery must have parental approval. The oldest patient on whom I have operated was 76 years old. If an older woman is in good health and desires the procedure, it should be offered to her.

Once the decision is made to perform an augmentation mammoplasty, there are several important details to be worked out in preparation for the surgery. Because the breast prosthesis is an implanted device, which can cause future problems, a complete preoperative discussion is necessary so that informed consent may be obtained. The patient also must know who has financial responsibility in case of problems. Despite what the patient is told before the surgery, she will recall, months or years later, that you told her you would correct it for her at no cost if anything goes wrong. Her husband will remember it that way also. I discuss the details of the procedure thoroughly with the patient. I then tell her all the potential problems, and who pays for them if they occur. I give her a booklet that describes the procedure and its problems, and also discusses financial responsibilities for the problems that might arise. She is then asked to sign a statement at the end of the operative permit that she has read the booklet, understands it, and has had an opportunity to ask any question. I have often found that months or years later when the patient needs further surgery as a result of complications, she is reminded of her financial responsibility only when I ask her to reread the booklet. Also during this meeting, I give the patient any preoperative instructions, such as a light diet the day of surgery, and I request that she not take aspirin for 2 weeks before surgery to minimize aspirin-related bleeding problems.

PROCEDURE AND ANCILLARY MEASURES

In planning the procedure, the surgeon must decide on the appropriate incision site, implant type, placement of the implant in relation to the pectoralis major muscle, and anesthesia. The three most common sites for the incision are in the axillary, submammary, and periareolar regions. Because the submammary incision, which gives better exposure, produces a visible scar, I use a periareolar incision so that the scar will be less visible. Once one masters this procedure through the periareolar incision, it is just as easy as through the submammary incision. The axillary incision may be visible even with clothes on and can become hypertrophic, with an unpleasant scar. Very few perioareolar scars become hypertrophic.

Some reports indicate that periareolar incisions have a higher incidence of permanent nipple anesthesia, but my experience agrees with that of Hetter, who reports that this is untrue. I make an inferior periareolar incision, carry the dissection to the inferior pole of the breast, and then dissect superiorly in the retromammary plane, with very little disruption of the small nerves to the nipple. Nipple anesthesia, in my opinion, arises from disruption of the fourth, fifth, and sixth intercostal nerves to the breast during the lateral subglandular dissection.

I have used the Mentor style 1600 round inflatable implant for 15 years because I find, as do others, that it produces a greater number of soft, augmented breasts. The manufacturer reports a 0.5 percent leak rate, and my experience agrees with this figure. It is very important to fill the implant with the manufacturer's maximum recommended amount. An underfilled implant creates more folds, and it is in these folds that fatigue fractures occur and result in leakage. I place the implants in the subglandular space. If the implant is placed in the submuscular space, it creates an unpleasant appearance of the breast during pectoralis muscle contracture; especially noticeable under close-fitting clothes.

The procedure in almost all cases is performed in our office operating room, which has all the equipment necessary for safe performance of major cosmetic surgery under local anesthesia with intravenous sedation. We start an IV to give medication and keep it open during the operation. The patient is attached to an automatic blood pressure recording machine. We also use an electrocardiogram monitor and pulse oximeter. The patient is given meperidine (Demerol) 25 mg and midazolam (Versed) 2 to 5 mg as she is prepped for surgery. The arms are lightly restrained.

Gordon maintains that meperidine causes nausea. I have tried eliminating meperidine, but find that the required dose of ketamine is then much higher and less predictable. Patients seldom become nauseated on only 25 mg of meperidine, and I prefer to use the lowest possible dose of ketamine.

When the patient is prepped and draped and I am ready to begin, the nurse gives the patient 50 mg of ketamine. As soon as it has taken effect, I infiltrate the breasts with local anesthesia. I use bupivacaine (Marcaine) 0.25 percent with a 1:200,000 solution of epinephrine, 50 cc in each breast. This is a total of 250 mg of bupivacaine, the maximum recommended dose. Because the patient has been pretreated with midazolam, which protects the central nervous system from the convulsive effects of bupivacaine, 250 mg of bupivacaine is not as critical as in a nonpretreated patient. I then use 5 cc of xylocaine 1 percent with a 1:200,000 solution of epinephrine in the area of each periareolar incision. Our group of four surgeons has used this routine for 15 years without a local anesthetic reaction.

I use the Irons' rapid injector with a long spinal needle to inject the local anesthesia rapidly while the patient experiences the maximum effect of the ketamine (Fig. 1). This injector can be assembled from off-the-shelf parts, and once mastered, it is easy to use. The suction drainage silicone bulb is compressed and the suction used to draw the local anesthetic in the bulb, which holds 100 cc, just enough to infiltrate both breasts. The long silicone tube, occluded between the thumb and forefinger, is then attached to the side arm on the metal barrel. When the syringe is aspirated, it fills with solution and is then ready to be injected. I use a number 22 spinal needle. A small-gauge long needle bends easily and can puncture the lung, creating a pneumothorax. If the patient begins to cough or complain of chest pain other than at the surgery site, or if she complains of shortness of breath at any time, her breath sounds should be listened to with a stethoscope as she may have a pneumothorax and need a chest tube.

The nurse then scrubs in, ready to assist. We do not use circulating nurses, since the routine is set and the nurse can have everything ready before she scrubs in. An inferior periareolar incision is made and dissection is carried beneath the inferior pole of the breast and into the subglandular plane. This space is easily created with blunt and long scissor dissection. I use the small Deaver's for retraction and the Gram's headlight for illumination; this combination provides good exposure. The Gram's headlight, with a high-intensity light bulb and a rechargeable battery pack worn on the surgeon's belt, allows freedom of movement around the operating table. I use a bovie extension so that the bleeders high in the wound can be controlled. The Gram's headlight and small Deaver's for exposure are the trick to make this procedure easy. The style 1600 round Mentor implant is then prepared. The dissected pocket is irrigated with 30 cc of 5 percent povidone-iodine (Betadine) solution, and antibiotics are placed in the lumen of the implant. We have found the use of povidone-iodine irrigation and intraluminal antibiotics greatly decreases our incidence of capsular contracture. I use cephalothin (Keflin), 2 g, in the lumen of each implant unless the patient is allergic to penicillin; in which case, I use 80 mg of gentamicin. If cephalothin is used in the implant and there is need to reoperate at

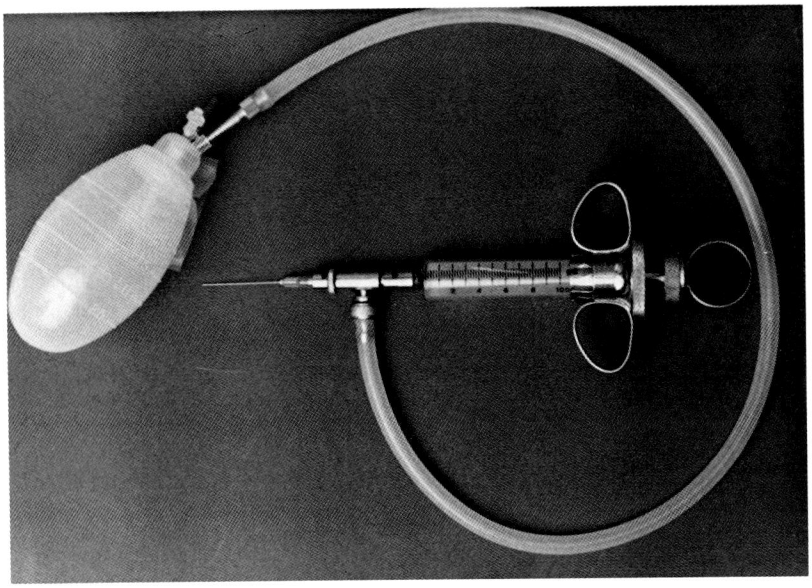

Figure 1 Irons' rapid injector, developed by Dr. George Irons of the Mayo Clinic.

a later time, the cephalothin solution will be found to have turned dark brown (Fig. 2).

The wound is closed with a pull-out subcuticular suture, and the patient is placed in an inexpensive sleeping brassiere that we keep in stock. This brassiere is quite adequate for support and is easier to use and less expensive than some of the stretch items that come from surgical supply houses. The patient then returns home with a responsible adult and is asked to stay in bed the day of surgery. The day following surgery, I place no restrictions on her. Most patients return to a normal, active life in 1 week, at which time the sutures are removed. We then instruct the patient in breast compression and ask her to do this for 6 months. Although some clinicians are convinced that this is an important preventive technique, I am not convinced that this alone prevents contracture, as I have seen patients who have been faithful in their compression develop firm capsular contracture.

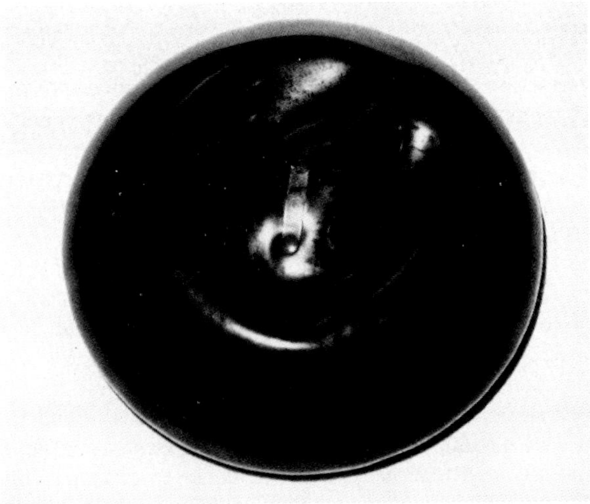

Figure 2 Inflatable implant with intraluminal cephalothin, removed 2 years after augmentation mammoplasty.

The patient is seen again in 3 months. If she has no complaints and both breasts are soft, she is discharged. If there are any problems, the patient is followed for a longer period. Usually, when patients develop problems in the future, they return to their original surgeon. Pre- and postoperative photographs are taken and copies are sent to the patient in a picture wallet (Figs. 3 and 4). Most patients enjoy seeing the difference, and this is good public relations for the surgeon.

BENEFITS AND PROBLEMS

There are many problems associated with augmentation mammoplasty. Aside from those that can occur during the operation, such as drug reactions, bleeding, and pneumothorax, many others can occur later. The most common problem is capsular contracture, resulting in a firm-to-hard breast that may be distorted and painful. Less frequent problems are implant failure, malposition, infection, and loss of sensation. Scars may be hypertrophic, and there may be long-term pain. Asymmetry may also be a problem.

The physical benefits of augmentation mammoplasty are breasts that are the proper size, soft, symmetrical, and have normal sensation. The scars are not visible and the implants are not palpable. The results last a long time.

SUGGESTED READING

Burkhardt BR, Dempsey PD, Schnur PL, Tofield JJ. Capsular contracture: a prospective study of the effect of local antibacterial agents. Plast Reconstr Surg 1986; 77:919–932.

Burkhardt BR, Fried M, Schnur PL, Tofield JJ. Capsules, infection and intraluminal antibiotics. Plast Reconstr Surg 1981; 68:43–49.

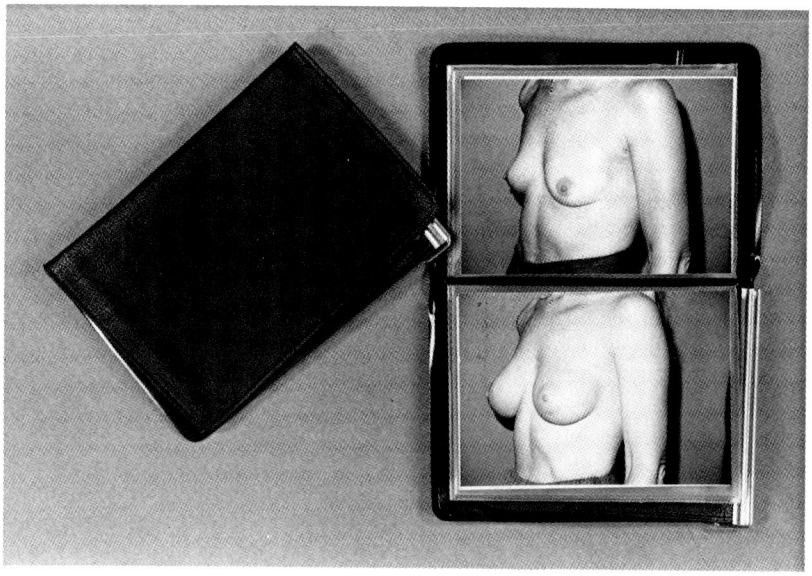

Figure 3 "Brag book" with pre- and postoperative photographs sent to patient.

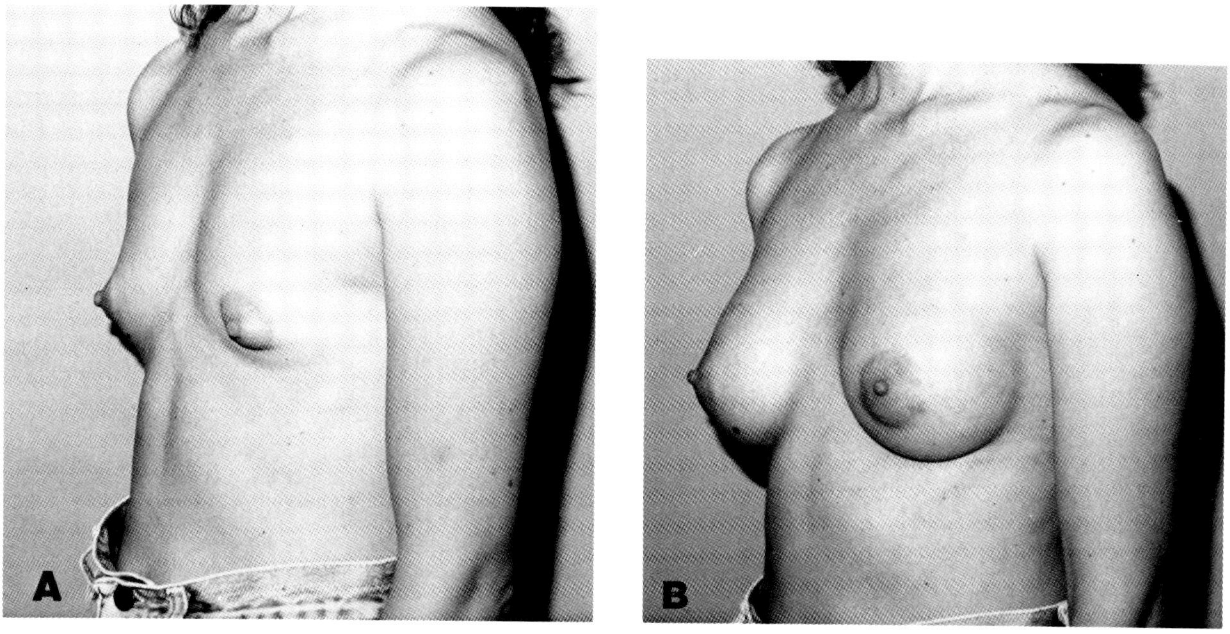

Figure 4 *A*, Preoperative patient for augmentation mammoplasty. *B*, Same patient following augmentation mammoplasty.

Cronin TD, Gerow F. Augmentation mammoplasty: a new "natural feel" prosthesis. In: Transactions of the Third International Congress of Plastic Surgery. Amsterdam: Excerpta Medica, 1964: 41–49.
Gordon HL. The selection of drugs in office surgery. Clin Plast Surg 1983; 10:277–284.
Hetter G. Satisfactions and dissatisfactions of patients with augmentation mammoplasty. Plast Reconstr Surg 1979; 64:151–155.
Reiffel RL, Rees TD, Guy CL, Aston SJ. A comparison of capsule formation following breast augmentation by saline or gelfilled implants. Aesthetic Plast Surg 1983; 7:113–116.
Vinnik C. Spherical contracture of fibrous capsules around breast implants. Plast Reconstr Surg 1976; 58:555–560.

AUGMENTATION MAMMOPLASTY: BIOLOGY OF CAPSULE CONTRACTURE

H. HOLLIS CAFFEE, M.D., F.A.C.S.

Breast augmentation is potentially the most gratifying of all the operations in the field of esthetic plastic surgery—for both surgeon and patient. The fact that some patients will experience some degree of capsule contracture has kept perfection just beyond the reach of this operation. In a specialty populated by perfectionists, it is not surprising that the problem of capsule contracture has generated an enormous amount of interest, literature, and ingenuity.

The etiology of capsule contracture is unknown. Although there is some evidence to implicate subclinical infection and silicone bleed, it is unlikely a single etiology can account for all cases. It is possible that capsule contracture is just part of the spectrum of normal wound healing. The therapeutic approaches to the problem, therefore, fall into two categories: those intended to eliminate a specific stimulus for capsule contracture, and those intended to modify the process of wound healing.

Therapy should be considered from two aspects: prevention of capsule contracture, and management of the established contracture. There is some overlap with certain therapeutic measures, but, in general, prevention and treatment are separate issues.

PREVENTION OF CAPSULE CONTRACTURE

Surgical Technique

There is only one sure way to prevent capsule contracture: implants should not be used. Those looking for a simple answer need not pursue the subject any further. For the rest of us, there are a number of measures that have varying degrees of scientific support, or at least theoretical merit.

The first principle for the prevention of capsule contracture is so simple as to be self-evident; yet it is usually not mentioned in discussions of the subject. Gentle technique, with minimal tissue trauma, is of vital importance in all areas of surgery and assumes greater significance in the specialty of plastic surgery. Just as the skin wounds have less scarring in the hands of the surgeon with greater skill, the implant pocket heals more kindly when it is spared from rough handling.

No-one could argue against the importance of good surgical technique, but consensus ends here, and the surgeon is faced with a number of difficult choices that include implant position (submuscular or retromammary), implant type, adjuvant drugs, and postoperative management.

Implant Position

There is general consensus that implants placed under the muscle are less likely to result in capsule contracture than are implants placed in the retromammary space. In spite of this consensus, the majority of surgeons continue to prefer the retromammary position for augmentation mammoplasty. There are several reasons for this apparent paradox. Although there is a general impression that submuscular implants are less vulnerable to contracture, this is by no means an established fact. At best, the use of the submuscular space reduces the contracture problem, but does not eliminate it. The reduction in contractures, if there is one, comes with several disadvantages. It is more difficult to obtain adequate local anesthesia for dissection of the submuscular space. The early results obtained with submuscular implants lack the projection found with retromammary implants; however, the problem is temporary and, eventually, the muscle will adapt to the presence of the implant and allow good projection. A long-term disadvantage with submuscular implants is that they are distorted by muscle contraction, but most patients accept the distortion problem if it is presented to them as a way to reduce the risk of contracture. The use of the submuscular position all but precludes closed capsulotomy. All these disadvantages are relative and are certainly acceptable if one believes submuscular implants significantly reduce contracture, if the patient is stoic or can afford general anesthesia, if she does not mind the temporary lack of projection or the intermittent distortion of her implants, or if one does not anticipate a need for closed capsulotomy. If one's practice does not meet any of the above conditions, the use of retromammary implants may be continued with a clear conscience.

The above remarks apply only to esthetic surgery. Breast reconstruction after mastectomy is in an entirely different category. In mastectomy reconstruction, retromammary placement is not an option; the choices are subcutaneous or submuscular. Subcutaneous implants have an extremely high risk of capsule contracture, which by itself is enough reason to use submuscular implants. Other equally valid reasons include the extra margin of safety when flap conditions are not optimal, and the use of submuscular implants in cancer patients allows, and possibly even enhances, the detection of local recurrence. Therefore, when an implant is used for mastectomy reconstruction, it should be placed under the pectoralis major and serratus muscles if they are present. If these muscles are absent, a muscle flap is indicated.

Implant Type

There are several types of implant available, and each has its advocates. The gel-filled implant in its original form is now obsolete. Saline-filled implants have been shown to result in fewer contractures, but their use adds the risk of eventual deflation. Low bleed gel implants have been shown to reduce contractures in experimental animals.

Double lumen implants probably do as well, but have not been as thoroughly studied. A specific application of the double lumen implant would be in those cases in which the use of intraprosthetic methylprednisolone is indicated.

The remaining category is the group of polyurethane foam-covered implants. The foam-covered implants have been purported to result in fewer contractures, but this has never been confirmed in controlled studies. One disadvantage is a high incidence of inflammation, which is temporary and apparently benign. The major disadvantage of the polyurethane foam is that it becomes incorporated in the capsule and can be difficult to remove if the implant must be changed later. This becomes a serious problem in the case of periprosthetic infection. The polyurethane ultimately disintegrates and is probably metabolized to some extent. The long-term effects of these implants are still uncertain.

Adjuvant Drugs

Adjuvant drugs fall into two general categories: those intended to combat infection, and those intended to modify the normal process of wound healing.

There is reason to believe that at least a few of the capsule contractures seen in breast augmentation patients are due to subclinical infection. Some form of antibacterial therapy should be employed and can be expected to reduce, but not eliminate, capsule contracture. Antibiotics or antiseptics have been put inside implants, but there is not enough known about the kinetics of these agents to recommend this route of administration. Topical administration by wound irrigation is a reasonable measure. Numerous antibiotics and povidone-iodine have been used for this purpose. The effect of any wound irrigant is necessarily transient, but very direct. Systemic administration of antibiotics delivers less of the drug to the implant pocket, but has the advantage of a more prolonged effect. A good approach is to combine perioperative systemic antibiotics and wound irrigation with half strength povidone-iodine.

The two classes of drugs used to modify the wound healing process are vitamin E and steroids. Both of these agents probably act by the same mechanism and interfere with fibroblast function; their differences are primarily in therapeutic index. Vitamin E is very safe, but not very effective; steroids are very effective, but not very safe. Vitamin E is recommended in a dose of 2,000 units a day and usually produces few side effects. The occasional incidence of nausea, or oily skin, can be reduced by the use of the synthetic form rather than the naturally occurring form, or by reducing the dose.

The use of steroids for contracture prevention was originally accomplished by injection of the drug into the wound pocket at the time of closure, but the effect is probably too brief to be of much benefit. Soluble steroids in a saline implant are very effective, but carry the risk of soft tissue atrophy that results in thin skin, implant ptosis, and even implant extrusion. Because of these risks, the routine use of steroids for capsule prevention is not recommended. It is possible that intraprosthetic steroids may be safer in submuscular implants, but this remains to be demonstrated.

Postoperative Management

When the implant space is dissected, it should be at least as large as the implant, and preferably larger. As long as this remains the case, the implant will remain soft. One concept has been that if the implant is periodically moved about within an oversized pocket, it can prevent the redundant space from closing. This is probably wishful thinking. A more rational concept is that scar, particularly while it is immature, can be stretched. This is the principle behind dynamic splinting in hand surgery and the dilation of strictures of hollow structures. Some form of implant massage, or compression, should be recommended, but one should not expect too much from it. Just as a successful tendolysis requires an extremely compulsive and tolerant patient, it is unlikely that many patients will be sufficiently compliant to have a significant effect on the implant capsule.

TREATMENT OF ESTABLISHED CONTRACTURE

Once a contracture develops, the only way to relieve it is by capsulotomy. Capsulotomy can be either open or closed, and each has a place. Closed capsulotomy has the obvious advantage of simplicity. It does not require an anesthetic or an operating room. The risks include implant rupture, bleeding, and physician hand trauma. In addition, the capsulotomy is often incomplete, and some capsules cannot be ruptured without excessive force. In experienced hands, closed capsulotomy is reasonably safe when restraint is exercised and if one is willing to accept failure and go to open capsulotomy if the capsule does not rupture easily. A good "rule of thumb" is that if one hurts one's thumb, one is squeezing too hard!

Open capsulotomy is quite safe, but obviously requires an anesthetic and an operating room. It is just as big an operation as the original surgery. Both closed and open capsulotomy carry a substantial chance of recurrence, but open capsulotomy gives one the chance to do something about it.

With open capsulotomy, some measure should be employed to reduce the risk of recurrence. At the very least, standard gel implants should be replaced with either low bleed or double lumen implants. If the patient has bilateral contracture and the implants are retromammary, new pockets in the submuscular position are recommended. A change to submuscular placement is much harder to recommend for the patient with unilateral contracture because of the asymmetry that would result. For those patients with unilateral contracture, the use of steroids is reasonable. The risk of steroid-related complications becomes more acceptable in the patient with a demonstrated tendency toward contracture. The other situation in which steroid use is attractive is after open capsulotomy for patients with submuscular implants.

The risk of steroid-related complications is dose-related, and the dosage should be considered in terms of concentration rather than the total dose. It is not known what concentration is both safe and effective, but most steroid-related complications have occurred in cases in which the concentration was greater than 20 mg per 100 milliliters. In addition, the reported complications have occurred late and in single lumen, saline-filled implants. The use of a double lumen implant allows the administration of a significant concentration in the outer lumen. This concentration decreases much more quickly than it would in a single lumen implant because the drug diffuses both into the tissue and into the inner gel compartment. For these reasons, the use of double lumen implants should make steroid use safer. There has not been sufficient experience to be sure of that, so steroids are recommended only for the capsulotomy patient.

For the future, there are some other options that are not yet perfected but are promising concepts. The development of a reliable self-sealing valve suggests the potential for percutaneous injection into the implant. This raises the possibilities of capsule expansion by overinflation, internal capsulotomy, and administration of steroids that can later be retrieved to avoid late complications. The entire field of capsule contracture management is filled with unexplored opportunities.

SUGGESTED READING

Asplund O. Capsule contracture in silicone gel and saline filled breast implants after reconstruction. Plast Reconstr Surg 1984; 73:270–275.

Burkhardt BR, Dempsey PD, Schnur PL, et al. Capsule contracture: a prospective study of the effect of local antibacterial agents. Plast Reconstr Surg 1986; 77:919–930.

Caffee HH. The influence of silicone bleed on capsule contracture. Ann Plast Surg 1986; 17:284–287.

Caffee HH. Vitamin E and capsule contracture. Ann Plast Surg 1988; 19:512–514.

Carrico TJ, Cohen IK. Capsular contracture and steroid-related complications after augmentation mammaplasty. Plast Reconstr Surg 1979; 64:377–380.

Helter GP. Satisfactions and dissatisfactions of patients with augmentation mammaplasty. Plast Reconstr Surg 1979; 64:151–155.

Nelson GD. Complications from the treatment of fibrous capsular contracture of the breast. Plast Reconstr Surg 1981; 66:969–970.

AUGMENTATION MAMMOPLASTY: POLYURETHANE-COVERED MAMMARY IMPLANT

T. RODERICK HESTER Jr., M.D.

Augmentation mammoplasty has become one of the most commonly performed procedures by plastic surgeons. To the end of 1986, over 1.5 million patients in North America had had implantation of breast prostheses. Since its introduction by Cronin and Gerow in 1962, the silicone gel implant has been by far the most commonly used prosthesis for augmentation mammoplasty. However, problems with capsular contracture that occurred with smooth-walled silicone gel-type prostheses have been significant, with rates of 0 to 74 percent reported. The polyurethane-covered silicone gel mammary prosthesis was introduced by Ashley in 1970, and since that time there have been sporadic reports of its use, primarily for postmastectomy breast reconstruction. These reports generally have been favorable and similar in their reporting of low capsular contracture rates in the complex surgical setting of breast reconstruction. However, because of the generally favorable results obtained in augmentation mammoplasty with smooth-walled silicone prostheses, surgeons have been slow to use the polyurethane-covered implant in this setting. I began using polyurethane-covered implants for augmentation mammoplasty in late 1983, after an encouraging experience with this type of prosthesis in the treatment of capsular contracture that followed the use of smooth-walled silicone devices.

THE IMPLANT

The Meme and Replicon* are the updated versions of polyurethane-covered silicone gel mammary implants that I have used for augmentation mammoplasty. Modern versions of these prostheses are said to have improved upon the original Ashley implant in that the polyurethane cover now is finer and biologically more stable. Also, the current implants incorporate a more highly cross-linked silicone gel, with an inherent memory that allows shaping for projection (Replicon, Meme mp), while maintaining weight and specific gravity that approximate normal breast tissue.

MECHANISM OF ACTION

Hester has summarized available data regarding the mechanism by which polyurethane foam inhibits spherical capsular contracture around mammary implants. This action appears to relate to a rather unique bioactive host response, both to the physical (textured) surface of the implant and to the chemical structure of the polyurethane itself. The foreign body response that occurs with implanted polyurethane foam apparently results in delayed fibrosis and inhibition of linear capsular contracture. The foreign body response to polyurethane is characterized by vascularity, hypercellularity (macrophages), and nonlinear

* Cooper Surgical/Natural Y, 17701 Cowan Avenue, Irvine, California, 92713

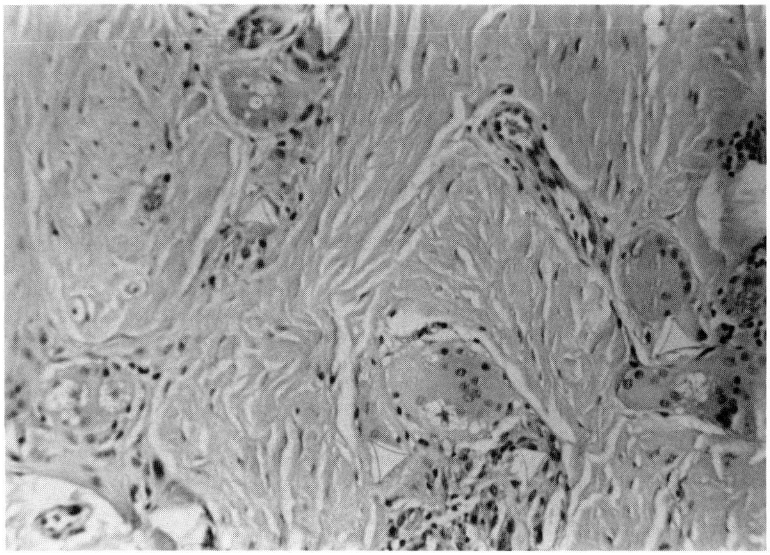

Figure 1 Histology of polyurethane capsule 3 years after insertion, shows triangular spicules of polyurethane, foreign body giant cells, and swirling, nonlinear fibrosis.

fibrosis (Fig. 1). Multiple polyurethane particles (triangular-shaped), surrounded by multinucleated giant cells and a complex, swirling pattern of collagen deposition, are noted histologically. This unique bioactive response of the host to implanted polyurethane results in a decreased tendency to form clinically significant concentric capsular contracture.

THE IMPLANTS

The Meme and Meme mp are the standard, lower profile implants, and the Replicon is the high profile variety. The Replicon more commonly is used for postmastectomy reconstruction but I have used it extensively for augmentation. For mammoplasties that require implants with a volume of 250 cc or less, the Meme is chosen; the reason being that the smaller Replicon implants have a slight resistance to total compression in the anteroposterior dimension. If an implant volume of 250 cc or more is needed, the Replicon is chosen. Larger Replicon implants have no resistance to anteroposterior compression, and their greater projection and narrower base than the larger Meme implants often give a definite esthetic advantage.

TECHNIQUE

Preoperative Evaluation

All patients who desire breast augmentation should have a complete history taken and a physical examination. Any familial history of breast cancer should be noted and the patient apprised of increased risk, if present. Careful breast examination for nodularity or masses, and mammography when indicated, must be done before the patient can be cleared for augmentation. Patients also should be informed of the need for yearly postaugmentation breast examination by a plastic surgeon who is familiar with the nuances of implanted mammary prostheses—if follow-up is to be ideal. In preparation for the surgery, the surgeon carefully should note patient desires regarding outcome and be sure that reality and patient expectations are compatible. Important anatomic points to be noted include presence of ptosis, thickness of subcutaneous fat and gland, areolar circumference, asymmetry of breast size, and differences in level of inframammary folds (Fig. 4). As will be seen, these findings are important to determine the incision to be used and the site into which the implant will be placed, and to assure as symmetrical and esthetically pleasing a result as possible.

Incision

Polyurethane-covered implants are best inserted through an incision of 4 to 6 cm in length, placed in the inframammary fold. The infra-areola incision can be used when areolar circumference is adequate. Proper placement of a polyurethane-covered implant through an axillary incision is awkward and therefore, this incision is not used.

Site

Low rates of occurrence of capsular contracture can be expected whether polyurethane-covered implants are placed in the subglandular or submuscular site. This knowledge allows the surgeon to choose the anatomic location most appropriate for a given patient. Patients who have adequate subcutaneous fat and glandular tissue and any degree of ptosis are ideal candidates for subglandular placement. Implants placed in the subglandular rather than the submuscular position are generally more efficacious in correcting moderate degrees of ptosis. Thin patients without ptosis are usually better served by submuscular placement, which assures adequate soft-tissue coverage of the prosthesis (Fig. 5). When a patient is athletically active, the subglandular site is preferred if any significant degree of native subcutaneous fat and glandular tissue is present, because some patients with submuscular implants (particularly if any degree of ptosis is present) will demonstrate an unattractive distortion of the breasts upon pectoralis major flexion.

Implant Insertion

The patient seen in Figure 2A, is seen immediately prior to augmentation mammoplasty. Her areolar circumference is adequate to allow a 5 cm incision and the infraareolar approach has been chosen. Careful marking of the inframammary folds documents the left as 2 cm higher than the right. At surgery, care will be taken to place the left implant a bit lower than the native fold in order to correct this discrepancy (arrow on left). It should be noted, however, that inframammary fold dystopias cannot always be totally corrected in this manner. The level of the nipple limits the inferior range of implant placement. The medial extensions of the inframammary fold lines mark the extent to which the pocket will be dissected. This dissection is shown in Figure 2B and is facilitated with the use of a lighted retractor and extended electrocautery unit. When one has chosen the submuscular site, it is essential that muscular attachments to the sternum be divided to the second rib interspace in order to allow sufficient medial placement of the implant to create cleavage and prevent an unnaturally wide sternal flatness between the breasts. The pocket is dissected superiorly to a point just below the clavicle and, laterally, to the anterior axillary line.

Because of the textured surface and resulting high friction coefficient between the polyurethane and tissues, actual implant insertion is more difficult than for smooth walled silicone devices. If the Replicon implant is to be used, it is also necessary that the seam remain at the inferior pole of the breast after prosthesis insertion (Fig. 2C). Although a Silastic sleeve can be used to aid implant insertion, the author prefers the method illustrated in Figure 2. The breast is retracted away from the chest wall and, with both hands lateral to the prosthesis, the index fingers are used to "milk" the implant gently into the pocket (Fig. 2D). Insertion is completed by placement of the index and long finger behind the implant, thereby facilitating superior placement and smoothing of the posterior wall of the implant (Fig. 2E). Finally, the anterior surface of the implant is freed of wrinkles by a finger or a curved, blunt dilator (Fig. 2F). The maneuvers illustrated in Figures 2D, E and F are necessary to place the implant correctly and prevent wrinkling, but should be done cautiously to prevent traumatic delamination of the polyurethane cover.

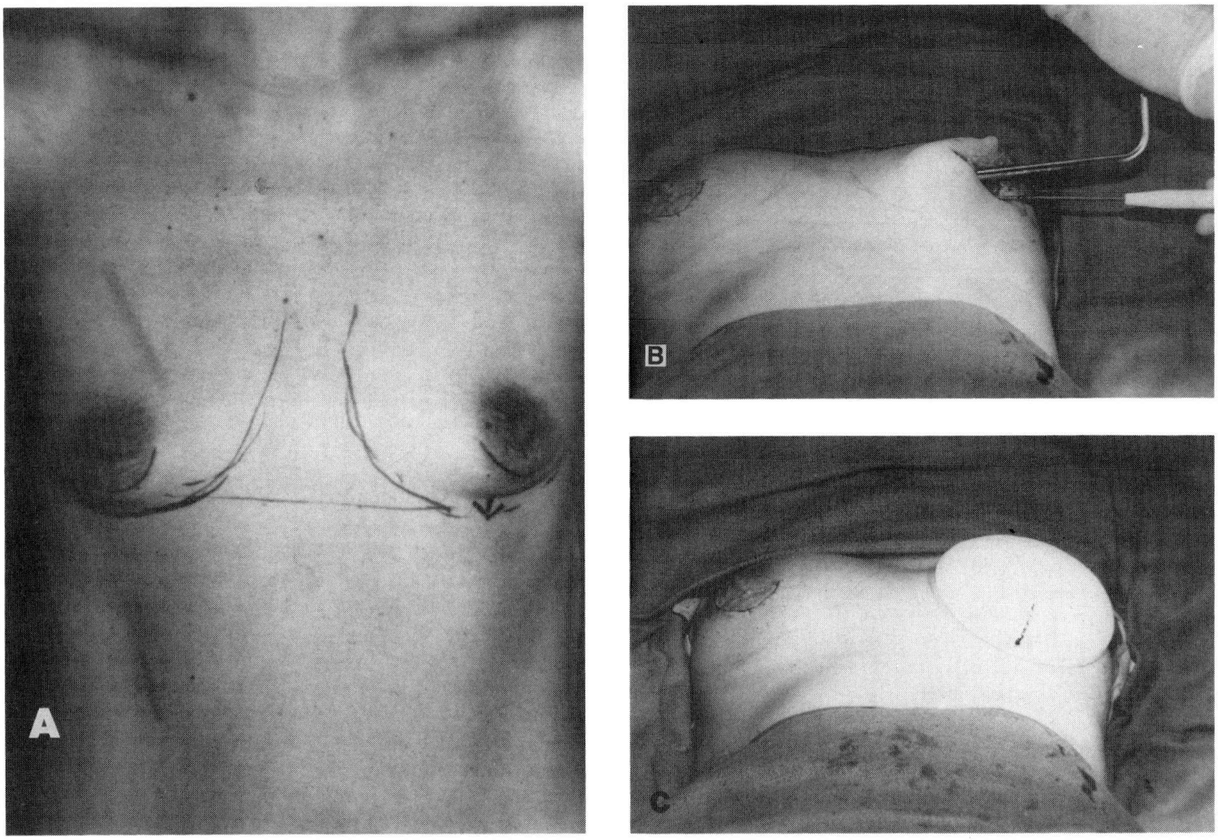

Figure 2 *A*, Preoperative markings for incision and extent of implant pocket dissection. *B*, Shows use of lighted retractor and extended electrocautery unit for dissection of pocket. *C*, Correct orientation of implant.

Figure continues on opposite page

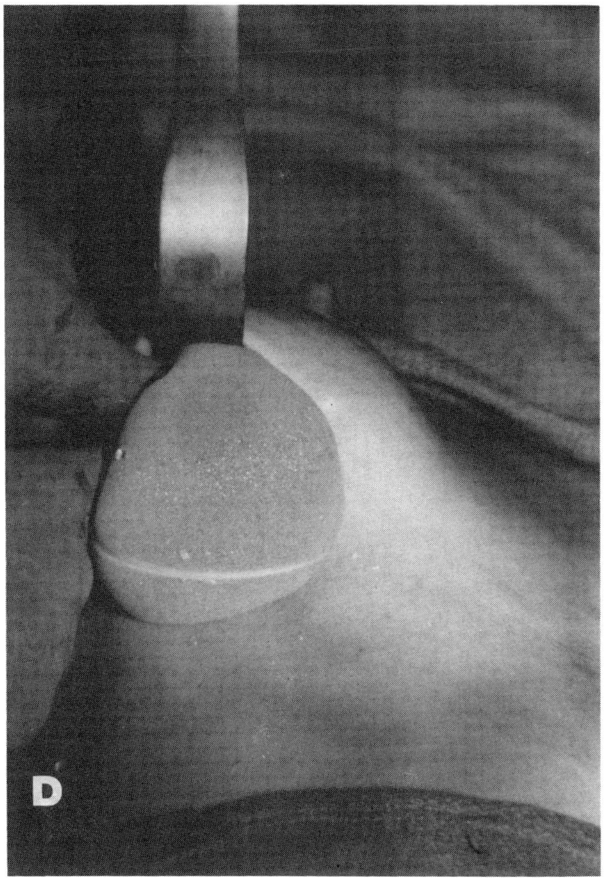

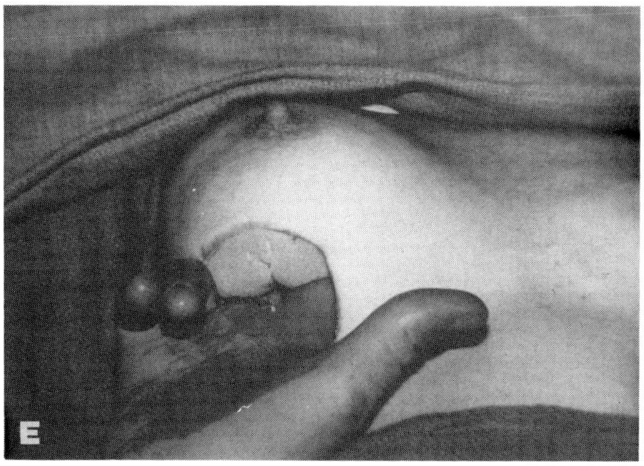

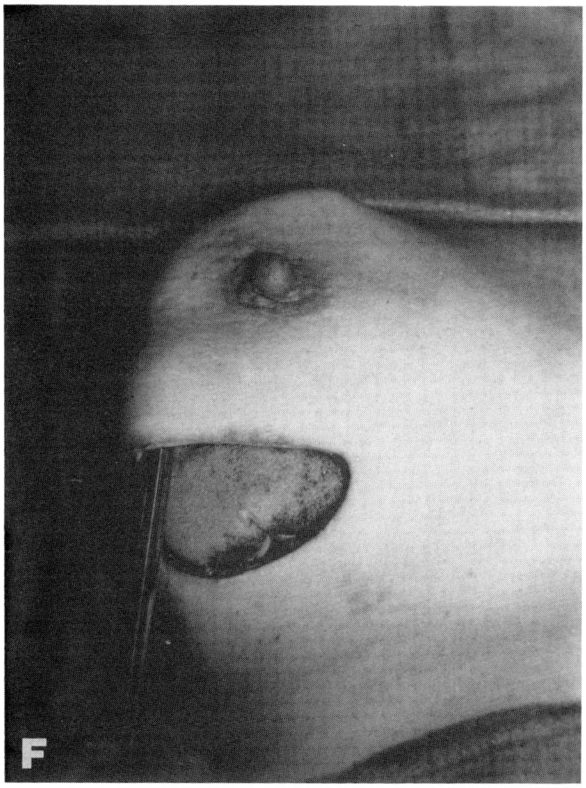

Figure 2 (continued) *D*, Bi-digital insertion of implant. *E*, Removal of wrinkles from posterior wall of implant. *F*, Removal of wrinkles from the anterior wall of the implant.

Postoperative Management

Sutures are removed at 5 to 7 days. Antibiotics are started prior to surgery and continued for 3 days. Swelling resolves rapidly, and most patients are comfortable, with relatively soft breasts, 1 month post surgery. However, patients should be aware that optimum softening of the breasts may not occur for 6 to 12 months.

RESULTS

My results with polyurethane-covered implants for primary augmentation mammoplasty have been gratifying (Table 1 and Fig. 6). Over 800 implants have been used during the past 4.5 years, with an identified rate of occurrence of clinically significant capsular contracture of 1.8 percent and infection of 0.2 percent. To describe capsular contracture as it relates to polyurethane-covered implants, a system that utilizes three classifications is used. This system allows the surgeon to identify the totally soft and compressible breast, the breast with minimal resistance to extremes of compression (clinically insignificant firmness), and the uncomfortable, noncompressible breast that

TABLE 1 Experience with Polyurethane-Covered Mammary Implants

Total Implants	*Capsules*	*Infections*
800	15 (1.8%)	2 (0.2%)

requires surgical correction. This classification is based on digital breast (implant) compressibility (Table 2). The breast is compressed at its base on the chest wall. Patients in Class I have breasts compressible to no more than 2 cm, fingertip to fingertip (Fig. 3). Patients in the Class II category have minimal resistance to extremes of implant compression (2 to 4 cm, fingertip to fingertip). Patients in the Class III category have obvious resistance to even minimal degrees of implant compression. In my experience, patients with Class II resistance to compression rarely perceive significant firmness and surgical revision has not been necessary for them. It is also important to note that Class I firmness may occur secondary to inherent minimal resistance to total compression of the implant itself and is more likely with the use of smaller (255 g or less) higher profile implants. Class III contractures have been distinctly rare, as noted in Table 3. Only one patient has required a unilateral capsulotomy to correct firmness over the 4.5 years of the study.

TABLE 2 Classification of Capsular Contracture

Class I	No resistance to implant compression
Class II	Minimal resistance to implant compression (2–4 cm)
Class III	Significant resistance to implant compression (<4 cm)

TABLE 3 Capsular Contracture with Polyurethane-Covered Implants

Total Implants	*Class II*	*Class III*
800	14 (1.2%)	1 (0.2%)

COMPLICATIONS

Infection

Infection has occurred in two breasts (0.2 percent). Although infection has been rare, all patients should be monitored closely in the perioperative period for its occurrence. In both patients, the presence of infection was apparent within 7 days of prosthesis insertion. *Staphylococcus aureus* and *S. epidermidis* were the pathogens. When identified early, infection easily can be managed with prompt removal of the implant and polyurethane cover, and appropriate antibiotic therapy. The longer that polyurethane-covered prostheses are left in contaminated pockets, the more likely it is that eradication of infection will require a more difficult surgical excision of bonded segments of the implant cover.

Rash

Less than 2 percent of the patients developed a rash. The rash developed usually in the inferior breast 1 to 3 weeks after implant insertion. The rash is more common in patients who have subcutaneous mastectomy, and in very thin patients who undergo augmentation. Scattered, raised erythematous patches occur, with varying degrees of itching. It is important for the surgeon who has used polyurethane-covered implants not to confuse this rash with an infectious process. The rash is distinguished from infection by its intense itching and the absence of systemic signs of infection. It is usually self-limiting; however, itching can be controlled more rapidly with topical or systemic steroids or both.

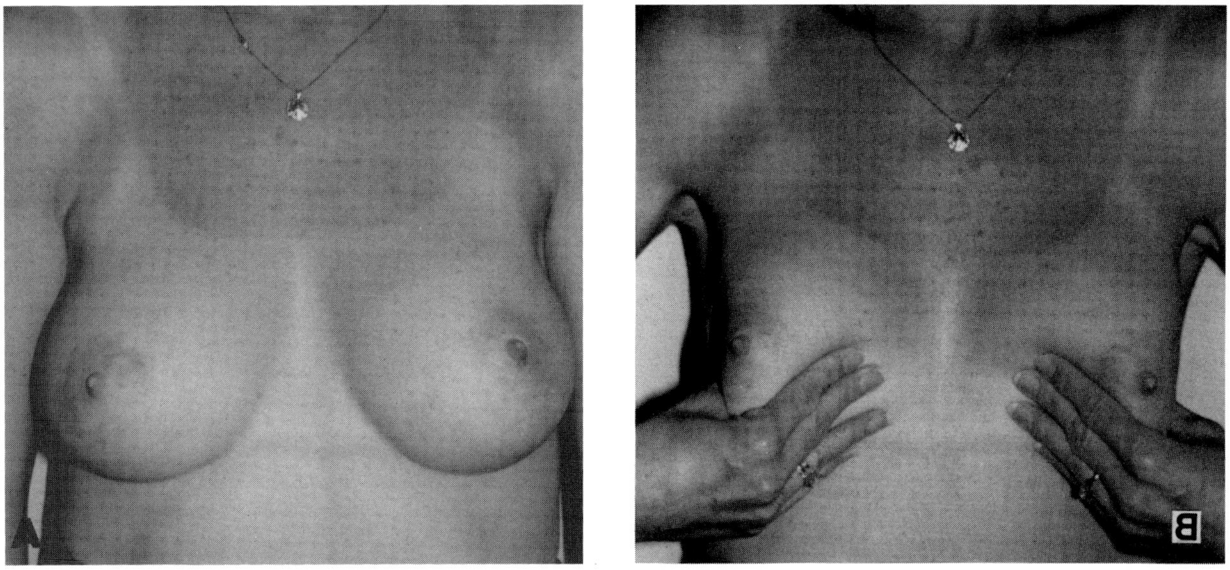

Figure 3 *A* and *B*, Two views of patient 2 years after augmentation mammoplasty, with Class I compressibility of the breasts.

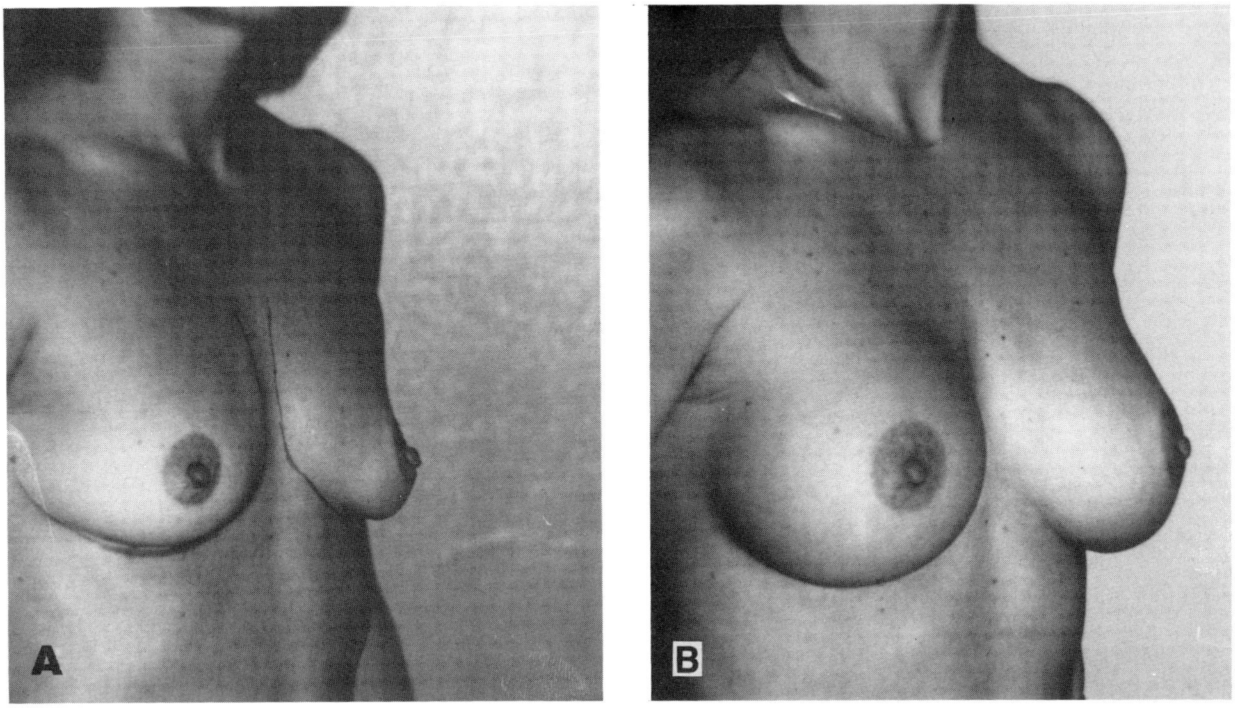

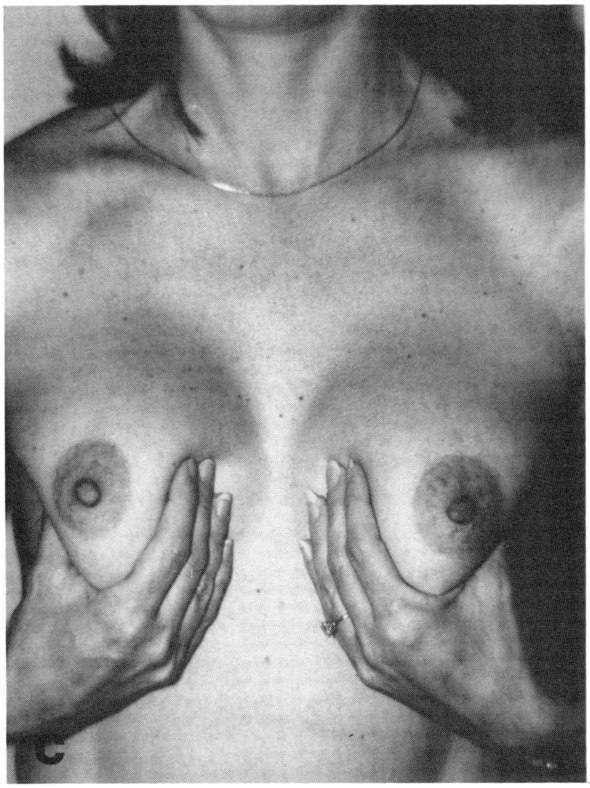

Figure 4 *A*, Shows preoperative view of patient with minimal ptosis, adequate gland and soft tissue for subglandular augmentation. *B*, The result 1 year postoperatively. *C*, Breast compressibility 1 year postoperatively.

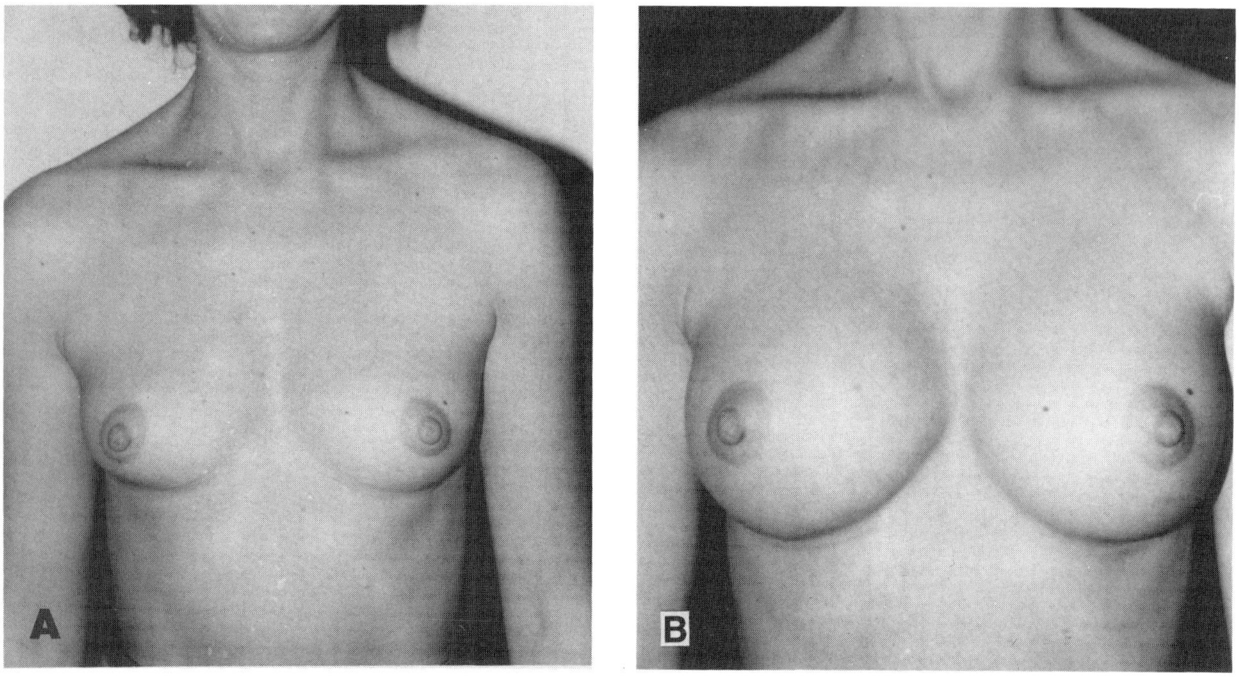

Figure 5 *A*, Preoperative view of thin patient who is better served by submuscular, rather than subglandular, augmentation, and *B*, The result at 1 year postoperatively.

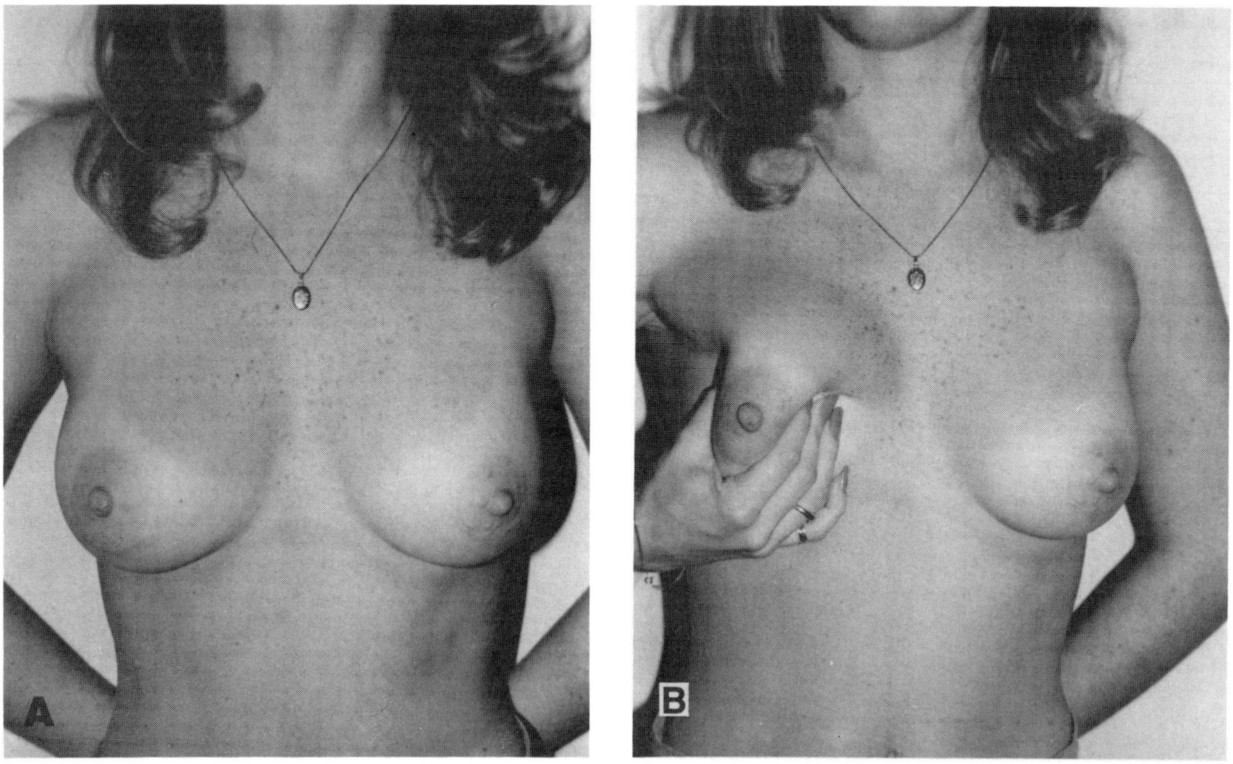

Figure 6 *A*, The patient has had polyurethane-covered implants in place for 4.5 years. *B*, Her breast compressibility at 4.5 years is shown.

Sensory Loss

Approximately 15 percent of patients notice sensory changes, most commonly over the medial breast. In most patients, this resolves in 6 to 12 months. Patients should be warned of the possibility of permanent sensory loss.

CONCLUSION

Polyurethane-covered mammary implants have been used successfully for 15 years now. Available clinical and research data fail to show any evidence that the polyurethane foam used in the construction of mammary prostheses is carcinogenic or otherwise toxic to the host. The implant is now being used more frequently for primary augmentation mammoplasty. Further experience and careful long-term follow-up of patients who have received polyurethane-covered prostheses will be necessary before it can be determined whether polyurethane-foam coating of prostheses prevents contracture for the short term (up to 5 years), for the long term (5 to 15 years), or can be expected to be a "permanent" solution to the problem.

SUGGESTED READING

Ashley FL. A new type of breast prosthesis: preliminary report. Plast Reconstr Surg 1970; 45:421–424.

Cronin TD, Gerow FJ. Augmentation mammoplasty: a new "natural feel" prosthesis. In: Transactions, Third International Congress of Plastic Surgery. (Excerpta Medica International Congress Series, No.66) Amsterdam: Excerpta Medica, 1964; 41–49.

Eyssen JE, von Werssowetz AJ, Middleton GD. Reconstruction of the breast using polyurethane-coated prostheses. Plast Reconstr Surg 1984; 73:415–419.

Herman S. The Même implant. Plast Reconstr Surg 1984; 73:411–414.

Hester TR. The polyurethane-covered mammary prosthesis: facts and fiction. In: Perspectives in Plastic Surgery. (In press).

McGrath MH, Burkhardt BR. The safety and efficacy of breast implants for augmentation mammaplasty. Plast Reconstr Surg 1984; 74:550–560.

Schatten WE, Reconstruction of the breasts following mastectomy with polyurethane-covered, gell-filled prosthesis. Ann Plast Surg 1984; 12:147–156.

Whidden PG. Augmentation mammoplasty. Transplantation/Implantation Today 1986; 3:43.

REDUCTION MAMMOPLASTY

ROBERT W. BERNARD, M.D.

The woman who desires breast reduction surgery has a strong motivation to be free of the physical and emotional disabilities associated with this problem. Reduction in breast volume can be accomplished with the inferior pedicle breast reduction technique. Many plastic surgeons attempt to relegate this method to antiquity. They cite unacceptable incisions and propose alternatives with supposedly superior results. As responsible physicians, we must continue to seek "perfection" in our results and, thus, we offer alternatives to the inferior pedicle breast reduction technique. Unfortunately, I have yet to find an acceptable alternative that provides such consistently excellent results. Some other procedures do leave fewer scars, but these are in more conspicuous areas of the breast, or else they produce a poor esthetic result, or can only be used with breasts of a given size, shape, or weight.

The inferior pedicle breast reduction procedure can be used with virtually every breast size and shape, and the results are predictable. We must keep in mind the bottom line—the patient finds the incisions acceptable. I presented a retrospective study at a national meeting in 1983, in which I indicated that 75 consecutive women who were polled were not bothered by the incisions and would undergo the surgery again. There was of course, the usual smattering of spread or hypertrophic scars, but, obviously, in the patient's mind, the trade-off is well worthwhile.

PATIENT SELECTION

Simultaneous with our patient selection process, the patient is making her own doctor selection. To this end the following takes you through one of my interviews and explains the virtues of my methodology.

Patient Weight and Other Problems

Patients are asked to disrobe and put on a gown before they are seen. They are first examined alone. It is important to obtain an idea of body habitus so that an intelligent decision may be made with respect to ultimate breast size. I put patient questions off until we are sitting in the consultation room. Many of these patients are overweight. I ask them to be practical. Have they lost the same 10 to 15 pounds and gained them back on several occasions? Is their present weight really their true "fighting weight" with anything less being wishful thinking? I tend to deal with weight as it exists. A 10 to 15 pound weight loss postoperatively will not affect breast size or contour. Additional postoperative weight loss may require secondary adjustment of the skin bra, although I have never had to do this. Preoperative attempts at weight loss usually are not long-lasting and may lead to significant negative nitrogen balance just prior to surgery.

I ask the patient what size bra she presently wears. This gives me a picture of the size she is starting with and ultimately helps me get her oriented toward a new bra size. I also obtain some information with respect to inframammary intertrigo, shoulder grooving, and low back pain. Questions are also asked about limitations in sport activities and about social problems.

These questions help me in decision making, and also indicate to the patient that I am knowledgeable about the problems shared by women with enlarged breasts. I can approach each of these subjects logically during the more formal aspect of the interview, and organize my responses so the patient is more apt to remember my answers.

This process takes only a few minutes. At this juncture, I ask the patient to remove the paper gown and sit in an upright position while I appraise the situation as follows:

1. How do the breasts look? Are they "boxy", ptotic, full laterally, do they meet in the midline, are they asymmetrical, which is larger and by how much?
2. How do the breasts feel? Are they cystic, firm, or soft and lacking substance?
3. I measure the midbreast line to the nipple.

Frontal, lateral and oblique photographs are obtained. If there is significant shoulder grooving, or inframammary intertrigo, this is photographed as well because it may help a patient sort out an insurance claim in the future.

While the patient dresses and while everything is still fresh in my mind, I make meticulous notes. She then joins me in the consultation room and I ask her if there is anyone in the waiting room with whom she would like to share the consultation.

Once settled in the consultation room, I describe in great detail my thoughts on breast reduction surgery. I follow a similar format with almost every patient and this assures me that I have given her as much information as possible and in an organized fashion.

I usually begin with a brief summary of my personal qualifications. If I do not leave the patient with a positive feeling about my abilities, she will go elsewhere, regardless of my skills. If the patient is indeed a good candidate for this procedure, I tell her so. I then describe some common misconceptions about the surgery and its outcome. For instance, I tell her that the surgery does not increase the chances of breast cancer; that it is quite possible she will be able to breastfeed after this surgery; that it is likely that nipple and areolar sensation will remain after surgery, and that it is possible to have breast biopsies, do breast examinations, and obtain mammograms after surgery.

I draw a picture of the incisions for the patient and show her pre- and postoperative photographs. I discuss anesthesia, length of hospital stay, postoperative convalescence, and possible complications such as infection, fat necrosis, tissue loss, and the uncertainty of the appearance of the scars.

It is unusual for the patient to have a clear idea of the breast size that she would like to have. Some patients desire a cup size far too small for their body habitus. I tell them that through careful measurements, we can determine a proper size at the time of surgery—although I give them a range at the time of consultation. Most patients are willing to leave a final size to my discretion. I have never had to operate secondarily to increase or reduce the size of a patient's breasts.

I then give the patient an opportunity to ask me any questions that she may have.

Contraindications

There are a few patients who are not good candidates for this type of surgery. They include patients with unrealistic expectations, and young women with breasts that are still enlarging. I prefer stabilization for a 6-month period before operating, but, even so, a secondary reduction might be needed a few years later, although I have never had to do this. Certain young patients, perhaps 12 or 13 years of age who are undergoing very rapid breast enlargement, may require the surgery for emotional and physical reasons, without meeting this stabilization criteria.

The truly obese patient is somewhat more problematic. My solution is simple. If the patient is a good medical risk, and she clearly understands that her breasts, while smaller, will not be in proportion to the rest of her body habitus, I will do a breast reduction. She must understand that, if she loses weight, she might need a readjustment in the skin envelope. These patients have trouble with inframammary intertrigo, breast pain from the sheer weight of their breasts, and difficulty with clothing; all of which are good reasons to undergo breast reduction in spite of excess weight elsewhere.

PRINCIPLES

Patients 35 years old, and older, must have a mammogram within one year prior to surgery. Postoperatively, patients whose breast pathology shows calcifications, cysts, or other abnormalities are asked to obtain a postoperative baseline mammogram.

I never do the preoperative markings in the operating room. They are completed before the patient is administered a sedative. The shape of the breasts, volume disparity, and ultimate size are considered. The patient sits straight, and the suprasternal notch is marked with an "X." The bra strap line is marked, and a short vertical mark is then made midway between these two points. This line is then extended vertically through the midbreast line and a tape measure is used to mark a short transverse line at 22.5 cm from the suprasternal notch to where it intersects the midbreast line. In very heavy breasts, this mark is made at 23.5 to 24 cm since the skin envelope has been pulled down. A McKissock keyhole pattern* is placed so that the center of the new areola site is at the "X." I make no attempt to make this site ovoid in a transverse dimension.

The length and width of the vertical portion of the keyhole need careful consideration. The distance between the lower points of the vertical limbs generally falls be-

* 38 mm diameter with centimeter markings. Catalog No. P4944, Padgett Instruments, Kansas City, Missouri

tween 6 and 9 cm (Fig. 1, points B and B^1). A breast that is short, fat, tense, and boxy requires a shorter distance between these two points. A breast that is long and involuted needs to have a wider distance between these two points. With the patient still sitting, the metal keyhole frame is opened or closed accordingly. I mark the vertical limbs for position only.

The inframammary crease is marked 1 cm cephalad to the anatomic crease. Laterally, it is gently curved cephalad, no further than the anterior axillary line and no higher than the new nipple areola site. Medially, the crease is marked short of the midline, even if a small dogear is to be left.

The patient is now placed flat in bed. The vertical limbs are marked at 4.5 cm on the stretch (see Fig. 1, A–B and A^1–B^1). If the breasts are tense or wide, they will need to be marked at 5 cm, or even 5.5 cm. Elongation of this line and narrowing of the distance between the inferior poles of these vertical limbs increases the size of the skin envelope.

A short transverse line is marked on the inframammary crease at 10 cm from the sternal midline. The distance from the lowest point of the vertical limb to the most lateral and medial points of the inframammary line should equal the distance from the mark at 10 cm along the inframammary crease to the most lateral point of this crease (at the anterior axillary line)(see Fig. 1 where C–B=C–E and B^1–D=D–E). If it does not, you may have to: (1) move the breast midpoint along the inframammary crease, and (2) make the vertical limbs wider or narrower.

The inferior pedicle is now drawn. This is marked at about 5 to 6 cm in width at the base and is gradually tapered superiorly. At the top of the pedicle, it is temporarily drawn to contact the lower aspect of the vertical limbs of the keyhole. This will be adjusted in surgery. The pedicle may appear narrow, but it is being de-epithelialized to make handling of the pedicle bulk easier, so that the less that needs to be done here, the faster surgery will go. In the operating room, the pedicle will be tapered outward from the dermis, thus making it wider at its base.

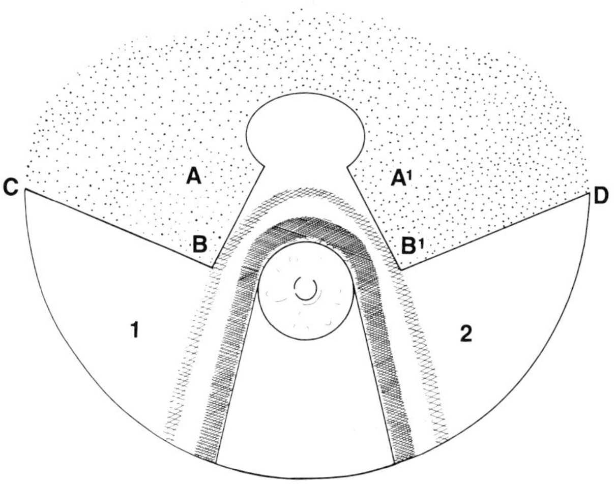

Figure 1 Breast with inferior pedicle. (Courtesy of Elizabeth Bernard.)

In the operating room, general anesthesia is administered. Systolic pressure is maintained at 80 mm of mercury, with no arterial line. (In several hundred cases of breast reduction, no blood has ever had to be administered.) The patient's arms are extended to 90 degrees. After preparation, the drapes are stapled in place, in particular laterally, where they tend to fall away from the patient's sides.

A hot knife is used for almost all the dissection and the power cord is led toward the patient's feet rather than off to the side, as is the suction tubing. A 12 to 14 mm metal suction cannula is used, which may be placed against a bleeding point and touched with the cautery.

A 4-cm washer is pressed into the areola while the assistant compresses the breast at its base. A No. 15 blade is used to circumscribe the washer imprint. Markings are then incised through dermis and four short hatch marks are made within the new areola to orient it on the pedicle. The inferior pedicle is adjusted so that its top is tangential to the upper portion of the circumference of the new areola, and this is incised.

A large Penrose drain is placed at the base of the compressed breast and clamped. De-epithelialization of the pedicle is then done with a No. 10 blade, after which the drain is removed and the hot knife used to dissect along the medial portion of the inferior pedicle. The surgeon holds a lap pad against the flap, and pulls toward himself, while the assistant places two Lahey clamps on the excess medial skin and lifts. This exposes a plane that tapers medially and is above the pectoralis fascia. It is impossible to dissect an inferior pedicle flap that is too broad at its base, but it is very easy to make one that is too narrow. Dissection is tapered superficial to serratus and pectoralis fascia at its most medial extent. The medial flap is then incised along its lower border to a depth of 1.5 cm. Two Lahey clamps are placed along the subcutaneous tissue of this border (the portion to be retained)—(see Fig. 1, A^1–B^1–D) and are held by the assistant. The surgeon countertracts, and constantly checks the thickness of his flaps. The tissue to be resected (see Fig. 1, No. 2) is incised full thickness from the medial border of the inferior pedicle to point D. The lateral flap is similarly dissected, and the specimen left attached superiorly.

The hot knife is used to incise the areola superiorly to a depth of 1.5 cm. Lahey clamps are placed on the superior border of the flap and tracted upwards. The inferior pedicle is cut with a slight "keel" superiorly. If the assistant places thumb and forefinger on either side of the pedicle and retracts downward while the surgeon cuts this keel, the pedicle is freed. It is protected by putting a towel clip through the dermis, and the flap is clamped to the medial chest skin to prevent avulsion at its base.

The tissue to be resected is still attached superiorly. The portion is frequently overresected, thus leaving a concavity, and this may be prevented by leaving thick upper flaps. The specimen is removed en bloc. A single staple marks the superior aspect of the resection, and two staples are placed laterally.

Hemostasis is checked. Skin staples are used temporarily to oppose skin edges. A suction drain is placed laterally and the specimen is weighed. Surgery to the opposite breast is now similarly performed, and one should keep possible size and weight differences in mind. The breasts are examined from both the top and bottom of the operating table at the completion of surgery.

Closure is done in a single layer. Four-0 interrupted Nylon sutures replace the staples. A running 3-0 intradermal Prolene suture completes the closure of the vertical limb and the inframammary incision. The areola incision is closed with interrupted half vertical mattress sutures of 4-0 Nylon. The drains are sutured in place and an antibiotic ointment and a single layer of sterile dressings are placed along the suture lines. A soft bra that clasps in the front is put on the patient.

The patient is generally discharged from the hospital 1 to 2 days after surgery and her drains are removed at that time. Rarely, a patient is sent home with the drains in place. Sutures are removed 1 and 2 weeks postoperatively. The patient is usually returned to full activities 2 to 3 weeks after surgery.

Any skin separation is allowed to heal by itself, and rarely requires revision. A patient might, on occasion, complain of decreased sensation in a nipple or areola. This will return in 2 to 4 months.

ANALYSIS OF APPROACH

This approach to breast reduction is straightforward. With a good assistant, surgery takes 2 hours or less. Complications are extremely rare and easily treated. I have never had nipple or areola loss or significant skin loss in a patient. Little artistic talent is needed to use this technique. Decisions are made before surgery, not during surgery, thus keeping the chances of error to a minimum.

SUGGESTED READING

Courtiss EH, Goldwyn RM. Reduction mammaplasty by the inferior pedicle technique. Plast Reconstr Surg 1977; 59:500–507.

Georgiade NG, Serafin D, Morris R, et al. Reduction mammoplasty utilizing an inferior pedicle nipple-areolar flap. Annals Plast Surg 1979; 3:211–218.

Robbins TH. A reduction mammaplasty with the areola-nipple based on the inferior dermal pedicle. Plast Reconstr Surg 1977; 59:64–67.

Robertson DC. The technique of inferior flap mammaplasty. Plast Reconstr Surg 1967; 40:372–377.

GYNECOMASTIA

RICHARD W. CLEMENT, M.D.

The term gynecomastia refers to development of abnormal hypertrophy and the appearance of female-like mammary glands in male patients. Estimates of the incidence of the problem range as high as 65 percent in otherwise normal adolescents and up to 40 percent of adults.

The causes of gynecomastia have been well described by numerous authors. Three general categories have been developed: exogenous (medications or hormonal), physiologic (neonatal, pubertal, or involutional), and endogenous (testicular, adrenal, thyroid, or pituitary). In the majority of patients, a cause cannot be found even with extensive work-up. Although a thorough history and physical examination are important, extensive laboratory tests are not indicated when the condition is of long duration, the patient is relatively asymptomatic, and is otherwise in good health. Surgical treatment remains the same regardless of the underlying cause. In patients in whom gynecomastia appears before puberty, or significantly later, the cause may be a serious condition that requires further investigation. Because over 50 percent of gynecomastia may be pharmacologically induced, a history of drug use is important to obtain.

Physical examination is important. Although carcinoma of the breast in males is rare, an irregular unilateral mass indicates the need for a breast biopsy. The testes should also be evaluated in every patient due to the fact that atrophy or enlargement may indicate an endogenous cause of gynecomastia. When testicular changes are present, laboratory studies may be of benefit. For the majority of patients, such tests rarely are necessary.

Prior to the development of suction lipectomy, all patients were treated with sharp excision of breast tissue and usually some excision of redundant skin. The use of suction lipectomy to contour the breasts has obviated the need for skin excision in all but the most extreme situations.

Patients may be assigned to four groups depending on the type of surgical procedure that is appropriate. Group I patients have glandular gynecomastia; they require open excision of breast parenchyma. Suction may be used for dissection and contouring. Group II patients have a predominance of glandular gynecomastia, with some breast ptosis. Although these patients can be treated with suction for dissection and fat removal, sharp excision of the parenchyma and destruction of the inframammary fold to correct ptosis are required for effective treatment. Group III patients primarily have fat in the breasts, which is managed by suction and sharp excision. Group IV patients require only removal of fat by suction.

Although the removal of breast parenchyma via suction alone, has been reported, this is not a reliable technique and often leaves residual breast parenchyma behind —a much less acceptable result.

Patients are marked preoperatively in the standing position to delineate the involved areas. The operation may be performed under either local anesthesia with sedation or under general anesthesia. The following locations for the incisions have been described: periareolar, axillary, inframammary, and mid-axillary line. The periareolar incision is preferred, especially when sharp excision of the breast parenchyma is required.

The procedure is begun with sharp dissection of the breast and removal of the breast parenchyma. The suction lipectomy cannulas are then utilized to contour any remaining fat and to disrupt the inframammary fold when ptosis is present. Many different cannulas can be used, however smaller diameter cannulas with internal diameters of less than 5 mm are preferred. After the breast parenchyma has been sharply removed, the procedure is essentially the same as any area that is treated with suction lipectomy. It is especially important to taper or feather the periphery of the involved area. After complete recontouring of the area has been achieved, the incision is closed in layers with an absorbable suture. Skin tapes are placed over the incision, and a bulky dressing is placed to achieve greater compression. The patient is placed in either a rib belt or a support bra without cups. The compression garment is worn for a minimum of 6 weeks after surgery. Suction drains are usually inserted before completion of the closure and are removed 2 to 4 days after surgery. At that time, the rib belt or bra is changed and the patient is allowed to shower. No less than 6 weeks of compression with the binder is required. Most patients are able to undergo the procedure on an outpatient basis. They require analgesics of moderate strength postoperatively.

With the advent of suction lipectomy techniques applied to patients with gynecomastia, complications and unfavorable results have decreased dramatically. The most common problem with this technique is the development of either an hematoma or a seroma. Fortunately, these are quite rare. The advantages of utilizing suction lipectomy for gynecomastia as compared to sharp excision alone are, better cosmetic results, more control of contour with fewer problems of over resection. In addition, it is a relatively easy and quick procedure to perform, and patients are able to return to normal activity in a much shorter time.

SUGGESTED READING

Carlson HE. Gynecomastia. N Engl J Med 1980; 303:795.

Cohen IK. Gynecomastia: suction lipectomy as a contemporary solution (discussion). Plast Reconstr Surg 1987; 80:386.

Courtiss EH. Gynecomastia: analysis of 159 patients and current recommendations for treatment. Plast Reconstr Surg 1987; 79:740–750.

Letterman G, Schurter M. Gynecomastia. In: Courtiss EH, ed. Male aesthetic surgery. St. Louis: CV Mosby, 1982:295–315.

Rosenberg GT. Gynecomastia: suction lipectomy as a contemporary solution. Plast Reconstr Surg 1987; 80:379–385.

Sarvin CT. Endocrine physiology and pathophysiology of the breast. In: Goldsyn RM, ed. Plastic and reconstructive surgery of the breast. Boston: Little Brown, 1976:83–102.

POSTMASTECTOMY RECONSTRUCTION

SURGICAL OPTIONS AND AESTHETIC CONSIDERATIONS

BENJAMIN E. COHEN, M.D., F.A.C.S.

Women seeking breast reconstruction are self-selected, highly-motivated individuals, who often become some of our most satisfied patients. The guidance of these patients along the path between their initial presentation and the completion of their reconstruction involves careful assessment and numerous decisions, both in the office and in the operating room. This chapter discusses the consultation process, the choice of surgical procedure, and the basics of achieving a good esthetic result by the methods most commonly used today. These methods will be more fully discussed and referenced in other chapters.

THE CONSULTATION

The first task is to form an alliance with the patient; to make her a collaborator in the exciting venture of creating a new breast. This alliance is forged by showing respect for the patient, demonstrating interest in her case, and spending the time and effort necessary to educate her so that she understands the potential benefits and pitfalls of the various methods and can participate in the decision-making process.

The patient is fully clothed during the first part of the consultation. Important basic general information is obtained, including the patient's age, weight, medical problems, smoking habits, previous operations, and family breast cancer history. In addition, I ask how her breast cancer was discovered and how the subsequent events in treatment unfolded. Information is obtained about tumor size and location, histologic type, nodal involvement, the surgical procedure, and any adjunctive chemotherapy or radiotherapy. This information is later supplemented by the operative and pathology reports and by direct contact with the patient's general surgeon or oncologist. This also allows me to confirm that there are no contraindications to breast reconstruction at this time, although most patients will not seek a plastic surgery consultation without first being cleared by their other physicians. I listen carefully for all the facts, and watch with equal care for residual depression, emotional instability, or displaced hostility which the patient may still have.

I next try to determine the patient's level of knowledge regarding breast reconstruction. The degree of self-education varies widely. Much has been written in the lay press and many of these patients have talked to one or more women who have had breast reconstruction. The growth of self-help groups such as the American Cancer Society's Reach to Recovery organization, with its Breast Reconstruction Information Service, has also increased the accessibility of this type of information. Many patients come with a bias, pro or con, towards a particular operation. All of this helps me conduct the remainder of the consultation at the appropriate plane, and also gives me a feeling for how much detail the patient wants and needs to know. Before I review the main breast reconstruction procedures, however, I examine the patient in order to see which methods are physically feasible. The ensuing discussion can then be kept to the relevant options. This keeps a long consultation from being even longer and too confusing.

The examination initiates the second phase of the consultation (Fig. 1). Factors to be ascertained include: (1) thickness and laxity of the remaining chest wall skin and subcutaneous tissues, (2) status of the pectoralis major muscle, i.e., its presence and whether there is any lower third denervation or fibrotic tightness, (3) quality and orientation of the mastectomy scar, (4) presence of any visible radiation damage, (5) shape, size, and nodularity of the opposite breast, (6) general body habitus, (7) amount and condition of lower abdominal skin and subcutaneous tissues, and any scars or abdominal wall weakness, (8) presence of a functioning latissimus dorsi muscle, and (9) size and color of the remaining areola, and bulk and projection of the remaining nipple. This information must be integrated with the history, emotional assessment, and any procedure bias that the patient may have. Conscious and unconscious mental flow sheets are employed by the surgeon to generate the best procedure for the particular patient.

The surgeon and patient then have a thorough discussion of the recommended method, including the possible complications. We also plan for a second meeting in the

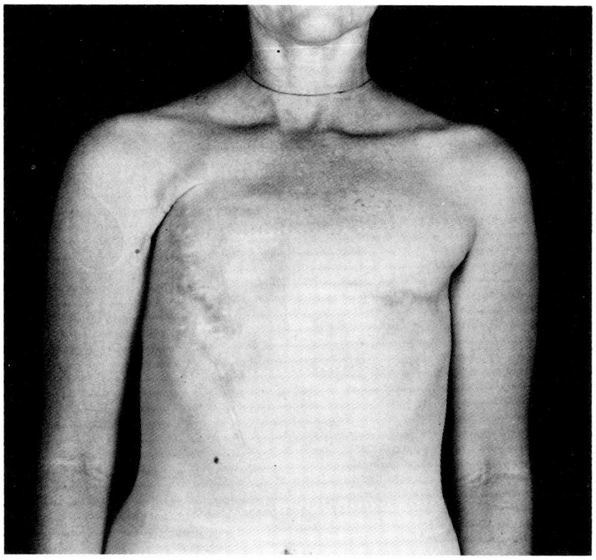

Figure 1 Two very different reconstruction problems are exhibited. The right radical mastectomy defect clearly requires transfer of a flap for reconstruction of the chest wall as well as the breast. The best treatment plan for the left modified radical defect is less clear. With the pectoralis major muscle present and good soft tissue coverage of the upper chest, she may or may not need a flap to effect a good reconstruction. Only one flap was used in this patient though an argument could be made for using flaps bilaterally in the interest of symmetry.

days prior to the operation. If the best choice is not clear in my own mind, I conduct a thorough discussion of the top two possibilities. When requested, I show anonymous photographs of my breast reconstruction results. This increases the patient's understanding and underscores the possibilities and limitations of these procedures. Often the final decision regarding the method to be used is deferred to a second consultation. In the interval, we each have time to think and reach a conclusion under more leisurely conditions. If she desires, I give access to completed patients (with their permission) as a source of additional information. To make a fair case, I try to provide the name of one woman whose reconstruction went well and one whose did not. The patient also has a chance to speak to her spouse if he has not been present at the first consultation. By the second consultation, all the pieces usually fall into place quite nicely, and firm plans for the reconstructive procedure are made.

THE OPTIONS

There are four major methods of breast reconstruction to be considered. Two make do with local tissues and two depend on flap transfers to the chest wall. They are not all equally applicable to each patient. Generally speaking, one must first decide whether a flap will be needed. If the local tissues are sufficient and the opposite breast is small, the choice is between insertion of an implant primarily, or after tissue expansion. If the chest wall skin is tight, or damaged by radiation, or there is a large opposite breast to be matched, then transfer of a latissimus dorsi or rectus abdominis musculocutaneous flap will be necessary. How much the patient is willing to go through, and the presence of any medical risk factors, also influence the operative decision. Reconstruction variations, such as the upper abdominal advancement flap or the thoracoepigastric flap, are infrequently chosen options that will not be considered here. The same is true for vertical or transverse upper rectus flaps as well as superior gluteal free flap transfers.

Implant Only

Initially the mainstay of the plastic surgeon, this method subsequently was overused for a time before the latissimus dorsi flap method, and then tissue expansion, were widely employed. It is only applicable to simple and modified radical mastectomy defects in which the chest wall skin is not too tight. The ideal candidate has unirradiated skin and thick, freely movable, almost slack, chest wall coverage. The opposite breast should be small and the torso small enough for good breast projection to be achieved with a moderate-sized implant. Though many results will be adequate, relatively few patients will have an outstanding esthetic result with this method. This is because few have enough tissue to obtain a nice rounding of the breast's lower pole, which would avoid a dome-like shape to the breast.

Tissue Expander

This method should be used for the same general group as discussed above. It has improved the final result in those patients who might have been reconstructed by primary implant placement alone, and has obviated the need for flap transfer in a transitional group of patients with modest tissue needs. The stretched skin, especially in the lower pole of the breast, allows it to drape more gracefully over the implant and to obtain a better final shape. Tissue expansion is not the panacea many seem to believe, however, and is not indicated in cases where the skin is quite tight or severely damaged by scars or radiation. This method requires an extra stage compared to the implant-only method, but it is not of great magnitude. While in place, there may be discomfort at the site of the injection port and after the expansions. Generally, the same complications occur as with any of the implant-requiring techniques. The large number of office visits makes it a less convenient choice for patients who live at a distance from their surgeon.

Latissimus Dorsi Flap

This reliable method can produce excellent results. It is useful in radical mastectomy cases, when there has been extensive radiation damage, a large opposite breast is to be matched, or more ptosis is needed than can be obtained with the implant-only method. The flap can be raised and transferred in a reasonable period of time without a great deal of surgical assistance, and has a robust circulation. Furthermore, the rudiments of its use are not difficult to learn. For these reasons, when a flap is needed, the latissimus dorsi is often the first-line choice, especially for the plastic surgeon who operates alone, or who does not do a lot of breast reconstruction surgery. Active muscle contraction should be checked preoperatively, even though it is rarely absent in this era of more conservative mastectomies. Compared to the lower transverse rectus abdominis musculocutaneous (TRAM) flap, the latissimus choice ranks higher for patients who have lower abdominal midline scars, are older, are more than moderately obese, or who will not completely stop smoking. The major latissimus complications have been esthetic and related to fibrous periprosthetic capsular contractures, whereas the TRAM flap can produce not only esthetic but comparably more severe complications.

Lower Transverse Rectus Abdominis Musculocutaneous (TRAM) Flap

This is an excellent technique, but is the most demanding for both patient and surgeon. The TRAM flap is very attractive, however, because a single-stage reconstruction can be achieved without an implant and with a simultaneous improvement in abdominal girth and contour. Unlike the implant-requiring methods, once completed there are no periprosthetic contracture problems to worry about. If the patient is too old, too thin, or too fat, has significant lower abdominal scarring, will not completely stop smoking, or is not willing to undergo a major operation with a 4 to 6 day hospitalization and significant potential complications, she should not have this procedure. Furthermore, the surgeon must also qualify. He or she should be well-versed in the operation and preferably have helped on, or observed, several procedures. The raising and transfer of the flap, the abdominal repair, and a method of fashioning a three-dimensional breast out of a two-dimensional flap without an implant should be thoroughly understood. In order for the case to go expeditiously, it helps to have two assistants, one of whom should be capable of closing the fascial and abdominal wounds while the surgeon's primary focus is turned towards shaping and insetting the flap. Experience with complicated tissue transfers is helpful in sometimes difficult intraoperative decisions regarding viability of portions of the flap. The quality of the results with any method are directly related to the surgeon's depth of experience, but more so with this technique than the others. The plastic surgeon who does the occasional breast reconstruction will not, and probably should not, choose this procedure. Provided strict patient selection and surgical ability criteria are met, this method is capable of producing outstanding results.

ESTHETIC ASPECTS OF THE SUCCESSFUL RECONSTRUCTION

We all can intuitively recognize a good breast reconstruction result. It has an attractive shape, matches the opposite breast, and any chest wall defect has been corrected. As surgical architects we should consciously be aware of the breast's integral elements and how to construct them, be prepared to make necessary alterations to the opposite breast, and consider deficits in the entire anterior hemithorax when planning the surgical reconstruction.

I have chosen certain of these basic esthetic elements for consideration here: the inframammary fold, fullness of the lower pole of the breast, the lateral curve and outline of the breast as seen in the anterior view, volume, skin scars and flap color match, softness and texture of the breast, sensibility, and donor defect. Symmetry, however, is probably our most important goal. This is probably most easily achieved in reconstruction of bilateral defects (Fig. 2). To this end, in the unilateral reconstruction case, some modification of the remaining breast is required more often than not. The following discussion is a supplement rather than a substitute for the in-depth discussion of method and nuance in other chapters.

Implant-Only Reconstruction

Inframammary Fold

The inframammary fold is one of the most important landmarks of the breast. It should be marked in the upright position with the opposite breast used as a reference. One can often see the inframammary fold in patients with enough lower tissues left behind to be good candidates for the operation (Fig. 3). I do not like to make a fresh incision at the inframammary fold but prefer to use the mastectomy scar and dissect down to, or slightly past, the proper level. It is sometimes useful to place sutures from within to help define the fold. It is important to check this and all other aspects of the reconstruction by bringing the patient to a sitting position during the operation. In secondary adjustments it is much easier to lower a fold than to raise one.

Lower Pole Fullness

Proper patient choice is critical in the achievement of lower pole fullness (Fig. 4). As noted, ideally the chest wall tissues should be lax and the opposite breast to be matched should be small. Even mild ptosis in the opposite breast may need correction to get a proper match. If the tissues are inadequate, fullness will never be achieved, although it does improve somewhat during the first few months as the implant stretches the skin. Lack of lower pole fullness is the greatest area of shortfall with the implant-only method and is the most common reason for selection of a tissue-adding (or stretching) technique. Loss of lower pole fullness and a rise in the inframammary fold are two of the earliest distortions associated with inferior fibrous capsule contracture.

Lateral Breast Outine

The pocket should be dissected towards the midaxillary line. Excision of excessive lateral tissue, and/or liposuction near the axilla or along the upper pectoral edge, may improve the breast-chest wall shape (see Fig. 3).

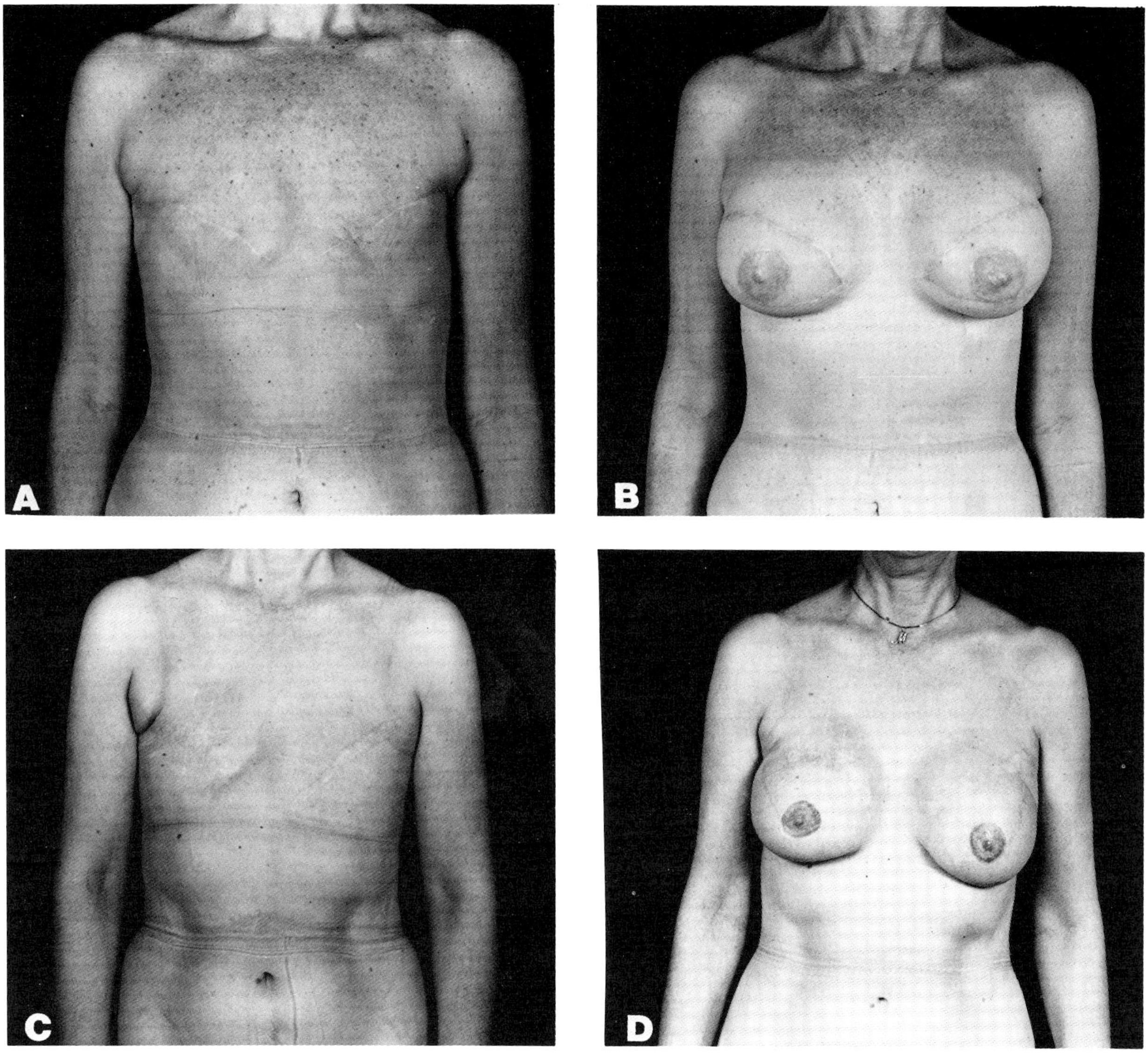

Figure 2 Some of the most symmetrical results are achieved in bilateral defects in which similar reconstruction methods are employed. Bilateral latissimus dorsi flaps and implants were used in these two cases. *A*, Represents the preoperative situation and *B*, the postoperative result. The flaps were placed in the oblique mastectomy scars. In the second case, *C*, is preoperative and *D*, postoperative. The flaps were placed in a curvilinear fashion beginning in the inframammary fold independent of the old scars. Grafts and local flaps were used for nipple-areola reconstruction in both cases. In the second case, tattoo coloration was added because of severe graft fading.

Volume

The need for similar volume on both sides is obvious, but not always easy to achieve. Preoperative volume studies are of variable help and are not frequently used. A set of breast implant sizers for intraoperative use, with the patient flexed and viewed in the sitting position, is helpful in implant selection. The double lumen gel-saline implant allows a certain leeway for fine tuning in this regard. Unfortunately, the tissues cannot always comfortably accommodate the necessary implant. This may necessitate acceptance of a smaller than ideal implant for an interval while the tissues stretch, or an intraoperative shift to a tissue expander.

Permission to adjust the opposite breast aids in achievement of symmetry with this and all breast reconstruction methods. Opposite breasts subjected to reduction-mastopexy procedures tend initially to be more conical and projecting than the reconstructed breast. With time, the reduced and/or lifted breast tends to flatten somewhat, which results in a better match.

Scars and Flap Color Match

The best option in this regard is to use an implant only, as no new scars are added and the color match is ideal.

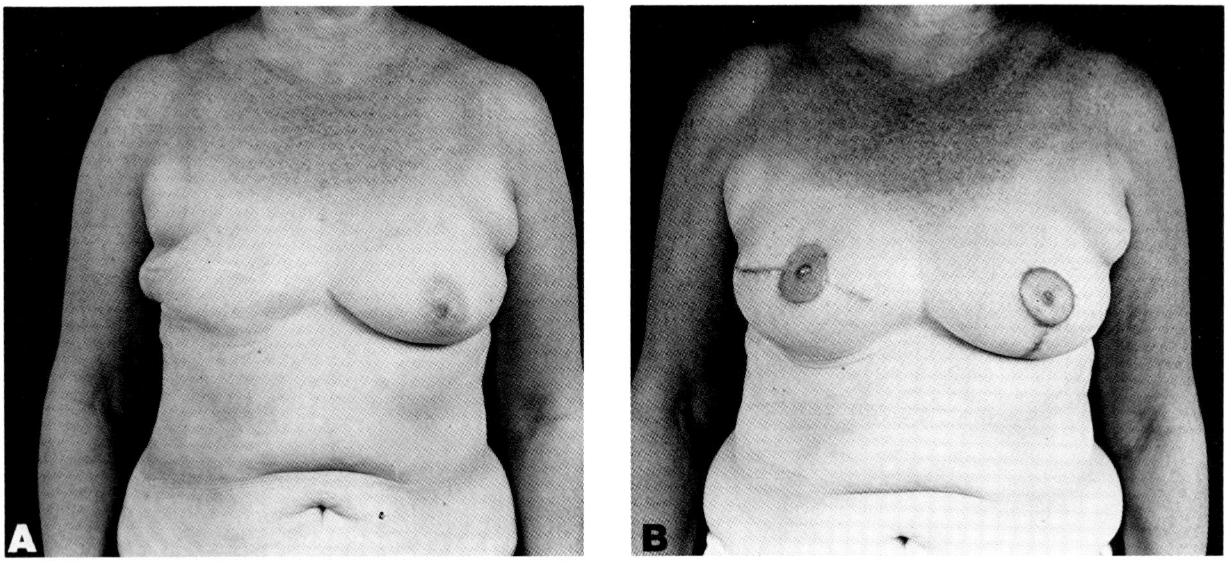

Figure 3 *A,* Chest wall tissues are so thick and lax that the inframammary fold position is obvious. There is skin excess at the lateral end of the mastectomy scar. *B,* Placement of an implant in the subpectoral position on the right and mastopexy on the left resulted in reasonable breast symmetry. Excision of the excess lateral skin present preoperatively on the right, helps the result by making the lateral breast outlines similar. Axillary fat suction on the left would have further improved this. High placement of the right nipple-areolar complex detracts from the final result.

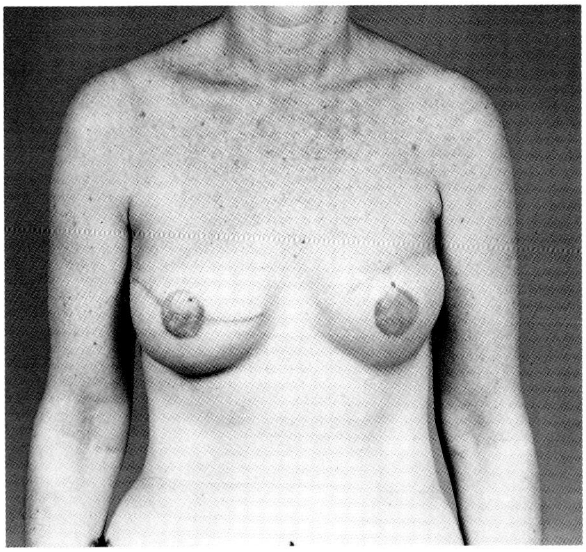

Figure 4 Patient demonstrates the difference that extra skin makes in an implant-only reconstruction. Submuscular silicone implants were placed bilaterally at the same operation. This was at an interval after a left modified radical mastectomy for cancer was performed and immediately following a right prophylactic simple mastectomy in which more skin was left behind. Both reconstructions are soft and reasonably symmetric, but the extra skin on the right provides for more fullness in the lower pole and a smoother inframammary fold, which blends into a more natural lateral outline. Perhaps preliminary tissue expansion on the left side would have improved the result. Direct tattooing of the breast has been used for areola reconstruction; the nipple has yet to be formed.

Sensibility

Sensation is quite good; better than with any method that employs a flap transfer.

Tissue Expander Reconstruction

Inframammary Fold

See above. Expander placement is critical in this regard.

Lower Pole Fullness

The lower aspect of the breast needs to project most and this is precisely where the chest wall skin is in shortest supply. Therefore, it is important to limit superior dissection when the expander is being placed and to center it in a low position. It is particularly easy to overdissect superiorly when subpectoral placement of the expander is chosen. If this occurs, the expansion tends to take place above, where there is less resistance but where additional tissue is least needed (Fig. 5). To concentrate expansion in the lower pole area even more, I sometimes choose the 400 cc tissue expander, which has a smaller base, rather than the larger expanders. If one over-stretches the skin and holds it for a month or two, the final result is probably improved.

Lateral Breast Outline

Same as implant-only reconstruction. The pocket is opened considerably when the expander is exchanged for the permanent implant.

Volume

An idea of the final implant size can be obtained by noting the point in the expansion where the opposite breast volume is closely matched.

Scars and Flap Color Match, Sensibility, Donor Defect

Same as implant only.

Latissimus Dorsi Flap Reconstruction

Inframammary Fold

Usually, I ignore the mastectomy scar and inset the flap in a fresh curvilinear incision at the lower pole of the breast. This incision begins along the desired inframammary fold and curves upward at the anterior axillary line thereby giving it a "J" shape (Fig. 6). If one does not start medially enough and continues too long along the inframammary line, the final breast placement will be too lateral (Fig. 7).

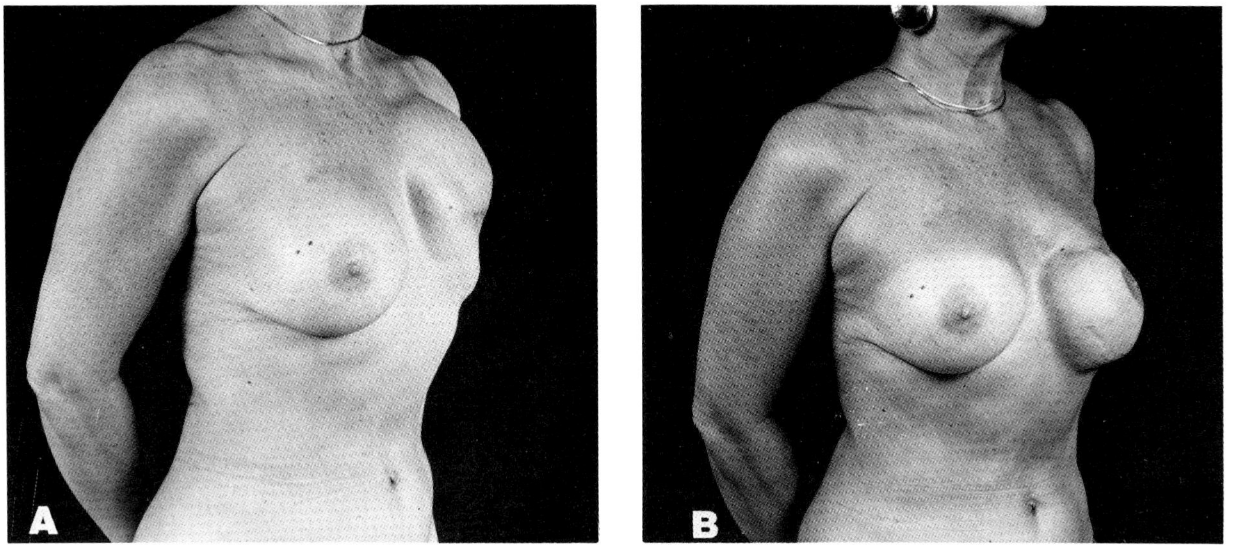

Figure 5 *A,* This patient underwent a left modified radical mastectomy. Elsewhere she had undergone placement of a tissue expander after an implant extrusion. She sought consultation because the tissue expansion was not occurring in the proper area. The right breast had been previously augmented. *B,* Because of poor lower pole tissue expansion, the expander was removed and a latissimus dorsi flap was placed in this area where fullness was needed. Nipple-areolar reconstruction was effected by a local flap plus direct breast tattoo.

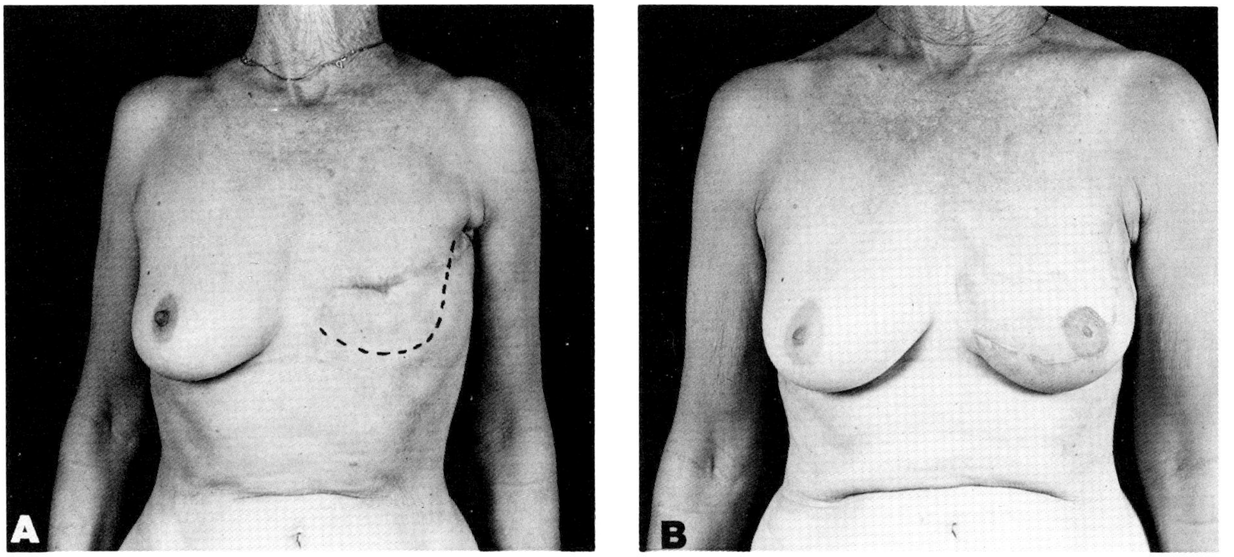

Figure 6 *A,* Patient had a left modified radical mastectomy with preservation of the upper chest wall structures but fairly tight tissues below the mastectomy scar. The planned "J" shaped curvilinear incision for insetting a latissimus dorsi flap is shown. *B,* The flap is placed in the inframammary fold and curves upward at the anterior axillary fold. Crossing the mastectomy scar helps relieve skin tightness at that level. This flap, however, may be slightly too anterior in that area.

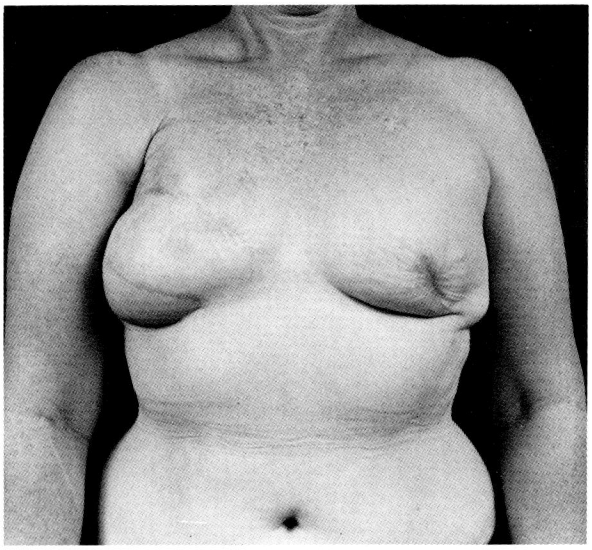

Figure 7 The right latissimus dorsi reconstruction, done elsewhere, suffers because of the too-lateral placement of the flap causing the breast to project in a lateral and inferior direction. The patient also had had a left prophylactic simple mastectomy with reconstruction.

Lower Pole Fullness

Placement of the flap as noted above, or with variously-shaped flaps, puts the flap tissue in the lower portion of the breast where it is most needed. This is not the case when a transversely-oriented mastectomy scar is simply opened to receive the flap. Use of the curvilinear inset with its more reliably obtained rounded lower pole, coupled with a strong circulation, served to boost the popularity of this method enormously.

Lateral Breast Outline

With flap placement as noted above, an ideal lateral breast outline can be created. This is a significant esthetic plus of the method. The proximal end of the flap (cephalic limb of the "J") should not be so long as to blunt the normal indentation between the breast and the anterior axillary fold. Also, the axillary tunnel should be high so as to avoid a visible unsightly bulge.

Volume

It is easier to achieve a proper match than with implant-only reconstruction because the additional tissue allows more choice among the larger implants. A broad-based, i.e., low profile, round implant usually works best as it gives a more natural blending of the breast shape with the chest wall. Too small a base may make the reconstructed breast look unnatural, especially if the opposite breast is even moderately large.

Scars and Flap Color Match

The color match with the chest wall is usually excellent, and the join line with the surrounding chest wall skin is usually smooth and natural. Flap placement in the inframammary fold with the "J" shaped curvilinear inset shows the upper flap scar, but much of the flap and the lower scar remains hidden, thereby avoiding a patch effect.

Sensibility

Sensation is less than with the implant-only and expander methods, but usually is not absent. It is often vaguely referred to the back.

Donor Defect

The scar is often wide and unattractive. The typical oblique scar allows the patient to expose the upper back to meet the needs of most clothing. Sometimes the scar can be placed horizontally and in the brassière line (especially when a vertical inset is needed anteriorly). Few complain of this out-of-sight dorsal scar, although it is not a plus for the procedure.

Lower Transverse Rectus Abdominis Flap

Inframammary Fold

The chest wall is usually incised so that the lower portion of the flap will be inset at the desired inframammary fold. This incision should be 2 to 3 cm above the desired level, and fairly straight. This allows for a significant downward displacement that occurs when the abdominal wound is closed. With time, the weight of the breast tends to cause even more descent. The funnel for flap passage and muscle pedicle should come in obliquely, thereby disrupting the inframammary fold as little as possible.

Lower Pole Fullness

This can be achieved very nicely with this method unless the patient is too thin. Over time, the lower pole improves as the weight of the new breast causes it to settle and the lower skin is stretched.

Lateral Breast Outline

It is important to limit lateral dissection of the chest wall so as not to end up with a laterally displaced, inadequately projecting breast. An oblique (30 to 45 degree rotation) or transverse (180 degree rotation) position of the flap gives good control over breast width, though the latter inset may cause problems with circulation. These rotations do not leave much flap to fill any upper chest wall defect. If the flap is rotated 90 degrees, good upper filling can be achieved, but care must be taken that the flap is wide enough to give adequate width to the new breast. The underside of the chest wall skin flaps and the abdominal flap should be tailored and thinned to achieve a smooth join, thereby enhancing the blend between the new breast and the chest wall.

Volume

One can get great projection and create a breast that fully fills out a brassière with this method (Fig. 8). A pa-

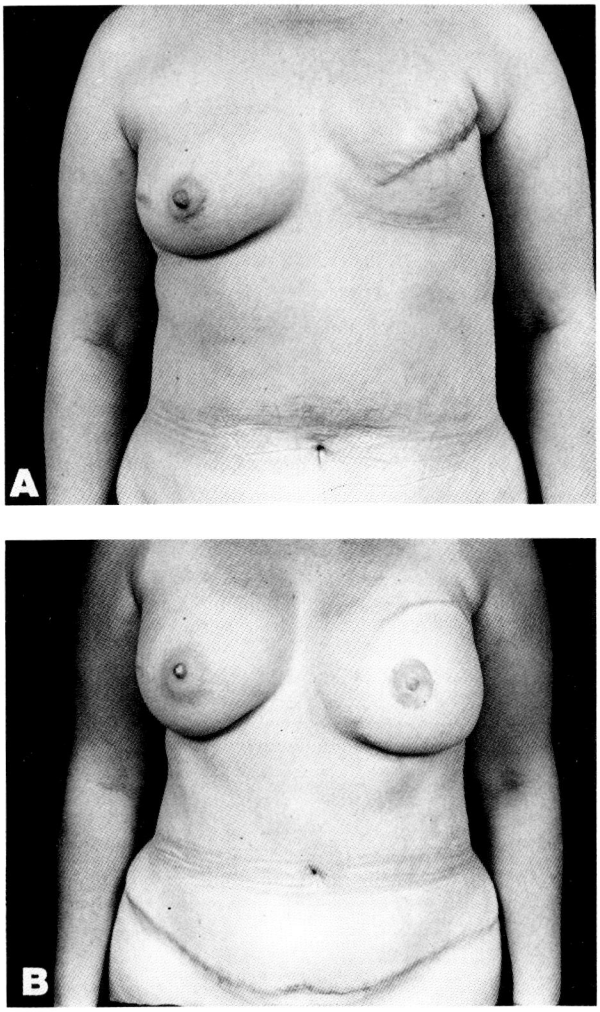

Figure 8 *A*, This patient was unhappy with the left implant-only reconstruction performed elsewhere. She desired larger breasts bilaterally if possible. *B*, The patient is more symmetrical following right breast augmentation and removal of the left breast implant and reconstruction with a rectus abdominis flap. The lateral outline of the breast-chest wall has been corrected from the preoperative state by placing a portion of the flap up towards the axilla. Nipple-areolar reconstruction consisted of a composite graft from the right nipple plus direct tattoo for the areola.

tient can be too thin when it comes to this operation. If this is the case, an implant is necessary and some of the benefit of the operation is lost. In very obese patients the incidence of flap necrosis rises sharply.

Natural Feel

Of all the methods, this comes closest to reproducing the natural feel, texture, and motion of the normal breast. This is something revealed more by physical examination than by photographs. All of the other methods, based on implants, will have a certain incidence of firmness and shape distortion. (The polyurethane-coated implant may offer some improvement in this regard.) The rectus reconstruction seems to improve with time and to become more natural.

Scars and Flap Color Match

The abdominal flap skin may have stretch marks and is often paler than the surrounding chest wall skin. The circumferential scars tend to be prominent for a long time and work against a blend with the surrounding chest wall.

Sensibility

The rectus flap regains only minimal, if any, sensation.

Donor Defect

The donor scar is long and often higher than that of the typical abdominoplasty. There is often some distortion of the umbilicus. The removal of the lower abdominal fat is an esthetic plus in most patients.

SUGGESTED READING

Bostwick J III. Reconstruction with the latissimus dorsi flap. In: Bostwick J III, ed. Aesthetic and reconstructive breast surgery. St. Louis: CV Mosby, 1983:379.

Cohen BE, Cronin ED. Breast reconstruction with the latissimus dorsi musculocutaneous flap. Clin Plast Surg 1984; 11:287–302.

Cronin TD, Cronin ED. The thoracoepigastric flap. In: Gant T, Vasconez L, eds. Postmastectomy reconstruction. Baltimore: Williams & Wilkins, 1981:91.

Hartrampf CR, Scheflan M, Black PM. Breast reconstruction with a transverse abdominal flap. Plast Reconstr Surg 1982; 69:216–225.

Millard DR Jr. Breast aesthetics when reconstructing with the latissimus dorsi musculocutaneous flap. Plast Reconstr Surg 1982; 70:161–172.

Ryan JJ. A lower thoracic advancement flap in breast reconstruction after mastectomy. Plast Reconstr Surg 1982; 70:153–159.

Shaw W. Breast reconstruction by superior gluteal microvascular free flaps without silicone implants. Plast Reconstr Surg 1983; 72:490–501.

Wolf LE, Biggs TM. Aesthetic refinements in the use of the latissimus dorsi flap in breast reconstruction. Plast Reconstr Surg 1982; 69:788–793.

IMMEDIATE BREAST RECONSTRUCTION

I. KELMAN COHEN, M.D.

The majority of patients who undergo modified radical mastectomy for carcinoma of the breast are now candidates for primary breast reconstruction because of the development of tissue expansion devices. Prior to these advances, primary reconstructions were carried out with silicone breast implants, which often required replacement because of size discrepancy or breast firmness. Patients underwent multiple procedures, often with only modest results. Transverse rectus abdominis myocutaneous (TRAM) flaps used primarily may produce excellent results, but operative time and blood loss make this a questionable procedure in the majority of primary cases. In contrast, the use of expansion devices at the time of modified radical mastectomy allows the reconstructive surgeon to place a submuscular device in undamaged tissues and, usually, obtain a reconstructed breast of size, shape, contour, and softness similar to the opposite breast.

Selection of patients for immediate reconstruction with expansion devices has few restrictions. Contraindications include implant phobia, radical mastectomy, and some patients with previous radiation to the breast. Serious consideration for delayed reconstruction must be given to those with large primary lesions and those with a strong suspicion of axillary or distant metastasis. In selected cases, primary reconstruction may be indicated in these poor risk groups because the quality of remaining life may be improved.

All patients who are smokers must be warned that they are at increased risk of skin loss and failure of primary reconstruction, and that the procedure will be abandoned if these risks are considered too great during surgery.

There are basically two types of expansion devices: the simple expanders, first described by Radovan, which must be replaced by a permanent breast implant, and the implant–expander, described by Becker, which need not be replaced and serves both as expander and implant as it has a removable filler valve.

The selection of procedures and type of device is quite clear (Fig. 1). When the patient has a nonptotic opposite breast, then an implant–expander is used because it is permanent and does not require replacement. When the opposite breast is ptotic, the surgeon and patient must collaborate to make a decision. When ptosis reduction is to be performed on the opposite side, then the implant–expander is utilized. When the opposite ptotic breast is not corrected then one must create ptosis in the reconstructed breast. This can only be done via a two-stage procedure with an expander placed low on the chest wall, which, when expanded, provides expanded abdominal skin. This can easily be advanced up from the abdomen to the breast, thus providing the extra skin required to produce the ptotic look to match the opposite breast.

The technique of immediate reconstruction is straightforward. Antibiotics are begun prior to surgery. The inframammary fold is marked, as well as the extent of abdominal dissection if the creation of ptosis is necessary. The drapes are stapled or sewn in place to avoid contamination. Usually, I first assist any general surgeon who is not accustomed to working with me. When possible, I mark out the mastectomy incision to ensure a good esthetic result. When the lesions are distant from the lower pectoralis fascia, I attempt to guide the general surgeon into preserving these tissues because they add to the support of the muscle closure over the expander. When this is impossible, and there is division of the pectoralis major muscle at the rectus insertion, then I simply raise up rectus fascia and advance it to the lower border of the detached pectoralis major. This is closed with a running heavy PDS suture. As an alternative, the lower free border of the pectoralis can be attached to skin.

The pectoralis major is undermined and retracted medially so that I can raise up all the serratus insertions from the ribs. This submuscular dissection is carried laterally to about the anterior axillary line (I mark the extent of the lateral dissection preoperatively). If even more muscle is needed the pectoralis minor may be suitable. At times, I have brought up a turnover flap of rectus abdominis to provide inferior muscle coverage. The latissimus dorsi muscle can be harvested through the same

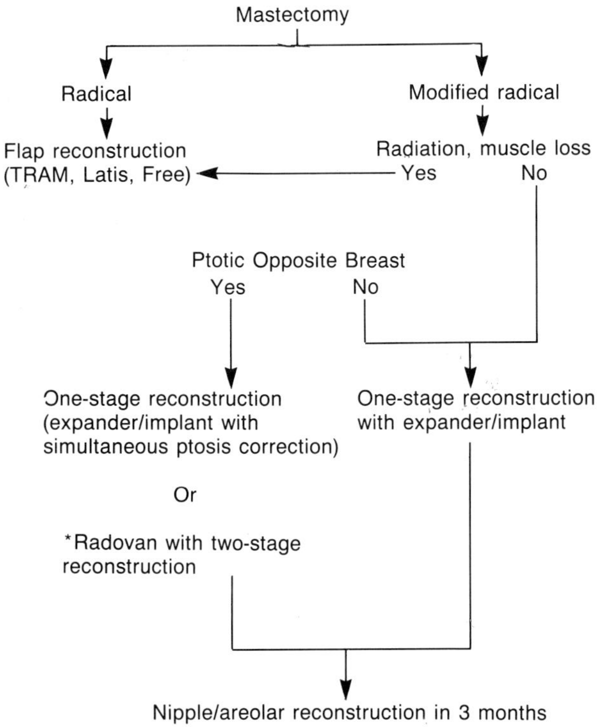

* 1. Insert Radovan below inframammary fold.
2. Two-degree creation of ptosis by removal of Radovan and Ryan ptosis correction.

Figure 1 Algorithm for postmastectomy breast reconstruction. (From Cohen IK, Turner D. Immediate breast reconstruction with tissue expanders. Clin Plast Surg 1987; 14:492.)

incision and used either laterally or inferiorly. Additional muscle is usually unnecessary.

When I use an implant–expander and the opposite side requires ptosis and reduction, I usually do this at the same time. However, care must be taken to avoid excessive blood loss and need for transfusion. Autologous blood transfusions are often used at the time of mastectomy.

Following surgery, the wound is covered with a clear dressing so that the suture line can be observed at all times. The drain site is covered with antibiotic ointment and an occlusive dressing.

Expansion is begun as soon as feasible, often within 48 hours of surgery, and continued as rapidly as possible (usually once a week for patient convenience) until a reasonable state of overexpansion is created. This is variable and depends on the matching problems with the opposite breast. Filling volumes have varied from simple filling to the final desired volume to putting in over 1,000 cc greater than the expected final volume. The expansion device is usually left inflated for 2 to 3 months but this time interval is quite variable. Softness is a good indicator that deflation can be accomplished. An implant-expander can be deflated until the patient is pleased with breast's appearance and its match with the opposite side. The situation for an expander is quite different. I usually deflate it in the office 24 to 48 hours prior to surgery so that I know the size of permanent implant to use. Recently, rather than use a permanent silicone implant as the final device, I have been replacing the expander with an expander–implant. This allows me to get near perfect size adjustment, which may not be obtained with a simple implant. Valve removal can be done in the office when final size adjustment is satisfactory.

Clearly, immediate breast reconstruction with expander or expander–implants is not for every patient. However, in my experience over the past 4 years, the results have been excellent, with an acceptable low morbidity. Almost all breasts have remained soft and natural and patient satisfaction has been great.

SUGGESTED READING

Bailey MH, Smith JW, Cass L, et al. Immediate breast reconstruction—reducing the risks. Plast Surg Forum 1986; IX:17–18.

Becker H. Breast reconstruction following mastectomy using a permanent tissue expander. Plast Surg Forum 1986; IX:20–22.

Cohen IK, Turner D. Immediate breast reconstruction with tissue expanders. Clin Plast Surg 1987; 14:491.

Georgiade GS, Riefkohl R, Cox E, et al. Long-term clinical outcome of immediate reconstruction after mastectomy. Plast Reconstr Surg 1985; 76:415–420.

Noone RB, Murphy JB, Spear SL, et al. A 6-year experience with immediate reconstruction after mastectomy for cancer. Plast Reconstr Surg 1985; 76:258–268.

Stevens LA, McGrath MH, et al. The psychological impact of immediate breast reconstruction for women with early breast cancer. Plast Reconstr Surg 1984; 73:619–628.

Ward JD, Brown P, Knaysi G, Cohen IK. Immediate breast reconstruction with tissue expansion. Plast Reconstr Surg 1987; 80(4):559-566.

Wellisch AK, Schain WS, Noone RB, et al. Psychological correlates of immediate versus delayed reconstruction of the breast. Plast Reconstr Surg 1986; 76:713–718.

TRAM FLAP

CARL R. HARTRAMPF Jr., M.D.

The transverse abdominal island flap (TRAM or TAIF) is a versatile one-stage operation designed to transfer a large quantity of well-vascularized tissue from the abdomen to the chest, where it can be used to reconstruct an autogenous breast or to repair a thoracic defect. We now have seven years of experience with this operation. A review of our first 357 patients who have had this procedure provides some insight into its benefits, its indications, and its contraindications.

THE OPERATIVE PROCEDURE

The transverse abdominal island flap (TAIF) method of breast reconstruction has undergone some modifications since its inception. Details of the operative technique can be gained by viewing the video on the subject available through the Educational Foundation of the American Society of Plastic and Reconstructive Surgery, or in selected readings. The basic procedure involves raising a large transverse ellipse of abdominal skin and subcutaneous fat on one or two rectus muscle pedicles that carry the superior epigastric vessels. The flap is then delivered through a subcutaneous tunnel into the recreated mastectomy defect, where it is tailored into the breast shape. With experience, the amount of muscle and fascia that is harvested with the vascular pedicle has been reduced. Unilateral patients with a single muscle harvest have a direct closure of the anterior rectus sheath. Nonabsorbable suture is used for the anterior rectus sheath closure. After bilateral rectus muscle harvest, the abdominal wall donor areas are closed on each side as in a unilateral procedure. Prolene mesh overlay is used as a reinforcement only when the direct repair is too tight or is inadequate.

INDICATIONS

Salvage Procedures of the Breast and Chest Wall

Extensive bony and soft tissue defects of the chest wall resulting from radical procedures for breast cancer can be reconstructed with the TRAM flap, often with spectacular results. Frequently, these extensive chest wall problems are accompanied by heavy irradiation damage and even by frank skin ulceration. Such patients usually have no other reconstructive options available to them, either because the latissimus dorsi is denervated or because other procedures have failed to correct the problem. The TRAM flap can provide the necessary coverage for even the most extensive defects and introduces badly needed revascularization to the area. In these extensive chest wall defects, it is prudent to use the blood supply from both superior epigastric vessels to vascularize one large flap to be used in the unilateral reconstruction.

Reconstruction Following Radical Mastectomy

There is no other procedure available that can reconstruct the radical mastectomy defect as completely as this operation (Fig. 1). This method reproduces the anterior axillary fold (the pectoralis major muscle), fills the infraclavicular hollow, and at the same time produces a nice breast that often matches the opposite side. As a rule of thumb, it takes one-half of the lower abdominal flap to reconstruct the infraclavicular and axillary defect, and one-half to reconstruct the breast. It is extremely important that both halves be well vascularized. This can be accomplished either by using both rectus muscle pedicles or by using one rectus muscle pedicle and one microvascular hook-up by the axilla.

Reconstruction Following Modified Radical Mastectomy

There are a number of acceptable options open to the individual who has undergone a modified radical mastectomy, but the TRAM flap usually produces the most remarkable results (Fig. 2). The new breast often matches the opposite side and has a natural shape with permanent softness.

Bilateral Reconstruction

This flap is especially suited to the bilateral breast reconstruction. The patient remains in the supine position throughout the operation. Both deep superior epigastric vascular pedicles are elevated, and each pedicle carries one-half of the lower abdominal flap. This is a dramatic procedure, but is in fact extremely safe. Each flap is passed through the common epigastric tunnel and used to fashion a breast on the ipsilateral side.

The Subcutaneous Mastectomy Cripple

Distressingly large numbers of women have significant complications following what is often an ill-advised subcutaneous mastectomy with silicone implant reconstruction. Most of these individuals have had multiple attempts to correct the problem with the same disappointing result. These women can be rehabilitated by removing the silicone implants and by placing well-vascularized autogenous fat flaps from the lower abdomen into a subcutaneous pocket.

Congenital and Traumatic Chest Wall Defects

The TAIF is useful in reconstructing defects of Poland's syndrome, pectus excavatum, massive sternal resections for neoplasm, and osteomyelitis following coronary bypass surgery.

DISADVANTAGES OF THIS PROCEDURE

Because of the relative newness of this operation, the surgeon's experience may be limited, and the exact indications and contraindications may be unclear in his or her mind. Therefore, the complication rate may be higher than with other myocutaneous flaps. The chance of a major complication is significant if the procedure is improperly performed. The operation is fairly long and demands the surgeon's constant attention. The procedure requires an intense preoperative, operative, and postoperative commitment from the surgeon if it is to be consistently successful. The patient's abdominal recovery time may be prolonged, and the operation should not be presented to the patient as an abdominoplasty.

PATIENT SELECTION

This operation is indicated for breast reconstruction only in women who are in good health, are well-motivated, and are adequately informed regarding the nuances of this operation. Careful patient selection is the critical determinant in attaining a successful outcome. I have assigned the risk factors for this operation a rating on a scale of 1 to 10 (Table 1). Potential patients with a cumulative score of greater than 5 are not candidates for this operation.

FORMING THE BREAST MOUND

Herein lies the essence of the procedure; the shaping of an esthetically pleasing breast. Time spent here will be directly reflected in the beauty of the final product. The major steps in the production of a breast from autogenous tissue are as follows:

I. Conceptualization
   A. Repeated exposures of the surgeon's mind to the patient's problem is necessary for a clear mental imprint, which is basic to the forming and shaping process.

II. Transforming the mental image to the physical form
   A. Planning on the day before surgery should include the following:
      1. Mark reference points on chest and abdomen with patient standing.
      2. Plan chest wall pocket and scar tissue excision.
      3. Design the flap to fit the chest wall defect:
         a) position the presenting portion (exposed skin) of new breast over vascular perforators; and

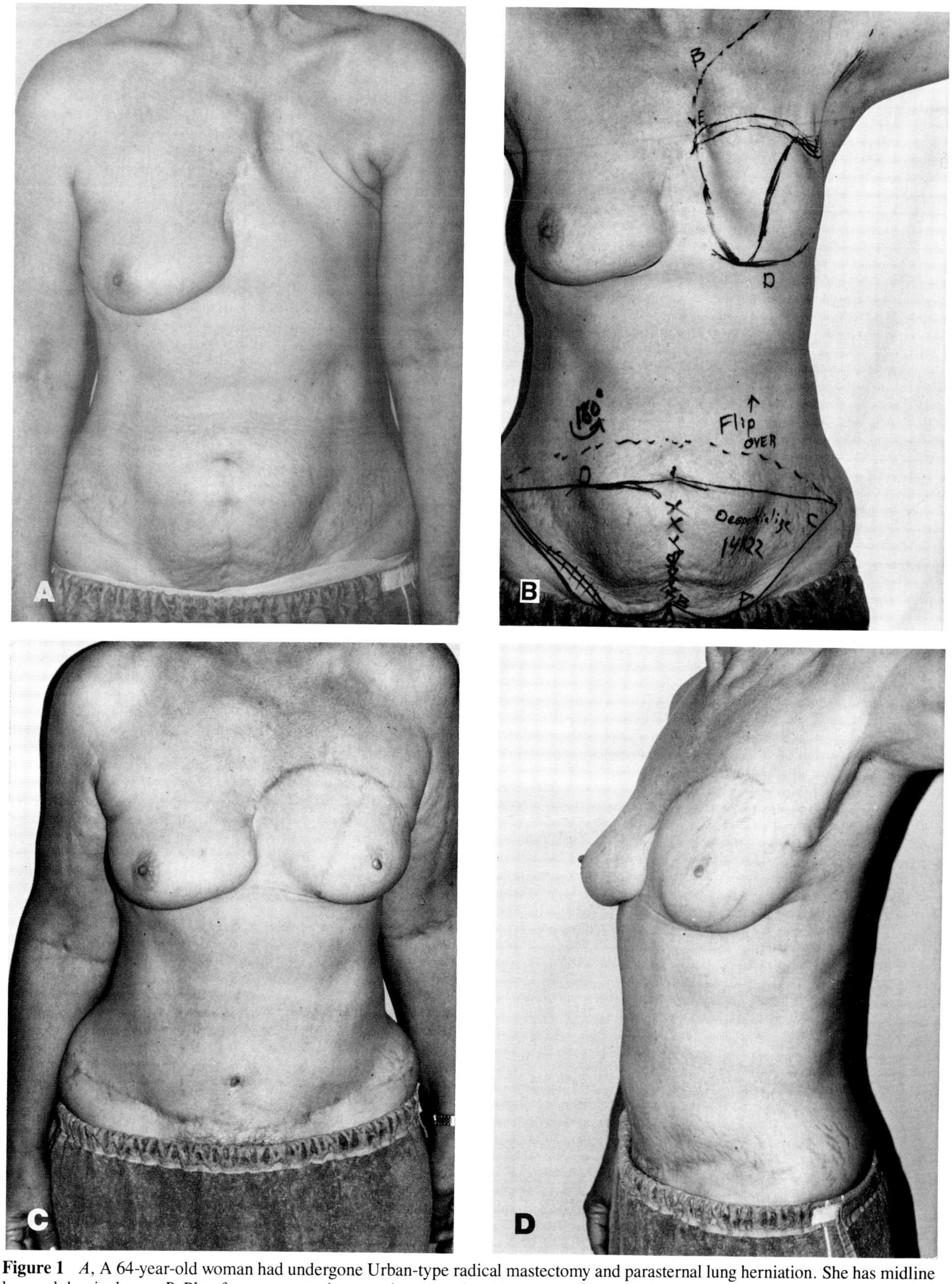

Figure 1 *A*, A 64-year-old woman had undergone Urban-type radical mastectomy and parasternal lung herniation. She has midline lower abdominal scar. *B*, Plan for reconstruction was drawn on the skin. Two abdominal flaps on separate rectus muscle (vascular) pedicles are shown. The left flap (patient's left) was used to fill the parasternal defect, the infraclavicular hollow, and form the anterior axillary fold. The right flap (contralateral pedicle) was used to reconstruct the breast. *C*, The patient one year following reconstruction with all autogenous material, and *D*, lateral view showing axillary and upper chest reconstruction.

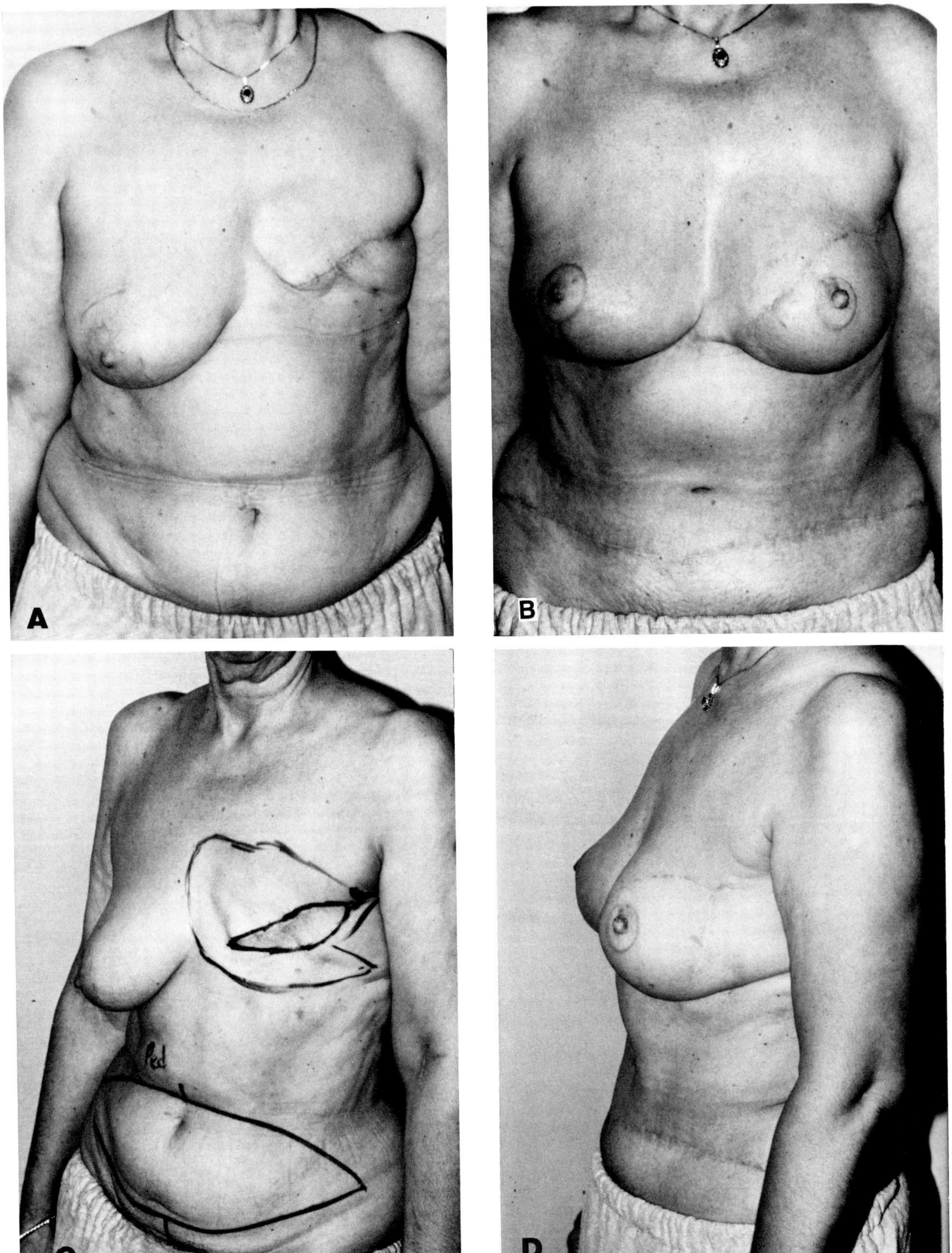

Figure 2 *A*, A 60-year-old woman had left modified radical mastectomy. *B*, She is shown 6 months after reconstruction of the breast followed by reduction of the opposite breast and nipple areolar reconstruction. *C*, Lateral view of the same patient shows abdominal flap that was designed higher than usual to avoid right lower quadrant scar. *D*, Lateral view at 6 months after reconstruction.

TABLE 1 Risk Factors for TRAM/TAIF Procedure

Risk Factor	*Rating Estimate*
Obesity	
Moderate (<25% above IBW)	2
Severe (>25% over IBW)	6
Small vessel disease	
Chronic heavy smoking (10–20 pack years)	4–6
Light to moderate smoking (1+ pack/day for 2–10 years)	2
Autoimmune disease (scleroderma, Raynaud's, etc.)	8
Diabetes mellitus	8
Psychosocial problems	
Unstable emotional state (life crisis)	1 or more
Personality disorder	2–6
Substance abuse	6–8
Abdominal scars	
If planned out of flap design	0–0.5
Disruption of vascular perforators or transection of superior epigastric vessels (Chevron incision, adominoplasty, etc.)	10
Patient cooperation	
Patient unable or unwilling to invest time required for healing	10
Surgeon's inexperience (less than 10 TAIF cases)	1–2
Problems inherent with this operation	0.5

b) discard as much tissue as necessary to give the desired size (a compromise toward a smaller breast may be prudent in cases with marginal vascularizaiton, i.e., in the smoker).

B. Intraoperative:
1. The surgeon must be schooled, skilled, and experienced in this procedure to allow his or her hands to create what has been conceptualized. Optimal results will be achieved only when technique and hand movements have become totally integrated and automatic.
2. *Do not roll, fold, or suture the flap into a cone for shaping.* Instead, utilize the chest wall skin as a natural brassiere (pocket) that will retain the fat in the form of a breast.
   a) If necessary for support, tack the dermis of the flap or Scarpa's fascia at the upper limit of the mastectomy defect.
   b) Support the bulk of the transferred flap on the preserved inframammary shelf.
   c) Avoid suturing on both sides of the pedicle that creates a bridle effect accross the pedicle because any tissue edema or a small hematoma in this restricted area will cause strangulation and obstruct venous return.
   d) Position the inferior tip of the flap in the lower outer quadrant of the new breast pocket for increased size and projection.

III. Cautions
A. Know your limits:
1. There is a critical balance between artistic license and the judicious handling of tissue necessary to preserve vascularity.
2. Do not jeopardize an overall successful result by straining for absolute perfection in the shaping process; a slight modification is easily accomplished when needed at a later time when nipple and areola are reconstructed.

B. Know the flap's limits:
1. When using one vascular pedicle, *do not count on tissue viability from flank to flank even in healthy patients.* To be safe when reconstructing after radical mastectomy, heavy irradiation to the axilla and upper chest, or in some cases when making a very large breast, *two* vascular pedicles should be used for one breast. In the younger, non-smoking patient, the safe area of the flap is from midline to the anterior superior iliac spine on the pedicle side, and from midline to lateral border of the rectus (linea semilunaris, SIEA) on the nonpedicle side. Midline vessels that cross in the subdermis must be protected, i.e., no cutting or binding at the site of the mastectomy scar.

EVALUATION OF THE RECONSTRUCTED BREAST

In a review of the first 300 patients, the surgical shaping of the new breast was completed in one operation in 221 patients (58 percent), and these breasts have been trouble-free for the length of this follow-up. Forty-eight percent required some revision of the reconstructed breast, but only 18 patients (6 percent) required a revision after their first postoperative year. A small silicone breast prosthesis was placed beneath the flap as a secondary procedure in 29 cases (7 percent).

Flap Failures

There were two complete flap losses in 444 breast reconstructions performed on 357 patients (0.45 percent). At least 50 percent loss occurred in three patients, 25 to 50 percent in four and less than 25 percent in 13 patients. With the exception of three patients, all patients with flap loss eventually achieved a satisfactory result. Eight of these patients required flap revision; three others required a latissimus dorsi flap; a silicone implant was used in five patients. In retrospect, there was a preventable cause of flap loss in every case. Inappropriate patient selection and use of the flap beyond reasonable limits were the cause of failure in 12 patients (six each). Partial flap loss requiring debridement has remained fairly constant at approximately 5 percent. There have been areas of induration (fat necrosis) in the reconstructed breast in 21 patients. This problem has become less frequent as increased experience has preserved vascularity of all the tissue used.

Major Causes of Flap Failure

1. Use of tissue beyond safe limits of the flap: the use of poorly vascularized tissue on the contralateral wing of the flap and the use of tissue distal to abdominal scars in the flap are major causes of fat necrosis and partial flap loss.
2. Venous obstruction at the level of the major vascular pedicle, caused either by tension on the vascular pedicle, or kinking or folding of the pedicle as a result of improper rotation of the flap on the chest wall.
3. Improper shaping of the flap into the breast mound. The delicate vascular system within the fat does not tolerate shaping by rolling, coning, or folding, or the maintenance of this shape by sutures. The flap skin does not tolerate tension on the suture line.
4. Vasospasm: the microcirculation in this island flap is subject to vasospasm. This phenomenon when it occurs is difficult to reverse and may lead to fat necrosis or areas of flap loss. Measures that aid in the prevention of vasospasm are:
   a. Avoid operating on chronic heavy smokers. There are other safer methods for these patients. If you must use this procedure, then cessation of smoking for 3 to 6 months before surgery is a must. In these cases, plan a conservative operation; use only tissue over the periumbilical vascular perforators and design the flap higher on the abdomen.
   b. Administer Sol-U Medrol 250 mg intravenously 6 hours preoperatively, again at the beginning of surgery, and two more doses given hourly, for a total dose of 1 gram.
   c. Use a calcium-channel blocker (Procardia), especially on reformed smokers. I use Procardia 10 mg sublingually 6 hours before surgery, at the beginning of surgery, and every 6 hours postoperatively.
   d. Replace blood loss with autologous blood *as it is lost*. (It may be too late after the first sign of central vascular system shock.)
   e. Begin intravenous hydration of patient the night before surgery and continue to keep patient well hydrated during and after surgery.

ABDOMINAL WALL COMPETENCE WITH RECTUS ABDOMINIS MYOCUTANEOUS FLAPS

This type of flap is of little value as a method of breast and chest wall reconstruction if the patient simply exchanges a chest defect for an abdominal wall problem. There are three supporting structures (the resultant forces) that are sacrosanct in the performance of this operation. These are the two linea semilunaris ligaments and the linea alba. When these structures are violated, a competent repair is difficult or impossible even with the aid of the synthetic mesh materials.

An unnecessarily radical resection of the rectus muscle with overlying sheath (including the linea alba in bilateral cases) may create such a residual abdominal wall defect that repair by any means may not reestablish abdominal wall integrity. The anatomic studies of Milloy et al, Taylor et al, and Boyd et al have clearly demonstrated that a more selective harvest of the rectus muscle and sheath can be accomplished and can still safely include the deep epigastric vessels with the important periumbilical vascular perforators.

The abdominal wall closure by synthetic mesh alone severely weakens the anterior abdominal wall and may lead to laxity or even frank herniation. Instead, the repair should be directed toward centralization of the remaining abdominal musculature, thereby reestablishing its mechanical advantage in the midabdomen, a position necessary for good posture and torso flexion. The balancing of the abdominal wall forces is also important. After I observed that this balance was best reestablished after bilateral reconstructions, I began to plicate the anterior rectus sheath on the nonpedicle side in the unilateral repair. This reefing of the normal side also serves to centralize the umbilicus.

A more conservative harvest of rectus muscle begins by using a sterile doppler to determine the exact location of the superior epigastric vessels. Only the portion of rectus muscle and sheath that includes the important periumbilical vascular perforators with the superior epigastric vessels is removed. This disturbs very little of the support below the arcuate line (at most, a narrow tongue of anterior rectus sheath and a small triangle of muscle) and preserves rectus abdominis muscle with overlying sheath from ribs to pubis, lateral to the large lateral vascular perforating vessels.

After completion of a conservative rectus muscle harvest, a straightforward, direct repair of the anterior rectus sheath should be possible in every unilateral muscle harvest and in most bilateral cases. I always use a three-layer closure. The first layer loosely approximates the remaining rectus muscle to the midline. With this muscle repair, each pass of the needle should include a bite of overlying sheath to avoid cutting and tearing the delicate muscle. The anterior sheath is then repaired with a double layer of continuous No. 1 Nylon. Interrupted sutures have no place in this repair for they concentrate the suture tension at specific points and will tear through the tissue.

The first tie in the Nylon suture is placed in a region of minimal tension (usually the epigastrium of the pubic region). Generous bites of tissue are taken with each pass of the needle, and tension is gradually increased on the suture to approximate the tighter area of the abdominal wall. Excessive pull on the suture will tear tissue, and this should be avoided by gradual increase of tension by sliding the slick Nylon along after several passes of the needle. A second continuous layer completes the approximation of the sheath edges and distributes the tension over the full length of the wound. A suitable synthetic mesh used as an overlay reinforcement is necessary in approximately 30 percent of cases of bilateral muscle harvest.

It should be emphasized that synthetic mesh is used only after the best possible direct repair is accomplished.

Use of the Entire Width of Rectus Muscle

If one feels uncomfortable with this intramuscular dissection, then the full width of rectus muscle may be taken, but only cephalad to the caudally located transverse tendinous inscription, which occurs most often at or just below the umbilicus. The full width of the rectus muscle and sheath should never be taken below the lowest transverse tendinous inscription, for without this fixation point the internal oblique and transversus muscles will retract laterally and downward, thus starting the erosion that leads to lower abdominal weakness and herniation. *In this circumstance, these complications cannot be prevented by using synthetic mesh.* When this upper full-muscle harvest is selected the transverse abdominal skin island should be designed higher on the abdomen (i.e., the upper incision of the skin island should be placed 3 cm or more above the umbilicicus). Another good choice in this situation is the upper transverse abdominal island flap. In this case, the lower incision of the flap is made at the umbilicus and the muscle is divided above the lowest transverse tendinous inscription. I find that this upper flap is highly reliable, safe, and very satisfactory in every respect and the higher midabdominal scar is only a minor disadvantage.

POSTOPERATIVE EVALUATION OF THE ABDOMEN

Abdominal herniation should be an infrequent occurrence if a conservative rectus muscle and sheath harvest and a multilayered direct closure are practiced. In bilateral and double pedicle cases, direct closure has been possible in 70 percent of the cases, and synthetic mesh as an overlay support was required in the remaining 30 percent. The only lower abdominal hernia occurred in patient 26. There is some loss of abdominal wall strength, especially in the bilateral muscle harvest cases, but this partial loss is not incapacitating to the patient. In a survey of the first 300 patients, 116 patients could perform sit-ups before their reconstruction. Of this number, 83 percent of the unilaterals and 36 percent of the bilaterals regained their ability to perform sit-ups after surgery. It is of interest that of the 114 patients who stated that they could not do sit-ups before reconstruction, 28 (40 percent) of the unilaterals and 8 (18 percent) of the bilaterals report they can now perform them. Twenty-five percent of the unilateral reconstructions and 43 percent of the bilateral reconstructions report that their abdominal strength decreased after surgery. Eighty percent judged the appearance of the abdominal wall to be improved after surgery. Postoperative back pain was not a problem. It is noteworthy that 30 percent of the bilateral reconstructions who reported back pain before surgery did not have back pain after surgery. A tandem finding was improved posture after reconstruction in 42 percent. Sports activity after reconstruction was the same or improved in 92 percent, and workday performance was the same or improved in 99 percent of the respondents.

PATIENT SATISFACTION

Photographs alone cannot convey the true worth of the breast produced by this method of reconstruction. The natural softness and shape of the reconstructed breast give postmastectomy patients a feeling of being genuine that is difficult for them to describe.

The response rate to a patient questionnaire submitted to the first 300 patients was 97.6 percent (290 out of 297). Questions that were not answered objectively (yes or no or multiple choice) were not tabulated. Patients generally perceived their sense of well-being and general appearance to be improved postoperatively (94 percent in unilateral reconstruction and 90 percent in bilateral). The answers to the final two questions reflect the patients' opinion of the procedure. The question, "Was your breast reconstruction worth the time and effort you devoted to it?" was answered "Yes" 266 times (98 percent) by 272 respondents. The last question, "Would you recommend this method of breast reconstruction to other mastectomy patients?" was answered "Yes" by 270 out of 274 respondents (98.5 percent).

CONCLUSION

The transverse abdominal island flap is complex and more demanding than the usual procedure performed in plastic surgery today. However, it is a reliable operation when strict lines are followed in patient selection, operative performance, and patient perioperative management. In order to perform the operation well, the surgeon must be well grounded in general surgery, should prepare himself by studying the experience of others, and then gain his experience cautiously in a self-critical manner. The poorly prepared surgeon who performs the operation only occasionally will have limited success and his complications are likely to be major ones, which will be difficult to repair. On the other hand, the prudent surgeon who takes the time to master the technique and perform it frequently can assure the mastectomy patient a breast reconstruction that will have a natural shape, will remain soft, and will be trouble-free.

SUGGESTED READING

Boyd JB, Taylor GI, Corlett R. The vascular territories of the superior epigastric and the deep inferior epigastric systems. Plast Reconstr Surg 1984; 73:1–16.

Hartrampf CR. Abdominal wall competence and the transverse abdominal island flap operations. Ann Plast Surg 1984; 12(2):139–146.

Hartrampf CR. Transverse abdominal island flap technique for breast reconstruction after mastectomy. Baltimore: University Park Press, 1984; 113.

Hartrampf CR, Bennett GK. Autogenous tissue reconstruction in the mastectomy patient; a critical review of 300 patients. Ann Surg 1987; 205 (5):508–519.

Hartrampf CR, Scheflan M, Black PW. Breast reconstruction with a transverse abdominal island flap. Plast Reconstr Surg 1982; 69:216–224.

Ishii CH, Bostwick J, Raine TJ, et al. Double-pedicle transverse rectus abdominis myocutaneous flap for unilateral breast and chest wall reconstruction. Plast Reconstr Surg 1985; 76:901–907.

McCraw JB, Arnold PG. McCraw and Arnold's atlas of muscle and musculocutaneous flaps. Norfolk: Hampton Press, 1986:735.

Milloy FG, Anson BJ, McAfee DK. The rectus abdominis muscle and the epigastric arteries. Surg Gynecol Obstet 1960; 110:293–302.
Shaw W, Feng L. A comparison of the superior vs inferior pedicles of the transverse rectus abdominis myocutaneous flap: implications in breast reconstruction. Plast Reconstr Surg. To be published.

LATISSIMUS DORSI

G. PATRICK MAXWELL, M.D.

The latissimus dorsi musculocutaneous flap technique of postmastectomy reconstruction has for the last 12 years been the standard by which other techniques are measured. Its main virtue is its reliability, which, when coupled with its inherent capability to produce an excellent aesthetic result, accounts for its popularity. This chapter focuses in detail on the use of this flap in immediate breast reconstruction and in the more standard delayed (or secondary) setting.

IMMEDIATE BREAST RECONSTRUCTION

Surgical Alternatives

Most plastic surgeons consider immediate breast reconstruction to be the submuscular insertion of a silicone prosthesis or tissue expander after the general surgeon has completed a modified radical mastectomy. While this may be the most popular and frequently preferable approach, it is not best suited for all occasions. It is best suited for thin patients with smaller-to-moderate-sized breasts where the general surgeon is able to preserve all of the pectoralis major muscle and the fascia over its lower portion and its continuity with the rectus abdominis and external oblique muscles. When the lower pectoral fascia has been removed, a turnover rectus abdominis fascial flap may be considered as a "patch" to maintain coverage over the prosthesis or expander. In patients with larger or more pendulous breasts, an immediate transverse rectus abdominis (TRAM) flap may be considered.

Indications

There are two specific situations in which a latissimus dorsi flap may be indicated in immediate breast reconstruction. The first is when the lower portion of the pectoralis major muscle has been removed, or its inferior fascial continuity destroyed, and especially when the size of this defect is larger than can be filled by a turnover rectus fascial flap. The surgical options in this setting are: (1) to accept lack of muscle cover beneath the thin inferior mastectomy flap over the lower portion of the prosthesis, (2) to abandon the planned immediate reconstruction, or (3) to harvest an island latissimus dorsi muscle as a lower pole patch to maintain total muscle coverage over the implant or expander.

The other indication is in women with larger, more full breasts, especially when the inframammary fold is very tight and the patient's desire is to match the opposite breast. The general surgeon can preserve the prethoracic attachments of the inframammary fold, and a latissimus dorsi muscle or myocutaneous flap can be placed in the lower pole of the breast over an expander (or implant) to allow the achievement of the desired breast shape.

Surgical Technique

Latissimus Dorsi Muscle Flap Patch

Every patient selected to undergo immediate reconstruction following mastectomy with an implant or expander should be advised preoperatively of the possible intraoperative need to harvest the anterior portion of the latissimus dorsi muscle through the lateral aspect of the mastectomy incision. The chances of this being necessary, of course, depend on the size and location of the tumor and the method of mastectomy employed by the general surgeon. Since these are variables that may not be alterable, the prudent plastic surgeon should always be prepared.

No special preoperative markings are made. On entering the operative procedure after completion of the mastectomy, and when the intraoperative decision is made that a latissimus dorsi muscle flap is necessary, the integrity of the thoracodorsal vasculature is first accessed. This is easily established by looking along the undersurface of the latissimus muscle in the posterior aspect of the axilla that has been cleared by the axillary dissection. If this is intact, one dissects the skin and subcutaneous tissue off the superficial aspect of the latissimus muscle at the fascial level for the distance necessary to fill the defect. At this point, the muscle is divided longitudinally in the division of its fibers. The origin of the anterior muscle slip is then divided, which creates a muscle flap attached superiorly by its muscular insertion into the humerus and its neurovascular leash. Division of the muscle superiorly as it approaches its insertion converts the flap into a true island muscle flap that has more mobility and, at the same time, prevents an axillary fullness or bulge that may occur with an intact muscle flap. When there is no question about the integrity of the thoracodorsal vascular leash, the serratus branch (or branches) may be divided if this provides some needed mobility. A branch of the thoracodorsal nerve may sometimes be preserved to the residual muscle. When it is totally contained within the flap, it is probably best transected to prevent inappropriate distortional movement of the resultant breast mound.

The muscle flap is rotated as a sling into the mastectomy wound. The superior edge is sutured to the inferior border of the pectoralis major muscle, and the inferior border is sutured to the serratus anterior and rectus abdominis muscle or fascia. The distal edge of the flap that lies closest to the sternum is secured to available parasternal soft tissue. An implant or expander is inserted laterally beneath this intact muscle sling before the lateral edge of the muscle flap is sutured to the serratus anterior muscle fibers in the anterior axillary area. Drains are placed in the anterior submuscular and subcutaneous spaces, the axilla, and the donor muscle area.

Latissimus Dorsi Musculocutaneous Flap for Larger Breasts

In women with larger, more full breasts who desire the reconstructed breast to match the opposite breast (without surgical alteration of the latter) a latissimus dorsi flap may be planned for the immediate reconstruction.

With the patient in the upright position preoperatively, the inframammary fold is marked on the involved breast along with the planned ellipse of skin to be removed. The patient is asked to put her hands on her hips and exert pressure, which defines the anterior border of the latissimus dorsi muscle. An ellipse of approximately the same dimensions as that on the breast is drawn on the patient's back. A paper or cloth pattern cut to the shape of the latissimus dorsi muscle and held to the apex of the axilla helps position the skin island design on the back in the location that will meet the reconstructive needs when transferred to the chest. The size and location of this skin island may be adjusted (smaller and more transverse in direction) to improve the donor back scar yet still meet the functional needs.

The arm on the mastectomy side is prepped free, and the patient's side and back is prepped to the midline. Sterile sheets are laid under her on this side. Since most larger breasts have tight inframammary folds, the general surgeon is asked to preserve these subcutaneous to prethoracic attachments. The modified radical mastectomy is then carried out in the otherwise standard fashion.

When the mastectomy has been completed, the integrity of the thoracodorsal vascular leash is first confirmed. The patient is then turned onto her side by passing the prepped free arm across her chest to the opposite side. There should be no need to reprep and drape. The previously-marked skin island is incised and skin flaps elevated. The dissection is aided also by the approach from the lateral mastectomy wound. The origin and posterior aspect of the muscle are divided. The insertion of the muscle can finally be divided to convert the flap into an island flap as described above. The donor site is closed in two layers, and the patient is turned back into the supine position.

The origin of the pectoralis major muscle is divided at the level of the inframammary fold, and the latissimus dorsi flap is draped into that position. The superior border of the latissimus muscle is sutured to the inferior border of the pectoralis muscle, while the inferior border of the latissimus muscle is sutured to the rectus abdominis muscle or fascia and the serratus anterior muscle in the inframammary fold. The distal portion of the latissimus muscle is sutured to the peristernal soft tissue. An expander (or implant) is positioned beneath this muscle drape and the lateral edge of the latissimus muscle is secured in the anterior axillary fold. Drains are placed as described above, and the skin island is carefully tailored before closure.

The use of an expander beneath this musculocutaneous flap lends more versatility from this point. The breast can be expanded as needed to match the opposite breast, or it can be overexpanded to allow the removal of the latissimus skin island if so desired.

SECONDARY (DELAYED) BREAST RECONSTRUCTION

Surgical Alternatives

There are four basic technical approaches to postmastectomy breast reconstruction available today: (1) subpectoral implantation, (2) tissue expansion, (3) TRAM flap reconstruction, and (4) latissimus dorsi flap reconstruction. The experienced plastic surgeon should be versatile in all of these techniques and able to match the appropriate operation to the appropriate patient in any given situation. Nonobese patients with adequate soft tissue present may be candidates for the placement of a silicone prosthesis. Patients with qualitatively good soft tissue but quantitative deficiency may be candidates for tissue expansion. Patients with pouchy but nonpendulous lower abdominal soft tissue may be good candidates for a TRAM flap. There may perhaps be an occasional patient who needs a microvascular flap reconstruction. Careful patient individualization is the obvious key to success in this decision.

Indications

Although it is difficult to define specific indications, latissimus dorsi flap breast reconstruction is a consideration for: (1) any patient without ample prethoracic soft tissue (for implant alone), (2) patients not desirous of tissue expansion, (3) patients with irradiated chests, (4) patients not desirous of a TRAM flap or in whom a TRAM flap is contraindicated, or (5) any patient where it is predicted to give the best aesthetic result as compared to the other options.

Patients should be carefully assessed preoperatively by noting the color and texture of the back skin as compared to the chest skin. Some patients have a very thick dermis and darkly-pigmented, freckled back skin that is not a good skin match on the breast mound. The innervation to the latissimus dorsi muscle should be evaluated by having the patient place her hands on her hips and exert pressure. An innervated latissimus muscle will be visibly apparent in the posterior axillary line on contraction. Although a denervated latissimus muscle does not preclude a viable flap transfer, there is less bulk and a smaller flap. The thoracodorsal blood supply has probably been divided in a patient with a denervated muscle, and one cannot be certain of its integrity in the patient with a contractile muscle. Our previous laboratory and clinical studies, however, have borne out the ability to utilize this flap even when the vasculature has been altered. The only relative contraindication to the use of a latissimus dorsi flap is a previous high-transverse thoracotomy incision that totally transected the latissimus muscle.

Preoperative Planning

Through clinical experience it has become apparent that in most cases the resultant breast mound has a better appearance when the latissimus dorsi skin island is placed in the inferolateral position (Fig. 1). This produces a sling or cradle-like soft-tissue envelope into which a prosthesis is placed. Additionally, the lateral and inferior incisions are hidden in the anterior axillary line and inframammary fold, thereby minimizing the patch-like quality that a latissimus reconstructed breast can have. A low, oblique, mastectomy scar allows this placement. Mastectomy scars in other locations (transverse or vertical) do not. In these latter situations, if the quality of the mastectomy scar is acceptable, it may be best to make a new incision that slopes low and obliquely to approach the inframammary fold for the placement of the latissimus skin island (Fig. 2).

The size, shape, and location of the planned skin island on the back depend on the chest requirements of skin relative to muscle, the location on the resultant breast mound when the skin is positioned (as discussed above), and the patient's acceptance of the back scar position. If one assumes the skin island is to be positioned inferolaterally, a portion of the latissimus dorsi muscle may be needed superiorly for suture to the remaining pectoralis major muscle. The more pectoralis major muscle that is removed, the more latissimus muscle will be needed superior to the skin island once transported. The higher the skin island is placed on the back, the more latissimus muscle will be present superior to it following transposition. Thus, in radical mastectomy reconstruction, the skin island is designed high on the back, while in modified mastectomy reconstruction it may be placed more low and obliquely (Fig. 3). Within these guidelines, the patient may have input as to what is more acceptable—a high transverse scar that is covered by a two-piece bathing suit; a medium transverse or slightly oblique scar covered by the bra line; or a low oblique scar that allows a low-back bathing suit or evening dress to be worn.

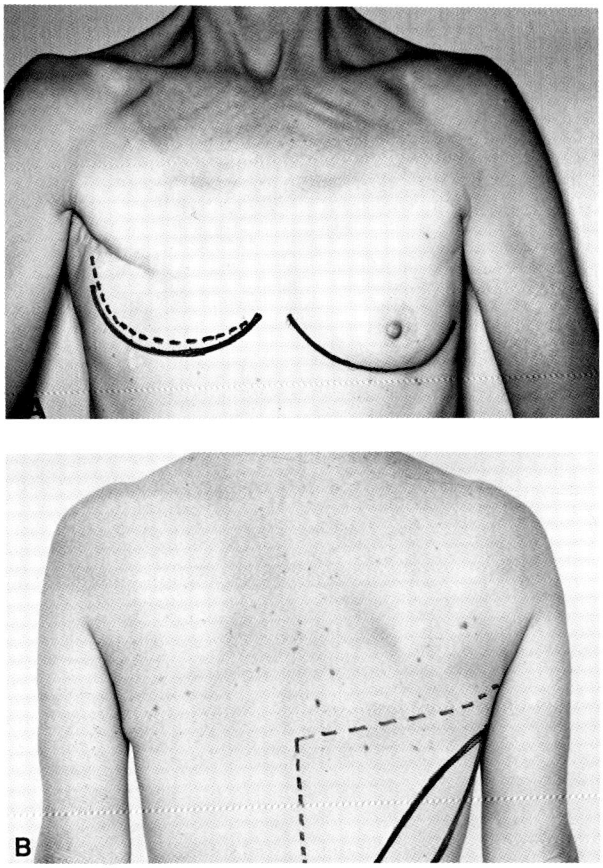

Figure 2 *A*, A patient is shown following modified radical mastectomy. Preoperative marking of the left inframammary fold and its transposition to the right chest are shown by solid lines. The dotted line is the planned incision rather than the higher mastectomy scar. *B*, Based on these chest requirements, the skin island is designed in the low-oblique position.

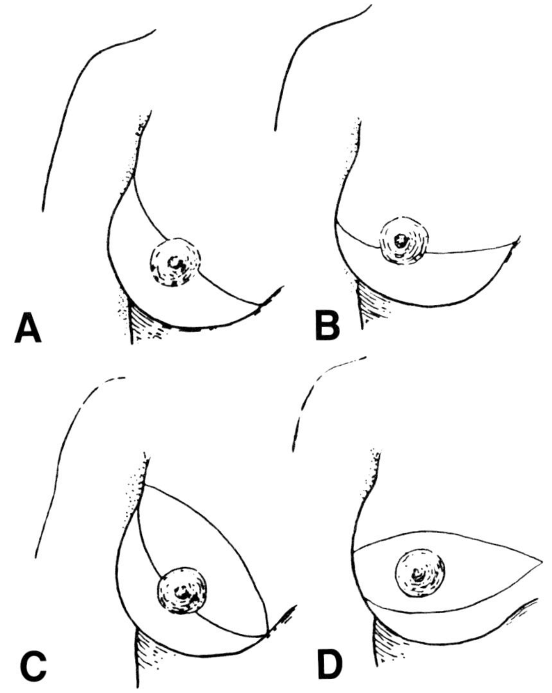

Figure 1 *A*, The preferred position for the latissimus dorsi skin island is in the inferolateral position on the removed breast. *B*, When a transverse position is necessary, it is preferable to compose the entire lower pole. *C*, Less desirable placement may be necessitated by the mastectomy scar, while *D*, transverse placement across the center of the breast is least desirable.

Surgical Technique

The patient is placed on the operating table in the supine position with the opposite arm out on an armboard.

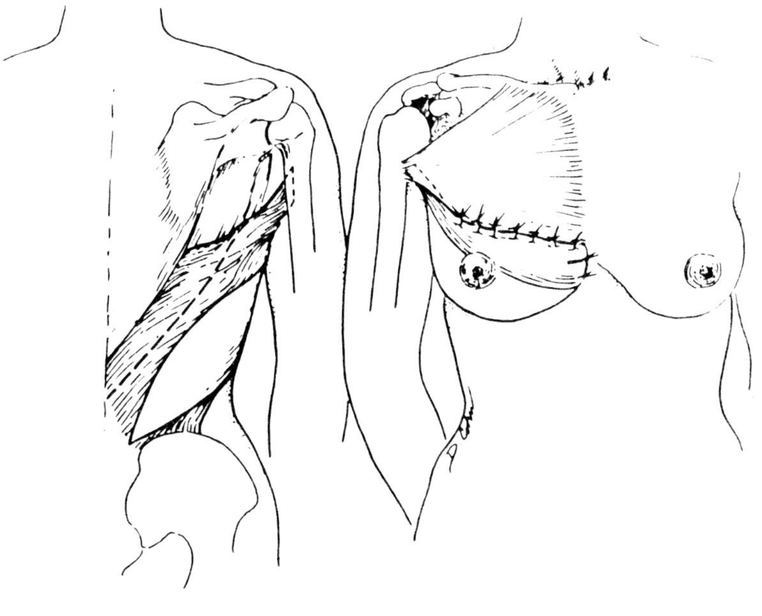

Figure 3 In modified radical mastectomy reconstruction the skin island can be placed low and obliquely on the back (and only a portion of latissimus muscle removed) since little muscle is needed above or below it when transported to the chest. This also places it in the preferred inferolateral position.

She is then totally prepped and the drapes placed on the opposite side. She is then turned into the lateral decubitus position and secured with a pillow between the legs, tape across the hips, and an axillary roll if needed. The side and back are prepped, with the involved arm prepped free. A padded ether stand is well secured, and the arm attached by towel clips. After the flap has been harvested, passed to the chest wound (or stuffed into the axilla), and the back closed, the circulator can remove the pillow, tape, and axillary roll, and the patient can be repositioned superiorly without the need to reprep or drape. An armboard is added on the mastectomy side for symmetrical patient position.

The skin island is incised and skin flaps elevated by peripheral beveling to maintain all possible perforators. The anterosuperior edge of the muscle is identified, and the dissection is carried in the fascial plane deep to the muscle. The origin of the muscle is then divided inferiorly and the paravertical or posterior edge of the muscle cut free. This dissection elevates the flap, based on its superior muscular insertion and blood supply. As the dissection is carried superiorly, one looks on the under surface of the muscle to see the thoracodorsal vessels that lead to the serratus branch (or branches). The latter should be left intact unless one is certain that the thoracodorsal vessel is intact above this and was not damaged in any way during the axillary dissection. Dissection is carried posterior to the serratus branch and elevates the latissimus off the teres major muscle. This is carried all the way to the tendinous insertion into the humerus, which can be divided if so desired. The axilla is freed subcutaneously to allow easy passage of the flap from the back to the chest. Two suction drains are placed in the back, and the donor site closed in two layers.

With the patient repositioned superiorly, the flap is positioned. The chest incision has been made and the subpectoral pocket dissected above. The superior edge of the latissimus muscle is sutured to the lower edge of the pec-

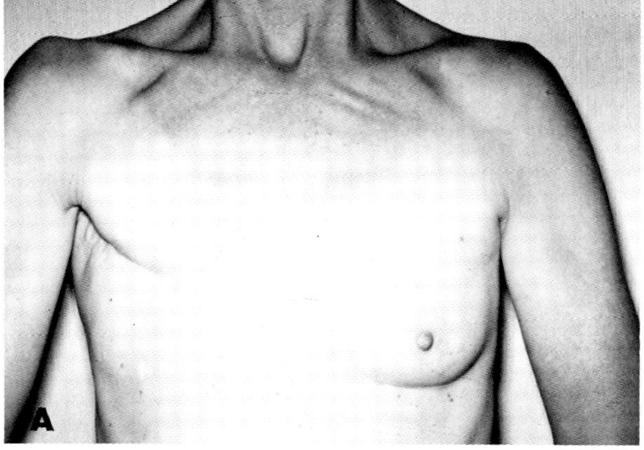

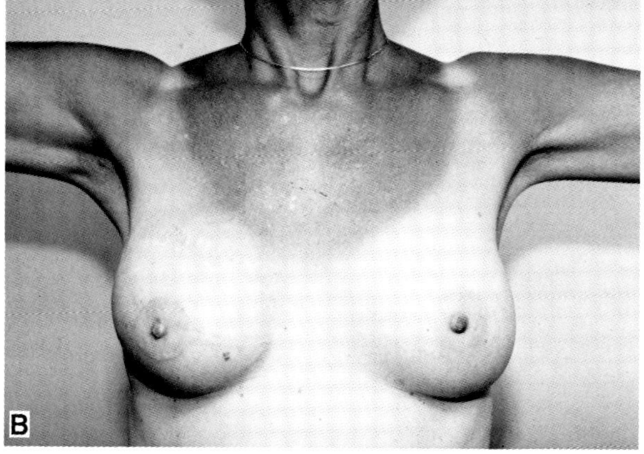

Figure 4 *A*, Preoperative appearance and *B*, postoperative result. The nipple-areola reconstruction was performed in a second operative procedure.

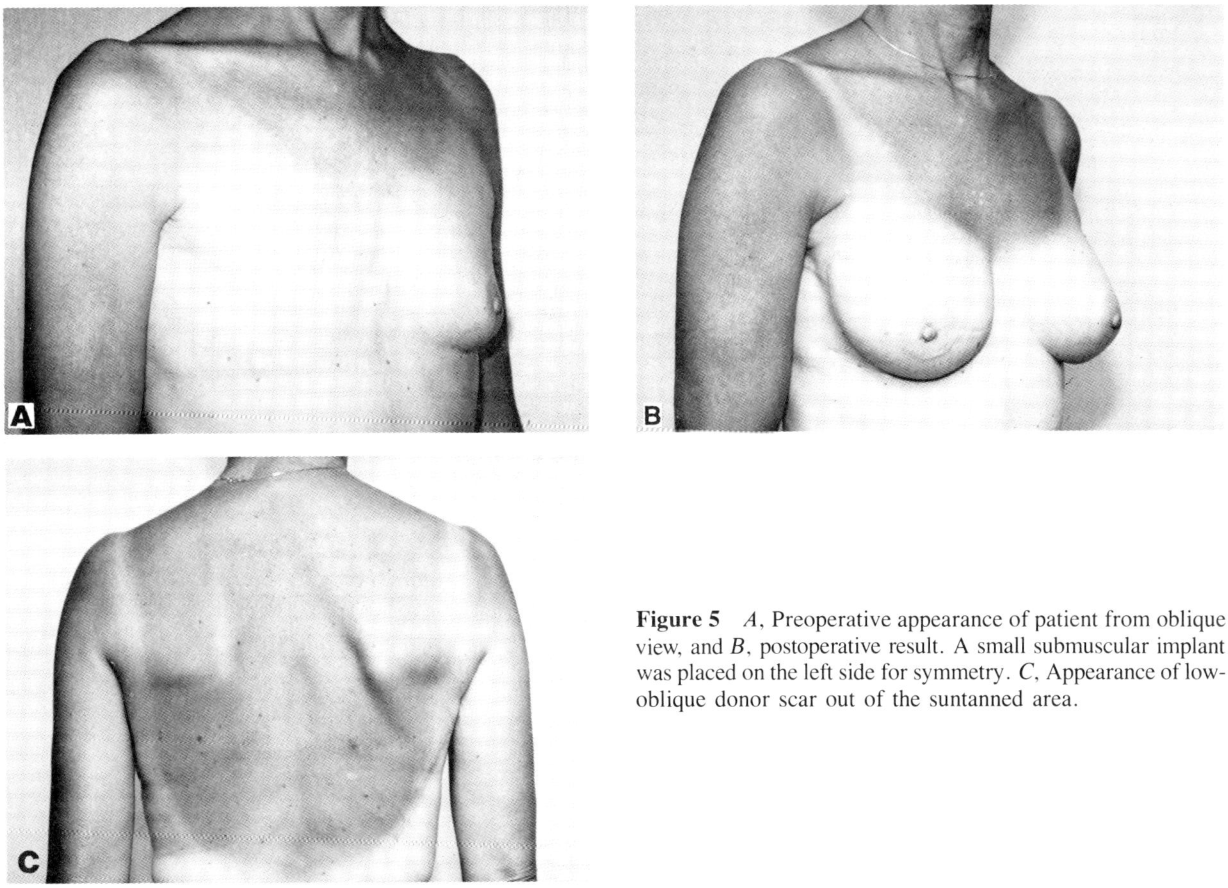

Figure 5 *A*, Preoperative appearance of patient from oblique view, and *B*, postoperative result. A small submuscular implant was placed on the left side for symmetry. *C*, Appearance of low-oblique donor scar out of the suntanned area.

toralis major. In a radical mastectomy reconstruction, the upper edge of the latissimus is sutured to the periosteum of the clavicle. Inferiorly, the latissimus muscle and skin island are positioned and sutured in the inframammary fold. The skin island is carefully tailored as necessary.

The operating table is cranked into a 90-degree angle to put the patient in an upright position. Any necessary adjustments in inframammary fold level, pocket dissection, etc., are now made. Sizer prostheses are inserted to determine the exact size and shape necessary. The patient is placed back in the supine position, the prosthesis is inserted, and lateral muscle is sutured to the chest wall to recreate the anterior axillary fold. Two drains are inserted, and skin closure completed. Drains are generally left in for 5 days and antibiotics are given.

ASSESSMENT

The latissimus dorsi flap, utilized in either the primary or secondary setting for postmastectomy reconstruction, has a proven record of reliability. It is extremely rare to incur any problems with flap viability, and wound-healing problems are rare. Donor site arm or shoulder disability is minimal, and the back scar is generally well-accepted by patients. The most frequent complication with the operation is the occurrence of a seroma in the back. This is due to the large, raw surface area from which the flap has been removed and which, perhaps, has several axillary lymphatics draining therein. The seromas may require aspiration, but generally resolve without serious consequence. The resultant reconstructed breast usually has an excellent esthetic quality (Figs. 4 and 5). Some have questioned a long-term, higher capsule rate with this technique as compared to others, but this has never been confirmed.

SUGGESTED READING

Bostwick J, Vasconez LD, Jurkiewicz ME. Breast reconstruction after a radical mastectomy. Plast Reconstr Surg 1978; 61:682–693.

Maxwell GP. Breast reconstruction following mastectomy. In: Grabb WC, Smith JW, Aston, eds. Plastic surgery. 4th ed. Boston: Little, Brown, (in press).

Maxwell GP. Selection of secondary breast reconstructive procedures. Clin Plast Surg 1984; 11:253–256.

Maxwell GP, McMibbon BM, Hoopes JE. Vascular consideration in the use of the latissimus dorsi myocutaneous flap following mastectomy with axillary dissection. Plast Reconstr Surg 1979; 64:771–780.

Maxwell GP. Latissimus dorsi breast reconstruction: aesthetic considerations. Clin Plast Surg 1981; 8:373–387.

MICROVASCULAR FREE FLAPS

WILLIAM W. SHAW, M.D., F.A.C.S.

Mastectomy deformities result from losses of skin surface, breast volume, nipple-areolar complex, symmetry, and, at times, specific contour defects. The initial step in breast reconstruction is invariably the formation of a suitable breast mound. The methods described generally fall into two groups: (1) the use of some kind of silicone implant to stretch the skin into shape and maintain the desired volume, or (2) the use of autologous tissue to replace the skin and the volume.

Because of the simplicity, an overwhelming number of reconstructions are done with silicone implants or expanders. Although most patients are grateful for the improvement achieved by implants, there are several fundamental limitations. As is true for any synthetic material, implants may become infected, extruded, or ruptured all of which result in the loss of the reconstruction and require additional surgery. A second inherent problem is the unavoidable foreign body reaction toward the implants that results in "capsule formations." The intensity of this normal response is unpredictable and often results in subsequent hard capsular contractures with shifting or distortion of the reconstructed breast mound. Finally, it is difficult to use available preformed implants to fully restore symmetry or to fill out specific contour defects.

Autogenous reconstruction methods require the transplantation of suitable skin and bulk from a different part of the body to create the breast mound. Once successfully transplanted, the tissue becomes a permanent reconstruction without the complications of implants. The living tissue can be sculpted to achieve optimal shape and size. In time, the warm and soft reconstructed breast becomes easily accepted by the patient. Many patients have also described a spontaneous restoration of sensation in the autogenous transplanted tissue, thereby adding to the sense of wholeness. The main disadvantages of autogenous reconstructions are the additional scars in the donor area and the more complex surgery required.

The methods employed to move a large block of skin and tissue for autologous breast reconstruction more or less parallel developments in flap surgery. Originally, multistaged, laborious operations were required to move abdominal skin and fat to the chest to allow the final shaping of the breast. As the myocutaneous flaps came along, small autologous breasts could be reconstructed with latissimus dorsi flaps. Variations of the superiorly-based rectus abdominis myocutaneous flap have become the main vehicle to transplant excess abdominal tissue to the breast area. Finally, free flaps, which were initially used only in difficult cases, have recently become utilized for elective reconstructions as well. As our confidence in free flap surgery becomes more secure this type of surgery is likely to become a standard method of autologous breast reconstruction.

INDICATIONS FOR FREE FLAPS

Difficult Surface or Contour Problems

Fortunately for today's surgeons and patients, the once-common, tight-skinned "washboard-like" chests with infraclavicular hollows have largely disappeared along with the formerly popular Halsted radical mastectomy. Occasionally, however, the surgeon is still faced with problems of skin shortage as a result of large fixed tumors, small breasts, or breast cancer recurrence after radiation. When implants or expanders are inserted under tight, irradiated skin, not only is the resultant shape often disappointing, but the reconstruction is also highly vulnerable to implant-related complications. Satisfactory breast mound reconstruction, therefore, requires addition of skin surface. When the pectoral muscle is fibrotic and contracted, its release or resection results in a deformity that cannot be corrected without additional autologous tissue. When this is not available from adjacent flaps, free flap transfer is the only solution.

Unsuitable Regional Flaps

Superiorly-based transverse rectus abdominis myocutaneous (TRAM) flaps are unsuitable in a significant number of patients who seek autologous reconstructions. Previous abdominoplasty, upper abdominal surgical scars, vertical midline scars, or other abdominal procedures preclude safe use of the abdominal tissue. In a thin patient with large breasts, the volume harvest from the abdomen may not be sufficient to achieve breast symmetry. The loss of the rectus abdominis muscle on one or both sides is generally well tolerated with no significant disability. For athletic patients, this minor loss of muscle function, along with an increased weakness of the abdominal wall, may be a serious concern. In women of childbearing age, the potential risk of pregnancy on the weakened abdominal wall is not yet fully evaluated. Finally, in patients with tight, attractive abdomens, the addition of the anterior scar together with a small asymmetry represent significant distractions.

Failures from Other Reconstructions

Every known method of reconstruction is associated with occasional failures. It is well-known that patients reconstructed with expanders or implants can have failures or disappointing results and these may occur years later as well. Many of these patients seek repeated procedures and, eventually, alternative methods of reconstruction. When all else fails, autologous methods represent the only permanent solution. Free flaps provide the greatest versatility in salvaging such cases.

Patient Preference

As experience is gained with different reconstructions, it is obvious that each has a different set of merits and problems. Simple implant procedures may be costly later in terms of reoperations and limited results. Pedicled TRAM flaps avoid microvascular anastomoses but are more limited in the size of flap available and the freedom of design. Free flaps have the greatest versatility but require specialized experience and bring worries over the possibility of thrombosis. Increasingly, well-informed patients prefer to have a voice in the selection of the method. Patients with unsightly abdomens may prefer to use the TRAM flap and get something of an abdominoplasty out of it. Others prefer to leave the abdomen alone and have the scar on the buttock where it is not generally seen.

Immediate Reconstructions

With increased numbers of lumpectomy and radiation cases being performed, many patients are now coming back with recurrences that require a wider skin excision than usual. Wound closure at the time of mastectomy may require immediate autologous tissue reconstruction. Also, some mastectomy patients desire immediate reconstructions with autologous tissue. Such reconstructions can be accomplished relatively easily in that the reconstructive surgeon has the opportunity to influence the skin incision and to anticipate the reconstruction needed. Also, the wound is already widely opened by the mastectomy surgeon and the recipient vessels are already partially exposed. The convenience and economic savings of such a combined procedure are greatly appreciated by the patient.

RECIPIENT VESSELS FOR FREE FLAPS

It is essential to find recipient vessels of suitable size, location, length, and expendability in any free flap operation. Preferably, the vessels should also be outside the zone of injury from severe radiation or previous surgical scar. The axillary vessels and their branches are most commonly used, but due to previous axillary dissections, they may be absent or scarred. Furthermore, the resultant breast mound tends to be too high if the flap pedicle is short. With the TRAM free flap and its long pedicle, this is not a problem. For gluteal free flaps, the internal mammary vessels provide the best insetting. The vein however, is too small for the gluteal vein in about 25 percent of cases, thus making anastomoses very difficult and prone to thrombosis. In these cases, use of the external jugular vein or the cephalic vein should be considered. When no easy local vessels are available, vein grafts can be tapped to the axillary vessels.

DONOR TISSUES FOR BREAST RECONSTRUCTION

Groin Flap

Serafin used the free groin flap to resurface chest wall skin to facilitate placement of implants. This was often necessary in the past due to large areas of skin-grafted chest from radical mastectomy. With the groin flap, the donor site scar is well concealed and no muscle is taken. The vessels, however, are small and short, which makes anastomosis more difficult and vein grafts are often required. Since the skin on the side of the abdomen tends to be flatter than in the central portion, it is not as easy to achieve a central projection with the groin flap as with the TRAM flap. Implants beneath the groin flap are generally required to produce a satisfactory breast mound. This free flap has been made obsolete by the introduction of the TRAM flap.

Contralateral Latissimus Dorsi Flap

When muscle and skin are needed but the ipsilateral latissimus is not available or sufficient, the contralateral-latissimus dorsi flap can be used. The awkward position and the redraping of the patient needed during the operation make this procedure not a first line choice. Because of its familiarity to most surgeons and the occasional need for extra skin and muscle, which are not available locally, this free flap may still be a useful procedure in selected patients.

Superior Gluteal Free Flap

The upper gluteus maximus myocutaneous free flap, based on the superior gluteal artery and vein, was first used by Fujino for breast reconstruction. It achieved an excellent breast mound, although the position was a little high because of the short vascular pedicle attached to the axilla. Shaw modified the procedure by using the internal mammary vessel to allow proper setting of the breast mound. The results have been highly gratifying to the extent that it is now increasingly used for elective reconstructions (Fig. 1). The muscle cuff taken represents approximately less than 20 percent of the gluteus maximus muscle and the functional loss is not noticeable. Skin widths of up to 13 cm have been taken without any difficulty in primary closure, or significant deformity. Indeed, even in thin patients, a generous amount of tissue is available for breast reconstruction. The main limitation with this procedure is that it is one of the more difficult free flaps in terms of flap dissection and vessel anastomoses.

Transverse Rectus Abdominis Myocutaneous Free Flap (TRAM Flap)

The experience gained with the pedicled TRAM flap confirmed the abdomen as a highly desirable source of donor tissue for the breast. Sometimes, however, the superior pedicle is not suitable due to previous surgery. At other times, the circulation to the skin flap is not vigorous and the result is partial flap loss. Studies on the relative importance of the superior versus the inferior pedicles clearly pointed out the dominance of the inferior epigastric system. Since the results of the inferiorly-based free flaps to the lower extremity were excellent, TRAM flaps are gradually being used as free flaps rather than as pedicle flaps. The long vascular pedicle allows easy anastomosis with either the thoracodorsal or the thoracoacromial vessels. Since the entire muscle no longer need be taken, the upper muscle dissection and the tunnelling of the pedicle is no longer needed. The abdominal closure and postoperative care seem much easier. The more immediate source of skin blood supply provides for a more generous skin flap and greater versatility in design (Fig. 2).

Inferior Gluteal Free Flap

The skin and subcutaneous tissue over the lower buttock can be harvested as a myocutaneous free flap based

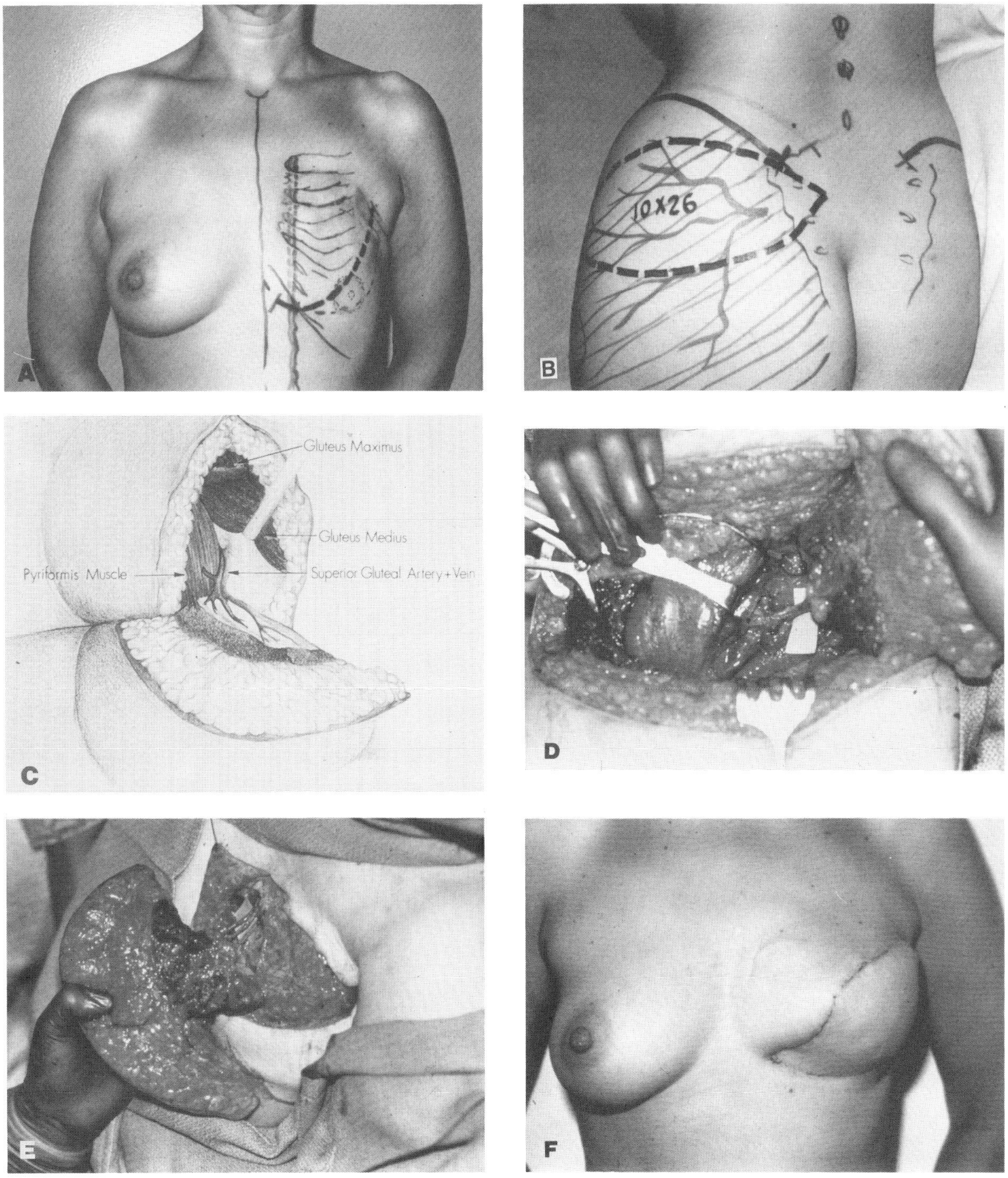

Figure 1 Shows breast reconstruction with superior gluteal free flap. *A,* Skin drawing of the incision and the location of the recipient internal mammary vessels. *B,* Skin markings of the 10 by 26 cm skin flap. *C* and *D,* Diagram and surgical dissection of the superior gluteal flap. *E,* Gluteal flap after anastomosis to the mammary vessels. *F,* Two weeks postoperatively.

Figure continues on following page

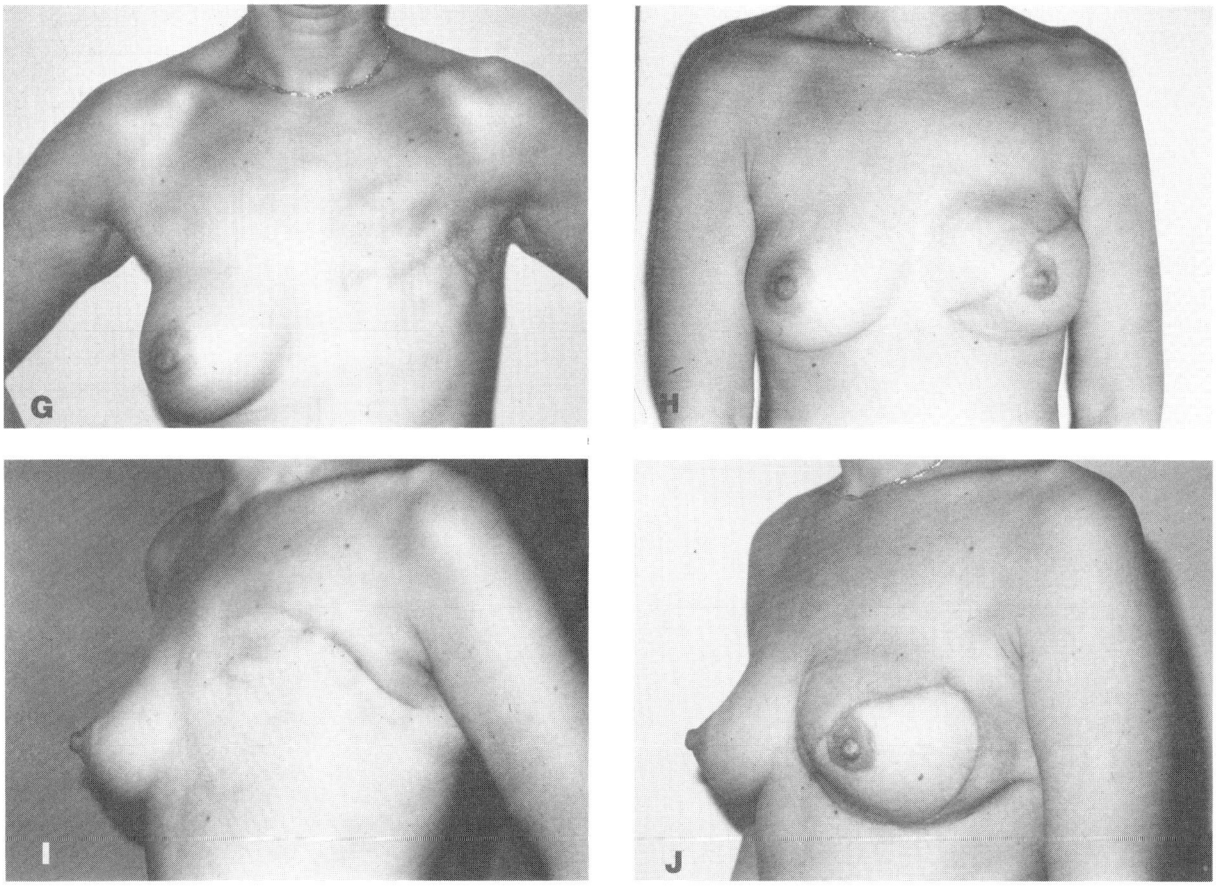

Figure 1 (continued) *G* to *J*, are views preoperatively and 1 year after second stage nipple-areolar reconstruction.

on the lower gluteus maximus muscle and the inferior gluteal vessels. The vascular pedicle is slightly longer than the superior system; however, the sciatic nerve is in the immediate vicinity and requires careful preservation. Also, the donor scar is more visible in today's bathing suits. With more experience, this may be a useful alternative to the superior gluteal flap.

Contralateral Breast Wedge

Le-Quang reported utilizing the lateral half of the contralateral breast, based on the lateral thoracic artery and vein for free flap breast reconstruction and simultaneous breast reduction. The esthetic result achieved was excellent. Because of the increased risk of developing cancer in the remaining breast and the difficulty of monitoring the postoperative breasts, this is not a well-accepted alternative.

SELECTIONS OF METHODS

The initial step in the interview of breast reconstruction patients involves their education as to the different methods available for reconstruction and the relative merits. The surgeon, in the meantime, tries to establish the patient's overall risk factors and specific reconstructive needs. A careful assessment of the anatomic deformity and the suitable methods of correction are then determined. Based on all of these factors, the patient and the surgeon can then jointly establish a realistic reconstructive plan. The patient should be fully aware of her active participation in the selection of the procedure and, therefore accept the risk associated with either flaps or implants.

Two anatomic features are important in the planning and selection of free flap reconstructions. First, one needs to look at the opposite breast to determine the size, shape, and location of the breast mound to be reconstructed. If reduction, ptosis correction, or augmentation is desired, this should be anticipated. A firm and conical breast is best reconstructed with a gluteal flap, whereas a soft, slightly ptotic breast is more ideally reconstructed with the TRAM flap. If both flaps are equally suitable, the specific donor site anatomy may be important in making the decision. Secondly, one should review all the technical aspects of the free flap operation to plan the choice of recipient vessels, skin coverage, and insetting of the flap. Severe scarring of the axillae or denervation of the latissimus muscle would suggest that the thoracodorsal vessels are probably not suitable.

The surgeon's experience is another important factor in the selection of the preferred method and in the

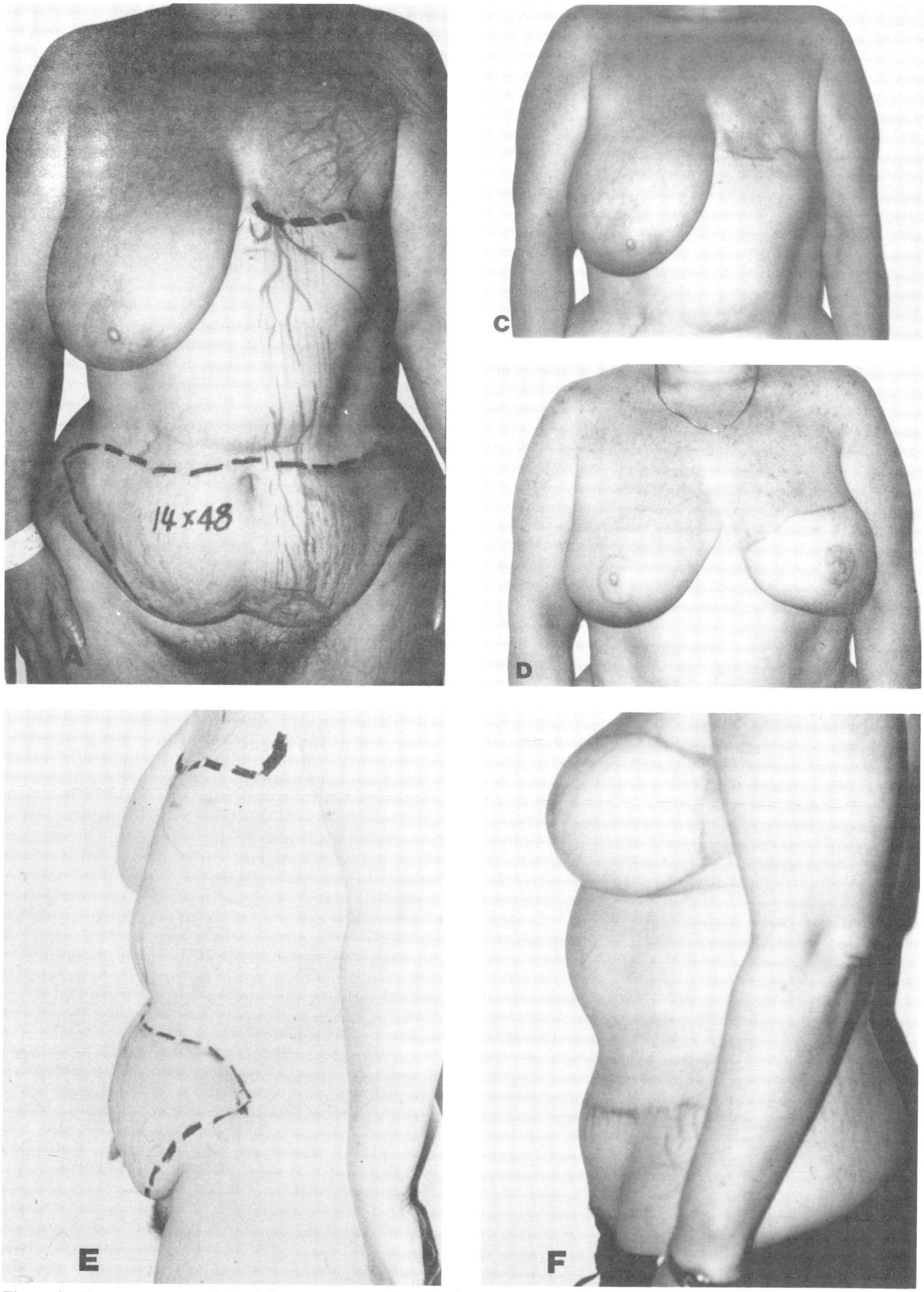

Figure 2 Transverse rectus abdominis myocutaneous free flap breast reconstruction shows *A*, The preoperative markings of the chest incision and abdominal skin island. *C*, and *D*, Preoperative and 6 months postoperative views. *E*, Lateral preoperative view. *F*, Lateral postoperative view.

Figure continues on following page

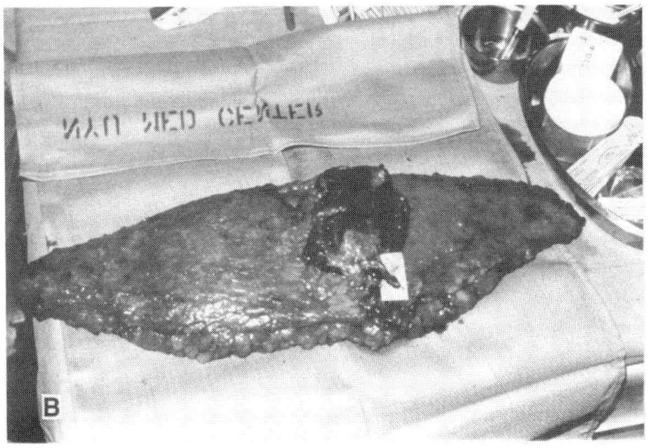

Figure 2(continued) *B*, The TRAM free flap and the small amount of muscle taken.

result achieved. The gluteal flap is technically quite difficult and requires considerable planning to achieve optimal results. It should not be attempted until the surgeon has had considerable microsurgical experience and has studied the specific anatomy carefully. The TRAM free flap is considerably easier and can be done with relative ease and safety by most surgeons with moderate microsurgical experience.

CONCLUSION

Despite the slightly longer initial operating time and the special microsurgical expertise required, free flaps are well accepted today because of their many inherent advantages, as important options for many patients who desire breast reconstruction. Patients who elect to have implant reconstructions must be willing to accept the possibility of late contracture (5 to 40 percent) and the need for future surgical revisions. Tissue expanders have provided valuable flexibility in the use of implants, but the complication rate is still considerable (40 percent with an ultimate failure rate of 4 percent). Hartrampf has produced excellent results with the pedicled TRAM flap, with a failure rate of only 2 percent and low incidence of complications. Others have experienced considerably more problems with partial flap necrosis or abdominal wall morbidities. My own experience with more than 114 free flaps for breast reconstruction has shown that the procedure can be done with a highly acceptable failure rate (1.8 percent) and, more importantly with gratifying results. With more cumulative experience in free flap breast reconstructions and more surgeons familiar with microsurgery, we are likely to see more and better free flap breast reconstructions.

SUGGESTED READING

Friedman RJ, Argenta LC, Anderson R. Deep inferior epigastric tree flap for breast reconstruction after radical mastectomy. Plast Reconstr Surg 1985; 76:454–458.

Fujino T, Harashina T, Enomoto K. Primary breast reconstruction after a standard radical mastectomy by a free flap transfer. Plast Reconstr Surg 1976; 58:372–374.

Le-Quang C. Microvascular tissue transfer in plastic surgery. In: Lie TS, ed. Microsurgery: Proceedings of the International Congress of the International Microsurgery Society. Amsterdam: Excerpta Medica 1979; 125.

Pennington DC, Pelly AD. The rectus abdominis myocutaneous free flap. Br J Plast Surg 1980; 33:277–282.

Serafin D, Georgiade NG, Given KS. Transfer of free flaps to provide well-vascularized thick cover for breast reconstructions after radical mastectomy. Plast Reconstr Surg 1978; 62:527–536.

Shaw W. Microvascular free flap breast reconstruction. Clin Plast Surg 1984; 11:333–341.

Shaw W. Breast reconstruction by superior gluteal microvascular free flaps without silicone implants. Plast Reconstr Surg 1983; 72: 490–499.

Shaw W. Discussion of deep inferior epigastric free flap for breast reconstruction. Plast Reconstr Surg 1985; 76:459–460.

Song RY, Yang PY, Yu HT, Huang HY. Breast reconstruction without a silicone implant. Clin Plast Surg 1982; 9:85–86.

NIPPLE-AREOLA RECONSTRUCTION

JOHN WILLIAM LITTLE III, M.D.

Realistic reconstruction of the nipple-areola is a low-investment, high-yield opportunity to dramatically enhance the result of prior breast mound reconstruction. Although I have suggested in the past that an artistic nipple-areolar reconstruction can be expected to do little to enhance the result of an unfavorable reconstruction of the mound, I no longer believe this to be true. Specifically, on a number of occasions I have witnessed an exciting nipple-areolar reconstruction bring patient acceptance of an otherwise mediocre breast mound reconstruction that had been disappointing overall (Fig. 1).

Nowadays, I hear less and less the statement that a certain percentage of the patients of any given surgeon does not wish nipple-areolar reconstruction or cannot be bothered. I see this as further evidence of maturation of the relatively young field of breast reconstruction. There will always be the occasional patient who, for any number of reasons, elects not to proceed with this further embellishment; just as there are patients who abandon other forms of multistaged reconstruction halfway through. But I find such a decision a missed opportunity for patient and surgeon alike. Surely, an ultimate benefit of breast reconstruction is the reversal of the physical stigma of having had a life-threatening cancer, with all that this implies. The woman with the completed reconstruction is more likely to enjoy this benefit when she catches a glimpse of her full and completed figure in the dressing room mirror than the patient who had breast mound reconstruction alone. The tasteful presentation of symmetrical nipple projection through the feminine fashions of today may be

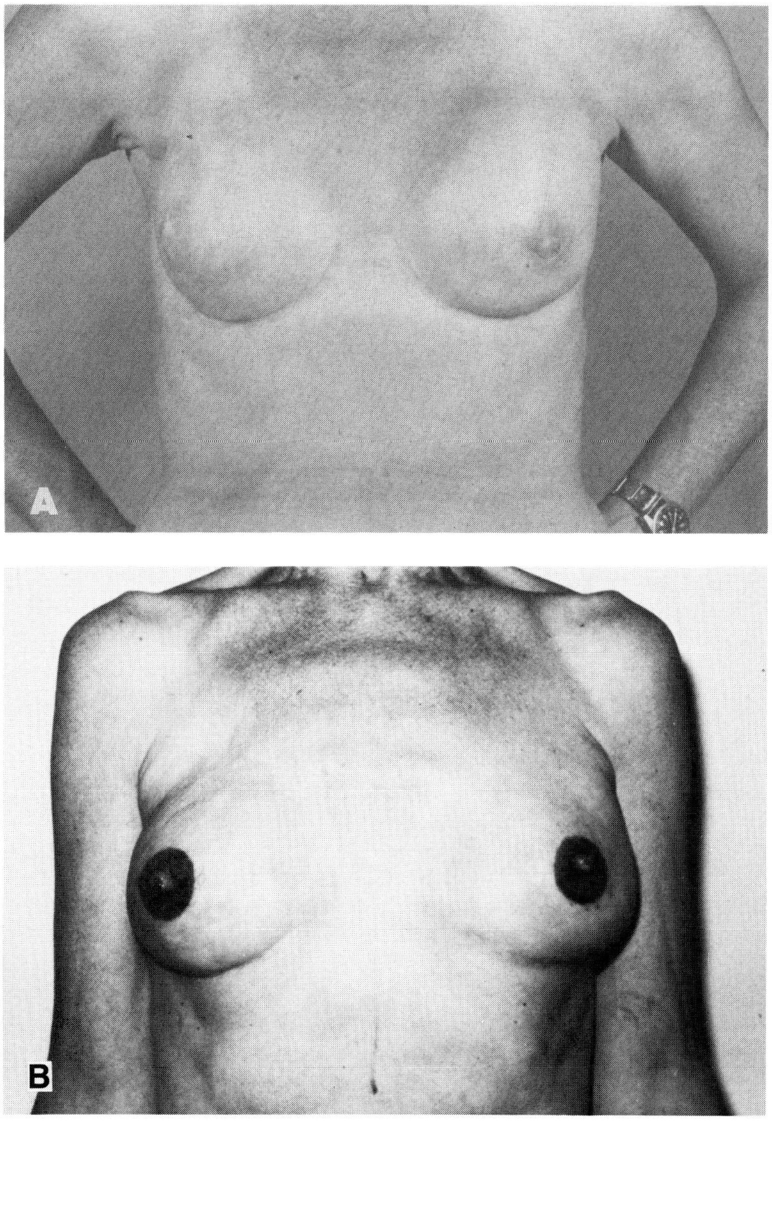

Figure 1 Secondary nipple-areolar reconstruction contributes to salvage of prior reconstruction elsewhere. *A*, Preoperative view 2 years following prophylactic mastectomies with subpectoral reconstruction and secondary capsulotomies. *B*, Postoperative view 6 months following total submuscular repositioning of implants and nipple-areolar reconstruction by skate technique.

the ultimate reassurance to a mastectomy patient that her life crisis is behind her. A personal retrospective psychological survey of patients who elected for and against nipple-areolar reconstruction tends to confirm these impressions; overall patient satisfaction with the breast reconstruction was significantly higher ($p = .004$) in the group that had elected the nipple-areolar addition than in those who had not.

For the past 10 years, I have considered breast reconstruction to be at the very least a two-stage reconstructive project and have presented it as such to my patients. Addition of the nipple-areola has been typically performed as a modest extension of the second stage that is necessary for balancing and fine tuning. As practiced today, it adds negligible morbidity in terms of either discomfort, scarring, or postoperative inconvenience. Lately, when the second stage has been more involved, as when significant alterations of both breasts are necessary, I have frequently postponed the nipple-areolar reconstruction to a third stage, because under such circumstances it is more difficult to select the proper nipple location. These are the only instances when nipple-areolar reconstruction does add some inconvenience to the overall reconstruction of a breast. Invariably, if no further significant revision is required of the breast mound itself, the third stage may be carried out in the office setting without premedication.

The reconstructive goals of nipple-areolar simulation are essentially four in number. The most important is accuracy of position: a two-edged requirement that may be difficult to accomplish. The reconstructed nipple-areolar complex must, in the first place, be sufficiently symmetrical with its opposite mate that, in or out of clothing, the presentation of projection is balanced. At the same time, the complex must also bear a centric relationship with its reconstructed breast mound and fall at the point of anterior convexity. Both aspects of proper positioning may be especially difficult to accomplish in breasts that are themselves innately different in terms of mass, shape, and constituent parts. A second goal is that of symmetrical nipple projection. Certainly, this has proven elusive in nearly all techniques of de novo nipple reconstruction, where late settling and flattening is the overwhelming rule. As will be seen, this need no longer be the case. A third goal has been symmetrical size or shape of the areolae. The fourth goal is symmetry of color and tone. These latter aims have proven essentially attainable through the introduction of coloring pigments by intradermal tattoo. Symmetry of texture and surface quality is of least importance and is discernible only at close distance.

AREOLAR RECONSTRUCTION

Areolar reconstruction has traditionally been available through banking, sharing, free graft, or tattoo. Today's technique of choice for areolar reconstruction per se is intradermal tattoo. It is true that the majority of nipple-areolar reconstructions performed require a skin graft to the areolar area prior to tattoo, but this maneuver does not, in general, enhance the final result of the areolar reconstruction. Rather, it is a necessary consequence of most effective techniques for nipple reconstruction in use today. Therefore, the size and shape of the graft to cover the nipple donor site need not correspond to or even approximate the desired final areola. Because coloration is provided by subsequent tattoo, skin graft donor sites may now be selected, without regard for local melanocyte populations, from any nonspecialized area that can be incorporated into existing scars. It is virtually unnecessary, therefore, to create a new and otherwise undesirable donor scar in order to provide a skin graft to cover the areolar defect. There is no justification for the harvesting of such areolar grafts from specialized tissue sources such as the genitalia, mucous membranes, or the paralabial tissues of the upper, inner thigh. Whatever color match can be expected from these specialized sources—and for however long—greater symmetry can be accomplished by tattoo. Typical donor sites are: (1) the border of the opposite areola as it undergoes reduction during mastopexy or reduction mammoplasty, (2) the low subaxillary skin fullness that typically remains following mastectomy, and which benefits from transverse excisional tailoring to enhance the shape of the reconstructed breast, (3) any area of slight redundancy along a prior scar from mastectomy or flap donation, and (4) dogears or excesses intentionally retained from the primary reconstructive operation, as when a portion of the unprofitable zone IV is retained as an abdominal dogear at the primary transverse rectus abdominal musculocutaneous (TRAM) flap transfer. Banking of pigmented tissues for later transfer in nipple-areolar reconstruction is unjustified for at least three reasons: the practice is inconvenient and creates unnecessary scars; twice-transferred composite tissues are vastly inferior in retention of both color and projection; and the potential for the dissemination of malignant cells is real and proven. Intradermal tattoo alone, then, is the treatment of choice in areolar reconstruction, while effective techniques in nipple reconstruction require a prior graft to the area that will receive the pigments. Finally, efforts to avoid such a graft by allowing secondary epithelialization of nipple donor sites will result in unacceptable amounts of scar epithelium if the primary nipple techniques have been properly carried out at the deep, split-thickness level.

NIPPLE RECONSTRUCTION

Nipple reconstruction has traditionally been accomplished by free graft or local flap. With respect to the former, only composite grafts from the remaining nipple have proven reliable, both in terms of initial take and lasting projection. Surely, the simplest nipple-areolar reconstruction occurs with the transfer of such a composite nipple graft to a tattooed areolar bed. Nevertheless, I argue against the routine use of this expedient as an unnecessary assault upon the final focus of erotic breast sensibility in these patients. In addition, there is a temptation for the surgeon who uses this technique routinely to extend it to donor nipples that are only average or less in bulk. The result may be virtual obliteration of the donor nipple, a situation that I have seen too many times in consultation. Finally, I would argue that if a woman has a highly projectile opposite nipple, creation of the same on the reconstructed breast goes a long way towards increasing the realism of the final result. If the patient has declined an autogenous reconstruction of the mound, for example, there may be little that can be done to enhance a disappointing lack of ptosis, inframammary fold, softness, or naturalness. Experience has taught me, however, that an impressive and realistic nipple-areolar reconstruction in such a circumstance may significantly diminish the patient's eventual overall disappointment. This beneficial effect increases in proportion to the greater prominence or visibility of the nipple reconstruction.

With respect to local flap techniques of de novo reconstruction, the current plethora of designs can be interpreted as evidence of the elusiveness of lasting projection. Despite long-term use of a quadrapod design based on a central subcutaneous pedicle, I have abandoned this in virtually all cases where significant projection is required. I utilize it only rarely (and mostly from nostalgia) in cases where the degree of opposite nipple projection is modest. Instead, I prefer a nonisland technique based on conventional subdermal, as well assubcutaneous, blood supply.

I find this "skate" technique unmatched for reliability, ease and rapidity of execution, simplicity of aftercare, and degree of long-term projection. Virtually all my initial efforts with this method, when carried out to its full potential, required major reductions (Fig. 2). I now use a modified technique that avoids the excessive projection of my earliest cases. Finally, secondary boosting of inadequate results is available through a simple pull-out technique with wrap-around graft, a simple office procedure accomplished in 15 minutes.

TATTOO

Intradermal tattoo must be seen as the coloring method of choice for the areola and nipple. Although there is a wide range of alternatives available, I prefer commercially available alcohol suspensions of conventional earth pigments to be embedded with the heavy-duty, inexpensive equipment used by lay tattoo artists. Pigments that simulate the range of normal areolar skin tones are increasingly available, although custom mixing with four basic pigment groups usually suffices, i.e., light brown, dark brown, white, and red. I delay tattoo of the nipple-areolar complex until some 3 or 4 months after the nipple-areolar reconstruction. This is performed as a simple office procedure that takes 10 or 15 minutes. The areola is tattooed to match the shape, position, and color tone of the opposite side, and, specifically, is not restricted to the pattern of skin graft that was a necessary consequence of the nipple reconstruction procedure. The nipple is often tattooed with a contrasting, brighter red pigment to simulate its erectile tissue component.

TECHNIQUE

My own preferred technique is to perform nipple-areolar reconstruction under local anesthesia on an outpatient basis, usually as a component of the second (but occasionally the third) stage of breast reconstruction during which further refinements of the two breast mounds are accomplished. The premedicated patient is seated on the operating room table while specific measurements are taken of the normal nipple position and transposed to the reconstructed breast. The artistic sensibilities of the surgeon then take over and guide further adjustments from this measured site to produce the best effect. In my experience with the occasional eccentric nipple, the position has invariably been too lateral and, occasionally, too high. The patient is then placed supine on the table and, after prepping and draping, the size and pattern of the normal areola is transferred to the reconstructive site, generally as a circle with a 4 cm diameter (Fig. 3). An inner concentric nipple circle is then placed to approximate the diameter of the opposite nipple. A tangent line is placed across the areolar pattern and touches the nipple circle at 12 o'clock. This orientation ensures that the nipple's seam falls on the undersurface of that structure. The pat-

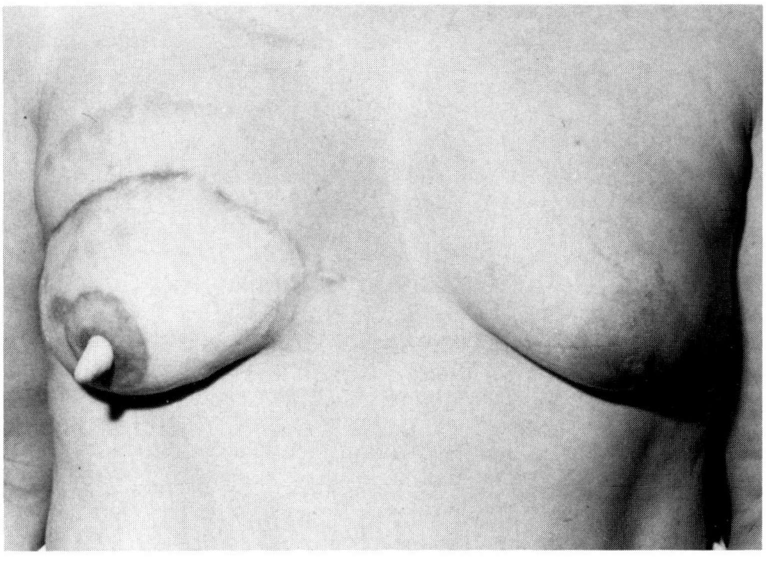

Figure 2 Excessive projection of skate nipple at 4 months is typical of earlier results executed to full potential. (From Little JW. Nipple-areolar reconstruction. Adv Plast Reconstr Surg 1987; 3:75.)

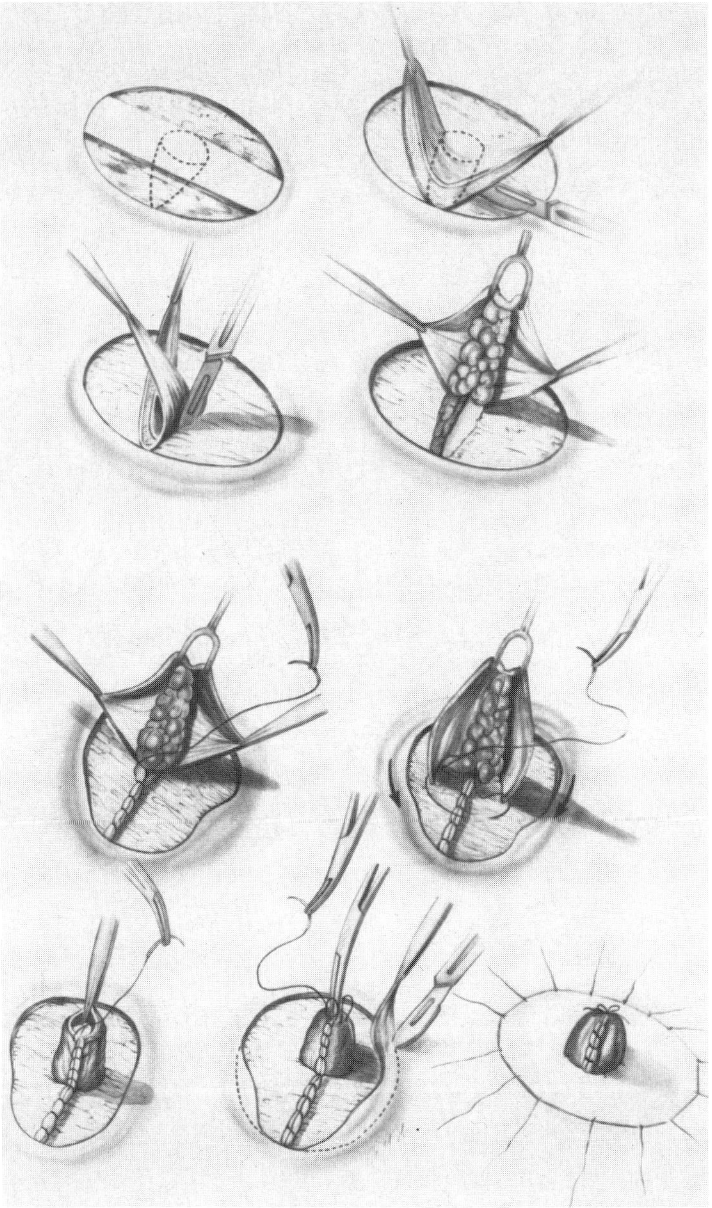

Figure 3 The skate flap. *Top row, left,* Markings, with areas above tangent and at design apex de-epithelialized. *Right,* Wings elevated at deepest split-thickness level up to lines of the body. *Second row, left,* Dissection changes at the dotted line from horizontal to vertical, and, *right,* composite body elevated with full component of deep subcutaneous tissue; trough defect remains. *Third row, left,* The defect is approximated with running suture, and, *right,* the running suture now incorporates tips of wings and wraps them around the underbody to each other. *Bottom, left,* Wings are approximated and de-epithelialized apex is inverted into the nipple cone. *Center,* Running suture finishes as purse string stitch and the areolar pattern is trued. *Right,* Doughnut graft from nonspecialized source covers split-thickness defect. (From: Little JW, Spear SL. Nipple-areolar reconstruction. Perspect Plast Surg 1988; 2(1):8.)

tern may be rotated, however, to accommodate either scars that cross its pattern or differential axes of tension and laxity at the breast apex. Dotted lines are now dropped from the 3 and 9 o'clock positions on the nipple circle to the 6 o'clock position in the areolar circle. The area confined within these dotted lines, including the nipple circle, is considered the composite body of the skate flap. The areas external to the dotted lines are considered the partial thickness wings of the skate. The area above and external to the tangent line, which is de-epithelialized and discarded, is the only area within the areolar pattern that does not contribute to final nipple projection and bulk. If the pattern, as it now exists, is executed to the full height of the design from the tangent base to the pattern apex at 6 o'clock, the resulting nipple will be an impressive conical structure that will exceed a match with most opposite nipples. The full execution of design, therefore, is reserved for especially large opposite structures. Most often, the design height is truncated by the placement of a second transverse line, parallel to the tangent line, which falls at some variable distance from the tangent base to the apex—most commonly one-half to two-thirds of this distance. A good rule of thumb suggests that this distance be twice the height of the opposite stimulated nipple. The area of the design apex beyond this second line is also de-epithelialized, meticulously and at the most superficial level possible. As many dermal elements as possible should be left for inclusion in the final nipple. This area with its underlying composite component will be inverted into the nipple body and will borrow from excessive height to contribute to final bulk.

The two wings are now elevated at the deepest possible split-thickness level, and only the finest reticular pattern of dermis is retained over the subcutaneous tissues of the areolar area. Upon reaching the exact limit of the dotted line of the composite body, the opposite wing is similarly elevated. If both these structures are grasped with forceps at this point and flapped rhythmically, one can appreciate the inspiration for the fanciful title "skate": one is reminded of the family of stingrays and devilfish. Now the two wings are held in an elevated position and the remaining dermis is incised exactly at the dotted lines of the composite body. This incision is deepened into the underlying subcutaneous tissue for a variable distance, usually at least 0.5 cm. The composite portion of the flap is then elevated by working centrally from the apex, taking care to retain a uniform and significant tongue of subcutaneous tissue attached to the body at all times. It is usually necessary to pursue this dissection centrally to the level of the tangent baseline. It is important, however, not to undercut the subcutaneous stalk at the central position of the areolar base where the nipple will fall, thus preserving a significant subcutaneous base to augment the conventional subdermal circulation that enters the flap at 12 o'clock. Insufficient dissection of the composite body results in a flap that resists an easy vertical position and, eventually, a nipple that lists inferiorly. The most likely error in the execution of this rapid and simple technique is the inclusion of too little subcutaneous or deep composite tissue with the body of the flap. A true, three-dimensional trough should be present as an areolar defect at the completion of elevation. This flap remains reliable even when subcutaneous tissues are scant. The underlying muscle that covers a breast prosthesis may be included in the composite portion of the flap, and so may the actual prosthetic capsule itself as I have done on a few occasions.

Closure of the defect is begun by a single running 5–0 Vicryl suture that approximates the dermal margins of the defect at the design apex and runs rapidly up the design to the desired 6 o'clock point of the new nipple, where it is locked. The same suture then picks up the extremity points at the tips of the two wings, approximating the wings as they wrap around the exposed, composite underbody of the skate. The suture then continues in a running fashion up the wings as far as the de-epithelialized zone. Here it is completed as a purse string cinch that invaginates the dermal and subcutaneous tissues of the design apex into the body of the nipple. The same suture material is then used to stabilize the nipple further at the 3 and 9 o'clock positions to the areolar dermal bed. Should closure of the areolar defect produce a distortion of the circular areolar pattern, this area is re-inked with the areolar marker. Any margin beyond the pattern is pulled into place with fine sutures and any areas within are further de-epithelialized to recreate a circle. The dermal areolar bed is then grafted from any convenient, nonspecialized site. The graft is sutured in place with 5–0 silk sutures, left long for tie-over, and further secured with a running, locking 6–0 Nylon suture that approximates any gaps between the tie-over stitches. The entire complex is covered with a greasy gauze dressing. The nipple flap is then protected within the rigid sleeve of the end of a plastic syringe barrel that has been detached with a disposable ophthalmic cautery. Wet cotton is wrapped around the sleeve to provide conventional tie-over pressure to the areolar graft, while the flap remains protected within. The dressing is removed at 4 days, along with the silk tie-over sutures. The area is recovered with a simple greasy dressing. At the end of a week, the 6–0 Nylon suture is removed and the dressing discontinued. Patients are allowed full activity, including bathing and swimming. In the event of partial loss of either the nipple or the areolar graft, greasy dressings may be continued and changed daily by the patient.

The reliability of this flap is excellent, even in the irradiated breast. Occasionally partial necrosis occurs along the margin or closure line of the nipple. Such areas are generally ignored and allowed to heal secondarily. Only rarely should such partial necrosis result in projection inadequate to the other nipple. Almost invariably, such inadequacy is the result of improper planning or execution. The original skate design in the hands of the first time practitioner should err on the side of excessive height, until he or she can judge the amount of shrinkage that will accompany execution of the technique. One should equally resist the temptation to reduce prematurely what appears to be an exuberant nipple. The most significant error in execution involves the incorporation of inadequate amounts of subcutaneous or muscular composite tissue within the composite body of the flap, or, equally serious, rough handling that detaches the composite tongue from the dermal undersurface, thereby producing apical necrosis, which should otherwise not be seen. Finally, inadequate dissection of the composite body centrally produces nipples that list and lean in the direction of the areolar donor site.

Some months after nipple-areolar reconstruction, color is added to the complex through intradermal tattoo with conventional pigments. At this time, a mirror image areola is simulated by tattoo, irrespective of the exact pattern or size of the prior areolar graft (Fig. 4). Thus, subtle degrees of malposition can be corrected by nudging the areolar pattern in the appropriate direction. Wide nipples can be sculpted and excessive nipples reduced be-

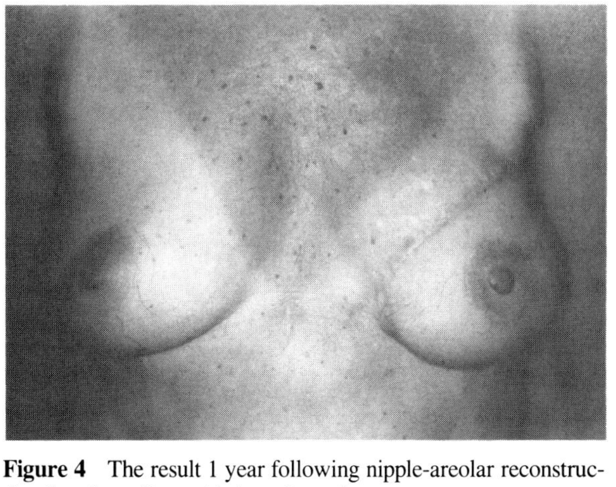

Figure 4 The result 1 year following nipple-areolar reconstruction by skate flap with intradermal tattoo.

fore the application of tattoo. The nipple and the areola are often treated with different pigments.

If the nipple appears wanting in terms of projection—a rare event following skate reconstruction—the complex may first be tattooed and immediately thereafter boosted by nipple pull-out with wrap-around graft. The circumference of the inadequate nipple is incised through the dermis and the incision deepened in an outward, tapering, conical fashion until the nipple cap elevates without resistance. The widest portion of the mastectomy scar is then identified and a 40 mm by 5 mm-deep split-thickness graft is taken from the scar and then thinned of excessive deep elements. The donor site is closed, thus producing concomitant scar revision. The graft is then wrapped around the exposed subcutaneous margins of the nipple column and sewn around to itself under slight tension. This maneuver produces a phimosis effect that maintains the nipple in the projected position without the need for mechanical assistance. The graft is then secured to both the areolar and nipple margins with fine absorbable sutures. A greasy dressing is added. While much of the initial gain will be lost during maturation, this simple expedient frequently produces a boost in the range of 20 to 50 percent, and may be repeated in the office as often as desired. When the nipple is thoroughly inadequate, on the other hand, the best practice is to exercise the full skate technique on top of existing remnants.

SUGGESTED READING

Little JW, Munasafi T, McCullough DT. One-stage reconstruction of a projecting nipple: the quadrapod flap. Plast Reconstr Surg 1983; 71:126–132.

Little JW. Nipple reconstruction by quadrapod flap (letter). Plast Reconstr Surg 1983; 72:422.

Little JW. Nipple-areolar reconstruction. Clin Plast Surg 1984; 11:351–364.

Little JW. Discussion of Becker H: the use of intradermal tattoo to enhance the final result of nipple-areolar reconstruction. Plast Reconstr Surg 1986; 77:676.

Little JW. Discussion of Cohen IK, Ward JA, Chandrasetchar B: the pinwheel flap nipple and barrier areolar graft reconstruction. Plast Reconstr Surg 1986; 77:999.

Little JW. Nipple-areolar reconstruction. Adv Plast Reconstr Surg 1987; 3:43–78.

Little JW, Spear SL. Nipple-areolar reconstruction. Perspect Plast Surg 1988; 2:1–22.

Wellisch DK, Schain, WS, Noone RB, Little JW. The psychological contribution of nipple addition in breast reconstruction. Plast Reconstr Surg 1987; 80:699–704.

INTRADERMAL TATTOOING

SCOTT L. SPEAR, M.D., F.A.C.S.

Intradermal tattooing has remained on the fringe of plastic surgery despite its clear efficacy in coloring skin for decorative and other purposes. Recent increased interest in tattooing stems from better equipment, safer pigments, and widening medical application. While intradermal tattoo was tried previously for port wine stain hemangiomas, discolored flaps and grafts, and restoration of eyebrows, eyelashes, and vermilion, it is now much more widely used for reconstruction of the nipple-areola and for eyeliner. Although theoretically useful for eyebrow, eyelid, lip, and scar purposes, our experience has been limited largely to the nipple-areola, which is the focus of this chapter.

Reconstruction of the nipple-areola is delayed until after breast reconstruction, whether by autogenous tissue, implant, or expander. Although advocated by some, nipple-areola reconstruction should not be solely or predominately by tattoo. Rather the nipple should be fashioned to create the most symmetrical and lasting projection possible, usually by the "skate" or "quadrapod" flap, or more rarely by composite nipple graft when the contralateral nipple is truly hypertrophied. Nipple-areola reconstruction with tattoo alone or combined with secondary nipple pull-out procedures simply cannot consistently produce significant, reliable, and long-term nipple projection. The areola is preferably fashioned from a full-thickness skin graft from the contralateral areola (when it can spare it), or from random skin, which is usually centered on a previous scar. In those rare cases where the contralateral nipple lacks any projection whatsoever, an exception can be made, and the nipple can be reconstructed by tattoo alone, with color used to create the optical illusion of both a nipple and an areola.

PATIENT SELECTION

As early as 6 to 12 weeks after nipple-areola reconstruction, the nipple and areola begin to fade from their initial darkened early postoperative appearance (Fig. 1). Although this fading process may take as long as 12 months, one may tattoo at this early stage. Similarly, although the reconstructed nipple may continue to flatten, and the grafted areola may continue to contract, tattooing may be undertaken at this point. This clearly represents a compromise rather than waiting for complete maturation of the reconstructed nipple-areola, in perhaps 12 months or even later.

Only the patient with a perfect nipple-areola reconstruction, using a composite nipple graft for the nipple and a full-thickness areola graft for the areola, would not benefit from subsequent intradermal tattoo. All other patients with otherwise attractive breast and nipple-areola reconstructions can benefit at this point either from coloring the nipple, coloring the areola, enlarging the areola, reshaping the areola, or reconstructing the areola all with the aid of intradermal tattooing.

METHOD

In the office or operating room, with the patient in a symmetrical sitting position, the reconstructed nipple-

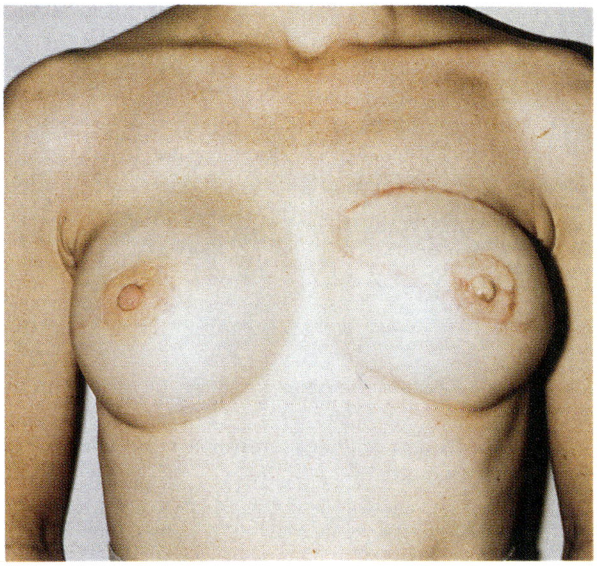

Figure 1 Faded nipple areola. A 40-year-old woman 6 months after left breast reconstruction with a Hartrampf-type transverse abdominis musculocutaneous flap and a right simple implant reconstruction after subcutaneous mastectomy. The right nipple-areola is the original; the left was fashioned 6 weeks before the photograph from a "skate" flap and a random skin graft. Note the left nipple and areola have already begun to fade.

areola is examined for position, shape, size, and color. Minor discrepancies in nipple position can be corrected by "V to Y" or somersault shifts of the nipple alone, combined with redefinition of the areola margins by tattoo. In a similar fashion, the entire nipple-areola complex can be moved as a flap either using a subcutaneous pedicle and "V to Y" technique or as a transposition flap. If the nipple position is suitable, the reconstructed areola is carefully compared to the normal for size, shape, and location. With the patient still sitting, ideal symmetrical areola borders are drawn on the reconstructed breast. The resulting plan often is neither a perfect circle nor match of the previous areola graft margins. With the tattoo and surgical plan indelibly marked, the patient is placed in a supine position and prepped as for any plastic surgical procedure.

Local anesthetic with Adrenalin is optional, but may help with excess dermal bleeding, which often obscures the degree of effective pigment penetration. If the nipple or nipple-areola complex requires surgical adjustment, that portion of the procedure is performed first. Bacitracin ointment is then lightly applied to the tattoo site to assist in wiping off excess pigment that has not penetrated the dermis during tattooing. All of the currently available machines are adequate for successful nipple-areola tattooing. Among the medical quality instruments, I prefer those from Permark* and Cooper Vision.† The commercial device manufactured by Spaulding and Rogers‡ also performs very well. Medical quality instruments are simpler, more convenient, and approved for hospital use, but they are considerably more expensive. The commercial tattoo machine, although very effective (perhaps more effective) is more crude, inconvenient, and complicated, but considerably less expensive. With increased medical interest in tattoos, I expect significant changes in equipment, pigments, and prices in the next several years.

The quality and variety of available tattoo pigments has increased dramatically during 1986 and 1987. Prior to that time, many of the pigments were made from derivatives of sulfur or mercury, and were prone to undesirable local reactions. At this point, most manufactured pigments are FDA-approved pigments derived from titanium or iron oxides. Whereas all of the tattoo needles either come sterilized or may be sterilized, not all of the pigments have that feature. Currently we can recommend the sterile pigments provided by Permark or Cooper Vision, but are cautious in endorsing Spaulding and Rogers' colors, which are premixed but not specifically sterile. This reservation may eventually change as our early tests suggest that the 70 percent isopropyl alcohol diluent used by Spaulding and Rogers may yield this mixture sterile in practice. In the meantime, we recommend that each lot of Spaulding and Rogers' pigments be cultured before using.

A sterile cotton swab is used to paint a palette of color choices around the nonreconstructed areola (Fig. 2). From these choices, the best match is selected, preferably *slightly* darker than the normal side. The selected color is transferred sterilely in a 1-cc tuberculin syringe or other sterile utensil (e.g., cotton swab) and delivered into a small sterile medicine cup or similar reservoir. If needed, the selected color can be further adjusted by selectively mixing white, brown, or other colors.

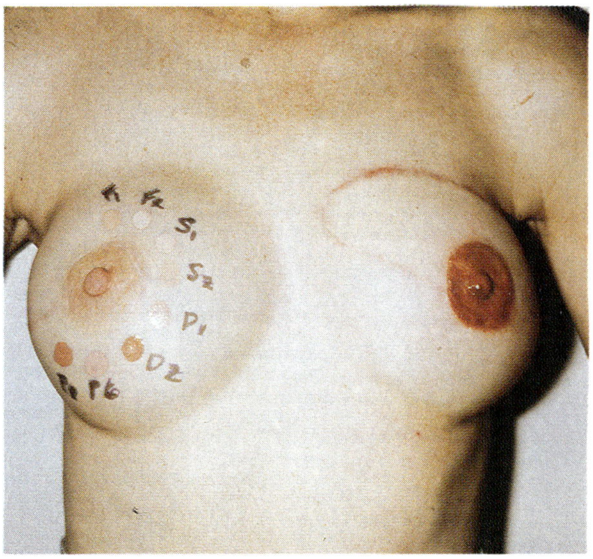

Figure 2 Palette of color choices. On the same patient as Figure 1, an array of possible colors has been sterilely painted adjacent to the right areola to help select the best match. In this case D2 was chosen with additional red added for the nipple. The immediate blood-stained result is apparent on the left.

* Permark, Glenpointe Center East, Teaneck, NJ. (201) 692-7755.
† Cooper Vision, P.O. Box 19587, Irvine CA 92713. (714) 474-5900.
‡ Spaulding & Rogers, Rt. 85, New Scotland Road, Voorheesville, NY 12186. (518) 768-2070.

Wearing sterile gloves, the surgeon immerses the sterile tattoo needle 2 or 3 mm deep into the tattoo pigment and the procedure begun. I prefer to tattoo the new margins of the areola first and then *slowly* fill in the areola contents (Fig. 3A and 3B). Although it is possible to tattoo the nipple only, I rarely do this in practice, preferring to tattoo the areola as well, either to redefine it, to blend it in with the nipple, or to insure against late fading of the areola graft. Reliable dermal penetration of the pigment requires a slow methodical technique and patience on the part of the operator. As the procedure progresses, excess pigment should be frequently wiped from the field using disposable alcohol sponges. As one gains experience, additional efforts can be made to feather the edges of the tattoo by lightly tattooing this region, while the central areola may be given a variegated color by using a second color.

Tattooing the grafted areola may be difficult, depending on the amount of scar present within the target area—the more scar, the more difficult the tattoo. The nipple may be even more difficult to color, in part due to the scar, and in part due to its mobility which can be controlled by pinching the nipple between thumb and index finger or by holding it gently in the jaws of an opened small hemostat. Rarely should the nipple be tattooed the same color as the areola, rather it should mimic the normal nipple, being redder or darker. Although it may be possible to get this effect by adding red or dark brown to the areola color mix, it often requires mixing an entirely new color.

At the completion of the tattoo, the tattooed nipple-areola should appear somewhat darker than the normal side (Fig. 4A and 4B). A sterile Xeroform gauze is applied and changed daily for 5 to 7 days. During that time, the tattooed site, except for the greasy dressing, should be kept dry. In most cases, the tattoo fades over 2 to 3 months. Should the color become lighter than the normal side with time, then the reconstructed nipple-areola can be easily tattooed a second time to achieve a better color match.

DISCUSSION

I was first introduced to tattooing by Bill Little at Georgetown University in 1981 or 1982, after it had become clear to him that a pale miscolored nipple-areola was the rate-limiting step in many of his breast reconstructions. Continued improvements in both results and techniques of nipple-areola and breast reconstruction have made this fact even more clear. Our combined experience in literally hundreds of tattoos has shown the procedure to be not only safe, but effective. As of this writing, we have not experienced significant complications with tattooing, although some degree of tattoo fading is common. Rarely, the entire tattoo disappears in the first week or two; this is associated with a slough of the superficial skin, presumably a result of excess tissue trauma from dull or barbed needles or of poor technique with skin tearing. To minimize loss or fading of the tattoo, I emphasize again the importance of slow methodical technique and the use

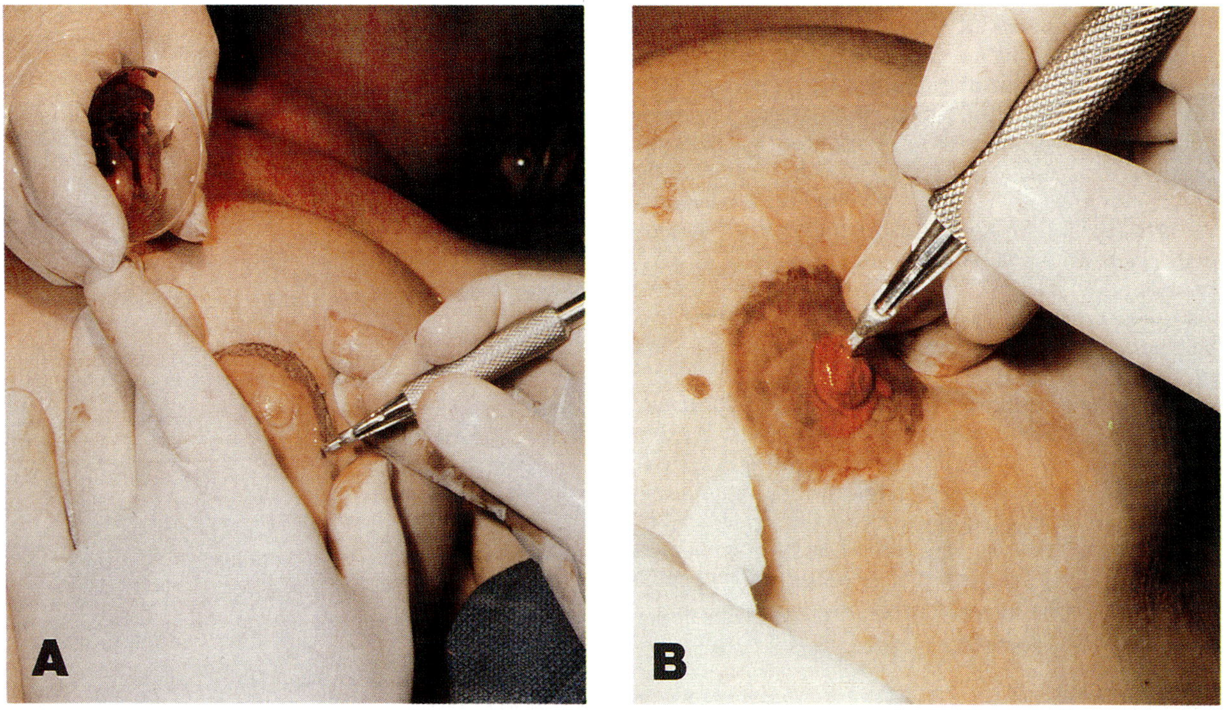

Figure 3 Technique: *A*, the tattoo of the areola is begun at the margins with the device held at approximately 60 degrees to the plane of the skin. The skin is held taught (as for a dermabrasion), and the operator works from side to side. *B*, the nipple is tattooed next, preferably with a distinctly redder or browner color. To steady the nipple, fingertip or gentle hemostat grasp may be required.

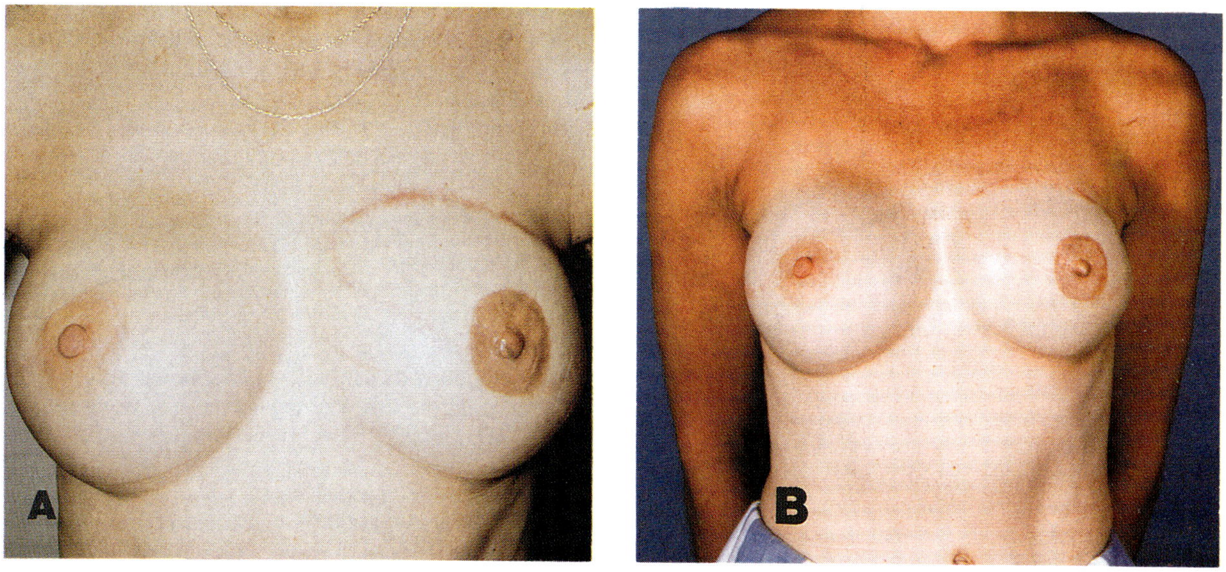

Figure 4 Early results: *A*, on the same patient as shown in Figures 1 and 3, the tattoo is seen as it appears 2 weeks after the procedure. While already appreciably lighter, it can be expected to fade still more over the next several months. *B*, Six months after tattooing with additional fading.

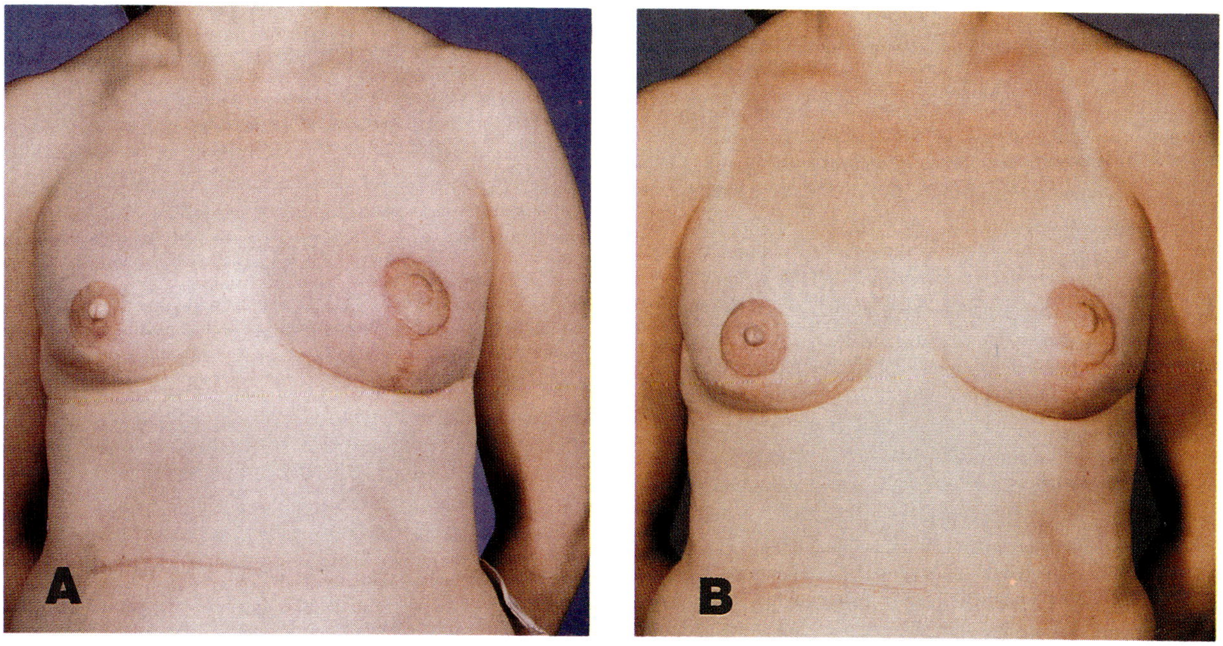

Figure 5 Late results: *A*, a 55-year-old woman 1 year after right simple immediate reconstruction with an implant after mastectomy and 3 months after right ''skate'' flap nipple reconstruction and areola reconstruction from excess left breast areola after mastopexy. Note the ''neon-light'' effect of the pale right nipple, as well as the disparity in areola sizes due to stretching of the left and contracting of the right. *B*, Same patient as seen 6 months after tattooing of the nipple-areola using brown, red, and white pigments prior to the availability of more recent flesh tones. Despite the unnaturally brown result, the pigmented and enlarged nipple-areola is already a better match, and the tattoo can be expected to fade slightly more with time.

of sharp needles and effective equipment. Although many tattoo needles may be reused and resterilized, I personally advise using new needles for each procedure, thereby ensuring their sharpness as much as possible. Although tattooing is typically the final touch in achieving an authentic breast reconstruction, even more remarkably it will often enhance the breast to such an extent that an otherwise mediocre or poor result suddenly achieves surprising authenticity and attractiveness (Fig. 5A and 5B).

SUGGESTED READING

Becker H. The uses of intradermal tattoo to enhance the final result of nipple-aerola reconstruction. Plast Reconstr Surg 1986; 77:673–677.

Hance G, Brown JB, Byars LT, McDowell F. Color matching of skin grafts and flaps with permanent pigment injection. Surg Gynecol Obstet 1944; 79:624–630.

Liltle JW. Nipple-areola reconstruction. Adv Plast Surg 1986; 3:43–58.

PROPHYLACTIC MASTECTOMY

JOHN R. JARRETT, M.D., F.A.C.S.

In January of 1987, the American Cancer Society released statistics indicating that the incidence of breast carcinoma in American women has increased to 10 percent and that 41,000 new cases of breast carcinoma would be diagnosed in the United States in 1987. Because of increased ability to identify patients who are at high risk for developing breast carcinoma, a mastectomy that is truly prophylactic could be extremely beneficial for these patients. Surgeons performing this operation are doing so in the belief that removal of 95 to 98 percent of the breast tissue will significantly reduce or eliminate the patient's chance of developing breast carcinoma. Although this opinion cannot at this time be substantiated by empiric data, preliminary reports of two large series seem to indicate that some forms of mastectomy may offer an effective prophylaxis against carcinoma. My personal series of more than 500 patients, representing more than 750 breasts, followed from 1 to 13 years with a mean follow-up of slightly more than 5 years, includes a zero incidence of subsequent carcinoma. The Mayo Clinic has recently reported a series of 1,700 patients followed up to a maximum of 20 years, with three cases of subsequent carcinoma. All three cases were diagnosed early as small subcutaneous nodules and are living and well with excellent prognoses.

Although subcutaneous mastectomies have been reported since the 1920s, the operation was not commonly performed until the introduction of a reliably satisfactory mammary prosthesis in the early 1960s. Throughout the 1960s and 1970s, surgeons performing this operation commonly left fairly thick skin flaps in order to offer better protection for the mammary prostheses that were placed subcutaneously. Because of problems relating to ischemic skin necrosis and implant loss, some surgeons recommended a two-stage procedure, wherein the mastectomy was followed several months later by delayed placement of implants. Even with this approach, complications of ischemic necrosis with loss of implant and severe capsular contractures remained extremely common. The introduction in 1977 of immediate submuscular reconstruction following prophylactic subcutaneous mastectomy allowed surgeons to eliminate or greatly reduce most of these problems. With complete muscle cover of the implants, it became possible to skeletonize the skin flaps during the adenomammectomy to a thickness comparable to flaps created in modified radical mastectomies, thereby improving the completeness of the resection.

RISK ASSESSMENT

Prophylactic mastectomy should be reserved for those patients who are identified as being at high risk. The only exceptions are the occasional patients suffering either from severe mastodynia associated with fibrocystic disease or from silicone mastopathy caused by liquid silicone injections. The two most significant cancer risk elevating factors are genetics and personal history of breast biopsy pathology; x-ray patterns, physical findings, and hormonal history are less significant factors.

Genetics

A woman who has a first degree relative (mother, sister, or daughter) with premenopausal breast carcinoma is at 3 times normal risk and thus has a 30 percent lifetime risk of developing invasive carcinoma. The term "familial breast carcinoma," which results in a risk factor of 6 times normal, is reserved for patients with two or more first degree relatives with premenopausal breast carcinoma. Additionally, breast carcinoma is diagnosed an average of 10 to 15 years earlier in patients with familial breast carcinoma than in patients with sporadically occurring disease and is also associated with an incidence of bilaterality at least 3 times greater.

The presence of invasive carcinoma in a postmenopausal first degree relative increases a patient's risk by 1.5 to 2 times normal. Likewise, the presence of carcinoma in a second degree relative, such as maternal grandmother, aunt, or cousin, is considered to be a minimal risk elevator of no more than 1.5 times normal. Little additional risk is incurred by paternal relatives with breast carcinoma. Even though geneticists have not been able to prove significant risk increases to those patients with history of carcinoma in second degree relatives or in paternal relatives, high anxiety or true cancer phobia may exist in patients who have observed suffering and/or death from breast carcinoma in such relatives. This fear is attributable in part to the public's incomplete knowledge of the hereditary aspects of breast carcinoma, thereby giving women the assumption that its occurrence in any relative places them at high risk. Unfortunately, most physicians are also unaware of the details of the newest genetic information and are thus unable to provide proper counsel.

History

The second major risk factor is the patient's individual history. Invasive lobular carcinoma carries a 30 percent risk of simultaneous bilaterality, whereas the risk of contralateral carcinoma increases 1 percent per year of survival for patients with invasive ductal carcinoma.

Biopsy-proven fibrocystic disease includes numerous pathologic entities, many of which impart no increased rate of carcinoma development (duct ectasia, blunt adenosis, apocrine metaplasia, and sclerosing adenosis). Likewise, the presence of fibroadenomas is not associated with increased risk of cancer development. However, most pathologists agree that biopsy-proven ductal or lobular carcinoma in situ, ductal or lobular hyperplasia with atypia, multiple papillomatosis with atypia, and ductal epithelial hyperplasia occurring in a postmenopausal patient are associated with a significant increase in carcinoma risk.

Minor Risk Elevators

Radiographic factors are often of assistance in assessing risk of carcinoma. Wolfe classified mammograms according to the prominence of their ductal pattern in a retrospective study of 7,214 patients. Patients with his dysplastic pattern (DY) constituted 7 percent of the total series, but eventually produced 30 percent of the carcinomas. When patients with slightly less dysplasia, but very prominent duct pattern (P2) were included, the two groups contained as many as 80 percent of the patients who developed carcinoma. Because other investigators have not been able to duplicate these figures, Wolfe's classification is not universally accepted.

However, the most troublesome aspect of dense dysplasia is the fact that early (and thus potentially curable) malignancies may be masked by these x-ray patterns. Likewise, physical examination is inaccurate in patients with the severity of nodular tissue that is associated with dense dysplastic patterns on x-ray film. This combination often raises patient and primary physician anxiety, particularly if any other risk elevators persist.

Nulliparity is associated with a slight increased risk of carcinoma, as are the late onset of menses and menopause.

INDICATIONS

Based on the previously discussed factors influencing risk, the following is a list of very strong indications for prophylactic mastectomy:

1. Familial breast carcinoma (two or more first degree relatives with premenopausal breast carcinoma) combined with even minimal evidence of fibrocystic mastopathy.
2. Premenopausal breast carcinoma in one first degree relative (mother, sister, or daughter) combined with significant fibrocystic mastopathy.
3. Biopsy-proven high risk tissue including:
   A. lobular or ductal carcinoma in situ;
   B. lobular or ductal epithelial hyperplasia with atypia; and
   C. papillomatosis with atypia.
4. History of carcinoma in one breast when associated with a history of one or more first degree relatives with premenopausal breast cancer.

There is another group of patients that have to be considered at higher than normal risk and are thus deserving of consideration for surgery based on an individual assessment of their risks and personal anxieties:

1. Previous carcinoma of the other breast without a positive family history, but with severe clinical mastopathy and Wolfe's high risk x-ray patterns in the contralateral breast.
2. Previous carcinoma of the other breast without a family history in a patient less than 50 years of age, in good health, with early carcinoma (stage 0 or I) that is either noninvasive or, if invasive, of a good prognostic type.
3. Severe fibrocystic mastopathy making physical examination extremely difficult or impossible when combined with one of two conditions:
   A. mammography interpreted as either Wolfe's DY or P2 category, or—
   B. severe patient anxiety or cancer phobia and unwillingness to continue conservative management.
4. Biopsy-proven ductal epithelial hyperplasia in a postmenopausal patient.
5. Multiple, persistent, or recurrent breast nodules requiring frequent biopsy, when biopsies show only routine fibrocystic changes, and associated with patient and physician anxiety.
6. Incapacitating mastodynia not controllable by routine conservative management when combined with significant fibrocystic mastopathy.
7. Silicone or paraffin mastopathy (secondary to injections of liquid silicone or paraffin).

SURGICAL TECHNIQUE

Preoperative Preparation

Preoperative preparation should include a very complete informed consent discussion with the patient that should definitely include, but not be limited to, the following items:

1. Description of incision choices and where final scars will be located.
2. The breast skin and nipple-areolar complexes will be completely numb for several months after surgery. Most patients regain protective sensation within 6 to 9 months, and at least one-third of patients without nipple grafts regain erotic sensation.
3. The compressive force of the muscle cover over the implants will tend to flatten the breasts, thereby causing them to bulge superiorly until satisfactory muscle stretching has occurred.
4. Early postoperative breast asymmetry is common, as a result of varying forces of muscle compression and stretching.
5. Discomfort along the sternal border and laterally along the fifth and sixth rib secondary to muscle elevation should be anticipated.
6. Decreased pectoralis muscle strength in the early postoperative period should be anticipated.
7. Skin and nipple ischemia or frank necrosis may require skin excision and grafting onto muscle tissue and may also lead to loss of the prosthesis if it is not adequately protected by muscle tissue.

All patients should have mammograms within 6 months of surgery. Anti-inflammatory drugs must be discontinued at least 2 weeks prior to surgery. Smoking should be eliminated at least 2 (and preferably 4) weeks prior to and following surgery in order to improve skin flap viability.

In anticipation of an average blood loss of one to two U, surgery should be scheduled in order to allow sufficient time for the patient to donate at least 1 U of autologous blood.

Incisions

Because of superior esthetic results, I prefer the inframammary incision for all patients not requiring a surgical mastopexy (Fig. 1). The inframammary incision allows excellent exposure for thorough glandular resection, including exposure of the axillary tail of the breast. This excision can be extended several centimeters laterally to allow improved axillary exposure for lymph node sampling, if desired.

Nonsurgical reduction of a small to moderate amount of skin redundancy can be accomplished with skin taping in the postoperative period (Fig. 2). I use 4-inch-wide Conform tape* for 2 to 6 weeks to allow the skin to adhere to the muscle tissue with the nipple in the appropriate position. This tape is a hypoallergenic stretchy tape that is porous enough to not macerate the skin. It is possible to elevate a nipple between 2.5 and 3 cm using this technique if the skin has good elasticity. Mild amounts of nipple-areolar ptosis following the use of taping can be corrected by a crescent-shaped skin excision above the areolar margin.

A mastopexy type of skin incision is used for the mastectomy of breasts that are extremely large or ptotic, along with nipple grafting on a de-epithelialized dermal bed of skin overlying the muscle-covered implant (Fig. 3). Transferring the nipple on a dermal pedicle is not recommended because of almost certain ischemia or necrosis. The Wise skin pattern, which results in an inverted T scar with free nipple graft, has produced satisfactory results in patients with sufficient skin to allow excision of skin in both the vertical and horizontal dimension that occurs with that skin pattern. Vertical limbs of the Wise pattern should be kept immediately adjacent to the areolar margins if one is to achieve a closure without tension.

Patients with only a moderate degree of ptosis or those with tubular breasts or with extremely stretched areolae probably do not have enough skin in the horizontal dimension to allow use of the Wise pattern. These patients should be treated by an oblique or transverse elliptical excision of the nipple-areolar complex and adjacent skin. This type

* Kendall Hospital Products, Boston, MA 02110

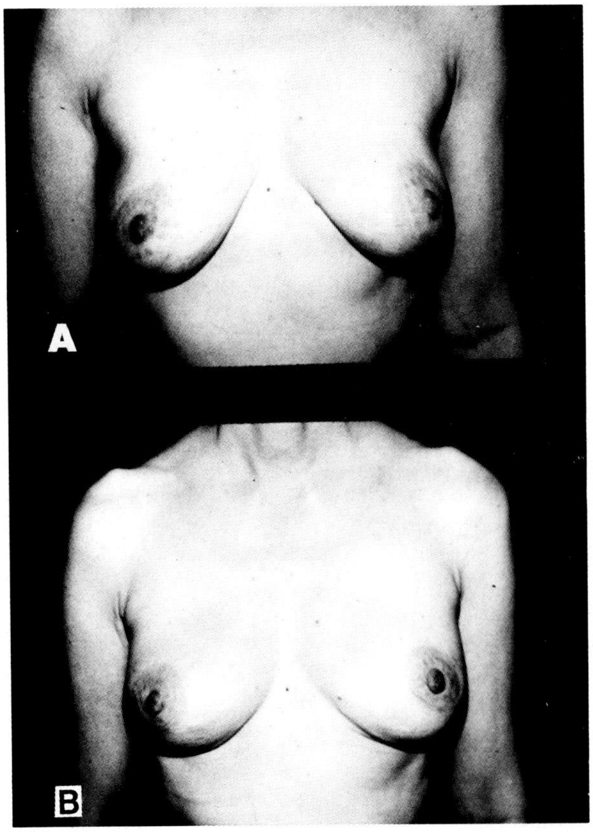

Figure 1 Patient with moderate ptosis *A*, before and *B*, 1 year after prophylactic mastectomy through inframammary incisions and nonsurgical mastopexy with skin taping utilizing 300 cc bilumen implants.

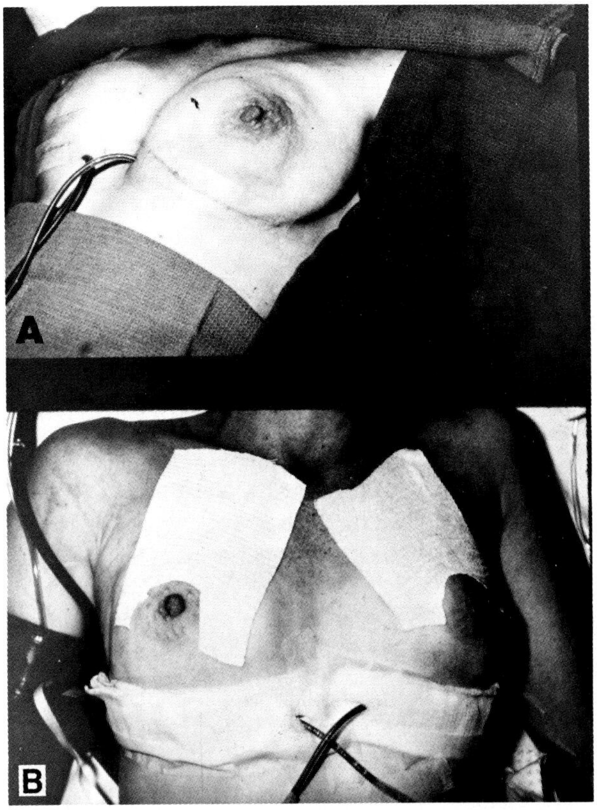

Figure 2 Intraoperative photographs of patient with moderate ptosis where inframammary incision was utilized and submuscular reconstruction performed with 310 cc implants. *A*, Redundant skin draping laterally; *B*, nipples properly positioned with Conform tape.

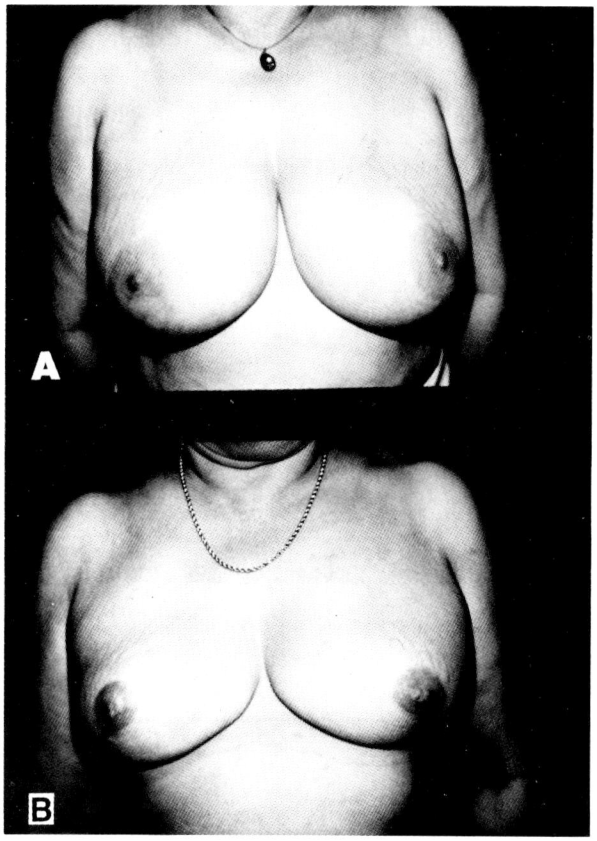

Figure 3 Large breasted patient with significant ptosis *A*, before and *B*, 1 year after prophylactic mastectomy utilizing Wise skin reduction pattern, nipple grafting, and 390 cc bilumen implants.

of incision can limit the skin resection to only the vertical dimension, thereby leaving sufficient skin for a well-rounded inframammary area. Using the inverted T skin pattern in such breasts results in extremely tight inframammary closures that, in addition to producing ischemia, produces a tightness across the lower part of the muscle pocket and results in a "pinched" final appearance of the inframammary area. Final determination of the site for nipple-areolar grafting is more difficult with the transverse elliptical skin excision technique as compared to the Wise pattern, where the nipple position is incorporated into the preoperative incision markings. The transverse elliptical skin incision is also preferred in patients that have a heavy smoking history, even if the patient has been able to stop smoking, because this incision interrupts less skin blood flow to the flaps.

Mastectomy Technique (Glandular Resection)

Mild hypotensive anesthesia is used for selected patients in order to minimize blood loss. Using the incision of choice, the initial dissection proceeds directly on the serratus and pectoralis muscle fascia from the inframammary line to the second rib and from the lateral edge of the sternum to the anterior border of the latissimus dorsi. My preference is to begin this dissection with a scalpel while retracting the breast tissue cephalad with large rake retractors; I switch to dissection with 9-inch scissors as soon as a well-defined plane on the pectoralis fascia is obtained. A fiberoptic retractor and a long hand-actuated cautery forceps have proven extremely useful in this dissection. The patient should not be paralyzed in order that serratus anterior muscle contraction will warn the surgeon of dissection close to the long thoracic nerve. Internal mammary perforating arteries along the sternal border in the third, fourth, and fifth interspaces are usually divided in the process of thinning the medial portion of the skin flap. The integrity of the pectoralis and serratus fascia must be maintained in order to provide complete muscle cover of the implant.

A scalpel is next used for sharp dissection from the inframammary line to the superior areolar margin, while maintaining countertraction on the parenchymal tissue. Scissor dissection is then used to finish this subcutaneous dissection in the plane between the ill-defined breast capsule and the skin. Dissection must extend under axillary hair bearing skin in order to ensure complete removal of the axillary tail and lower fat pad, which commonly includes several low axillary lymph nodes.

Following specimen removal, the skin flap is carefully examined and cleaned of any protruding fat globules or fibrous bands. If the nipple-areolar complex was not removed with the initial incision, the skin flap is inverted and the subareolar area cleaned of all tissue down to the subareolar dermal vessels, thereby leaving only ductal tissue within the nipple papilla. The periphery of the dissection, as well as the axilla, should then be carefully inspected to ensure that no shelf of fatty tissue has been left.

After weighing the specimens (often helpful in determining implant size), the specimen is sent to pathology for prompt inspection, with the subareolar and axillary tail portion of the breasts identified by sutures. Submuscular reconstruction is not begun until the pathologist has reported the absence of malignant tissue.

Submuscular Reconstruction

Since initially describing the term and technique of submuscular reconstruction in 1977, I have continued to enter the space from a 6 to 7 cm incision through serratus anterior and portions of the rectus abdominis and external oblique onto the sixth rib. Figure 4A illustrates this entry into the submuscular space with a drawing oriented identically with the photograph in Figure 4B. This muscle incision is kept as medial as possible in order to avoid an incision in the lateral serratus fascia, which is often thin and difficult to close, thus creating the possibility of implant herniation into the subcutaneous space. The direct approach on the sixth rib also facilitates creation of sharp inframammary definition. The serratus and rectus abdominis are then elevated by sharp dissection directly on top of the intercostal muscles until the subpectoral space is entered, where blunt dissection with scissors and/or fingers is usually adequate. It is important to release all pectoralis major insertions onto the anterior portion of the fourth

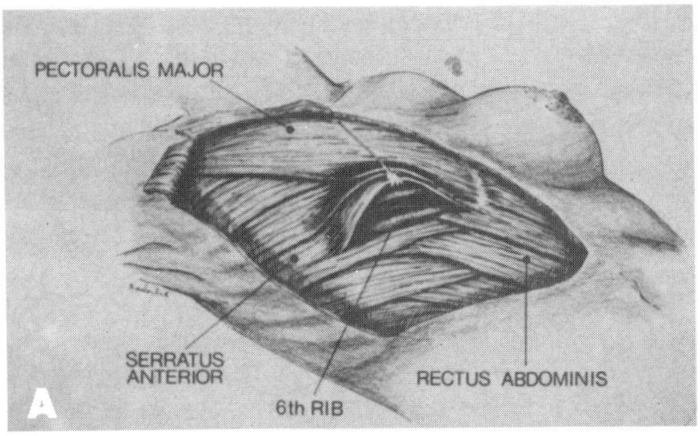

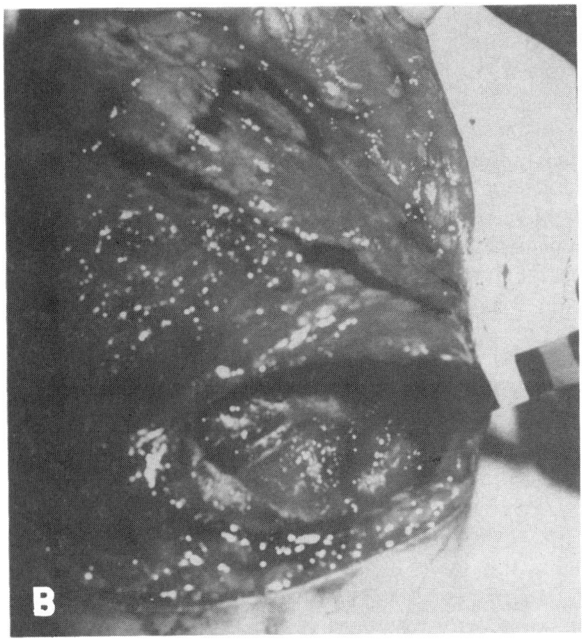

Figure 4 *A*, Drawing illustrating site of incision through serratus anterior and rectus abdominis to the sixth rib; *B*, intraoperative view showing the submuscular pocket, oriented as in *A*, ready to receive the implant.

and fifth ribs and to continue the superior portion of the dissection in a plane superficial to the pectoralis minor. Sternal attachments of the pectoralis must be maintained. The inferior dissection usually frees serratus and rectus to the lower border of the sixth rib or to the top of the seventh rib to a point that is 1 to 2 cm inferior to the desired inframammary line. Sizer implants are then utilized both in determining muscle pocket symmetry and in choosing the final implant size. Complete muscle enclosure of the implant is then obtained after placing suction catheters to drain both the subcutaneous and submuscular spaces.

It is far better to obtain good muscle closure over an implant that is slightly smaller than the patient might desire than to have a tenuous or incomplete closure over a larger implant. My patients are informed that the initial implant may be viewed as a tissue expander, to be exchanged for a considerably larger one in a very simple operation under local anesthesia following complete muscle stretching. Strict adherence to this philosophy has helped produce a zero incidence of implant herniation or extrusion through muscle tissue into the subcutaneous space.

Submuscular pocket preparation is facilitated by totally paralyzing the patient during that part of the dissection. Small defects in the muscle cover are easily sutured and do not compromise implant coverage. Larger openings should be well-sutured, followed by utilization of an implant that is small enough to allow complete muscle enclosure of the implant without excessive tension. Hypotensive agents, such as sodium nitroprusside, should be stopped and blood placement started as soon as the blunt dissection under the pectoralis begins. This practice greatly reduces the incidence of postoperative hematomas by allowing final hemostasis to be obtained with the patient in a normotensive state.

The average implant size used in my series is 325 cc, with implants ranging from 250 to 400 cc. I have used only double lumen implants for the past 8 years, currently preferring those with a "low bleed" inner bag. My preference for double lumen implants is related to the fact that I like to use the outer saline-filled bag as a vehicle for a small dose of Solu-Medrol. I routinely insert 12 mg of Solu-Medrol into the outer lumen in addition to the recommended amount of saline. Although I don't have any controlled study to prove that Solu-Medrol reduces the incidence of capsule formation, I have been so pleased with my results that I hesitate to change. I have not seen complications of cortisone atrophy from this dose of Solu-Medrol in a double lumen implant covered with muscle and skin.

I have no experience with polyurethane-covered implants, but I don't consider them suitable for submuscular reconstruction, particularly in view of the excellent results that can be achieved with regular implants that are totally covered with muscle tissue for compression and capsule prevention.

Postoperative Care

Early postoperative care is focused on observation for excessive bleeding, promoting satisfactory drainage, and doing everything possible to enhance skin blood supply. Postoperative bleeding and hematoma formation is lessened by closing incisions with the patient in a normotensive state, which requires blood transfusion (if used) and stopping hypotensive drugs well in advance of skin closure. Postoperative bleeding is also reduced by eliminating the hypertension sometimes associated with postoperative anxiety, excessive coughing, or unrelieved surgical pain. I prefer to have my patients receive intratracheal Xylocaine prior to extubation as well as intravenous narcotics prior to the end of the procedure in order to promote a smooth recovery.

Satisfactory drainage is enhanced by having a separate Jackson-Pratt reservoir for each breast; this is based on the philosophy that when two drain tubes are hooked up to one suction, the drain tube pulling against the least amount of resistance produces most of the drainage, thereby leaving the opposite breast with inadequate drainage. Double reservoirs have the additional advantage of allowing each breast to have maximum suction in the event that the reservoirs are not emptied frequently enough. Vacuum pressure studies of Jackson-Pratt reservoirs show that they are ineffective when they are even 50 percent filled with fluid or air. I instruct the nurses to check the reservoirs at least every 30 minutes to empty them whenever they appear even one-third full. Drain tubes are left in until they are draining approximately 1 cc per hour and the fluid is serous in nature. The average drain is left in place for 3 to 5 days.

Skin vascularity is enhanced by avoiding undue skin tension that results from large implants or excessive bleeding. Compression dressings are likewise avoided. If the patient's skin vascularity is questioned, particularly in patients who have a history of smoking, I use 10 mg nitroglycerin transderm patches changed at 24-hour intervals. Very light gauze dressings are placed over the incisions and all taping is kept inferior to the muscle pockets to avoid compression of the lower muscle pocket. I insist that the patient not wear any type of bra for at least 3 months in order to avoid obliteration of the lower portion of the submuscular pocket by the pressure of a bra. Most patients are comfortable wearing only a camisole under their clothing and report that the "living bra" created by the muscle cover is extremely effective in simulating the feel of a bra.

Arm activity is restricted for the first 3 to 5 days after surgery or until there is little evidence of surgical bleeding. This is followed by a program of gentle stretching exercises and isometric contractures of the pectorals, progressing to full range of motion 7 to 10 days after surgery. Strenuous exercises are avoided for 3 to 4 weeks.

If the skin has been taped in surgery to hold the nipple-areolar complex in the ideal position, the tape is readjusted 24 to 48 hours postoperatively with the patient standing at the bedside.

Implant massage is begun following removal of the drains. The patient is instructed to use very gentle compression of her implants for the first 3 to 5 days, followed by more vigorous compression. She is instructed to continue vigorous massage for 3 months, after which she is asked to massage her breasts once a day for the rest of her life, in order to maintain a large periprosthetic space.

Complications

Early postoperative hemorrhage producing hematoma is the first problem that may occur, usually caused by excessive bleeding in the subcutaneous space. Patients should be returned to surgery as soon as a definite hematoma is diagnosed in order to stop excessive hemorrhage and to save the already partially ischemic skin flap from the added problems of excessive tightness and the toxic effects of the subcutaneous blood.

Although early postoperative skin ischemia is common in properly thinned skin flaps, actual necrosis is extremely rare unless the patient has been a heavy cigarette smoker. Avoidance of any type of compressive bandage, rapid evacuation of any significant subcutaneous hematoma, and strict adherence to a no smoking policy in the pre- and postoperative period should produce an extremely low incidence of actual necrosis. With adequate muscle enclosure of the implants, small areas of full-thickness necrosis may be treated by slow debridement, followed by secondary healing without any sequelae other than extra scar tissue on the skin. Large areas of full-thickness necrosis (more than 3 cm in diameter) will probably need to be excised and replaced with a skin graft directly on the muscle tissue. In the absence of complete muscle cover, even the smallest area of skin necrosis will probably result in implant loss.

The combination of complete muscle cover over implants plus diligent breast massage has made capsular contracture around double lumen implants an infrequent complication. Should contracture occur, capsulotomy, including thorough scoring of the dome of the capsule to allow expansion in all directions, combined with placement of a new double lumen prosthesis containing 12 mg of Solu-Medrol plus saline in the outer lumen, has usually been successful. Compression Ace bandages are worn on a 24-hour basis during the first week following capsulotomy, followed by vigorous implant massage, with both treatments intended to assist in maintenance of a large periprosthetic space.

In summary, the techniques described in this chapter have produced breast reconstructive results free from significant complications and with a high degree of patient satisfaction. Due to the fact that the term "total" mastectomy is a misnomer other than for Halsted radical mastectomies, the operation should be called prophylactic subcutaneous mastectomy when inframammary incisions are used or prophylactic simple mastectomy if some form of surgical reduction of the skin envelope is performed. There is no available data to suggest that subcutaneous mastectomies through inframammary incisions with skeletonized skin flaps, including the subareolar area, offer less cancer prophylaxis than do simple mastectomies, with or without using the nipple-areolar tissue as grafts. In view of this fact, the superior esthetic results obtained with the inframammary incision mandate continued usage whenever possible, with skin resection performed only when anatomically necessary.

Although preliminary data from accurate follow-up of my personal series tend to indicate that the mastectomy described herein may be an effective prophylaxis against breast cancer, nothing short of a long-term follow-up (10 or more years) of a group of these patients who are proven to be in at least a 3 times normal risk category will substantiate the true effectiveness of the operation. Such a study is currently in progress.

SUGGESTED READING

Anderson DE. A genetic study of human breast cancer. J Natl Cancer Inst 1972; 48:1029–1034.

Azzopardi JG. The histogenesis of "early" carcinoma. In: Azzopardi JD, ed. Problems in breast pathology. Philadelphia: WB Saunders, 1979; 92.

Jarrett JR, et al. Subcutaneous mastectomy in small, large or ptotic breasts

with immediate submuscular placement of implants. Plast Reconstr Surg 1978; 62:702–705.
Jarrett JR, et al. Aesthetic refinements in prophylactic subcutaneous mastectomy with submuscular reconstruction. Plast Reconstr Surg 1982; 69:624–631.
Leis HP, et al. Bilateral breast cancer. Breast, Dis Breast 1981; 7:13–17.
Lynch HT, et al. Genetic counseling, familial breast cancer and surgeon's responsibility. Plast Reconstr Surg 1980; 66:303–309.
Wise RJ, Gannon JP, Hill JR. Further experience with reduction mammoplasty. Plast Reconstr Surg 1963; 32:12–20.
Wolfe JN. Breast patterns as an index of risk for developing breast cancer. AJR 1976; 126:1130–1139.
Woods JE. Detailed technique of subcutaneous mastectomy with and without mastopexy. Ann Plast Surg 1987; 18:51—62.

WHO CAN BENEFIT FROM PROPHYLACTIC MASTECTOMY?

JACK C. FISHER, M.D., F.A.C.S.

The problem, as I see it, is too many mastectomies for cancer prophylaxis without adequate medical justification.

This is an issue made worse by surgeons with an outdated understanding of breast cancer, or an unwillingness to define risks and represent accurately to patients the probable outcome of mastectomy. Perhaps our highly competitive professional environment also contributes to the problem.

Some of us are uncomfortable recommending mastectomy for increased risk of breast carcinoma because definition of risk depends on so many different variables. The purpose of this discussion is to organize known risk categories in a manner easily understood by surgeons and readily explainable to patients.

BACKGROUND RISK

Very few discussions of subcutaneous mastectomy begin with a consideration of what I call background risk. The indicators of increased risk cannot possibly be placed into context until the risk for all patients is defined.

Today, the lifetime risk for development of breast carcinoma is approximately one in eleven (9 percent). This risk is somewhat higher for women who waited until later in life to bear children, and it is slightly lower for women who bore children early. Therefore, a survey of cancer in a more prosperous (and presumably longer-educated) neighborhood could be expected to yield slightly more breast cancer. Women in a lower socioeconomic neighborhood would experience less breast cancer.

Risk of breast cancer is greatest in the fifth and sixth decades of life. A woman in her sixties is past the worse part of her risk exposure.

Family History

No longer is it sufficient to just ask for past occurrence of breast cancer in *any* family member. Knowledge that an aunt dying some time after a mastectomy does not allow for accurate determination of risk. We must focus on parents and siblings.

Three questions need to be asked about every instance of breast cancer that has affected siblings, parents, and grandparents. Premenopausal or postmenopausal? Bilateral or unilateral? What kind of cancer was it? Some of this information may prove difficult to find but an effort must be made.

Either a sibling or a parent (but not both) with breast cancer doubles the lifetime risk (18 percent). This figure will vary somewhat according to age of onset, bilaterality, etc. For example, prior history of bilateral disease appearing early in life is a more significant indicator of added risk.

Whenever breast cancer affects successive generations within the same family, the risk to additional members of that family rises sharply. A condition known as familial breast cancer does exist. The risk in these families exceeds 50 percent, and may approach 100 percent when there is regular successive generation occurrence or else appearance in multiple siblings, especially when malignancy occurs prior to menopause or in both breasts.

The significance of an isolated aunt or grandparent with breast cancer is not clearly defined but the risk is probably not much more than background (9 percent).

Histologic Markers

Too many names have been assigned to the benign pathologic changes affecting a woman's breasts. These names no longer make any semantic sense to surgeons who must evaluate the prognostic significance of a given histologic pattern.

Fibrocystic disease is a catch-all phrase that does not mean very much by itself. Some physicians have even questioned use of the word "disease" for a condition that affects far more than half of all women over 45.

In the past, arguments have been made for and against the premalignant status of fibrocystic disease. Today, we must know more about the specific histologic nature of the fibrocystic condition present.

Two particular words are gaining importance and should be watched for by the surgeon when evaluating the pathologist's report. These key words are "proliferative disease" and "atypia."

Little significance should be assigned to such time-honored designations as apocrine metaplasia or the myriad of other diagnostic headings. What the surgeon needs to know is whether ductal proliferation is seen or whether atypical cells are present. If this is not apparent after reading the written report, then your pathologist should be asked for clarification.

When patients with fibrocystic disease are categorized, those with ordinary fibrocystic disease bear no increased risk for malignancy over background risk (9 percent). On the other hand, patients with proliferative changes and atypia experience a very significant added risk—in excess of 50 percent.

Noninvasive Cancer

There are two kinds of breast cancer, ductal and lobular; and each has its invasive and noninvasive form. Sometimes a breast tissue biopsy will show evidence of noninvasive ductal (intraductal) carcinoma or noninvasive lobular (lobular-in-situ) carcinoma. By convention, we do not ordinarily say intralobular or ductal-in-situ.

Two questions to be asked by the patient whenever a biopsy shows noninvasive malignancy are: "What are my chances that invasive cancer will develop—and when?" The answers are only partially known, and they are different for intraductal and noninvasive lobular carcinoma.

Intraductal carcinoma is essentially a unilateral disease. It can be multifocal and it can lead to invasive carcinoma relatively quickly: 35 to 50 percent within 10 years.

Lobular-in-situ is both multifocal and bilateral. A decision to reduce risk for development of invasive carcinoma must, therefore, include both breasts. Lobular-in-situ carries a similar risk but it is spread over a long interval (20 to 30 years).

Not often remembered or well understood is the fact that each form of noninvasive malignancy can precede both kinds of invasive carcinoma. In other words, intraductal does not always precede ductal carcinoma; it can lead to lobular carcinoma as well.

Contralateral Malignancy

A woman who has already experienced invasive carcinoma bears increased risk for cancer in the remaining breast, but not as much as many of us think. Older reports of contralateral cancer incidence failed to differentiate between the many different categories of risk.

Prior ductal carcinoma is associated with a 12 percent incidence of another ductal carcinoma in the other breast. Contralateral incidence for lobular carcinoma has been reported as 22 percent.

Patients should be told either of a modest increase or of a doubling of risk over background, depending on the histology of the prior malignancy.

WHAT IS PROPHYLACTIC MASTECTOMY?

Two kinds of mastectomy are recognized for their prophylactic potential: the subcutaneous and the total (simple) mastectomy. They are defined as follows:

A total mastectomy is neither total nor simple. By convention, total mastectomy includes removal of the entire nipple and areola. It involves removal of nearly all of the glandular breast (95 to 99 percent), but not every bit of it.

The subcutaneous mastectomy was conceived to preserve the nipple, areola, and overlying breast skin. It removes a very great portion of the glandular breast itself. Opinions vary but the resection is believed to be within the range of 75 to 95 percent, depending on the surgeon's technique. Surgeons with the fewest complications have probably removed less breast tissue.

In neither instance is every cell at risk for carcinogenesis removed, which leads many to question the validity of any mastectomy being truly prophylactic.

Is Any Mastectomy Prophylactic?

No valid evidence has ever been offered to prove that mastectomy can in fact prevent cancer. A controlled prospective study is probably not feasible any longer, nor would it be ethical to structure a study that omits mastectomy in the presence of high risk for malignancy.

Whenever important clinical issues remain unanswered or are difficult to study, an experimental model can be designed. Miller et al has done this, removing some or all of the identifiable breast tissue prior to introduction of a carcinogenetic influence. Unfortunately, experimental mastectomy does not appear to reduce the frequency of induced tumors. Residual cells presumably serve as a more focused or intensive target for the carcinogen.

Proponents of prophylactic mastectomy tend to discount the significance of this animal-derived data. They may be correct. However, if the same model had shown a sharp reduction in cancers in the mastectomy group, doubtless this finding would have been offered as evidence in favor of the procedure.

One way to generate valid evidence in support of prophylactic mastectomy would be to focus on a very high risk population, for example, individuals in the familial breast carcinoma category. Then, looking either prospectively or retrospectively, the rate of appearance of cancer could be determined among patients who have or have not chosen mastectomy. Such a study would take several years to complete. Studies of this type are not easy to complete, but are more worthwhile than scrutiny of a population that has experienced subcutaneous mastectomy for several different reasons.

What Should I Tell My Patients?

There is no easy answer to the question, "Who needs prophylactic mastectomy?" Until more tangible information is forwarded for our consideration, we are forced to act on empiric evidence. What this means to me is that *no surgeon should tell a patient she ought to have her breasts removed.* What surgeons can and should do is help patients define their particular risk category, and this can be done with reasonable accuracy after obtaining a very thorough history.

After asking about prior family experience with breast carcinoma, inquire about histology, age of onset, bilaterality, and, of course, response to therapy. We must also know about any prior biopsies or prior cancers. Patients should be asked to find results of any histologic exams done previously.

With an adequate history in hand, the only additional evidence that might be obtained is a mammogram, perhaps also a biopsy in the presence of fibrocystic disease not previously biopsied.

Provided none of the aforementioned measures yield evidence of invasive malignancy, the decision for mastectomy must be a joint effort by the patient and her surgeon. In other words, a decision for mastectomy should mean the patient does not want to accept the risk as defined by her surgeon.

Indications for Prophylactic Mastectomy

To restate the important principle defined above—no surgeon should unilaterally insist that a patient ought to have a mastectomy! The physician is a teacher who tells the patient in straightforward terms what the risk is. The patient decides in favor of mastectomy based on her willingness or reluctance to accept a given risk.

Patients with the highest defined risk for development of invasive cancer include those with familial breast cancer, those with histologically proven noninvasive cancer (intraductal or lobular-in-situ), and those with a proliferative form of fibrocystic disease. Patients in these categories experience lifetime risks in excess of 50 percent, a greater than ever chance of developing cancer. In my experience most patients will not accept that risk, although some will.

Patients with ordinary fibrocystic disease, with a single relative with breast cancer, or with a past history of breast cancer do not share much more than background risk. Most patients in these latter categories are unwilling to give up their breasts. A few however will be.

Subjective Indications for Prophylactic Mastectomy

Medical indications aside, there are a few subjective reasons to proceed with a mastectomy in the absence of biologic risk. These include long-standing misery associated with chronic persistent fibrocystic disease, often repeated biopsies, or an exaggerated fear of cancer. In addition the patient who feels guilty about having had silicone injected into her breasts has probably lost the ability to self-examine and perceive early the development of a cancer.

Regrettably the subjective indications for mastectomy are seized upon by surgeon-advocates of prophylactic mastectomy. Far too often, patients are preprogrammed for subcutaneous mastectomy even before they have been given enough facts to balance risks against probable surgical outcome.

Patients Already Programmed for Mastectomy

Patients often arrive for plastic surgery consultation already convinced that they must have subcutaneous mastectomy. Sometimes, they cannot be easily dissuaded despite absence of medical or subjective indication.

The prudent surgeon-advisor must begin with an assessment of risk, then a discussion of mastectomy, its variations, and its probable outcome. The decision for mastectomy is a mutual one, with the surgeon serving as teacher, not advocate. The patient must balance risk versus outcome, and the surgeon must describe realistically what the patient's reconstructed breasts will be like after surgery.

The Outcome of Prophylactic Mastectomy?

Our journals are filled with postoperative assessments of both subcutaneous mastectomy and total mastectomy. Sufficient emphasis is placed on the postoperative appearance of the breast, the frequency of tissue loss, and the incidence of capsule contraction. Less well-emphasized is the likelihood that these breasts are, more often than not, anesthetic to touch, especially when an adequate excision of breast tissue has been achieved. Patients need to be warned of this in advance. The breast is a sexual organ for a lifetime. Following mastectomy, this sexual function is very often lost.

Who Needs Prophylactic Mastectomy?

If we assume that a surgical removal in breast tissue at risk can reduce the risk of cancer (and nobody knows for sure whether that is in fact true), the patients most likely to benefit from either total mastectomy or subcutaneous mastectomy are those with an extra risk over and above background risk.

A few patients will reach a threshold of chronic annoyance or fear, based on unusually persistent cystic breasts. Some of these will, in fact, be better off after mastectomy even though their risk of cancer was no different from the general female population. But, these patients must be selected very, very carefully.

Mastectomy is never a procedure to be taken lightly or to be applied indiscriminately. The benefits and the resulting deformity should be in balance with the known risk.

SUGGESTED READING

Buehler PK. Patient selection for prophylactic mastectomy: who is at risk? Plast Reconstr Surg 1983; 72(3):324–334.

Goodnight JE Jr, Quagliana JM; Morton DL. Failure of subcutaneous mastectomy to prevent the development of breast cancer. J Surg Oncol 1984; 26(3):198–201.

Rubin LR. Prophylactic mastectomy with immediate reconstruction for the high risk woman. Clin Plast Surg 1984; 11(2):369–381.

Schecthter MT. Breast cancer risk factors: can we select women for prophylactic mastectomy? Can J Surg 1985; 28(3):242–244, 247.

Snyderman RK. Prophylactic mastectomy: pros and cons. Cancer 1984; 53(3):806–808.

THE TRUNK

ABDOMINOPLASTY

JOHN R. LEWIS Jr., M.D.

Abdominoplasty is one of the more common procedures carried out as part of body contouring. The specific problems that may be indications for abdominoplasty are: (1) striae, (2) dermatochalasis, (3) lipodystrophy, (4) ptosis, (5) a panniculus of skin and fat, (6) diastasis recti, (7) ventral hernia, (8) umbilical hernia, (9) generalized laxity of the muscles and fascia of the abdominal wall and, (10) abdominal scars.

ETIOLOGY

Etiologic factors that cause or contribute to the above problems are:

1. Inherited characteristics, particularly inherited hernias and weaknesses, type of abdomen, and type of fat distribution.
2. Congenital characteristics, primarily problems present at birth such as a wide umbilical ring or an inguinal weakness, which may be neither a family characteristic nor an inherited trait.
3. Obesity and weight loss. Rapid weight gain is particularly likely to cause striae and localized, as well as generalized, fat collections. Longstanding obesity is more likely to be characterized by generalized obesity and ptosis, varying from mild to marked panniculus.
4. Pregnancy causes problems due to weight gain as well as the stretching of the tissues of the abdominal wall. This is more likely to occur with multiple pregnancies. Diastasis recti, striae, and loss of elasticity of the abdominal musculature, fascia, and skin may follow multiple pregnancies or marked enlargement of the abdominal cavity.
5. Chronic straining. Diastasis recti and hernias may occur with chronic straining.
6. Sedentary habitus. Patients with morbid obesity, or who pursue an inactive lifestyle, may have weakness and flaccidity of the muscles and fasciae, thereby predisposing to ptosis of the abdominal wall and/or a globular abdomen. There may also be a predisposition to hernias.
7. Injury. Injury to the abdomen may cause scars and also hernias.
8. Surgery. Abdominal surgery for the correction of intra-abdominal problems, or attempts to correct abdominal wall deformities, cause scars; these mar the appearance of the abdomen. A tight or depressed scar of the abdomen often gives an obvious depression with separation of the subcutaneous fat; it is made more obvious by the increased fullness at each side of the scar.
9. Chronic pulmonary disease. Problems such as emphysema from heavy smoking affect the shape of the abdomen because of the degree of abdominal respiration.

INDICATIONS FOR TREATMENT

Indications for treatment are generally: (1) appearance, (2) poor fitting of clothes, (3) disabilities related to the size of the abdomen or the ptosis of the abdominal tissues, (4) discomfort, as from tight adherent scars, and (5) hernias. The latter may occur through the umbilical ring, between the separated rectus muscles, through an enlarged inguinal ring, or through scar tissue following surgical procedures or injuries.

CONTRAINDICATIONS OF SURGERY

Contraindications include problems of general health, such as severe anemia, uncontrolled diabetes, severe emphysema, myasthenia gravis, and severe coronary artery disease. Problems of wound healing occur more frequently in patients who are heavy smokers. Frequent coughing, of course, also occurs more often in smokers and endangers a recently repaired hernia or diastasis recti. Patients should be advised to stop smoking or at least to cut down markedly.

Wide defects of muscle and fascia may indicate a supportive garment rather than surgery in the older patient in ill health.

MANAGEMENT

Before the popularity of suction-assisted lipectomy, the excess fat of the abdominal wall in lipodystrophies was usually surgically resected (Figs. 1 and 2). This operation left a thick abdominal flap of skin and fat that had to be pulled tightly and closed in the suprapubic area,

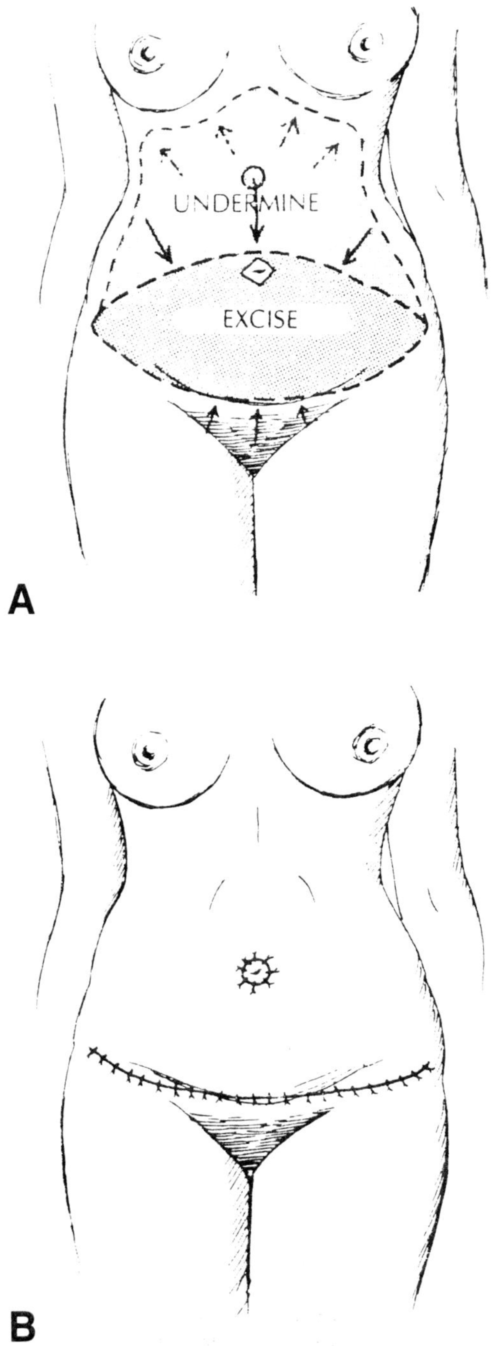

Figure 1 *A*, Undermining of the skin and subcutaneous tissue of the abdominal wall allows tightening downward to a suprapubic closure line. The amount of skin and subcutaneous fat that may be excised is outlined. *B*, The skin and fat of the abdomen is freed from the underlying fascia through the suprapubic incision. This flap is then pulled downward firmly and the excess resected to allow closure. A small vertical opening is made at the appropriate place to pull through the circumscribed umbilicus, which is sutured into its new location. This closure leaves the least obvious scars, for the umbilical repair heals with minimal scarring. The suprapubic incision line is closed in layers and the final scar is usually flat and narrow. Also, it falls below the panty line. (All drawings of technique used by permission and redrawn from Lewis JR. The atlas of aesthetic plastic surgery. Boston: Little, Brown, 1973.)

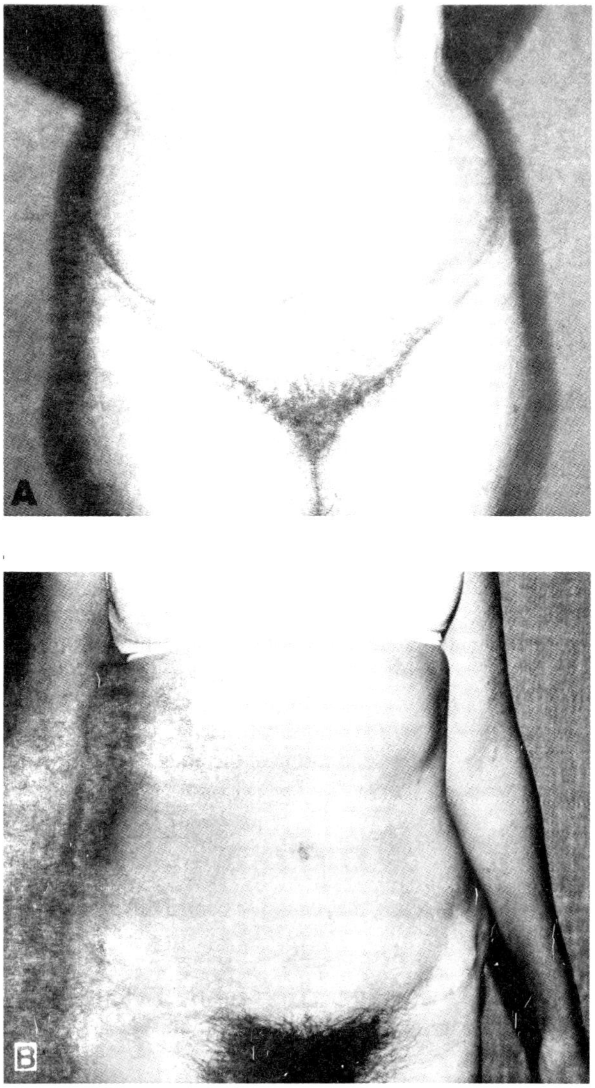

Figure 2 *A*, Preoperative patient with an obese abdomen and with relaxation of the subcutaneous tissues and skin. A lower midline abdominal scar is present with contracture above the pubis. *B*, Patient is shown following closure as in Figure 1.

usually with superior repositioning of the umbilicus. Lipodystrophy is now often corrected by suction lipectomy when it involves somewhat localized areas or if the skin is not relaxed and ptotic. If ptosis is notably present, skin resection is indicated as well, though this may be done at a subsequent procedure, thus allowing time for skin shrinking and retraction. For generalized obesity of the abdominal area with little relaxation of the skin, there is probably no indication for surgery. Instead, weight reduction and exercise are recommended to help achieve a trimmer figure.

For generalized fat excess and skin relaxation, or ptosis of the abdominal skin, the tissues may require an abdominoplasty with a wide skin-fat resection, repositioning of the umbilicus and closure along a suprapubic line (see Figs. 1 and 2). The resulting scar should fall under the panty line. A skin-fat panniculus should usually be resected and repaired in the same manner, though an "apron" of skin may be simply resected and the wound closed. Marked weight loss often results in marked ptosis of the skin and fat.

Management of abdominal striae is probably not indicated if the skin of the abdomen is snug. If striae are accompanied by a great deal of relaxation and loss of tone of the abdominal skin, a wide resection of skin may be indicated (Figs. 3 and 4). Tightening of the residual skin gives a flatter, snugger abdomen and a more pleasing appearance. Dermatochalasis with wrinkling and/or ptosis of the abdominal skin and fat is usually correctable in a similar fashion. Wide resection of the relaxed skin, with or without repositioning of the umbilicus, should allow the skin to be pulled downward for closure in the suprapubic area (Figs. 5 and 6).

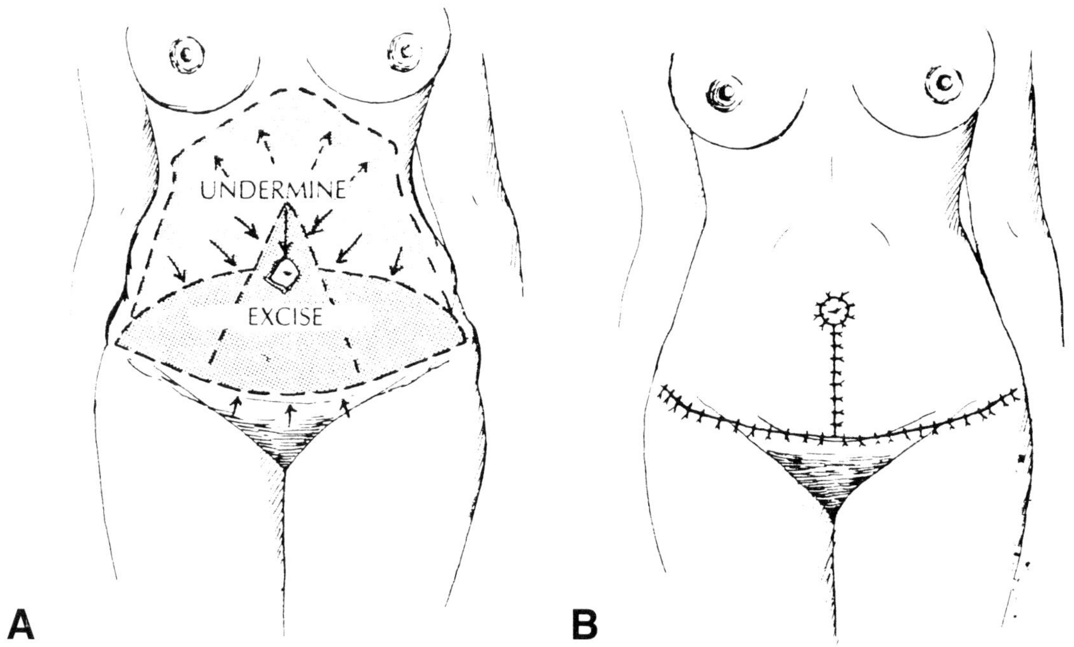

Figure 3 *A*, This type of resection allows for tightening in a vertical direction by pulling the superior flap downward to the suprapubic line for resection and closure as well as horizontal tightening by excision of a triangle of skin from the superior flap to be closed vertically. *B*, Final repair of the patient. The vertical midline scar is often more noticeable than the horizontal scar, but a layer closure and postoperative support of the wound will result in an acceptable scar.

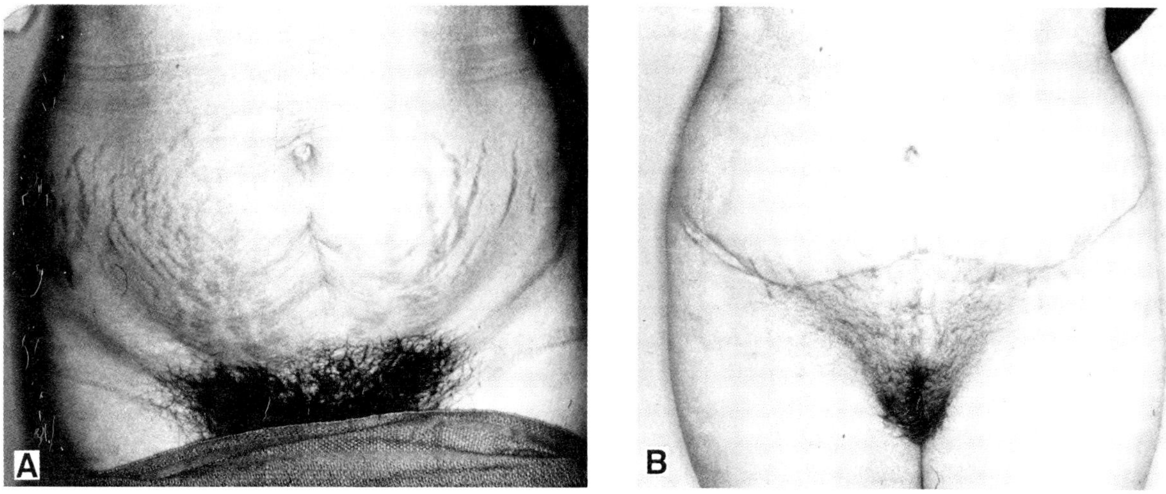

Figure 4 *A*, Ptotic relaxed abdomen with marked striae and with a midline vertical abdominal scar. *B*, The same patient following wide undermining and resection of a wide area of excessive skin and fat. Closure is around the umbilicus, which is brought out through a new opening in the abdominal flap, and vertically from the umbilicus down to the suprapubic incision line. The transverse suprapubic incision line has a modified "gull wing" shape to allow slightly more relaxation for repair in the midline area.

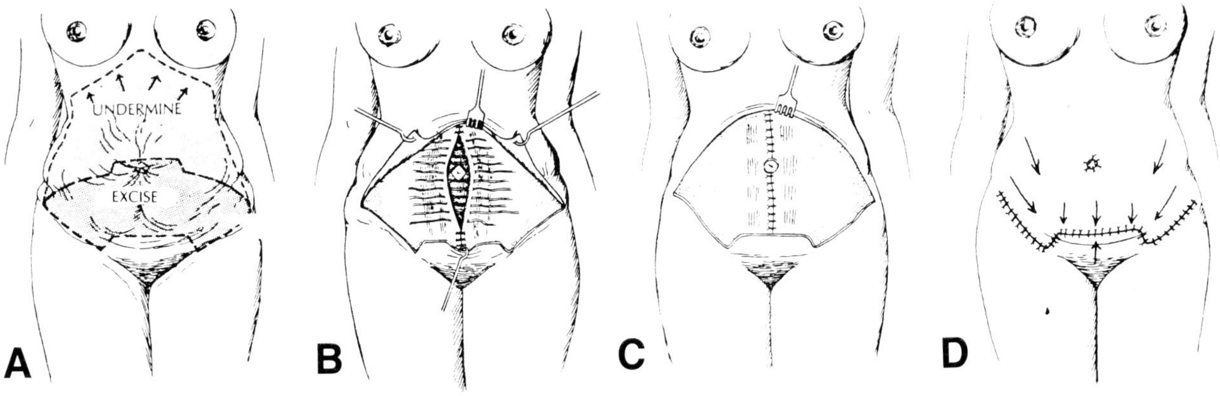

Figure 5 *A*, Another pattern of skin-fat resection following wide undermining of the abdominal subcutaneous tissue and skin. *B*, The deep closure is one of repair of the rectus sheath vertically beneath the flap that has been raised through the horizontal incision in the suprapubic area. For wide diastasis recti or true hernias, one may split the rectus sheaths and repair as a double-layer, overlapping closure of the rectus sheaths across the midline. *C*, Following repair of the rectus sheaths with correction of a wide diastasis recti, the abdominal flap is now ready to be pulled downward for resection and closure in the suprapubic area. *D*, The usual type of closure for the abdominal incision is a repair in layers with nonabsorbable sutures such as braided Nylon, or slowly absorbable sutures such as Maxon, with a final intracuticular single filament suture closure such as 3-0 Prolene. The pattern of this incision is more angled and less rounded to allow the incision to come across the top of the pubis and then lower on each side to be more easily hidden.

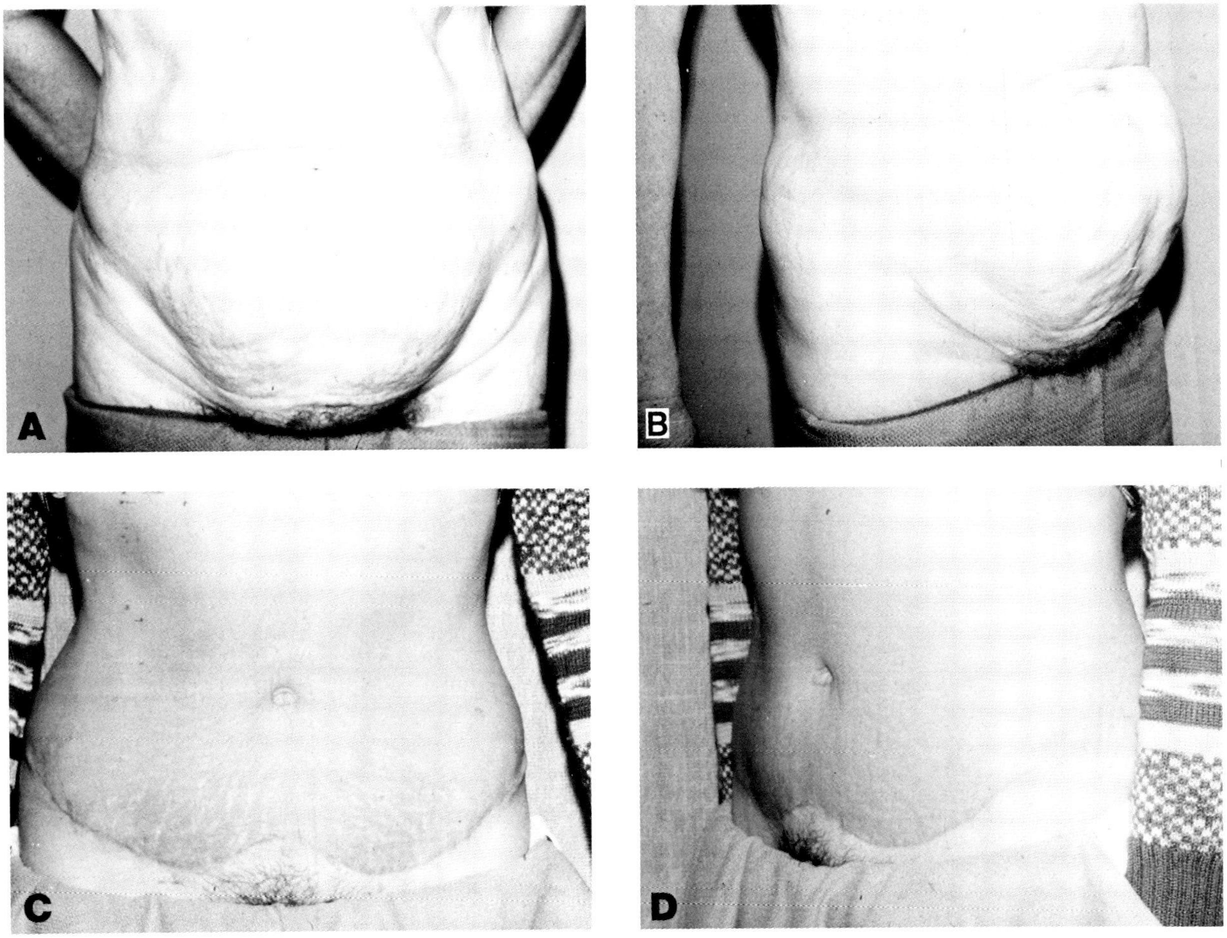

Figure 6 *A*, There is marked relaxation of the abdomen with subcutaneous tissue, skin, muscles, and fascia involved as well. *B*, Note the marked relaxation and protrusion of the abdomen, which produce a globular shape due to the weakness and stretching of the abdominal supportive structures. *C*, Following wide resection of skin and fat and vertical repair of the rectus sheaths, which are overlapped, there is support and correction of the diastasis recti and/or ventral hernias with resultant flatter, more pleasing abdomen. *D*, Lateral view of patient shows snugging and flattening of the abdomen.

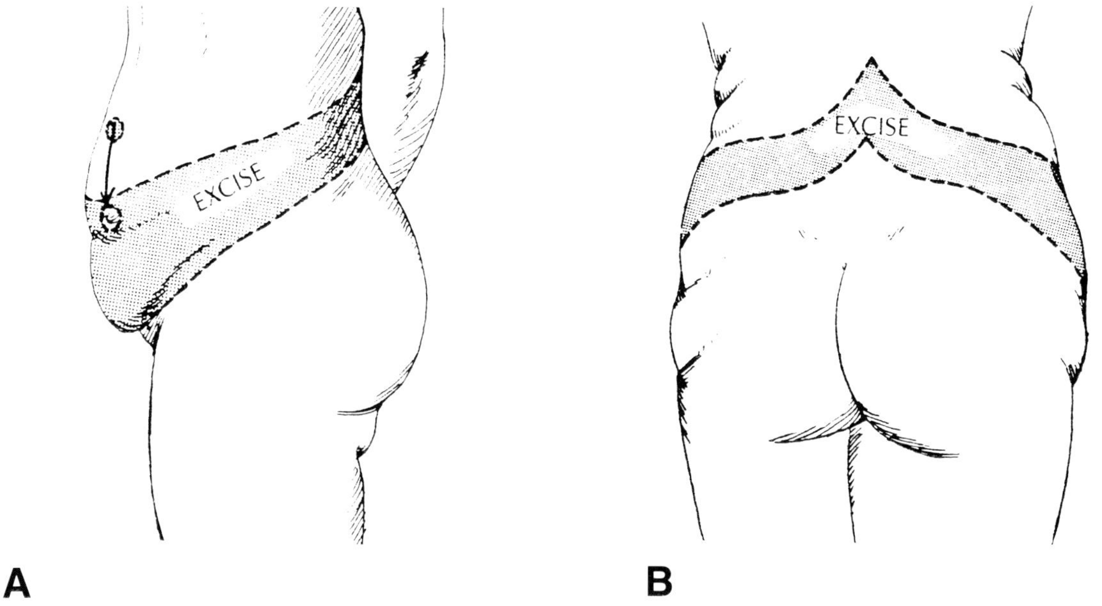

Figure 7 Extensive weight loss usually results in marked ptosis of subcutaneous tissue and skin of the abdomen, flanks, buttocks, thighs, breasts, and arms. It may prove advantageous to extend the resection circumferentially to the posterior midline as a belt dermatolipectomy.

For diastasis recti, support of the rectus muscles and rectus sheaths is indicated as well, for support and for snugging the abdomen; also to give a flatter, more attractive appearance.

The presence of a substantial diastasis recti and/or a ventral hernia indicates approximation of the rectus muscles by suture of the rectus sheaths as a vertical midline repair (Figs. 7 and 8). Nonabsorbable sutures are used for more longstanding support. If there is an enlargement of the umbilical ring, this is narrowed at the same operative procedure. Weaknesses and diastasis in the supraumbilical area are repaired in a similar fashion to those occurring between the umbilicus and the pubis.

Ventral hernias usually do not have a narrow-necked peritoneal sac that would indicate resection. Instead, one pushes the bulging sac inward as the defect is closed. If there is a wide area of laxity in the midabdomen, or a wide ventral hernia, the anterior rectus sheath is divided and overlapped for repair, also approximating the rectus muscles. For extremely wide defects, one may even elect to use a Dacron or Teflon sheet to suture over the defect as part of the strengthening of the anterior abdominal wall. The fibrous tissue reaction created by the mesh replaces the deficient fascial support when healing is complete.

Repair of scars of the abdomen is often combined with either suction lipectomy or an abdominal dermatolipectomy with repair. Lower abdominal scars often may be completely resected and the skin pulled downward for closure in the suprapubic area (see Figs. 2 and 4). For a scar with a hernia, the dissection is carried out carefully and the tissues repaired by layer closure or tissue overlap.

Scars of the upper abdomen may indicate a more conservative undermining and a less tight vertical pull of the skin for closure. It used to be thought that the skin must be made very tight to give a pleasing appearance to the abdomen. The tissues should be snug, but wide resection of skin with unduly tight closure is not necessary and, indeed, is often contraindicated.

Localized areas of fat hypertrophy without any great skin laxity are generally managed by suction lipectomy. Localized areas of fat hypertrophy, or fat limited to the lower portion of the abdominal wall, are often managed by suction lipectomy with a conservative skin-tightening procedure at the same operative stage; else the skin resection is performed at a later stage when the tissues have retracted and healed from the suction lipectomy. Obviously, skin laxity indicates skin resection, but one may often elect to perform a limited skin resection when the procedure is combined with suction lipectomy. For milder problems, or in older patients, this is often a wise choice of procedures.

The management of abdominal lipodystrophy or generalized obesity should usually first be by reasonable weight loss and exercise, with the muscles kept toned and strengthened while the excess weight is lost. This may help avoid an abdominal dermatolipectomy or at least minimize the degree of surgery. It may change the indication from a wide abdominal dermatolipectomy to that of a simpler suction lipectomy of the lower abdomen. The upper abdomen may also be suctioned in continuity with the lower abdomen, or separately through a small incision inside the rim of the umbilicus.

Marked weight loss may result in extensive ptosis of the skin. If the deformity is great, a circumferential resection may be needed to tighten the abdomen and the flanks and to support the thighs and the buttocks (Fig. 9, see also Figs. 7 and 8).

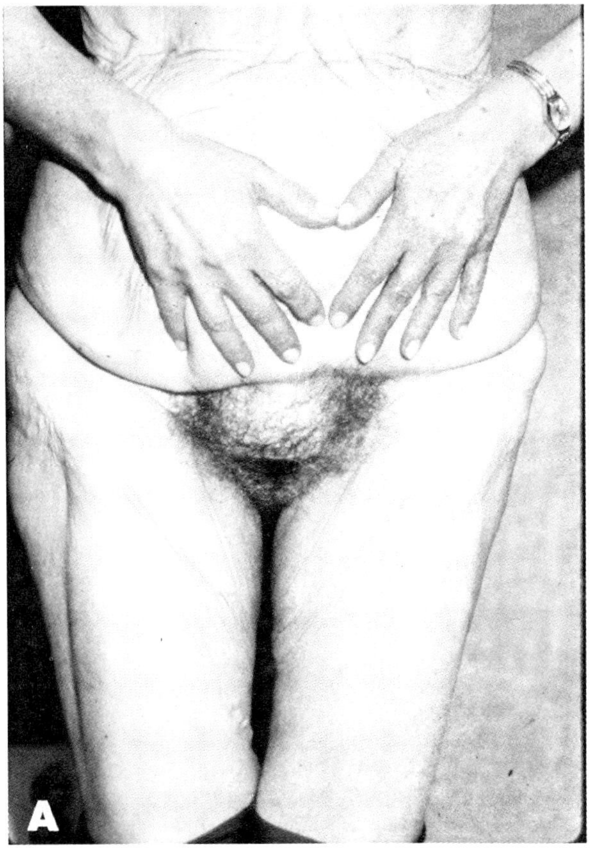

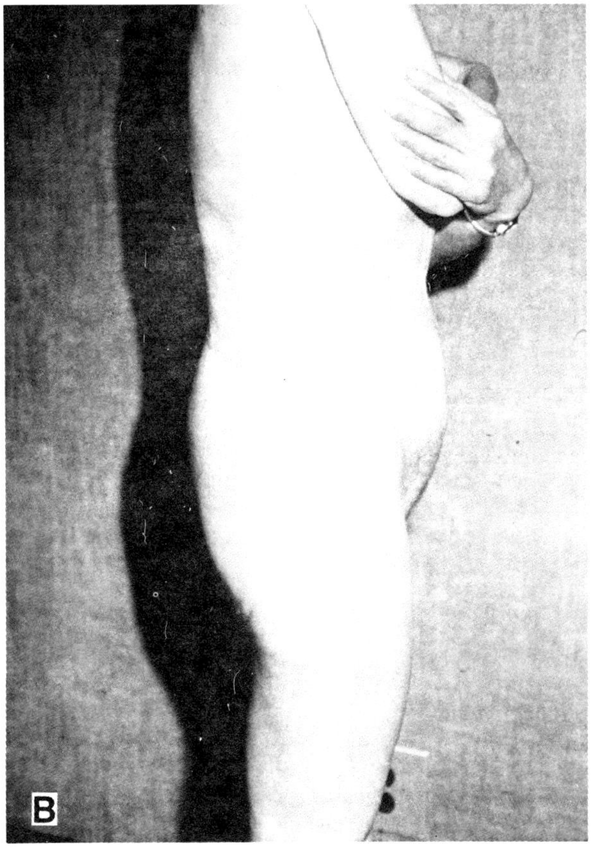

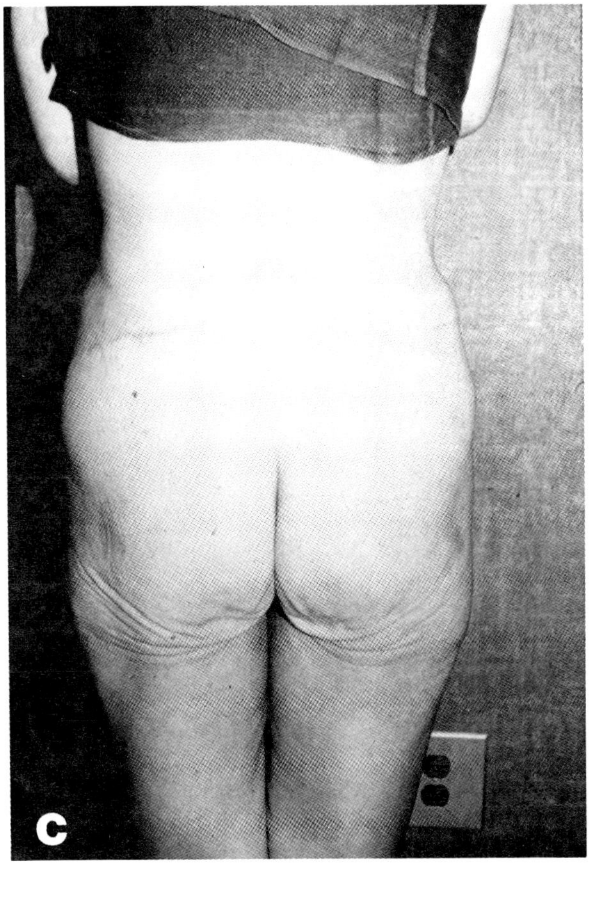

Figure 8 *A*, Patient following weight loss of approximately 100 pounds. Patient showed marked ptosis of subcutaneous tissue and skin of trunk, extremities, face, and neck. Her primary problem is one of the abdomen, flanks, and buttocks. *B* and *C*, The patient is shown following abdominoplasty, which was extended circumferentially as a belt lipectomy to support the buttocks posteriorly, the flanks laterally, and the abdomen anteriorly.

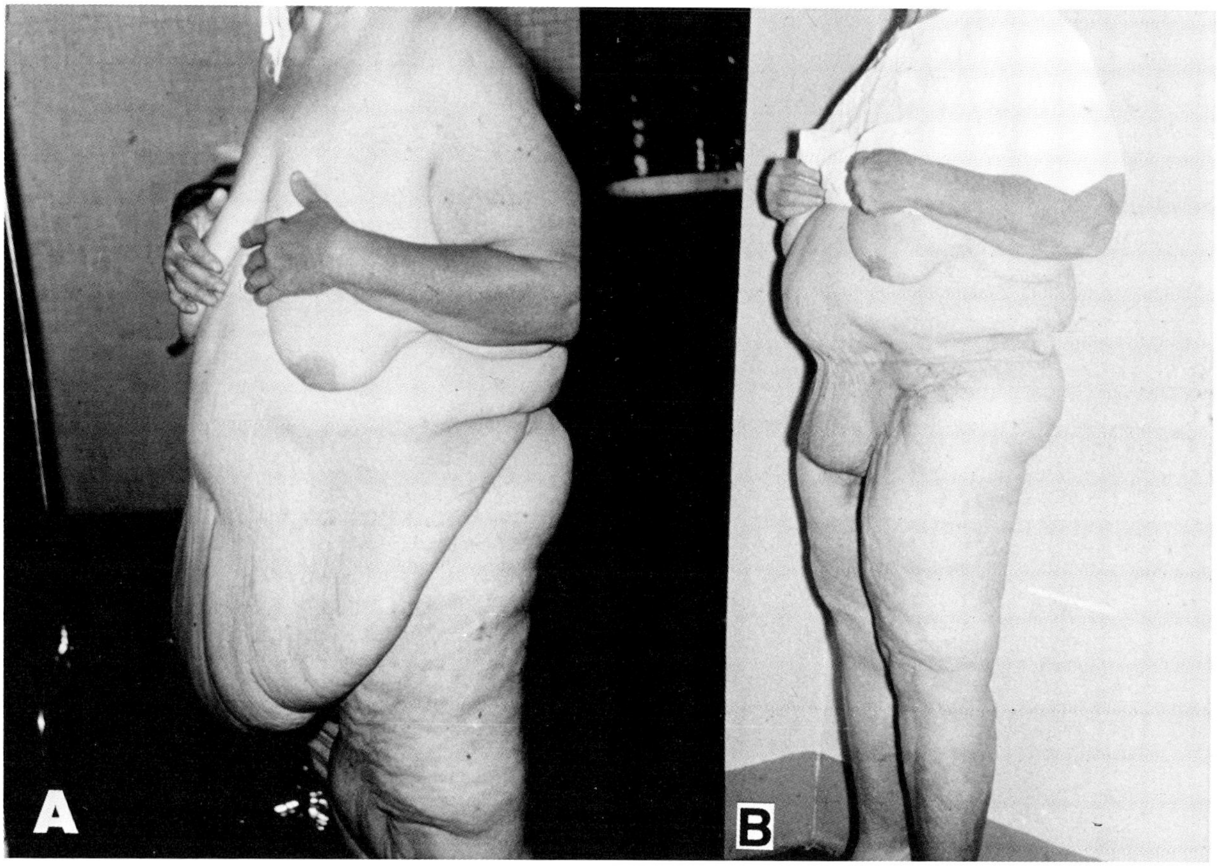

Figure 9 *A*, Patient had large panniculus of fat and skin with marked ptosis of the abdomen and flanks. This is a disabling condition. *B*, She is shown following wide resection of the large panniculus of the abdomen and flanks, which went well around to the back and excised approximately 40 pounds of tissue. Though the esthetic result leaves much to be desired, the patient can now wear normal clothing and can also get about much more easily.

AVOIDANCE OF COMPLICATIONS

The avoidance of complications in abdominoplasty is aided by proper patient selection, just as for other surgical procedures. The patient should be in reasonable health, of good general nutrition, should be in the general range of normal weight, and should be motivated to help him- or herself by trimming excess weight if indicated. The technique of the procedure should be appropriate for the particular case, and the surgical technique should be adapted to the patient rather than the patient to the technique.

The support of the tissues should be in layers for the wound repair, with a final intracuticular skin closure. The diastasis recti or hernias should be repaired by nonabsorbable sutures in an appropriate fashion to approximate the separated muscles and sheaths.

Hemostasis is just as important in abdominoplasty as in other areas of surgery. The wound is irrigated with an antibiotic solution to help avoid infection, and the patient is kept on antibiotics by mouth as an additional precaution for a few days following surgery.

The postoperative support of the wounds and of the abdominal wall is indicated. Snug dressings and an elastic support give more insurance against dehiscence of the abdominal wound and, in addition, aid in flattening the tissues of the abdomen, which have been reduced of fat by either surgical resection or suction lipectomy. A snug pressure support minimizes swelling and ecchymosis and speeds healing of the tissues, while at the same time a flattened contour is maintained.

The patient should be graduated as to activities and should avoid early vigorous active exercises and sports. There should be a gradual increase of activities to avoid undue pulling on an incompletely-healed skin incision line or deeper muscle and fascial repair. This does not mean that early ambulation is contraindicated, for it is not. The patient should be up and about early with proper support of the abdomen. The possibilities of hematoma and seroma are reduced by the use of pressure dressings and snug support, as well as by good surgical technique and careful hemostasis. The possibilities of thromboses and emboli are reduced also by good surgical technique, by early ambulation, by deep-breathing exercises, and by avoiding stasis in the extremities.

Although abdominoplasties have been blamed for a high incidence of vascular and pulmonary complications, I have not seen these problems. The general care of the patient is very important and attention to details helps avoid problems and ensure prompt healing and a rapid return to usual activities and work.

SUGGESTED READING

Baroudi R. Umbilicalplasty. Clin Plast Surg 1975; 2:431–448.
Carvalho CG, Baroudi R, Keppke EM. Anatomical and technical refinements for abdominoplasty. Aesthetic Plast Surg 1977; 1:217.
Grazer FM, Klingbeil JR. Body image: a surgical perspective. St. Louis: CV Mosby, 1980.
Lewis JR. Atlas of aesthetic plastic surgery. Boston: Little, Brown, 1973.
Lewis JR. Midabdominoplasty. Aesthetic Plast Surg 1979; 3:195–199.
Lewis JR, ed. The art of aesthetic plastic surgery. Boston: Little, Brown, (in press).
Pitanguy I. Abdominal lipectomy. Clin Plast Surg 1975; 2:401–410.
Planas J. The "vest-over-pants abdominoplasty." Plast Reconstr Surg 1978; 61:694–700.
Psillakis JM. Abdominoplasty: some ideas to improve results. Aesthetic Plast Surg 1978; 2:205.
Regnault P, Daniel RK, eds. Aesthetic plastic surgery. Boston: Little, Brown, 1984:617.

SUCTION LIPECTOMY: BODY CONTOURING—SUCTION VERSUS SCALPEL

BAHMAN TEIMOURIAN, M.D.

The emergence of suction lipectomy in the last 10 years as the most useful new technique to be developed for body contouring has consequences yet to be appreciated. Not only has it become well-known among plastic surgeons and physicians in many different disciplines, but the technique has also received considerable attention in the press. Healthy men and women now seek this surgery as a means to improve their self-image, thereby creating a demand that may be filled too rapidly. Suction lipectomy appears to be so simple to perform that physicians who would never have attempted body contouring with the scalpel are now agreeing to do the more complicated sculpturing by suction.

Perhaps we should reflect briefly on the surgical techniques that were still used up to the early 1980s for removing unsightly fat deposits. The scalpel, with the help of scissors, was the instrument of choice, and its action was observed under direct vision. Long incisions were made, the skin overlying the area to be treated was drawn back, and surplus fat was removed by gross dissection. Many areas of the body were not accessible to this treatment, and large areas of skin detached from the underlying fascia frequently led to necrosis and indentations. Because of this severing of blood vessels and consequent loss of blood, volumes of tissue that could be removed were very limited.

In retrospect, the achievements were remarkable. Contours were indeed improved, and since the body was usually clothed, at least in public, only the patient knew the real cost of the improvement in terms of the unsightly scars with dogears and the unwanted depressions that developed with the healing of necrotic areas. Because of these problems, body contouring did not gain wide popularity. In fact few patients were aware of the possibility that contouring might be for them. Facelifting and nose restructuring were well-known, but it was usually surgeons who suggested to patients that shape improvements could be brought about by surgery.

Now the scalpel has become secondary to the suction cannula in body contouring. Even in surgery where suction lipectomy is used as an adjunct to other techniques, as in dermatolipectomy of the thigh or upper arm, the fine contouring of the dermal flap is achieved by "open" suction rather than with the scalpel. Although routine "closed" suction lipectomy is performed "blind" in the sense that the tissue is hidden by the overlying skin while it is being treated, we nevertheless know the effect of the technique on the tissues and understand why it is so successful. During my early work with the suction cannula, I wanted to determine exactly what physical effect the suctioning had on the fat cells removed and on the tissue that remained. In studies with cadavers, I showed that, in contrast to the slicing effect of the scalpel, the suction pressure loosens the fat cells and detaches them from the connective tissues in which they lie. With careful handling, the cannula leaves undamaged a honeycomb of veins, arteries, and nerves connecting the fascia to the overlying skin, thus minimizing the possibility of necrosis. Careful handling must be emphasized, however, because without adequate training and skill the surgeon can easily remove too much tissue too quickly and cause unsightly depressions that in some instances can never be corrected.

In this chapter, the focus is on treatment of the thigh, which, prior to the development of suction lipectomy, was a common area for reduction by scalpel (Figs. 1, 2, and 3). My studies with cadavers led me to develop, for teaching and investigative purposes, an instrument that allows direct vision of the area being suctioned. This cannula (usual length of 25 cm) has three lumens, one for extracting tissue, one for introducing a medium such as saline or carbon dioxide, and a third that holds a telescope with a light at its tip. The telescope also permits display of the operative field on a television monitor.

While I was using this instrument to study the effects of suction lipectomy on thigh tissue, I was able to show that the shape of the tip of the cannula, provided that it is not sharp, is less important than cannula diameter. Much less damage can be done with a small diameter. I have since shown that a plastic cannula of 4.5 mm inner diameter, or a metal one of 1.5 to 4 mm, is sufficient for

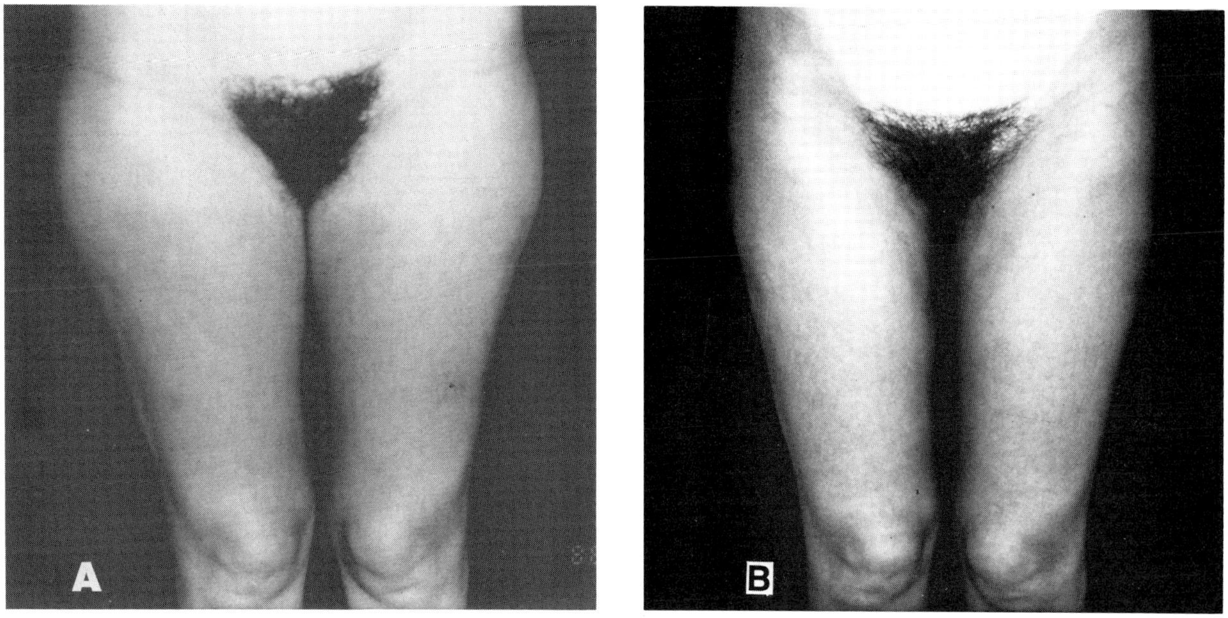

Figure 1 Frontal *A*, preoperative and *B*, postoperative view of a 33-year-old patient who underwent suction lipectomy of the medial and lateral thigh bilaterally. A total of 800 cc of fat was aspirated.

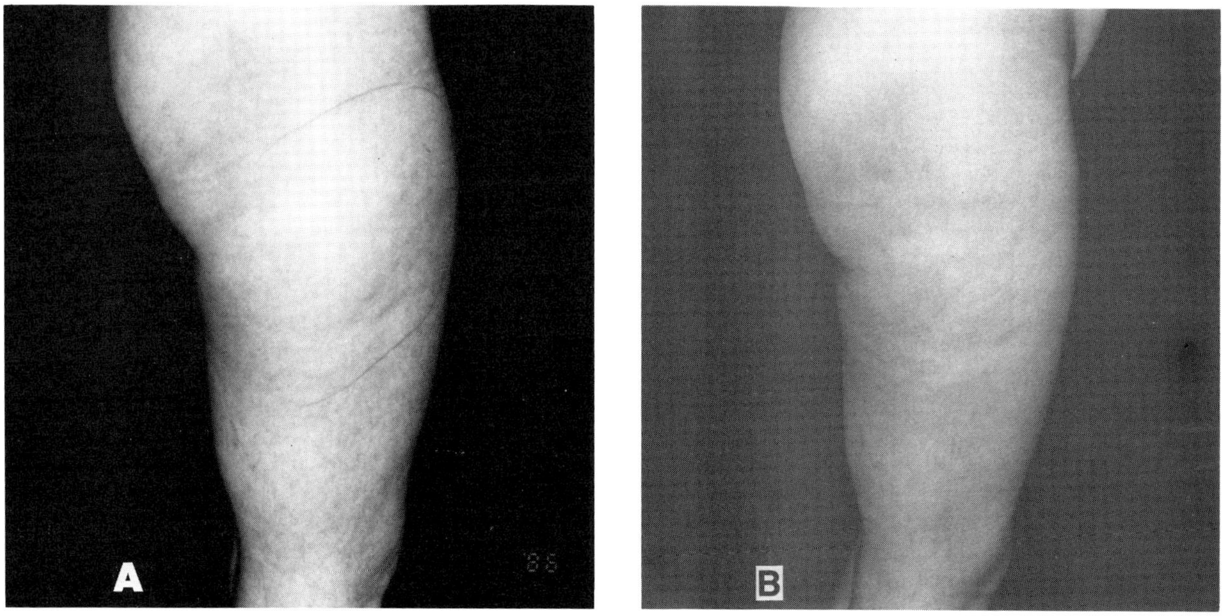

Figure 2 Lateral *A*, preoperative and *B*, postoperative view of same patient as in Figure 1.

most purposes. The cannula opening can be 2 cm or more from the tip or closer to it. Depressions in the skin can be avoided by not having the suction pressure turned on when the cannula is first inserted. Some cannulae have multiple openings, including openings on opposite sides (top and bottom), and these are also effective and now very popular.

Suction lipectomy of the thigh, as of any area of the body, requires great care in patient selection. In fact, with the rapid increase in the number of patients seeking suction lipectomy it is clear that more emphasis has to be placed on screening out those patients who will clearly not benefit from the operation. I have found that some patients with a poor self-image need psychological help as much as surgery, and these patients need to be guided toward qualified psychologists before plans are made for body contouring. All patients being considered for suction lipectomy need a thorough medical examination. Like

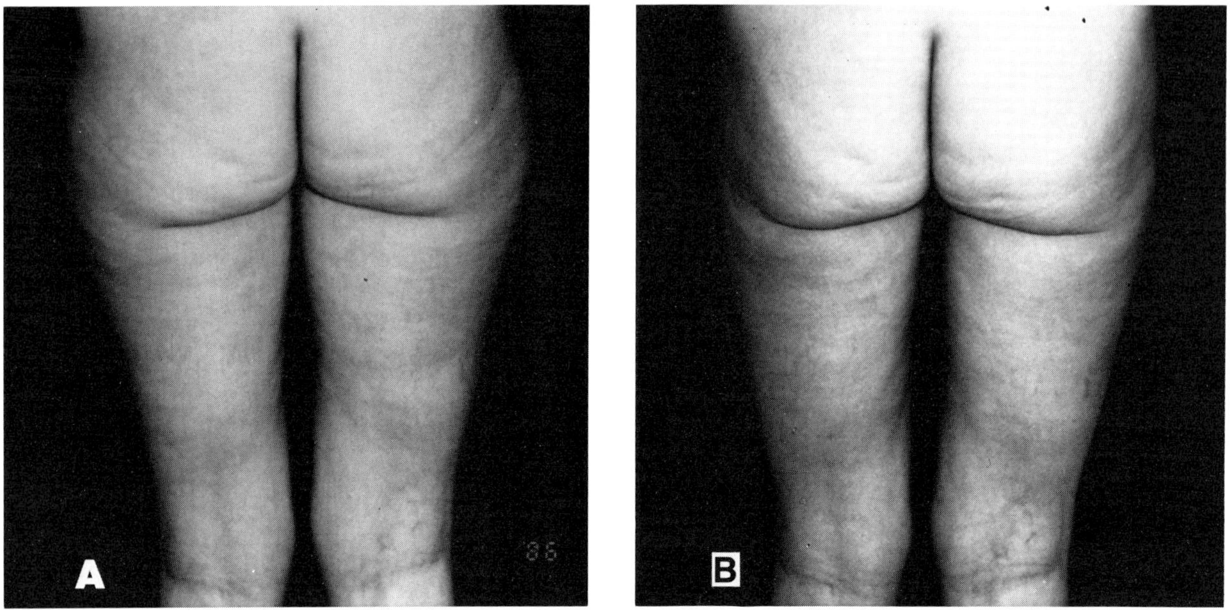

Figure 3 Dorsal *A*, preoperative and *B*, postoperative view of same patient as in Figure 1.

any other elective surgery, the operation may not be appropriate for patients with certain pre-existing medical conditions, such as heart disease, hypertension, diabetes, or allergies to anesthetics.

In evaluating a patient seeking thigh contouring, it is important to view the areas of concern from the patient's perspective. By standing close to the patient and looking down the surgeon may see a bulging area that is not obvious when viewed sideways from a few feet away. It is also helpful to ask the patient to stand in front of the mirror and point to those areas that worry her most. Some patients may have exaggerated ideas about the way they look. The surgeon should advise them honestly and sympathetically before agreeing to operate on them.

Next in importance, after patient evaluation, is patient preparation. I try to estimate, as closely as possible, how much tissue must be removed over what surface area to achieve the desired results, and how much blood will be lost. The volume of fat removed is not a true indication of the total amount of fluid lost. In addition to the fat and blood collected in the measured container, blood and fluid is lost during surgery from the whole area being treated, and all of these fluids need to be replaced. The average amount of blood lost during the removal of 1,500 cc of fat from the lateral thigh should be no more than 500 cc, but the removal of similar quantities of fat from the abdomen would result in far greater blood loss. Thus arrangements must be made for the patient to supply, several weeks preoperatively, the appropriate quantities of blood for autologous transfusion. A balanced electrolyte solution must also be infused during and after surgery.

With suction lipectomy of the thigh, the best results are obtained in young patients whose skin will readily contract over the newly contoured frame. In older patients, suction lipectomy may be used together with skin resection to achieve a pleasing result. Excessive thigh fat in some patients may be quite localized, for example, in the upper lateral area, and can be treated through a subgluteal or pubic incision. In many patients, however, circumferential reduction of the thighs gives the best results.

My approach to circumferential thigh reduction is to use a subgluteal incision for the upper lateral and posterior regions, and a pubic incision for the medial and anterior regions. Incisions in the upper and lateral aspects of the popliteal area are used for the lower and lateral regions of the thigh, respectively. Sites for incisions and contours to indicate the extent of treatment areas are all marked with the patient in a standing position. The patient then lies down on the operating table and is kept warm by means of a heating blanket placed under the sterile sheets and by keeping covered those areas not being treated. In addition to the general anesthesia, which I always use for extensive thigh surgery, I administer a local anesthetic, infiltrating the whole operative site with 0.125 percent bupivacaine (Marcaine) containing epinephrine (Adrenalin 1:400,000) to help reduce bleeding.

With the patient brought into a lateral position and the knee and hip brought forward, I make a subgluteal stab incision and, by means of angled scissors, make a short tunnel into which I insert the suction cannula. I then turn on the suction pressure and create multiple tunnels that radiate out from the site of insertion. I keep strictly within the areas that I have outlined, remembering to extract less fat as I progress toward the outer boundary so as to make a smooth transition between the treated and untreated areas. I use a metal cannula (2.4 to 4 mm) initially for preliminary probing and suctioning, and then a plastic one (4.5 mm inner diameter). The two can be used interchangeably in a cross-probing manner to get a more even surface. I use the pinch test to estimate the amount of fat remaining and make repeated comparisons with the opposite side to achieve the desired contours. In difficult cases I find that infiltrating the area with saline to expand it and then extracting the saline along with any loose tissue remaining can help in contour assessment. I then repeat these procedures on each area to be treated, keeping careful records of the volume of tissue collected from every area on each side of the body.

When using suction lipectomy on the thigh as an adjunct to dermatolipectomy, I do not always resect the skin during the same operation. In older patients it is not always easy to determine the degree of skin elasticity or the extent to which the skin will contract, without undue rippling, over the treated area. Suction lipectomy always precedes skin resection, thus resection can be delayed for several weeks if there is any doubt about its being needed. Incisions for dermatolipectomy should be marked, as usual, with the patient in a standing position, and they should be as high as possible without distorting the genitals because the scars may descend over time as a result of gravity.

Assuming that closed suction lipectomy has already been done, the next step in dermatolipectomy of the thigh is to develop a dermal suspension flap that extends as needed from the groin crease to the superior iliac spine. The incision is made and the flap is raised and contoured as necessary with the suction curette by the open method. The appropriate amount of skin to be resected is then determined by drawing the flap up and over the superior edge of the incision. At this point the entire leg should be raised with the knee so that it forms a 90-degree angle with the table. This gives an exaggerated view of the amount of surplus skin; the exact amount removed should be less than that indicated when the leg is raised, both because of possible scar descent after surgery and because of the possibility of necrosis occurring in tissue that is subjected to too much tension. The skin is resected and a section of the remaining skin along the lower edge of the incision, about 2 to 3 cm wide, is de-epithelialized. This flap is then suspended from the iliac crest, periosteum, and inguinal ligament by means of permanent sutures. The superior edge of the incision is then drawn down and sutured to the lower edge in the usual manner.

With careful planning and execution of the operation, the results should be satisfactory to patient and surgeon. A certain amount of skin rippling to the thighs is normal during aging, and is likely to increase after suction lipectomy of the thighs, but this should be pointed out to the patient before surgery. Accidents can happen, however, and unsightly depressions can remain if too much fat is removed with the suction cannula.

Some of these depressions can now be corrected. Studies of the effect of suction on the tissues have led to the development of a technique known as semiliquid fat grafting. The fat is extracted by suction from an appropriate area of the body, such as the iliac crest, and is collected in a container. Since fat obtained by suction is already in semiliquid form, it can be injected into the area that requires correction by means of a syringe with a 14- to 22-gauge needle. A slight excess of semiliquid fat is introduced into the depressed area to compensate for some reabsorption that will take place post surgery. The results to date have been encouraging. This grafting technique can also be used to correct post-traumatic deformities and to improve aging lines of the face.

Suction lipectomy at present is not used as a general remedy for obesity. In my office, an obese patient requesting suction lipectomy of the thighs, or of any part of the body, is asked to try dieting and exercising for several weeks before further consultation for surgery. In several hospitals investigations are now being directed toward the possibility of using suction lipectomy as part of the treatment for patients with diabetes and moderate obesity. Although it is too early to draw conclusions from the results, it does appear that fat removal from certain areas may be beneficial in reducing insulin dependency. Patients with morbid obesity can sometimes be helped by suction, but the cause of their condition must be established and dealt with appropriately before patients are subjected to surgical contouring. Great care is needed in planning surgery with these patients because the amount of tissue, including skin, that has to be removed generally necessitates several operations.

It seems clear that many more applications will be found for suction lipectomy in the future. Its utility, compared with fat removal by the scalpel, has been proved, but its safety depends entirely on the training and experience of the surgeon. Much damage can be done by the unskilled, and severe complications, in some instances leading to death, have already been reported in Europe as well as in the United States. If studies now in progress around the country show that this technique can be used in the treatment of moderate obesity in otherwise normal as well as diabetic patients, a great many more trained surgeons will be required than are now available. Perhaps it is time to start planning for this increase in the use of suction lipectomy so that patients are not tempted to seek the treatment from unqualified practitioners.

SUGGESTED READING

Hetter GP, ed. Lipoplasty. Boston: Little, Brown, 1984.

Illouz YG. Body contouring by lipolysis: a 5-year experience with over 3000 cases. Plast Reconstr Surg 1983; 72(5):591–597.

Shirakabe T. Japanese suction-assisted lipectomy. Clin Plast Surg 1984; II(3):549–565.

Teimourian B. Suction lipectomy and body sculpturing. St. Louis: CV Mosby, 1987.

Teimourian B, Fisher JB. Suction curettage to remove excess fat for body contouring. Plast Reconstr Surg 1981; 68(1):50–58.

RECONSTRUCTION OF BURNS OF THE TRUNK AND BREAST

HENRY W. NEALE, M.D., F.A.C.S.

Within the last 15 years, burn reconstruction of the trunk and chest has been a major challenge for the reconstructive plastic surgeon, due to much greater survival of acute burn patients. Sometimes, numerous reconstructive procedures, over literally generations of plastic surgeons, are required to restore the disfigured burn victim and enable the patient to accept his or her identity and be productive in society. Burns of the trunk and chest are particularly challenging, and the principles of the approach to their surgical restoration will be addressed in this chapter.

BURNS OF THE ABDOMEN

As a general rule, in third degree burns of the abdomen where the abdominal wall musculature and fascia are covered with split-thickness skin grafts (STSG), there is no interference with the expansion of this area of the body in the growing patient. In the past, questions have been raised about the possible interference with subsequent pregnancy from abdominal burns in nulliparous females. This has not proved to be a problem. Unburned areas of the abdomen, the general distention of the abdominal wall musculature, and perhaps elevation of the diaphragm accommodate the growing uterus during pregnancy. The unburned skin of the abdominal wall seems to distend more during pregnancy than the unyielding STSG, which lacks dermal elastic fibers, due to the path of least resistance in the distention phase of the abdomen (Fig. 1). If there are isolated areas of the abdominal soft tissue coverage with severe constriction, these can either be excised and replaced with full-thickness or very thick split-thickness skin grafts. If there is normal adjacent unburned skin, expanders can be placed at a young age beneath this normal skin. These areas can be stretched, and the adjacent restricted scarred areas can be excised with advancement of the normal skin envelope. It is usually preferable to place these tissue expanders over rigid structures such as ribs so that the resultant pressure is not downward toward the abdominal contents but rather distends the unburned skin. Unburned skin of infants and children seems to be more easily and quickly expanded than that of adults. In a review of some 30 pregnant females at our institution, with complete or almost complete full-thickness burns of the abdomen, there was no incidence of difficulty encountered in carrying a full-term pregnancy because of constrictive burn scar of the abdomen. No emergency surgical release of the burn scar abdominal contracture was required.

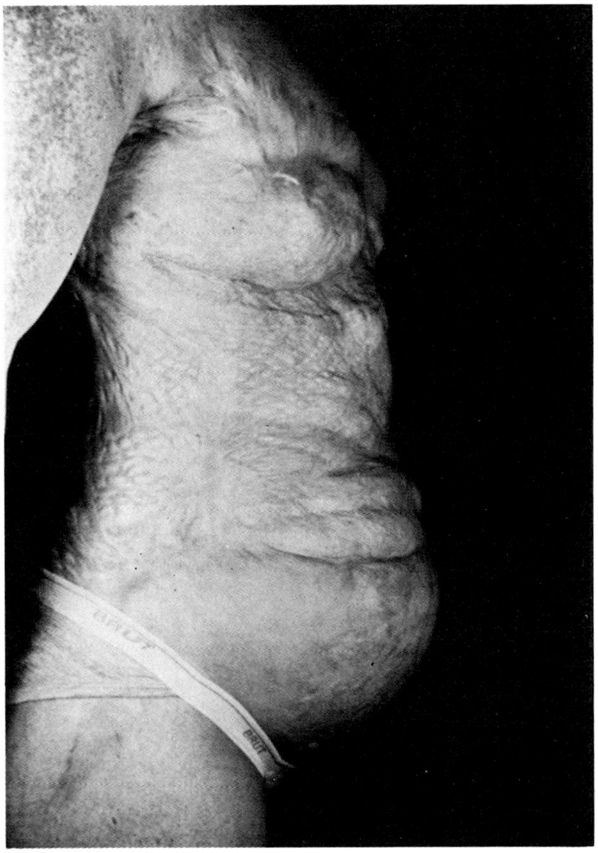

Figure 1 Appearance of an 18-year-old female whose upper two-thirds of the abdomen sustained third degree thermal burns 6 years previously and which were covered with meshed split-thickness skin graft. The patient is here 8 months pregnant and one can easily visualize the protruberance of the lower one-third of the abdomen with normal unburned skin and the relative constrictive split-thickness skin graft of the upper two-thirds of the abdomen with less expansion. Later, this patient delivered a normal full-term 7-1/2-pound healthy baby. The unburned skin of the pregnant female stretches and protrudes more with the enlarging uterus than the split-thickness skin graft over the abdominal fascia.

RECONSTRUCTION OF THE BURNED CHEST AND BREAST

Acute Burn

The management of the acute burn of the anterior chest can play a major role in future breast development of the female burn patient as she enters puberty. The initial burn surgeon must take great care to avoid early aggressive debridement of full-thickness injuries over the anticipated breast development area. Tangential excision of breast bud areas should be conservative and should not extend past nonviable tissue. The burn skin eschar should be allowed to demarcate over the breast buds in young females, and conservative debridement is the rule in these areas (Fig. 2). The acute burn defect, after tangential excision down to a viable bed, can be covered with a STSG. This principle of conservation of breast bud tissue will markedly facilitate future reconstruction of the breast and nipple areolar complex.

Preoperative Assessment and Timing of Surgical Reconstruction

Secondary reconstruction of the burned adolescent female chest is indicated when the burned skin envelope is insufficient and restricts the normal growth and development of the pubescent breast. Reconstruction should not begin until the burns are healed with autogenous skin and the scars are mature (Figs. 3 and 4). Instead of an exact age when reconstructive surgery of the breast is indicated, patient selection should be geared to release of the breast mound when bulging of the breast tissue and nonscarred areas is apparent, or when there is a definite impression of restriction of breast development because of burn scar envelope contracture that entraps the developing breast. When a normal unburned breast on the opposite side is present, comparison reveals when surgical release of the opposite burned breast is indicated. Examination of the burned breast should be performed preoperatively, with the patient standing, to reveal potentially palpable mammary structures that often serve as valuable landmarks for contracture release. The nipple areolar complex with the breast bud tissue crowded beneath it may be palpable but not visually noticeable. The anatomic configuration of the breast fat may be better realized by palpation than by sight. These palpable structures help the surgeon to set the breast within the anatomic configuration of the individual whose breast is being reconstructed. It may also help to ask the patient to identify the structure one is seeking, for she may be more facile than the surgeon in this respect, although in my experience, this has been of minimal help.

Breast Mound

The surgeon should strive for a single breast mound reconstructive operation if at all possible, but, in certain patients, a secondary release procedure may be indicated. In all cases, the mound should be reconstructed prior to nipple and areolar reconstruction, especially if the nipple remnant is not present on the burned breast. With the patient standing, the surgeon should determine the desired anatomic location for the incision for the contracture release and a mental attempt should be made to sculpt the breast in its proposed correct location so that it will look normal on the chest wall after an adequate release.

Operative Technique

The inframammary surgical release should be carried down to the deep fascia overlying the chest muscle. The depth on the incision of the inframammary release should

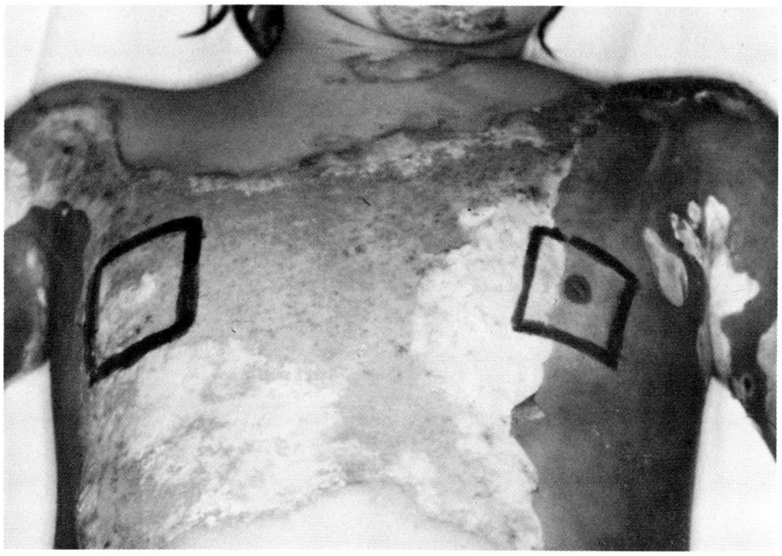

Figure 2 Appearance of an 11-year-old female 1 week after sustaining partial and full-thickness thermal burns to the anterior chest. The marked square boxes around her nipple and areolar complex depict areas of breast bud to be spared from primary burn eschar debridement.

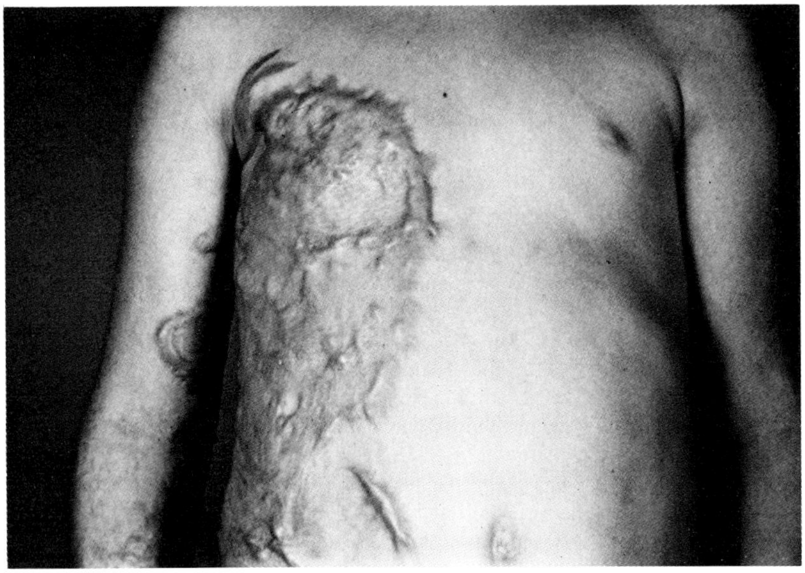

Figure 3 Appearance of the right chest and upper abdomen of a 4-year-old after sustaining a full-thickness thermal injury and 6 months after split-thickness nonexpanded mesh graft. The nipple has not been destroyed; however, this skin graft will inhibit adequate future development of the breast.

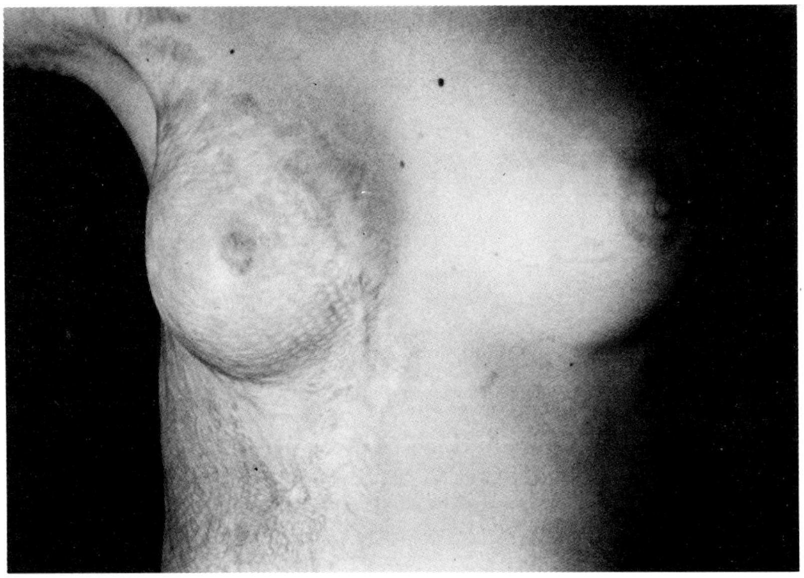

Figure 4 Shows loss of areola but presence of nipple and some inframammary constriction of the breast skin envelope of the burned right side of the teen-aged female shown in Figure 1.

be such that it lies at the correct anatomic level of the inframammary fold, thus necessitating skin graft on both the superior and inferior borders (Fig. 5). As the incision is made, fat intrinsic to the breast guides the incision by separating from adipose tissue *not* intrinsic to the breast, and this permits the surgeon to use this natural tendency to help sculpt the breast during the contracture release. Tacking sutures should be used to attach the STSG carefully to the newly-reconstructed inframammary crease. If the opposite breast is unburned, its inframammary crease level can be used as a comparison landmark. It is imperative that, even if a single burned breast is to be released, the patient's whole chest wall be prepped and draped into the surgical field.

Generally, breast mound release requires an inframammary incision approximately five-eighths of the palpable circumference of the breast, but this depends more on the individual depth and extent of the burn than on absolute measurement. This incision is often U-shaped and should be carried down into the normal unburned skin of the chest. Thick STSG should be applied superiorly and inferiorly to the inframammary crease release incision. No undermining and suturing of the breast envelope to the inframammary crease is indicated, as this often results in necrosis because of previously burned tissue and STSG being applied to this area. In addition to the inframammary incision, supermammary, intramammary, or intermammary incisions for contracture release may occasionally be necessary, especially when the extent of the burn involves the superior chest and the axilla. When both breast mounds are released, and there is considerable burn scar between the breasts, an extended intermammary release is often necessary. Overcorrection should be carried out in this area.

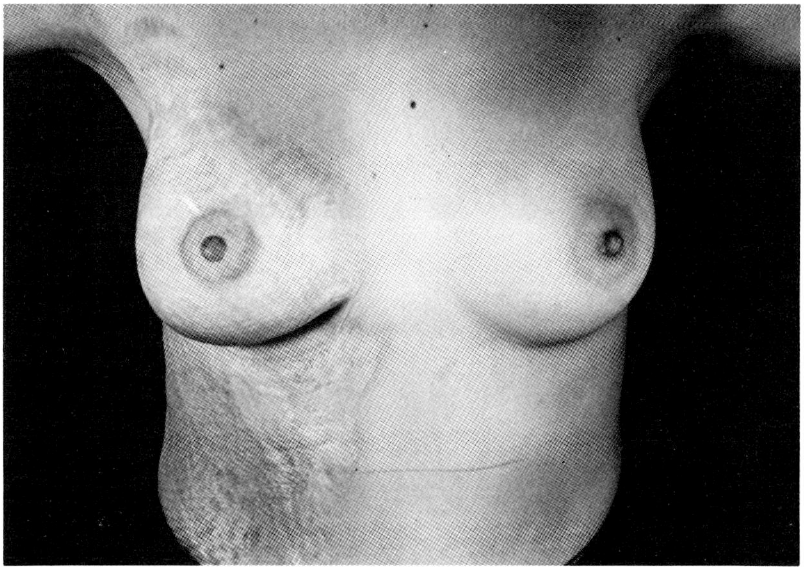

Figure 5 Appearance of the same girl 1 year after inframammary release with a thick split-thickness sheet graft applied to reconstruct the inframammary fold. The nipple has been released and the areola has been reconstructed with a full-thickness proximal inner thigh skin graft. Note symmetry of both breasts.

Complete contracture release is sought during a single operation to avoid the problems, expense, and inherent dangers of multiple surgical procedures. Occasionally, despite well-intentioned efforts, the tissue heals in a contracted state and requires a second operative release before further efforts at reconstruction are initiated.

In selected patients, the burn may be so extensive and the contraction and distortion so severe, that simple release is not adequate and a better esthetic result can be achieved if the entire scar tissue is excised en bloc and replaced with a thick split-thickness sheet graft. This occurrence is usually found in a burned chest where there is an isolated area with very thick scar, and adjacent normal unburned skin of the breast with severe distortion present.

A split-thickness sheet graft, at least .016 inch or greater, should be used to obtain a skin envelope with characteristics suitable for supporting the breast tissue. The donor site generally chosen for its thickness and cosmetic location is the buttock. Ultimately, the choice of donor site depends on available nonburned donor areas.

Additional Procedures

When severe burns produce a deficient, hypoplastic breast in addition to destruction of the skin envelope, augmentation can be achieved in carefully selected cases, either by inserting a mammary prosthesis subpectorally, or by transferring and inserting a latissimus dorsi musculocutaneous flap, with or without a prosthesis. Local chest wall skin flaps can also be used, and, in selected cases, the transverse rectus abdominis musculocutaneous flap may serve as an alternative if there is ablation of the breast tissue. This flap, although frequently chosen as a primary alternative in adult mastectomy reconstruction, has a limited role in the young nulliparous female because of insufficient laxity of abdominal skin. Infrequently, the free microvascular gluteal musculocutaneous flap may be utilized. If the opposite breast is unburned and has a significant degree of ptosis, or is exceedingly large, a mastopexy reduction of the normal breast may be indicated for purposes of symmetry.

Nipple and Areolar Complex

Surgical release of the scar contracture of the nipple and areolar complex should be complete and sufficiently deep to incise all burn scar tissue. The surgeon should proceed cautiously while he releases these delicate structures, for it is easy inadvertently to sever the blood supply that lies directly beneath their surface. There should be an examination for a preexisting nipple, and all reconstructive surgery should be centered upon a nipple if its existence is present. I have found preoperative mammograms generally do not help to determine the location of this structure. Also, there is the unnecessary danger of radiation exposure for this diagnostic purpose.

The reconstruction of the nipple areolar complex should be delayed until the breast mound has been reconstructed and fully settled from a previous release (6 to 12 months). If the nipple is present, but has surrounding burn scar, a circumvential release of the nipple itself can be carried out, thereby allowing for full protrusion and subsequent reconstruction of the areola. Dermal flaps may be used around the central core nipple, with its abundant vascular supply, if a preexisting nipple is present. In general, I have avoided local dermal flaps if no nipple exists, or if split-thickness burn scar is present in the nipple area, because of its inherent poor blood supply and risk of necrosis of the dermal flaps. If no nipple on the reconstructed burned breast is present, but there is adequate and protruding opposite normal nipple, my best results have been with composite tissue-sharing from the normal side.

Nipple reconstruction without an existing nipple has been carried out with numerous techniques. These include local dermal flaps, toe pulp, earlobe, postauricular cartilage and skin graft, rib cartilage, composite tongue tissue, and oral and vaginal mucosa full-thickness skin grafts. In general, long-term settling of the nipple height and its flattening effect have been observed; with a need for more than 1 year follow-up for permanent evaluation. It is important to overestimate the height of the nipple reconstruction if the procedure is performed with local dermal flaps.

Areolar reconstruction should be carried out at or after the time of nipple reconstruction, and my best results have been obtained with full-thickness areolar sharing procedures from the opposite normal areola, if present, through the outer donut sharing technique. Other procedures utilized have been full-thickness skin grafts (FTSG) from the proximal inner thigh with primary closure where the skin tends to be darker and thinner (see Fig. 5). In general, there have been poorer results from STSG, with resultant hypopigmentation on long-term follow-up. The use of labia minora has now been discontinued because of the resultant hyperpigmentation. Although I have had minimal experience to date, the alternative of tattooing is very promising if sufficient dermis is present to hold the pigment permanently in place. If there has been hypopigmentation in FTSG from the inner thigh for areolar reconstruction, secondary tattooing of this FTSG to match the opposite normal areola may give more satisfying color-matching results. In the male, reconstruction of the burned areola has been routinely and satisfactorily done with FTSG from the scrotum.

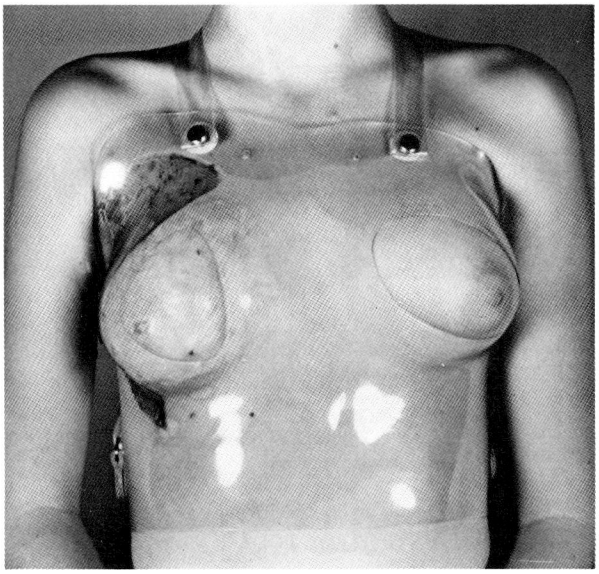

Figure 6 A different patient is wearing a Uvex chest shield to deliver pressure on a recent split-thickness skin graft that was applied to the superior and lateral aspect of the right breast. This transparent Uvex breastplate allows for appropriate pressure after skin grafting, as well as support of the breast, and permits observation through the clear plastic-type material to ensure that pressure is being applied to the appropriate area.

Postoperative Management

After breast contracture release, the skin grafts are stented for 7 to 10 days and protected by circumferential chest dressing. After complete epithelialization of the grafts (approximately 10 to 12 days), silicone molds that conform to the new breast contours are made to reduce graft contracture scar hypertrophy. If silicone molds are used, they are held in place by well-fitting brassières, which are worn continuously for approximately 6 to 12 months until the grafts have matured. Recently, the use of Uvex splints for pressure on the grafts has been increasingly successful in the control of the hypotrophic scar (Fig. 6). It is important to leave a central circular defect in the nipple-areolar area of the mold to permit protrusion of the nipple and decrease the effect pressure might have on lessening the final projection of this structure. If only nipple and areolar construction has been performed, foam rubber stents are sutured in place to immobilize the areolar and nipple graft. These are left in place for 1 week and no brassière for pressure is worn. Once the breast reconstruction molds have been removed and the patient resumes wearing a normal brassière, follow-up should continue for a minimum of 1 year to ensure that a relapse or a recurrence of skin graft contracture does not occur.

SUGGESTED READING

Broadbent TR, Woolf RM, Metz PS. Restoring the mammary areola by a skin graft from the upper inner thigh. Br J Plast Surg 1977; 30:220–222.

Dipirro E. Reconstruction of the nipple and areola after a burn. Plast Reconstr Surg 1970; 46:299–300.

Neale HW, Smith GL, Gregory, RO, MacMillan BG. Breast reconstruction in the burned adolescent female. Plast Reconst Surg 1982; 70:718–724.

Pensler JM, Haab RL, Parry SW. Reconstruction of the burned nipple-areola complex. Plast Reconstr Surg 1986; 78:480–484. Discussion: Chang WHJ. Plast Reconstr Surg 1986; 78:485.

Silversmith PE. Nipple reconstruction by quadropod flaps. Plast Reconstr Surg 1983; 72:422.

Wexler MR, Oneal RM. Areolar sharing to reconstruct the absent nipple. Plast Reconstr Surg 1973; 51:176–178.

CHEST RECONSTRUCTION

VERNON L. YOUNG, M.D.
BARRY FERNANDO, M.D.

Chest reconstruction requires a multidisciplinary team approach. To achieve a satisfactory end point, the plastic surgeon must be willing to work closely with his cardiothoracic colleagues. This chapter outlines the principles of chest reconstruction as they pertain to two of the most common problems encountered by the plastic surgeon: closure of the infected sternal wound, and radiation ulcers of the chest wall. Though the pathogenesis and initial care of these problems vary, the goals of reconstruction are essentially the same: (1) development of a stable wound with adequate soft-tissue coverage, and (2) reconstruction of the bony thorax, if necessary, to achieve normal pulmonary dynamics.

Many of these patients are either critically ill or have multiple medical problems. For this reason, the appropriate and the most expeditious means of reconstruction must be chosen. An understanding of the pathophysiology of the disease process and the available reconstructive options is essential.

SURGICAL MANAGEMENT OF THE INFECTED STERNAL WOUND

The median sternotomy is the most commonly used incision in cardiac surgery. Its popularity is secondary to the excellent exposure it provides to the heart and great vessels. Infections of this incision are uncommon, with major centers reporting an incidence of 0.5 to 5.9 percent. Unfortunately, the sequelae of this complication can be devastating. Untreated infections can extend to cardiac and aortic suture lines and prosthetic grafts. In addition, septic thrombosis of aortocoronary grafts can occur. The infected median sternotomy wound can present in several different ways. Initial treatment will often vary, depending on its early presentation. Mediastinitis can be an acute, fulminant process or a chronic, indolent infection.

Episodes of sternal dehiscence without mediastinal suppuration are commonly managed by the operating cardiac surgeon. This situation does not involve sternal instability or necrosis and is treated with systemic antibiotics and reclosure of the sternum over mediastinal drains. This problem is usually not brought to the attention of the plastic surgeon.

On the other hand, the development of suppurative mediastinitis can be life-threatening. These patients present with a fulminant infection within the first 2 weeks postoperatively. In our institution, the initial surgical care of this complication is handled by the cardiothoracic surgery team. Adequate debridement of necrotic bone, soft tissue, and cartilage is essential. Antibiotics specific for the infective organism, though of questionable merit, are used. Meticulous postdebridement wound care is more important. Frequent removal of necrotic debris and pooled exudate is the mainstay of treatment. The timing for closure depends on the appearance of the wound. A clean, healthy, granulating surface, devoid of purulent drainage, provides the ideal circumstances for reconstruction. Closure of these wounds as early as possible is optimal. The next step in treatment of these patients is obliteration of mediastinal dead space with a vascularized muscle flap. This will be discussed later in this chapter.

The chronically-infected sternotomy is another presentation in the spectrum of postoperative mediastinitis. The presence of a persistent draining sinus tract heralds the presence of an underlying bone or cartilage infection (Fig. 1.) Diagnosis is aided by the use of computed tomography. Treatment is essentially the same as the management of the acutely infected wound. The key to success is identification of the nidus of infection and adequate debridement of the involved bone and cartilage.

USE OF VASCULARIZED MUSCLE FLAPS

The plastic surgeon is frequently consulted at a time far removed from the patient's initial operation. Usually the patient has failed other more conservative means of therapy, i.e., systemic antibiotics and reclosure with mediastinal drainage. The substernal space under these circumstances is often a rigid cavity with a thick fibrinous peel. The principles of aggressive debridement, and obliteration of this mediastinal dead space with a vascularized muscle flap, have been well-established since the initial description by Jurkiewicz in 1980. Chang demonstrated the bactericidal effects of vascularized muscle and its ability to promote wound healing. In addition, concerns regarding sternal instability and respiratory decompensation after sternectomy without sternal reconstruction have proved to be unfounded. Therefore, the use of transposed, vascularized muscle is the cornerstone of surgical therapy.

The importance of adequate debridement cannot be overemphasized. Any necrotic bone must be resected. In addition, exposed cartilage, even if it is viable, should be excised, as this may become the source of a subsequent infection. The entire granulating surface of skin and soft tissue should be excised. Significant blood loss is not uncommon during this portion of the procedure, and meticulous hemostasis is essential.

Obliteration of the mediastinal dead space can then be accomplished with several different muscle flaps, either alone or in combination: (1) the pectoralis major, (2) the rectus abdominis, and (3) the latissimus dorsi (see Fig. 1).

The pectoralis major is the most commonly used muscle flap for closure of defects that involve the upper two-thirds of the sternum. This muscle has a dual blood supply, with the dominant pedicle based on the pectoral branch of the thoracoacromial artery and the secondary

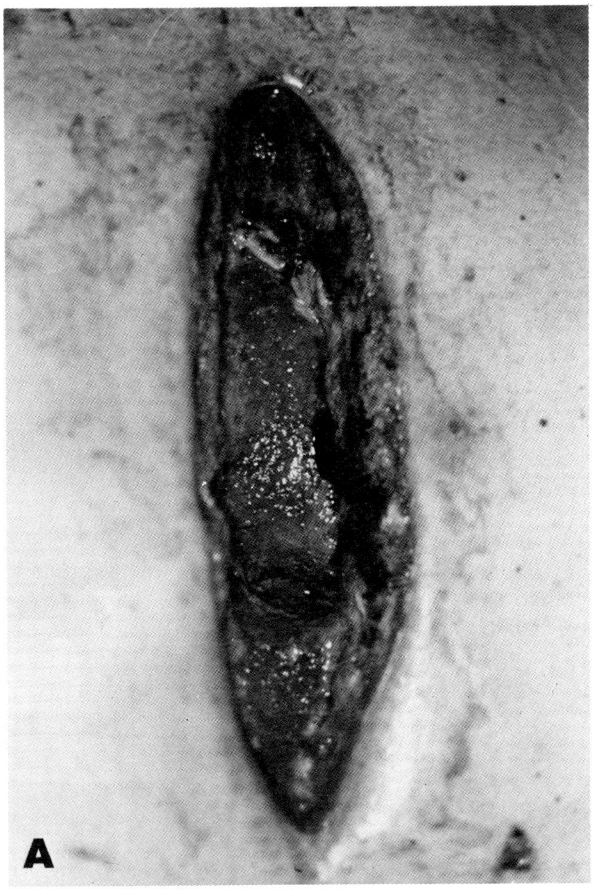

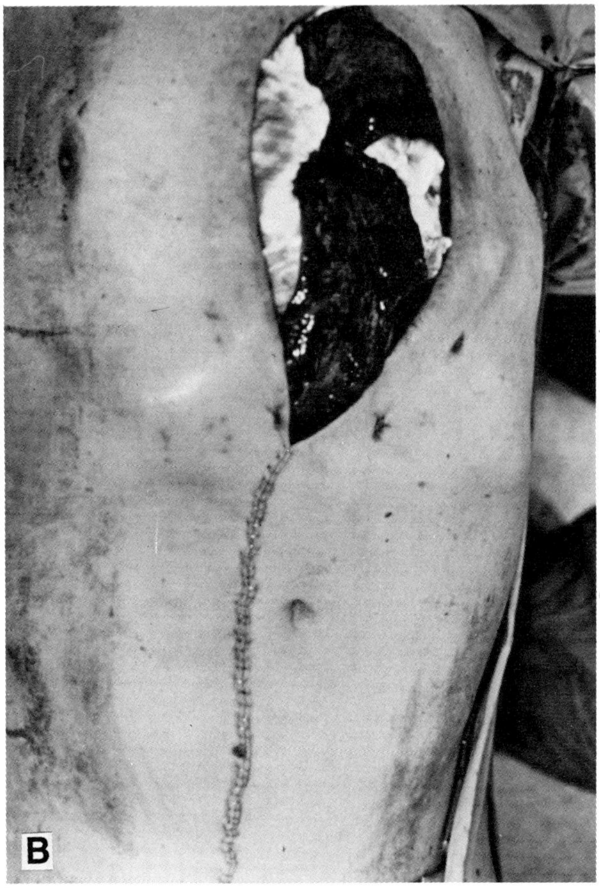

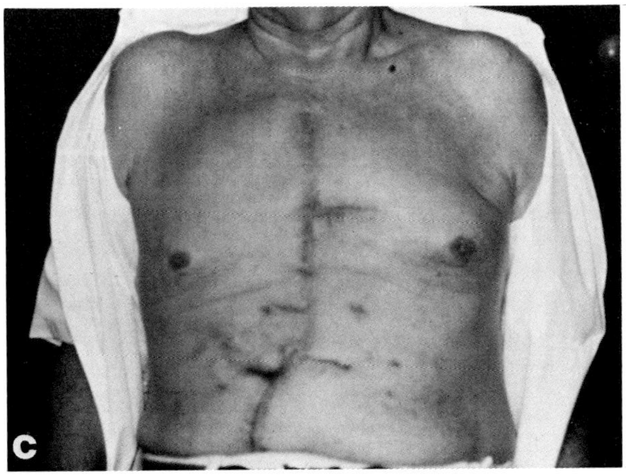

Figure 1 *A,* Open sternal wound with exposed mediastinum. *B,* Sternal wound after debridement of devitalized bone and cartilage and transposition of the pectoralis major and rectus abdominis muscle flaps. *C,* The healed sternal wound several months postoperatively.

pedicles arising from perforating branches of the internal mammary. The flap can be based on either pedicle. Our preference is to utilize the pectoralis major as a transposition rather than a turnover flap, as the patency of the internal mammary artery can be questionable in the presence of sternal infection, sternal debridement, or the prior use of internal mammary artery grafts. If the defect cannot be closed with the unilateral muscle, the contralateral pectoralis is also mobilized. Complete mobility of this muscle flap can be accomplished with detachment at its points of origin along the sternum, medial clavicle, and aponeurosis of the external oblique, and division of its tendinous insertion at the humerus. The use of the pectoralis in this fashion results in both the functional loss of the muscle and loss of the anterior axillary fold. Nahai has described a modification of the turnover flap that preserves the lateral one-third of the muscle and potentially circumvents these problems.

The rectus abdominis can be used alone, or in conjunction with the pectoralis. It is ideal for closure of defects that involve the lower one-third of the sternum. The viability of this flap is dependent on the patency of the internal mammary artery. Though the deep inferior epigastric artery is the dominant pedicle, the entire muscle can be transposed superiorly. After transposition of the pectoralis, if a large defect remains, the rectus is then mobilized.

The latissimus dorsi is not a primary choice for closure of sternal defects. When the pectoralis major muscle cannot be used, secondary to atrophy or fibrosis, or use of the rectus is contraindicated because of loss of both internal mammary arteries, the latissimus can be a viable option. Its significant muscle mass length and wide arc of rotation allow coverage of mediastinal organs. The muscle should be transposed beneath the pectoralis to achieve maximum length.

Another option under these circumstances is the use of free tissue transfer.

INTERNAL MAMMARY ARTERY GRAFTS

A Problem in Management

Over the last 10 years, the use of the internal mammary arteries as grafts for myocardial revascularization has increased. It has been demonstrated that these grafts enjoy an improved long-term patency rate as compared to their venous counterparts. Unfortunately, the use of bilateral internal mammary artery grafts is associated with an 8.5 percent increase in the incidence of postoperative sternal infection. The blood supply to the sternum is derived solely from segmental sternal branches of the internal mammary artery. No apparent intramedullary nutrient system is demonstrable. Development of postoperative sternal infection is probably caused by avascular necrosis of the sternum in combination with other risk factors. To date, this entity has been poorly studied. Loss of both internal mammary arteries severely limits the reconstructive options when dealing with lower sternal defects. The pectoralis major and the latissimus dorsi are unable to obliterate defects in this region adequately. Most authors feel that, under these circumstances, options are limited to the use of omental transposition flaps. Omental transposition is felt to be a relatively safe procedure. The omentum, with its rich blood supply and abundant lymphatic vessels, can promote healing in a manner similar to vascularized muscle. The problems with use of this flap lie in the contamination of the sterile visceral cavity, the risk of development of volvulus, and the necessary production of a ventral or diaphragmatic hernia for transposition. In critically ill patients, and those who have had a previous laparotomy, the use of an omental transposition flap is not ideal.

The use of the rectus under these circumstances is felt to be contraindicated. Fernando, however, described a case of successful transposition of the rectus based entirely on the intercostal perforators. He postulated that a long delay between the initial operation and sternal closure allowed these collateral vessels to play a more dominant role in the circulation to this muscle.

POTENTIAL POSTOPERATIVE PROBLEMS

After successful muscle transposition, the skin and subcutaneous tissue can usually be closed primarily. Certainly, if excessive tension exists with primary closure, a split-thickness skin graft can be substituted. Multiple suction drains, especially in the substernal region, are essential. In our patients, antibiotics specific to the initial offending organism are instituted preoperatively and continued postoperatively until the drains are removed. Premature drain removal can result in the development of a seroma or substernal abscess that can smoulder undetected for several weeks.

Meticulous control of the blood pressure, both intra- and postoperatively, is critical. Flap elevation and sternal debridement result in an extensive raw surface. Dramatic elevations in the systolic blood pressure increase the risk of a hematoma.

Another late complication is caused by inadequate sternal and costal cartilage debridement. These patients can present several months or years later with a draining sinus tract. The offending bone and cartilage must be excised to eradicate the infection (Fig. 2).

MANAGEMENT OF RADIATION ULCERS OF THE CHEST WALL

One of the most difficult problems encountered in reconstructive surgery is the treatment of the infected radiation ulcer of the chest wall. Radiation therapy is used as an adjuvant for treatment of malignancies involving the breast, chest wall, and the lung. The extent of radiation-induced tissue damage is dependent on the total dose administered. The amount of damage may not be obvious for several years. Irradiated skin and soft tissue demonstrate an inadequate host response to trauma. This is secondary to a combination of deep tissue involvement, poor vascularity, and marginal skin quality. The histopathology of radiation-induced skin and soft-tissue damage has been previously described. The response of the host tissue to radiation can be separated into the response of its individual components: skin, dermal appendages, subcutaneous tissue, blood vessels, and underlying muscle, bone, and cartilage. The epithelium, once it has regenerated, is thin and easily damaged by minor trauma. There is degeneration of elastic tissue and replacement of normal dermal collagen with an amorphous debris. Dermal appendages undergo atrophic changes. One of the most physiologically significant problems is the progressive obliterative endarteritis found in irradiated tissue. This alone can result in necrosis of the underlying muscle, bone, and cartilage. The combination of all of these dramatic changes results in the development of a wound that demonstrates diminished healing capabilities, an increased susceptibility to infection, and is extremely painful.

Surgical treatment of the chest wall radiation ulcer requires adherence to three important principles: (1) adequate debridement of involved skin and underlying structures, (2) coverage of the wound with a vascularized

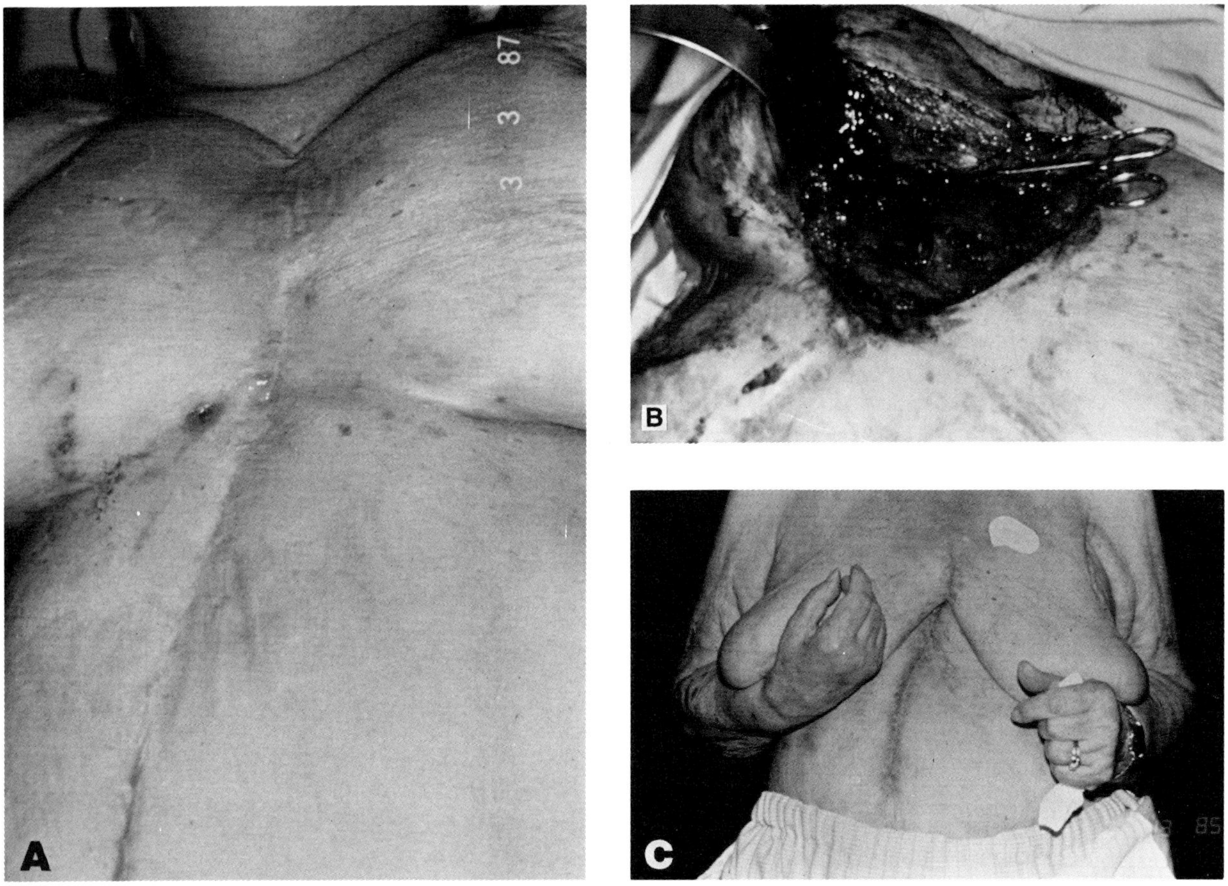

Figure 2 *A*, Patient several years after coronary artery bypass surgery presenting now with a persistently draining sinus tract. *B*, The sternal wound after extensive debridement of necrotic bone and cartilage. *C*, Final result several months after allowing the wound to close by secondary intention.

muscle or myocutaneous flap, and (3) when necessary, reconstruction of a bony thorax capable of maintaining normal pulmonary dynamics.

Debridement of the Radiation Ulcer

The patient with a radiation ulcer that involves the chest wall presents with a significant social, as well as surgical, problem. A normal existence is unlikely in the presence of a painful, draining chest wall ulcer (Fig. 3). Successful treatment of this problem results in a dramatic psychological, as well as physical, improvement.

The key to management of the radiation ulcer is adequate debridement of the involved tissue (Fig. 4). Unfortunately, radiation does not produce well-delineated boundaries of tissue damage. Often, complete excision of ischemic tissue is either impractical or impossible. As described earlier, radiation damage can extend through the soft tissue and involve the bony thorax and underlying pulmonary parenchyma. It is not an uncommon practice to resect a portion of the thoracic skeleton. Inadequate debridement results in a recurrence of the infection, often caused by an underlying osteomyelitis or chondritis. Under normal circumstances, extensive resection of the bony thorax can result in a significant physiologic pulmonary deficit. The amount of respiratory distress developed postoperatively is dependent on the preoperative pulmonary status and the number of ribs resected. Many authors feel that resection of more than four ribs with a portion of the sternum results in significant respiratory compromise. However, body plethysmography demonstrates that anterior chest wall resection only results in minor changes in respiratory function. The irradiated chest wall appears to be a different entity. The ischemic fibrosis produced by radiation allows even more extensive resection by imparting some degree of stability to the thorax. In Arnold's large series of patients who underwent resection and reconstruction after radiation injury, none experienced postoperative respiratory deterioration or required prolonged mechanical ventilation. Coverage of these defects is usually accomplished with muscle or myocutaneous flaps. The use of synthetic mesh for additional support has been described, but is uncommon in our experience.

Coverage of the Chest Wall Defect

The success of vascularized muscle for coverage of radiation-induced chest wall defects is well documented. Other methods of reconstruction have produced less than

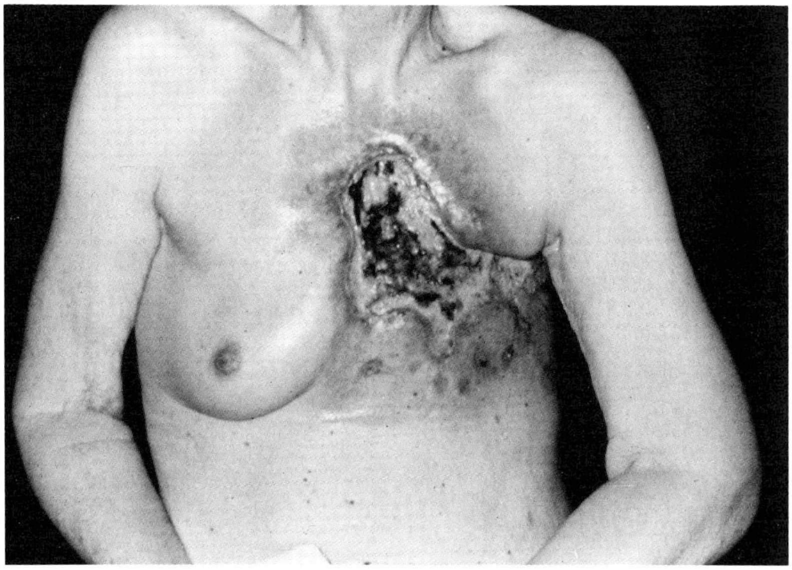

Figure 3 Severe radiation chest wall ulcer in a patient after mastectomy and postoperative radiation several years earlier.

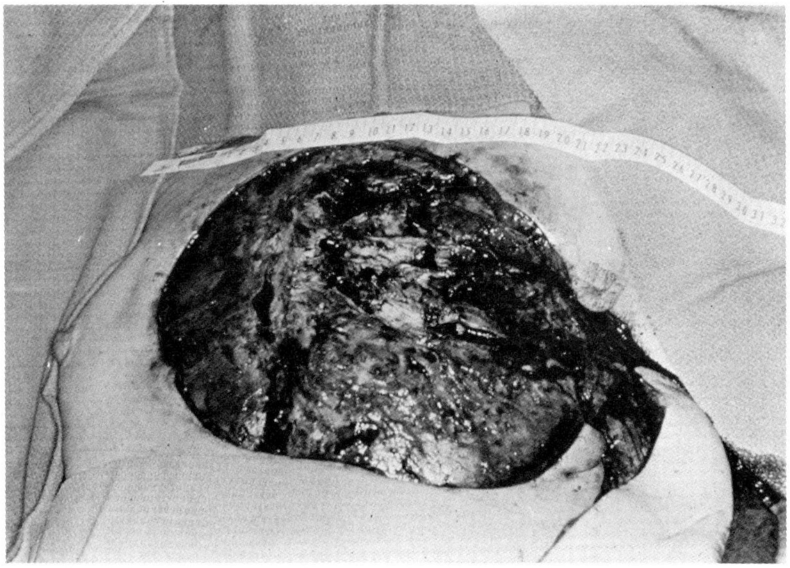

Figure 4 Appearance of the radiation ulcer after debridement to viable margins.

satisfactory results. The use of adjacent skin and subcutaneous tissue as random pattern flaps has a uniformly high incidence of complications. Coverage of radiation ulcers with split-thickness skin grafts has also been demonstrated to have a 50 percent failure rate.

Ideally, vascularized muscle, the pedicle of which is removed from the radiation port, should be used. The choice of muscle flaps is identical to those used to cover the open mediastinal wound: the contralateral pectoralis major, the rectus abdominis, and the latissimus dorsi. Unfortunately, these muscles may have been included in the field of radiation, thus making them inadequate for transposition, secondary to atrophy or fibrosis. A prior mastectomy may have rendered either the pectoralis or the latissimus atrophic, secondary to interruption of the nervous or vascular supply. Certainly, all of these factors must be considered during the preoperative planning stage. Microsurgical techniques have expanded the options for reconstruction when local muscle flaps are not feasible. It is important to perform the microvascular anastomosis in an area removed from the irradiated field. Though successful free tissue transfer can occur with utilization of irradiated vessels, there is a higher incidence of vascular thrombosis. This is felt to be secondary to a propensity for intimal dissection in irradiated vessels.

Another choice in coverage of extensive postradiation ulcers is the use of an omental transposition flap. The omentum can mold into large irregular contours more satisfactorily than muscle can. The use of this flap may require placement of an underlying synthetic mesh support, and carries all of the disadvantages mentioned previously in the section on sternal reconstruction.

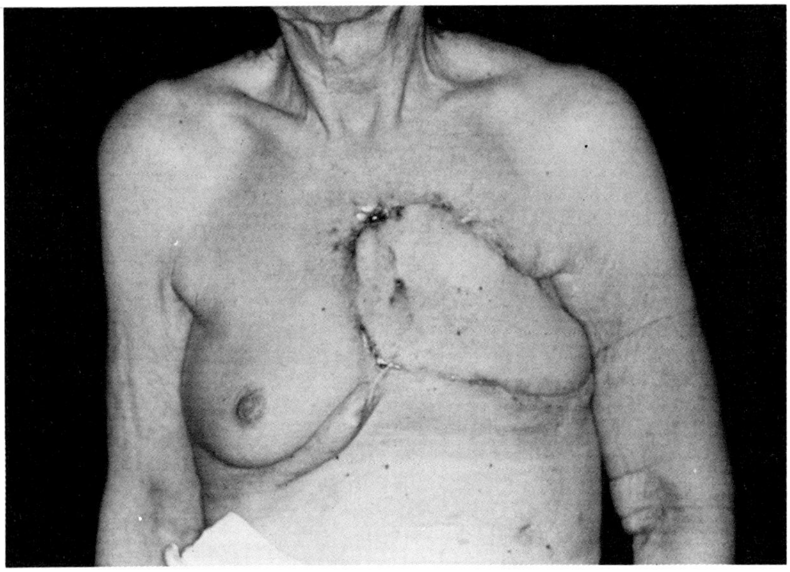

Figure 5 Closure of the defect with a latissimus myocutaneous transposition flap.

Conclusion

Our approach to the management of the radiation ulcer of the chest wall begins with a thorough preoperative discussion with the patient regarding all the surgical options. Often, these patients have been plagued with a painful, draining ulcer for a period of months or years. Any means of successful eradication of this problem is usually greatly appreciated. The patients must understand the extensive nature of their disease process and the potential for a significant resection of skin, soft tissue, and, possibly, bony thorax. A thorough understanding of the histopathology of radiation-damaged tissue is essential. An evaluation of the adequacy of local muscle flaps for coverage of the potential defect must be performed preoperatively. The cornerstone of successful treatment lies with adequate debridement of involved tissue. Though there is a potential for respiratory compromise after extensive chest wall resections, this problem in our experience is uncommon in the irradiated chest wall. Synthetic mesh can be used to provide stability in clean wounds.

The achievement of a cosmetically-appealing final result is important in any reconstructive procedure. The primary goal, however, in management of radiation ulcers is a stable, healed wound (Fig. 5).

SUGGESTED READING

Arnold M. The surgical anatomy of sternal blood supply. J Thorac Cardiovasc Surg 1972; 64:596–610.

Chang N, Mathes SJ. Comparison of the effect of bacterial inoculation in musculocutaneous and random pattern flaps. Plast Reconstr Surg 1982; 70:1–9.

Culliford AT, Cunninham JN Jr, Zeff RH. Sternal and costochondral infections following open heart surgery: a review of 2594 cases. J Thorac Surg 1976; 72:714–726.

Jurkiewicz MJ, Bostwick J, Hester TR, Bishop B, Craver J. Infected median sternotomy wound. Ann Surg 1980; 191:738–744.

Loop FD, Irarrazal MJ, Bredee JJ, et al. Internal mammary artery graft for ischemic heart disease: effect of revascularization on clinical status and survival. Am J Cardiol 1977; 39:516–522.

INFECTED VASCULAR PROSTHESES

RICHARD P. RAND, M.D.
FOAD NAHAI, M.D., F.A.C.S.

The evolution of modern vascular surgery began in 1912 when Alexis Carrel demonstrated the potential for long-term blood flow via a prosthetic conduit. Autogenous tissues were the first materials employed in arterial bypass surgery and, in 1951, a rapid advance in the field occurred with the introduction of synthetic bypass materials. Since then, numerous types of conduits have been produced that allow patients to undergo limb- or life-saving operations which would not otherwise have been possible.

Graft infection and exposure remain among the most feared and ominous complications in vascular surgery. This untoward outcome can result in organ dysfunction, amputation, and death. Indeed, the ultimate result of a prosthetic graft infection is often worse than the natural history of the condition for which the arterial surgery was performed.

As a result, much study of the pathogenesis and etiology of graft infection has been made in order to minimize the frequency of this complication. A review of the literature documents an overall incidence of 1 to 6 percent, with most series falling in the 2 to 3 percent range. The associated mortality statistics are from 20 to 75 percent and are highest when an aortic level anastomosis is involved. The incidence of limb amputation is approximately 30 percent when a graft becomes infected in an extremity.

Approximately 75 percent of graft infections occur in the femoral region. A two- to three-fold increased incidence of infection is seen in aortic surgery when femoral anastomoses are required, rather than when the surgery can be confined to the retroperitoneum. Local flora and the division of bacteria-laden lymph nodes in the groin are implicated in the infection rate, especially when contaminated and ischemic lower extremity lesions are present. The most commonly cultured organism is *Staphylococcus aureus.*

The consensus among most vascular surgeons is that the presence of a prosthetic conduit infection necessitates the removal of the graft. Arterial reconstruction could then be performed immediately via another route in a sterile field. Alternatively, a staged reconstruction may be elected while the resolution of infection after graft removal is awaited. This option, however, could expose the patient to a critical level of distal ischemia and an increased risk of amputation while the infection resolves.

Complete excision of prosthetic grafts and immediate reconstruction can be long and complex procedures in a patient who is compromised by infection and in whom there is often an associated component of coronary artery disease. Therefore, a more conservative approach to graft infection and exposure has been advocated by some surgeons. The ultimate success of this approach depends on proper assessment of the extent of graft involvement with infection. Grafts that are occluded should be removed as should those in which an anastomosis is involved or where there are signs of a systemic infection with positive blood cultures. Otherwise, specifically localized infection and graft exposure can be successfully managed by soft tissue debridement and coverage with well-vascularized muscle tissue. This treatment carries the obvious advantage of preserving a functioning bypass and may eliminate the need for an immediate or delayed graft revision. The muscle brings with it the blood-borne elements of host defense and systemic levels of antibiotic medication.

Graft infections may occur acutely, but the average onset is nearly 2 years after the initial surgery. Occasionally, thrombectomies or embolectomies must be performed in longstanding grafts in which complete tissue incorporation has previously taken place. Under these circumstances, a limited operative exposure of the graft is required. A wound infection is most likely to be locally confined and may thus be treated by muscle flap transposition, with good results.

The common sites of graft infection are reviewed next and available local muscle flaps are described.

FEMORAL

The femoral region represents the site of infection in 75 percent of patients with graft sepsis. Following adequate debridement, the sartorius muscle may be transposed to cover exposed vascular grafts in this region. This muscle has a type IV pattern of circulation and is supplied along its medial border with as many as ten segmental arterial branches that arise from the superficial femoral artery.

Chronic superficial femoral occlusion, as is often seen in patients with atherosclerotic disease, does not limit the utility of this flap because of the development of collateral circulation. Transposition of the sartorius is accomplished by division of the origin of the muscle from the anterior superior iliac spine and ligation of the proximal two arterial pedicles. This provides an adequate arc of rotation for coverage of grafts in the groin. The skin that overlies the proximal muscle may be carried with the flaps, but this is rarely indicated since the muscle will only cover adjacent defects.

When the sartorius does not provide adequate coverage, a rectus femoris or vastus lateralis flap may be performed (Fig. 1). While the sartorius is an expendable lateral rotator and flexor of the hip, use of these other muscles may result in some degree of limb impairment. This would seem to be justified, though, when faced with the alternative of limb loss.

The rectus femoris is a member of the quadriceps mechanism and is located anteromedially in the thigh. It is supplied by a single dominant vascular pedicle (type I), which is a branch of the lateral circumflex femoral artery. Transposition of the rectus femoris is accomplished by dividing it several centimeters above the knee and elevating the muscle until the pedicle is visualized in the vicinity of the sartorius muscle, approximately 8 to 10 cm below the anterior superior iliac spine. A skin island may be carried over the muscle, and primary closure of the donor site is generally accomplished.

The vastus lateralis is also a component of the quadriceps mechanism and is located deep to the fascia lata between the rectus femoris medially and the biceps femoris posteriorly. The muscle has a type II vascular pattern, with the dominant pedicle being the descending branch of the lateral circumflex femoral artery that enters the proximal third of the muscle. Elevation of the muscle flap is performed through a lateral thigh incision. After incision of the fascia lata, the vastus lateralis is divided above its insertion to the patella and mobilized to its proximal third. It is then rotated into the groin and covered by split skin grafts.

An inferiorly-based rectus abdominis flap may also be employed to cover exposed grafts in the femoral region. This flap carries a potential for abdominal wall laxity or herniation, but does not result in altered limb function. The muscle alone, or in conjunction with a vertical skin island, is transected superiorly and transposed on its deep inferior epigastric blood supply. Division and reconstruc-

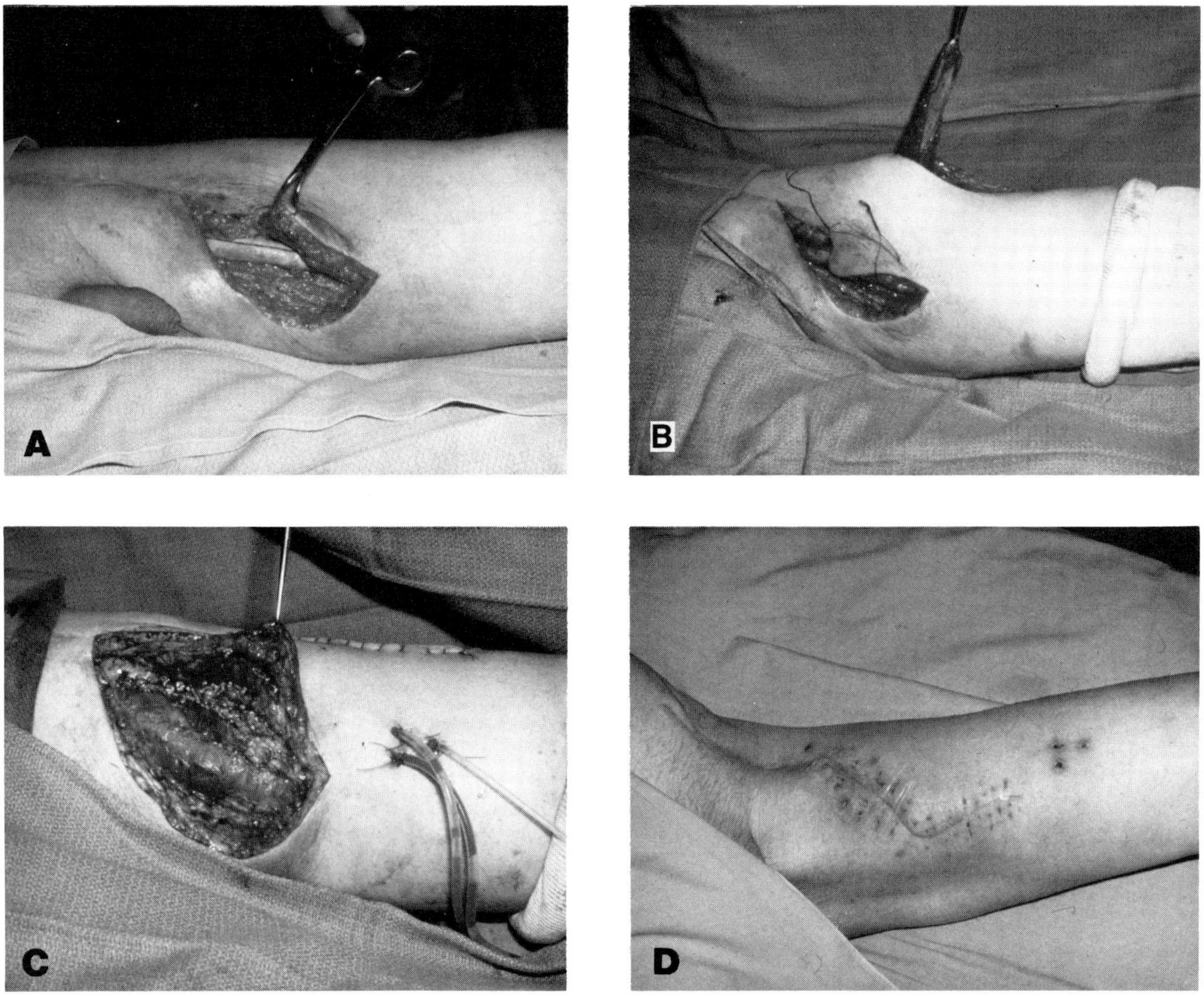

Figure 1 *A*, This 73-year-old male presented with an exposed, infected, dacron femoral prosthesis. *B*, The wound was debrided and a rectus femoris muscle flap was elevated. *C*, The rectus flap was transposed medially to cover the graft. Irrigation and drainage catheters were placed in the wound and removed after 2 weeks. *D*, The wound healed primarily and has not exhibited evidence of infection over a 7-year follow-up. (We would like to acknowledge Dr. P.G. Arnold for his contribution of this clinical case.)

tion of the inguinal ligament may facilitate transfer of the flap.

The tensor fascia lata (TFL) may also be rotated to provide coverage to the groin, but since fasciocutaneous flaps are less resistant to infection than muscle flaps, this is considered to be a secondary alternative. The TFL flap may best be used to provide additional coverage over a transposed sartorius flap.

POPLITEAL

It is presently believed that femoral to below-knee popliteal or tibial bypasses carry better long-term patency rates when performed with autogenous, reversed, or in situ saphenous vein. Therefore, distal prosthetic graft infection is generally seen only in the above-knee position. In this instance, a medial gastrocnemius flap may provide suitable coverage. Graft exposure that occurs more proximally in the thigh likely indicates infectious involvement of the tunnel in which the graft is situated and usually necessitates graft removal. If, however, the infection is believed to be truly localized, simple elevation and advancement of adjacent muscular tissue suffices.

AXILLAE

Extra-anatomic bypass via the axillofemoral route is often performed on high-risk patients and on those in whom aortic level infection has occurred. Obviously, all efforts should be made to salvage these grafts for they present among the last alternative means of revascularization available to these patients. Localized graft exposure in the axillary position may be managed by debridement and coverage with pectoralis major or latissimus dorsi flaps. The pectoralis flap has the advantage of proximity and may be rotated over the prosthetic graft after division of the humeral insertion. Adequate nutritional blood supply is provided by perforating branches of the internal mammary artery, even if the thoracoacromial pedicle has been previously divided during the arterial bypass surgery.

SUGGESTED READING

Bernhard VM, Towne JB. Complications in vascular surgery. In: Moore WS, ed. Vascular surgery—a comprehensive review. Orlando: Grune & Stratton, 1983.

Mathes SJ, Nahai F. Clinical Applications for muscle and musculocutaneous flaps. St. Louis: CV Mosby, 1982:421.

Poposky J, Singer S. Infected prosthetic grafts. Arch Surg 1980; 115:203-205.

Quarfordt PG, Reilly LM, Ehrenfeld WK, Stoney RJ. Surgical management of vascular graft infections—local treatment, graft excision, and methods of revascularization. In: Bernhard VM, Towne JB, eds. Complications in vascular surgery. Orlando: Grune & Stratton, 1985.

Szilagyi DE, Smith RF, Elliott JP, Vrandecic MP. Infection in arterial reconstruction with synthetic grafts. Ann Surg 1972; 176:320-333.

PRESSURE SORES

NEIL E. KLEIN, B.A., M.D.

Early in their training, most plastic surgeons develop a revulsion for pressure sores, perhaps during medical school or internship. I recall, as an intern, being sent to debride a large, foul-smelling, necrotic ulceration. A smirking senior resident sent me to a back bed in a dark ward to treat a near moribund patient whose only ability to respond was to whimper in pain as I touched any tissue that approached viability. Imagine the negative reinforcement as such a scene is replayed throughout the world of surgical training programs!

Thus negatively predisposed, I went on to learn that the initial care of a pressure sore was physically uncomfortable. In addition, the patients were usually difficult, uncooperative, predisposed to nonhealing, and determined to undo any good that I thought could be accomplished.

At the completion of my training, I was fortunate enough to be offered a position at Rancho Los Amigos Medical Center. This facility is the Los Angeles County rehabilitation hospital and deals with large numbers of patients who have had spinal cord injuries. Hence the hospital has a fairly large population of patients with pressure sores. It became obvious that a philosophy of treatment beyond that of a self-centered resident would need to be developed if any progress was to be made. It also seemed obvious that this philosophy would be diametrically opposed to that which I had been practising up to then; i.e., avoidance of the pressure sore patient.

Plastic surgery training teaches the value of teams for dealing with difficult problems. In the patient with pressure sores due to spinal cord injury, the overwhelming surgical problems, aside from the actual coverage of the defect, are orthopedic. Therefore, I felt that a team for care of these patients should be codirected by a plastic surgeon and an orthopedist. In fact, many of the judgment errors that cause tissue flaps to fail involve orthopedic problems being overlooked. Simultaneous rounds by a plastic surgical service as well as an orthopedic service could avoid these difficulties. A psychologist and social worker are essential to the team. Also required are nutritionists, neurologists, urologists, physical and occupational therapists, and a dedicated nursing staff. To this is added the availability of a cushion-manufacturing department and an administration eager to help in this difficult area. It may seem difficult to put together such a team; however, at Rancho Los Amigos Medical Center the team concept is the preferred form of treatment and it was an easy matter to find participants.

One other advantage of an institution of this type is that it represents the final common pathway for referrals of the most difficult patients. As a result, the team is able to attain a fairly good follow-up. Our patients have few other places to go.

PROBLEMS ASSOCIATED WITH PRESSURE SORES

A pressure sore rarely exists as a problem by itself. It is invariably associated with a multitude of problems. One must look not only at the pressure sore, but at the entire patient in whom the problem exists. The question which must always be answered is, "Why did the pressure sore occur?" We know that pressure sores occur mainly in patients with either congenital or acquired spinal cord pathology, the elderly, and the debilitated. However, none of these problems alone should lead to the development of a pressure sore.

In the spinal cord injury patient, difficulty with skin breakdown may begin within the first 24 to 48 hours following injury. Even in centers familiar with treatment of spinal cord injuries, patients develop pressure sores acutely in the postinjury period. Often, inadequate training and fear of causing iatrogenic injuries prevent physicians and other hospital personnel from giving adequate pressure relief to the patient with the acute spinal cord injury. Frequently, prolonged surgical procedures, or logistical difficulties following surgery, prevent patients from being turned. Patients who have developed pressure sores early are not necessarily of the hard core recidivist type, (i.e., patients who develop frequent recurrences of pressure sores, often long after their spinal cord injuries and despite attempts at training). The answer to the pressure sore that occurs early following spinal cord injury is education of the hospital staff. Physicians and nurses must learn safe effective methods of pressure relief while treating the acute spinal cord injury and related trauma.

Recidivist patients require the greatest patience and perhaps the greatest resources of the surgeon and pressure sore team. A history of drug or alcohol abuse may be the basic etiology of the recurrent pressure sore problem. Chronic depression, or acute bouts of depression with a self-destructive focus, may be the culprit. It is important to identify the problems before team resources are exhausted or one of a finite number of flaps is needlessly destroyed.

Treatment of these psychosocial ills is quite difficult and one should be certain that the patient will not go home and sit through a freshly-placed flap in an alcoholic stupor.

In the elderly or debilitated patient, we are often called upon to cover a pressure sore because "the patient can't get into a nursing home." This alone is not an adequate justification for surgery. If the patient is felt not to be a surgical candidate because of the lack of rehabilitation potential, he or she is not necessarily a candidate for pressure sore flap coverage. In this instance, the pressure sores should be debrided and kept clean with a careful regimen of redressings, but the patient should not be subjected to the unnecessary risk of surgery.

Patients may develop a pressure sore during an acute period of debilitation. Unless the pressure sore is very large, these ulcers will often close spontaneously as the patient begins to ambulate and improve nutritionally. Surgical debridement and observation often cure these wounds. If not, minor procedures such as skin grafts or simple closures are helpful.

Pediatric patients with pressure sores have different problems from adults. They may have been born with a meningomyelocele, have developed a spinal cord tumor, or had a spinal cord injury at an early age. Problems with pressure sores often develop as the child enters the teenage years. This period is difficult even for the most well-adjusted, but, in those with a physical disability, puberty seems to explode. Much of this difficulty is related to a distorted image of the portion of the body that has been paralyzed or is insensate. As expected, these children find it difficult to deal with the care of the skin in these areas. This pressure, added to the pressures of trying to cope with adolescence, leads to the development of pressure sores. Intensive education and therapy may be helpful for these young adults. In the patient with a low level meningomyelocele, sensory flaps such as the tensor fascia lata flap, including the lateral femoral cutaneous nerve, have been effective, but cooperation and patient education are needed. If self-destruction is the goal, it is a simple matter to move off the sensate area and create an ulceration immediately adjacent to the sensate pedicle. The answer lies not in the surgery itself, but in teaching that the sensory cue is a reminder—a signal to change position and relieve pressure.

In general, pressure sores should be thought of as a psychosocial rather than surgical disease. I do not believe that the ulcer can be closed when the patient or his circumstances do not allow it to be closed.

Nutrition is a major problem. Simple laboratory studies demonstrated that nearly 80 percent of the patients with whom our team dealt had some degree of malnutrition. Observation of patients showed that, despite beautifully filled out request menus, they often failed to eat. Ordered meals were consumed by family members or other patients. It is easy to obtain calorie counts and, in most cases, patients can be encouraged to increase their caloric intake. Protein supplements can augment the diet. Rarely is total parenteral nutrition necessary. History of weight loss, low serum albumin or serum cholesterol, altered transferrin levels and iron binding capacities, or an anergic response to skin tests demonstrate malnutrition. Malnourishment may frequently be present as a result of drug or alcohol abuse, or depression.

Urologic problems are often present in a spinal cord injury patient. These may not be directly related to the pressure sore; however, they may make dealing with the pressure sore more difficult. Amyloidosis is often mentioned as a reason for the repair of pressure sores. This problem is not usually seen unless the pressure sore is accompanied by chronic infection or an uncontrolled osteomyelitis.

Autonomic dysreflexia is rarely mentioned in the plastic surgical literature, but is a common problem. Spinal cord lesions above T-7 may result in this patient response. Symptomatically, a patient with a bout of autonomic dysreflexia may complain of headaches, severe sweating, chills, cutis anserina, chest tightness, or palpitations. Marked hypertension can result in myocardial insufficiency and retinal or cerebral hemorrhages. Eighty-five percent of patients with a spinal cord lesion at T-7 or above may exhibit this phenomenon, and it can be precipitated by distention of the bowel or bladder, cutting of the insensate skin, or stimulation of an internal viscus during surgery. Internal disease processes may also stimulate a bout of autonomic dysreflexia. When an episode occurs, it is an acute emergency, and treatment entails dealing with the cause. This may mean evacuation of the distended bowel or bladder, or masking of the surgical stimulus with the use of local, regional, or spinal anesthetic. Acute medical treatment of the high blood pressure with a rapid-acting antihypertensive agent is often required. Most patients who have this problem are aware of it and of the usual causes. They can tell the physician or the nurse what treatment has been historically effective.

Spasms must be controlled prior to surgical repair of an ulceration. Spasms affect the muscle flap directly as well as the extremities or truncal areas that are being operated upon. I have seen a tensor fascia lata flap literally jump from its bed during an acute spastic episode in the postoperative patient. Doses of antispasticity drugs must be adequate and, occasionally, doses greater than those recommended on package inserts may be required. Help from a neurologist can provide the surgeon with effective guidelines. If medication alone is inadequate, then the use of splints or even surgical release of spastic muscles may be needed. Intrathecal alcohol blocks may be helpful, but patients are often opposed to this measure. When a muscle flap is used, temporary denervation of the muscle simply by crushing the nerve to that muscle may prevent local spastic episodes. In certain extreme cases a body cast may be helpful, but this requires experienced specialized personnel for adequate management.

Contractures must certainly be treated prior to the closure of a pressure sore. Serial casts may be useful for the knee. Prone positioning helps hip flexion contractures. Severe contractures, or those complicated by heterotrophic ossification require surgical release. We attempt to teach all spinal cord injury patients to rest prone, and I would estimate that 90 percent or more of our patients are capable of lying prone nearly all the time while in bed. One must be wary of pressure ulcerations at the knee or chest in the prone patient, but with proper bolstering at the levels of the midthigh, lower leg, and abdomen or chest areas, these anterior ulcers should not develop. For the few patients who are unable to lie prone, the air-fluidized silicone bed seems to provide the best protection, but one should be aware that the type of mattress alone is not the answer.

PREPARING THE WOUND

The initial surgical intervention is usually debridement of the wound, removal of all nonviable tissue; either sharp surgical removal for large quantities or redressings for the small bits of debris. For day-to-day treatment of the wound, it does not matter whether simple redressings, topical antibiotics, or yogurt are used as long as the wound is inspected frequently and regularly. Osteomyelitis, if present, must be dealt with sternly. There is a feeling in plastic surgery that just "shaving a little bone" is the answer to the exposed bone at the base of a pressure sore—and often this is the case. A more severe osteomyelitis can be diagnosed only by bone biopsy and culture. The surgeon should have an increased level of awareness of this problem. If there is indeed a deep osteomyelitis, the involved bone must be debrided and a course of parenteral antibiotics should be given. When considering closure of an ulcer of this type, preference should be given to flaps where muscle directly contacts the debrided bony surface.

A frequent cause for recurrence of pressure sores about the hip joint is an unrecognized septic hip. It is quite easy for organisms to enter the hip through an occult opening in the joint capsule. Diagnostic taps or arthrograms are useful to exclude this problem, but the septic hip is easily overlooked if not kept in mind and, if present, removal of the proximal femur may be required.

BONE RESECTION

In the past, removal of large amounts of bone has been proposed with the idea that the pressure in a given area is due to a bony prominence and, therefore, removal of the bony prominence will eliminate the pressure. In some cases this is true. It must be remembered, however, that once a bony prominence is removed, the pressure will certainly be transferred to another area, perhaps with less desirable consequences. An example of this is the total ischial resection. This procedure was once viewed as a way to eliminate pressure over the ischial tuberosities. An unfavorable sequence of events often followed: the patient developed a unilateral ischial pressure sore; he would then be subjected to a total ischiectomy and flap closure on that side. This resulted in an abnormal transfer of pressure to the other ischial tuberosity, thus causing a breakdown on that side. With the same logic as for the first operation, a total ischiectomy would then be performed on the second side, and the patient left to sit on his unprotected perineum. The poor recipient of the bilateral total ischiectomy would then break down the perineum, enter into the urethra, and then reulcerate both ischial areas as well. This left a gigantic ulceration that extended from trochanter to trochanter with little hope of a simple cure.

When bone resection is being planned, thought must be given to the functional anatomy of the skeleton in relation to the chair. It is useful here to have help from an orthopedic colleague. We sit on our ischial tuberosities, but the thighs are extremely important in weight bearing, as is the integrity of the hip joint. The tilt of the pelvis and the presence of curvatures of the spine might add excessive pressures to a given area. These same skeletal analyses are required when one deals with the lying down ulcerations that occur on the sacrum or the trochanters. The removal of bone simply to reduce pressure in a given area should be eschewed. The outcome of such a maneuver can only be hazardous.

CLOSURE OF PRESSURE ULCERATIONS

The least important part of treating a pressure sore is the flap closure of the wound. There is such a fine assortment of healthy, large, well-vascularized flaps in the areas about the pelvis where most pressure sores occur, that the actual surgical closure has become minimally challenging. By the morning of surgery, the patient should have a biologically clean wound, free from infection and necrotic debris. (Small uncomplicated ulcerations may be debrided and closed in one stage, if the patient is ready for surgery from the other points of view). He should be in a positive nitrogen balance with spasms controlled. Contractures will have been released. Medical problems are stabilized and, if appropriate, the patient is able to lie prone or assume a safe position for several days postoperatively. Thought should be given to transfusion and, if the procedure is extensive, then blood should be prepared.

Most of the flaps the team uses are myocutaneous flaps. In many of the designs, muscle does not come into contact with the ulcer bed, but rather serves as a carrier for a healthy random paddle. The concept of muscle as a padding or cushion over a bony prominence is invalid and, in fact, muscle vitality is more sensitive to pressure than the skin and subcutaneous tissue. Muscle is effective when used directly over an ulcer bed to help in the treatment of osteomyelitis. Muscle under skin graft also acts as an effective pseudosubcutaneous tissue to allow shear relief.

The flaps used most frequently are as follows. For a sacral pressure sore, the gluteus maximus myocutaneous flap is favored. This flap may be designed so that no skin grafting of the donor site is necessary. The design is essentially the same as that used prior to the era of the myocutaneous flap; however, when dissecting from the random area into the portion of the flap that overlies the gluteus maximus muscle, the muscle is taken and a rather small random area of the flap is left, thus giving the flap its vigorous nature. In this flap the muscle does not lie over the ulceration, only the random portion of the flap.

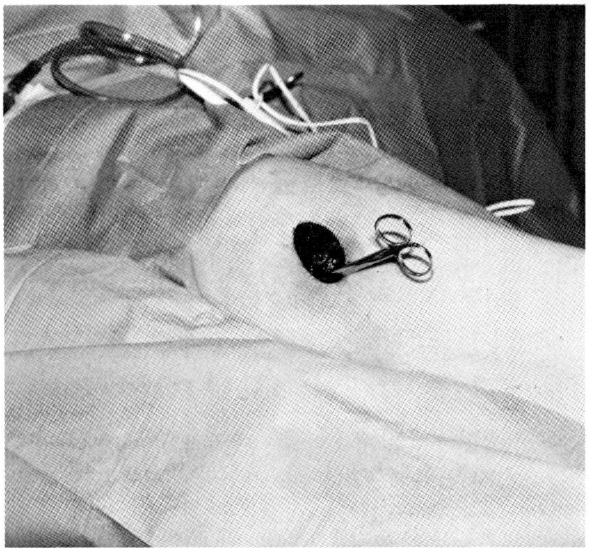

Figure 1 Right trochanteric ulceration. Wound is stained with methylene blue to facilitate excision.

For the ischial pressure sore, choice of flap depends upon the size and shape of the ulceration that overlies the ischial tuberosity. A large horizontal ulceration can be closed quite nicely by a V-Y advancement flap from a posterior thigh to incorporate the hamstring muscles. A small first-time ulceration may be easily closed by gluteus maximus myocutaneous rotation flap.

Our flap of choice for trochanteric ulceration is a tensor fascia lata myocutaneous flap, advanced proximally in a V-Y pattern. This flap is particularly effective because we can use a healthy portion of the flap for the actual closure, i.e., that area near the pedicle as opposed to the most ischemic area of the flap (Figs. 1, 2, and 3).

For more difficult closures and more difficult patients, heroic measures are required. Patients who have had removal of the proximal femur due to septic arthritis, or dislocation of the femoral head from the acetabulum, require careful evaluation. Remember the importance of the

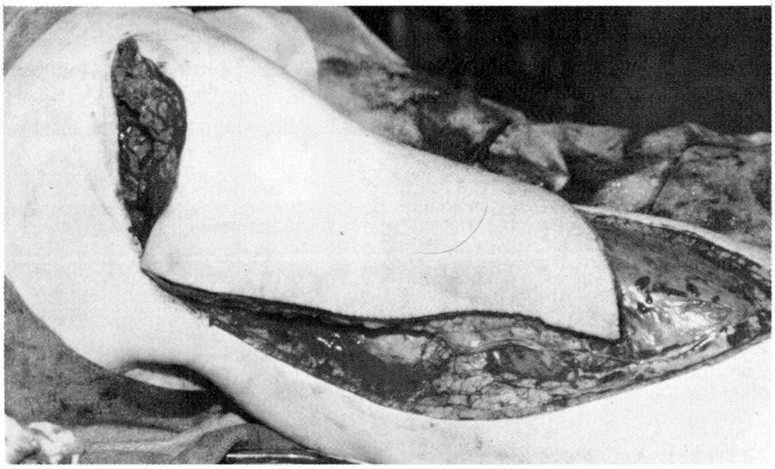

Figure 2 Tensor fasciae latae V-Y flap elevated from right lateral thigh. Ulceration has been completely excised.

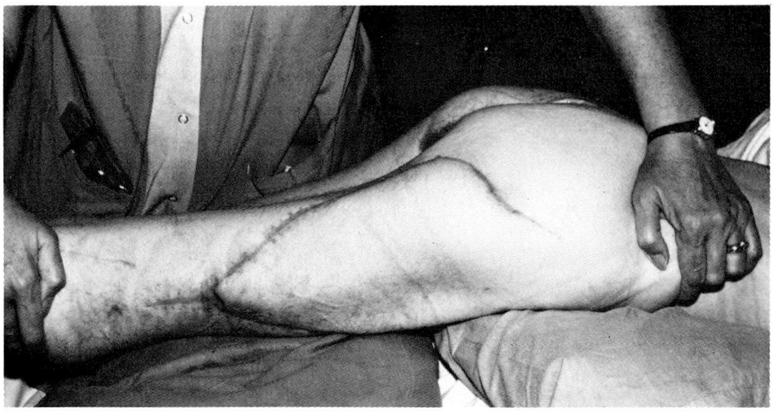

Figure 3 Healed tensor fasciae latae V-Y advancement flap.

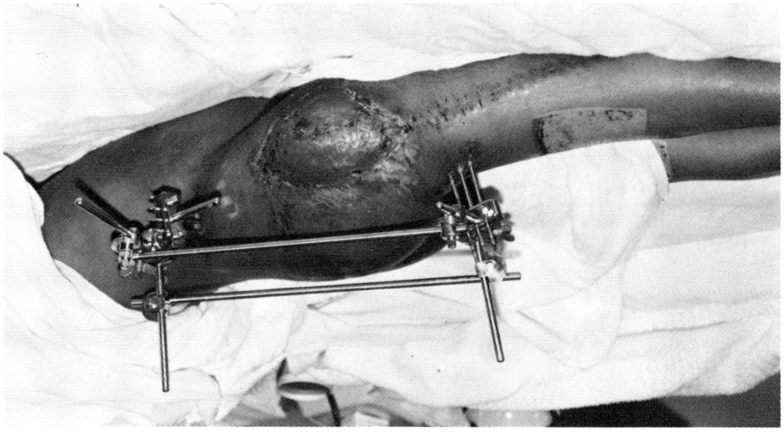

Figure 4 Proximal femoral resection defect closed with a vastus lateralis muscle flap and skin graft. External orthopedic fixation device is in place for stability.

thighs and the integrity of the hip joints for weight bearing in sitting! About half of our patients with this problem have had successful long-term closure of the ulcerations with the use of an orthopedic external fixation device to immobilize the unstable lower extremity (Fig. 4). The large and deep wound left by removal of the proximal femur is then closed with a vastus lateralis muscle flap and skin graft. These patients, if intensively prepared both physically and psychologically, can be rehabilitated to sitting.

The patient with an extremely large pressure ulceration requires removal of the bones of the lower extremity to allow the use of the skin and muscles of the leg to complete closures. Despite the apparent length obtained in these fillet procedures, it is often still impossible to reach the more proximal points of ulceration with the leg flap itself. In these instances, more proximal flaps from the hip area can be moved into the proximal reaches of the ulceration, and the flaps from the filleted leg can be used to close the donor sites of these primary flaps. Once again, it must be remembered that the patient who has reached this point of most serious ulceration is in need of more than surgical closure. Often, these complicated closures mark the beginning of the successful end of the patient's self-destructive behavior.

SUGGESTED READING

Constantian MB. Pressure ulcers: principles and techniques of management. Boston: Little, Brown, 1980.

Daniel RK, Hall EJ, MacLeod MK. Pressure sores: a reappraisal. Ann Plast Surg 1979; 3:53–63.

Fredricks S, Brody GS, eds. Symposium on the neurologic aspects of plastic surgery. St. Louis: CV Mosby, 1978.

Garber SL, Krouskop TA, Carter RE. A system for clinically evaluating wheelchair pressure-relief cushions. Am J Occup Ther 1978; 329:565–570.

Kenedi RM, Cowden JM, Scoles JT. Bed sore biomechanics. Baltimore: University Park Press, 1975.

Kenney JG, Edgerton MT, Edlich RF. Recurrent pressure sores: evaluation and treatment. Contemp Orthop 1984; 8(2):51–60.

Mathes SJ, Nahai F. Clinical atlas of muscle and musculocutaneous flaps. St. Louis: CV Mosby, 1979.

Minami RT, Mills R, Pardol R. Gluteus maximus myocutaneous flaps for repair of pressure sores. Plast Reconstr Surg 1977; 60:242–249.

PERINEAL DEFECTS

DENNIS J. HURWITZ, M.D.

Problematic acute and chronic wounds of the perineum and pelvic cavity are effectively treated with the advent of nearby muscle, musculocutaneous and skin fascial flaps. Over the past 10 years, a treatment protocol has been developed from experience gained in over 40 patients.

The perineum extends from the pubic arch to the coccyx, and between the inferior rami of the pubis and ischium. A line drawn transversely between the ischial tuberosities divides the space into two portions. The dorsal contains the termination of the anal canal and is known as the anal region; the ventral, which contains the external urogenital organs, is termed the urogenital region. The wounds considered in this discussion extend from the anal region to the presacral space, with sinus tracts up to the sacral promontory. The perineal center in the male or the vaginal introitus may be involved. However, the disorders of the urethra and the male genitalia are of a different nature and complexity and, as such, will not be discussed.

Surgical and/or irradiation treatment of carcinoma of the anus, rectum, and female genital tract are frequent etiologies for nonhealing wounds in this region. Malignancy of this region is so common that the rarity of chronic wounds is surprising. In fact, persistent wounds and fistulas more commonly follow the treatment of inflammatory bowel disease than carcinoma.

In either case, abdominoperineal resection leaves a pelvic space bounded by the pubis, the two ischia, the sacrum, and the coccyx. Anteriorly, the urogenital structures are fixed by firm fascial attachments to the pubis. Repair of the retroperitoneum limits the descent of the bowel. Below, the skin of the buttocks contracts into the cavity to meet the viscera from above. If the peritoneal descent is retarded by packing, serum, or hematoma, then subsequent fibrosis leaves the peritoneum high in the pelvis, unable to coapt to the contracting perineal wound. The perineal sinus has a relatively small opening and often has a bottleneck constriction leading to a second cavity (Fig. 1).

A perineal wound that fails to heal 6 months after a proctocolectomy is considered a perineal sinus. The incidence varies from 22 to 77 percent. The nonlethality of this complication, coupled with heretofore ineffective treatment, lent an air of resignation to general surgeons. These draining wounds are annoying and occasionally painful to the patient. The wound soaks perineal pads, soils undergarments, and lingers as a distasteful reminder of the original surgical disorder. If delayed healing occurs, a perineal hernia with bowel protuberance may result. Proctologists and most general surgeons have patients suffering from this condition, and all would appreciate its correction.

Conscientious wound hygiene and periodic debridement is the accepted and generally effective treatment. Small and shallow sinus tracts may respond to coccygeal and soft tissue debridement. These steps have usually already been executed by the referring general surgeon, gynecologist, or urologist. When these local measures have been unsuccessful, a thorough work-up is indicated. An unsubstantiated diagnosis from surgical colleagues should not be accepted. A gastrointestinal work-up, including barium contrast studies, computed tomography (CT) scan, and endoscopy, is indicated. The persistence of inflammatory bowel disease is considered and, if present, it is treated prior to an attempt at reconstruction. Under optimum treatment, relapsing inflammatory bowel disease is no contraindication to resection of the sinus tract and flap reconstruction. A genitourinary evaluation, including intravenous pyelogram, and cystoscopy with instillation of methylene blue to rule out bladder or seminal vesicle fistula, should be considered.

Therapeutic Alternatives

Superficial wounds with healthy granulation tissue are covered with split-thickness skin grafts by the exposure technique. Wounds too scarred to accept a skin graft can be closed with sliding island gluteus maximus myocutaneous flaps. Most wounds of the perineum extend into the sacral hollow; a location too remote for the gluteus maximus flap.

One or two gracili can fill smaller sinus tracts. The skin island flap that overlies the distal half of the gracilis is not reliable. The biceps femoris muscle has a point of rotation too low in the thigh to allow relocation into the pelvis. With the advent of the gluteal thigh flap, the biceps femoris flap became obsolete for this type of reconstruction. The rectus abdominis, rectus femoris, and/or omental flaps will reach the pelvis through an anterior approach. Often, the rectus abdominis is unavailable because of a colostomy. The rectus femoris muscle and omentum rarely have the reach to fill deep in the pelvic cavity. The large size and reliability of the gluteal thigh flap have made it the preferred flap (Fig. 2).

Preferred Approach

Extensive or nonhealing wounds of the perineum are repaired when wound hygiene is optimal. In the acute case,

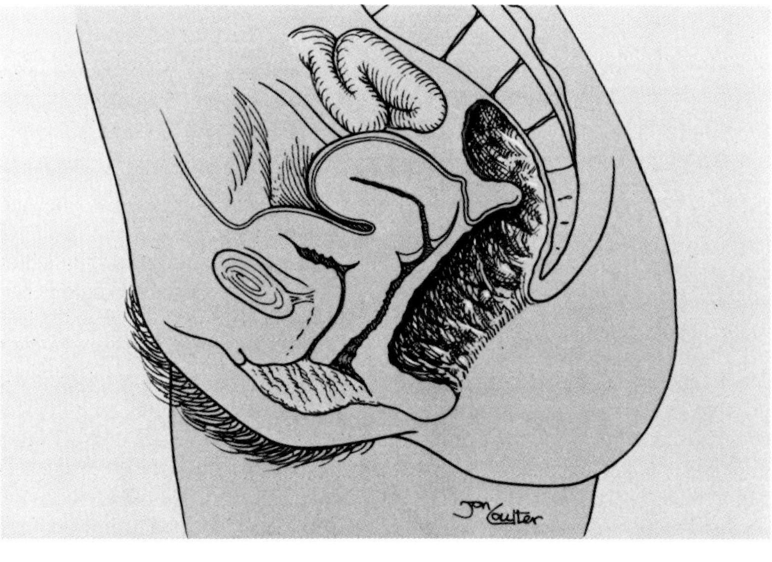

Figure 1 The most common perineal defect is the perineal/pelvic sinus that follows abdominoperineal resection of the rectum. This is a wound of the dorsal perineum with the anterior wall consisting of the posterior wall of the vagina in the female, and the bladder and seminal vesicles in the male. The sinus ends close to descending intestines, and often a slight constriction occurs, as diagrammed in this sagittal view.

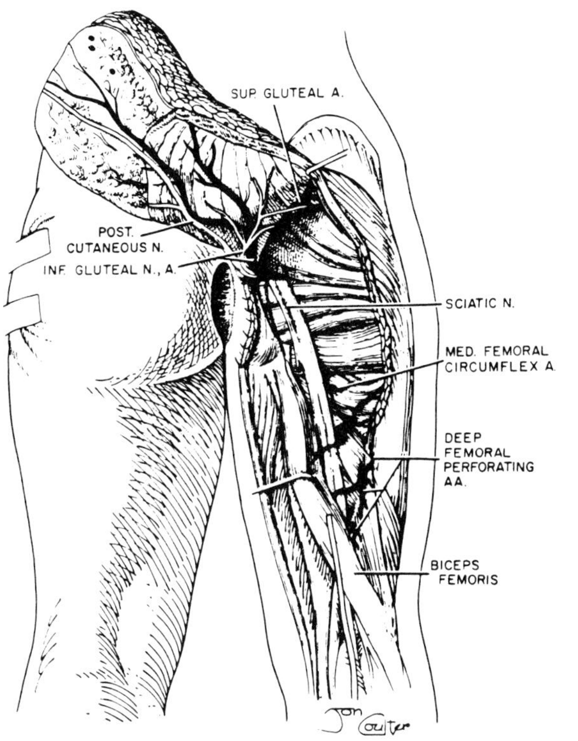

Figure 2 This is an anatomic dissection of the gluteal thigh flap. The fasciocutaneous branch of the inferior gluteal artery is a continuation of the main vessel on the undersurface of the gluteus maximus muscle. The posterior cutaneous nerve of the thigh is taken with the flap. The deep femoral perforating arteries are transsected as the flap is elevated. The sciatic nerve is under cover of the biceps femoris muscle, except in the most distal and proximal portions of the flap elevation.

that means at the time of resection, or some days thereafter. When there is no skin deficit, either the gracilis or gluteal thigh flap will do. Heavily scarred and contaminated chronic cavities, as can occur after irradiation therapy, may be packed with gracilis muscle and covered by gluteal thigh flaps.

If a patient can tolerate the extirpative therapy, then he or she is a candidate for reconstruction. The massive postoperative fluid and protein loss of draining pelvic cavities is reduced by the flap fill. Males are preferred gracilis flap donors because of the muscle bulk. Moreover, wide gluteal thigh flap donor sites in muscular patients are difficult to close. Conversely, females, particularly moderately obese ones, donate broad gluteal thigh flaps with little morbidity. The posterior thigh scar is inconspicuous. He or she must accept that sitting will be uncomfortable for weeks after the operation, and that numbness in the popliteal space and paresthesia in the thigh can last from months to years.

The flaps may be done immediately after the abdominoperineal resection, and their pelvic positioning is made safe and accurate by the anterior approach. The lithotomy position is required and care in orienting the skin, muscle, and bone must be taken (Fig. 3). Errors can be avoided by preoperative marking.

Consideration must be given to an exclusive posterior approach or to one combined with anterior abdominal exposure. After general anesthesia of the patient, the bladder is catheterized with a 30 cc balloon Foley to help identify the posterior bladder wall. The patient is turned prone, and the buttock skin distracted with three-inch adhesive tape. The operating room table is slightly jackknifed.

The perineal pelvic wound extends to the new peritoneal reflection with small and/or large bowel close by. The midline sinus tract is usually lined with pseudoepithelium. Sharp dissection of granulation tissue and sinus tract may inadvertently injure intestine or bladder. To avoid visceral damage, vigorous curettage of the wound bed with large, sharp orthopedic instruments has been helpful. If adequate debridement cannot be safely done through the perineum, then an anterior approach to retract vulnerable organs is chosen. This measure had to be taken in only one of our patients.

Once the surgical defect is created, the choice of flap and how many is made. Note that bilateral gluteal thigh flaps allow for narrower flaps, easier donor site closure, and thigh symmetry. If a gracilis muscle flap is indicated, then two medial thigh incisions are made; the longer one proximal, and the shorter one near the knee. Through the distal incision, the round, tendinous portion of the muscle is identified. Through the proximal incision, the broad, flat, and smooth contour of the gracilis in noted. The muscle runs to the pubic ramus and distinguishes it from the semimembranosus muscle, which goes to the ischium. The more medially situated sartorius has a rougher contour and multiple perforating blood supply. Midway in the thigh, the sartorius diverges anterolaterally towards the anterosuperior iliac spine. After the gracilis is dissected free to its dominant proximal pedicle, the distal two-thirds can be turned and tunneled beneath the medial thigh skin through the ischiorectal space to the pelvic wound. Even small sinus tracts should be closed with a muscle flap. The temptation should be avoided, particularly in obese patients, to close the debrided perineal pelvic defect with local tissue only.

Two gluteal thigh flaps are obligatory to cover large surface areas and any pelvic wound that extends to both the presacral and retropubic space. The jackknife position allows for two-team simultaneous harvesting of bilateral gluteal thigh flaps; for a significant reduction in operative time. Flap elevation in experienced hands takes approximately 30 minutes. (Before perineal reconstruction is undertaken, the surgeon should gain facility with the use of the gluteal thigh flap by treating pressure sores).

The cutaneous extension of the inferior gluteal artery lies beneath the fascia lata of the thigh on the line that starts between the middle and medial thirds of the distance between the ischial tuberosity and the lateral trochanter of the thigh, and ends in the midpoint of the popliteal fossa (Fig. 4). In thin patients, particularly males, this vessel can be easily visualized as it accompanies the posterior cutaneous nerve of the thigh, which bowstrings as tension is placed on the flap surface. In obese patients, both the vessel and nerve can be difficult to identify. When there is fatty atrophy of the hamstring muscles, such as in

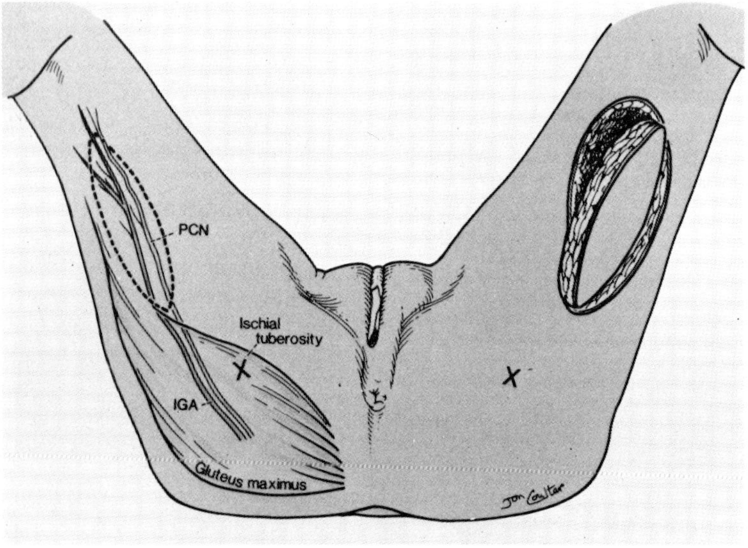

Figure 3 For vaginal reconstruction or flap elevation following abdominoperineal resection, the patient is in the lithotomy position. Flap islands should be marked prior to the procedure with the patient prone or standing for customary orientation. With the legs in stirrups, flaps lie lateral to the thigh midline.

chronic paraplegia, gauging dissection depth can be difficult, thereby making the sciatic nerve vulnerable to injury. With experience, one can confidently center the island skin paddle over the subfascial posterior thigh branch of the inferior gluteal artery. If the perineal sinus requires cavitary fill with no cutaneous coverage, as is the case in most wounds that result from abdominoperineal resection, then the flap is deeply de-epithelialized prior to elevation. At times, one de-epithelialized flap has been used for fill and another intact flap for coverage.

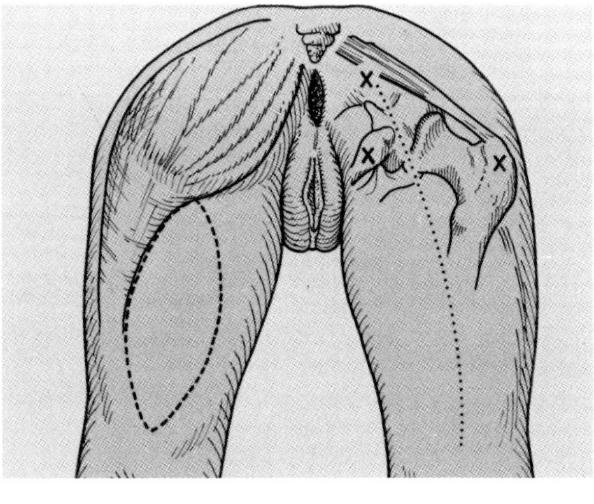

Figure 4 Jackknife position is the usual approach to perineal reconstruction. The midaxis of the flap is found by locating the three Xs noted on this diagram. The ischial tuberosity and the greater trochanter are easily palpated. Between the medial and middle thirds of a line between these two points, a perpendicular is drawn that extends from the inferior border of the piriformis muscle to the midportion of the popliteal muscle. The tip of the flap island is no higher than the gluteal fold, since a superior location would result in a tight closure over the ischial tuberosity.

The flap harvest is initiated by incision of the distal portion of the skin ellipse through the subcutaneous tissue, beveling slightly away from the skin edge of the flap. The fascia lata is first incised in the lateral thigh, where it is better developed. Loose areolar tissue is present beneath the fascia lata and is included with the flap by dissecting sharply onto the hamstring musculature. In women, particularly obese individuals, this layer will be thick. As soon as the tip of the flap has been elevated, a full-thickness holding suture, including fascia lata and skin, is secured to avoid shearing the vascularity. The middle portion of the flap is elevated by vigorous traction on the holding suture and firm countertraction on the bare muscular thigh. It is better to cut the hamstring muscles superficially than lacerate the vascular pedicle on the undersurface of the fascia lata. Perforators from the profundus system will be encountered periodically, and require transsection. As dissection proceeds towards the ischial tuberosity, a sweeping blunt push against the thigh muscles can be done since the soft tissues are less adherent to the flap at this level.

The caudal portion of the gluteus maximus muscle is identified with care so as to avoid injury to the flap pedicle, which has already been identified. A caudal cuff of gluteus muscle is usually left attached to the thigh flap (Fig. 5). When the fasciocutaneous branch of the inferior gluteal artery is well-developed, only the deep fascia of the gluteus maximus need be pedicled to the flap. When possible, the fasciocutaneous branch of the first deep femoral perforator, located near the lesser trochanter, should be preserved. It supplies generous posterior thigh skin blood supply, but will have to be transsected if it inhibits flap reach.

A tunnel is usually created under the inferior medial buttock skin to the ischiorectal space to relocate the de-epithelialized flap to the pelvic cavity (Fig. 6), or else a direct full-thickness incision can be made through the skin down through the ischiorectal space. After the flap is in position, it should be examined for dermal bleeding.

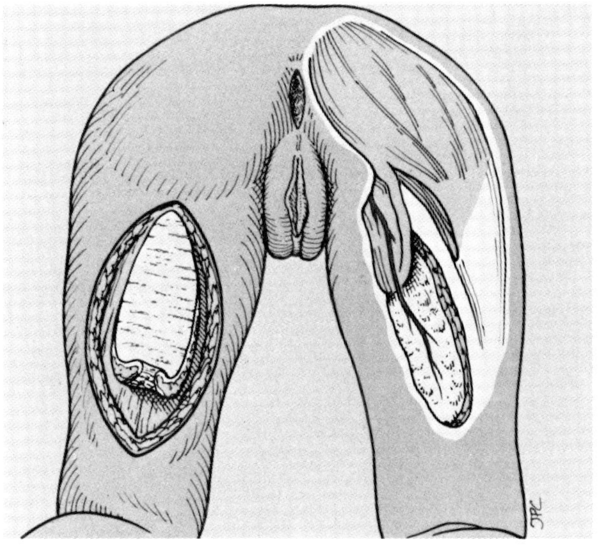

Figure 5 Shows the gluteal thigh flap in different stages of dissection. On the left, the flap has been deepithelialized and an elliptical beveled incision has been made down to the hamstring muscles. On the right, the undersurface of the flap is seen, and a cuff of the inferior border of the gluteus maximus muscle is included to avoid injury to the inferior gluteal artery.

When the traumatized distal tip of the flap is excised, wound edge bleeding is observed. Sluggish, dark venous ooze is not acceptable. The flap should be withdrawn and the approach revised.

When the distal extent of the pelvic cavity is too far for the tip of the flap to be secured to it, a dermal suture can be placed some distance from the tip and sewn to the presacral fascia (Fig. 7). After this stitch is tied, the tip of the flap can be flipped into position. Only a few key sutures need be placed to approximate the flap to its bed. The retracting adhesive tape is cut, and the buttock skin is sewn over the buried flap. Suction drains are placed in each of the donor sites and in the pelvic region, as postoperative drainage is expected (Fig. 8).

When a large flap is used, the donor site can be difficult to close without a skin graft. Primary closure may be impossible if the patient is obese. Liposuction of the

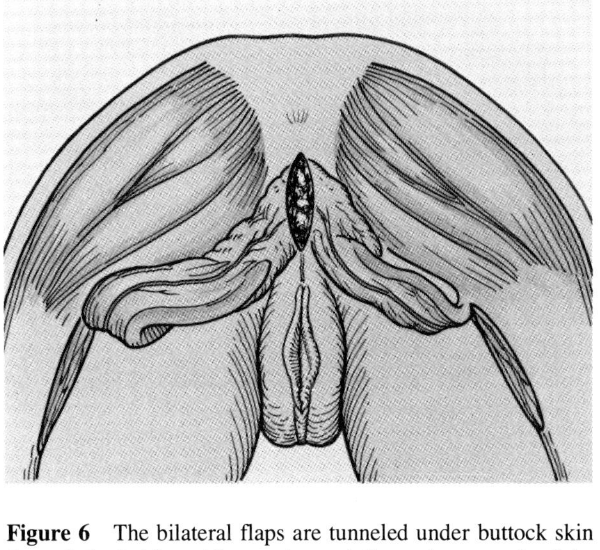

Figure 6 The bilateral flaps are tunneled under buttock skin through the ischiorectal space to reach the perineum and pelvis. Only a small portion of the inferior gluteus maximus need be taken with the flap.

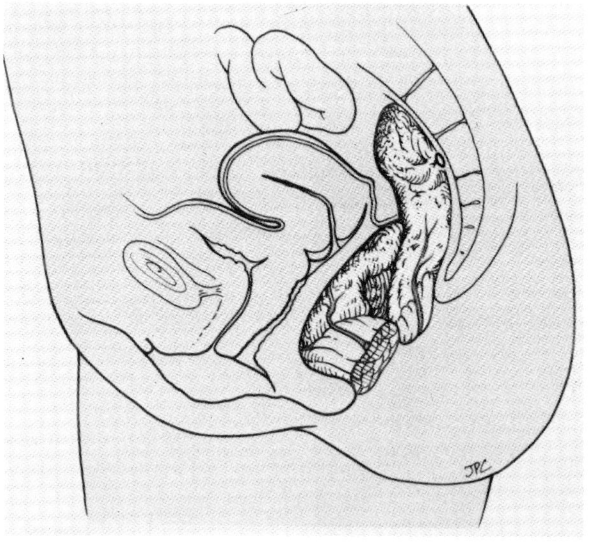

Figure 7 This sagittal view of the reconstruction shows why two flaps are necessary when the defect extends from near the retropubic space to the presacral space. To secure the flap towards the sacral promontory, a dermal suture is placed at as high a level as possible and sewn to the presacral fascia. The tip of the flap is then flipped into position.

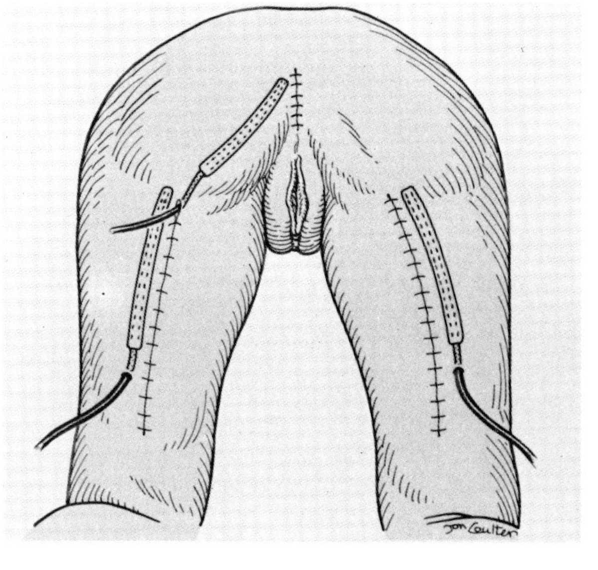

Figure 8 At closure, there is liberal use of suction drains. Skin replacement in the perineum is necessary only if a large amount of skin has been resected.

thigh assists in mobilizing the skin. The skin edges can be elevated above or below the level of the fascia lata. If the fascia lata is included, multiple longitudinal relaxing incisions are made to improve extensibility. The donor site is closed in two layers.

Patients are put on bedrest for several days if the closure is very tight. Otherwise, they are up the next day and allowed to sit after 4 days.

A de-epithelialized flap is buried only when the surgeon is confident of the blood supply. These flaps do not fail when properly raised from a well-vascularized extremity and carefully relocated into an adequately debrided cavity.

SUGGESTED READING

Cohen BE, Ryan JA. Gracilis muscle flap for closure of the persistent perineal sinus. Surg Gynecol Obstet 1969; 148:33–35.

Hurwitz DJ, Swartz WM, Mathes SJ. The gluteal thigh flap: a reliable, sensate flap for the closure of buttock and perineal wounds. Plast Reconstr Surg 1981; 68:521–529.

Hurwitz DJ, Walton RL. Closure of chronic wounds of the perineal and sacral regions using the gluteal thigh flap. Ann Plast Surg 1982; 8:375–386.

Hurwitz DJ, Zweibel PC. Gluteal thigh flap repair of chronic perineal wounds. Am J Surg 1985; 150:386–391.

Mathes SJ, Hurwitz DJ. Repair of chronic radiation wounds of the pelvis. World J Surg 1986; 10:269–280.

Mathes SJ, Nahai F. Clinical applications for muscle and musculocutaneous flaps. St. Louis: CV Mosby, 1982.

Silen W, Glotzer DS. The prevention and treatment of the perineal sinus. Surgery 1974; 75:535–542.

RECTAL SPHINCTER RECONSTRUCTION

MICHAEL G. ORGEL, M.D., F.A.C.S.

Reconstruction of the rectal sphincter may be indicated after disruptive trauma to or surgery of the anal region. When consideration is given to anal sphincter reconstruction, attention should be directed only to the external sphincter. The internal sphincter actually relaxes with rectal distention and, therefore, probably does not function in rectal continence. If possible, the external sphincter mechanism should be repaired by direct approximation. However, when a significant portion of this muscle is absent, severely scarred, or paralyzed, this method is doomed to failure. The presence of normal sensory nerve supply to the rectal ampulla is mandatory for any successful sphincter reconstruction. That is, the patient must be able to sense rectal distention and then contract the transferred voluntary muscle for temporary sphincter control.

THERAPEUTIC ALTERNATIVES

Therapeutic alternatives for rectal sphincter reconstruction utilize muscles from adjacent or more remote sites. Rectal continence has been achieved by reefing of the puborectalis sling above the destroyed rectal sphincter and this may be indicated when not injured by the original trauma. Part of the levator ani mechanism has also been used successfully for anal sphincter reconstruction. Since the motor nerve supply to the levator ani and external rectal sphincter are identical, the use of this muscle is somewhat limited.

Distant muscle transfers for rectal sphincter repair have concentrated on the gracilis muscle. However, successful control of rectal contents in children with myelomeningocele has not been uniformly repeated in the treatment of traumatic rectal incontinence in adults.

Gluteus maximus muscle transfer for rectal sphincter reconstruction predates the use of the gracilis muscle. Recent interest in this muscle for reconstructive problems in the perineal area has again directed attention to its use for sphincter reconstruction. Several case reports appeared in the literature prior to the use by my former colleague and myself of the gluteus maximus muscle for reconstruction of the anal sphincter. We modified reported techniques in order to transpose a well-vascularized innervated unit and ensure hip stability in the ambulatory patient.

Our preferred method for rectal sphincter reconstruction involves the use of the inferior half of one gluteus maximus muscle, detached from its insertion, transposed posteriorly, split longitudinally to surround the anus, and reinserted into the contralateral ischial tuberosity.

ANATOMY

The gluteus maximus muscle is a broad, flat muscle that originates on the gluteal line of the ilium and the sacrum and inserts into the gluteal tuberosity on the posterior aspect of the femur, and to the iliotibial tract (Fig. 1). The muscle functions as an extensor and lateral rotator of the femur and stabilizes the hip joint posteriorly. Either the superior or inferior half of the muscle should probably be left intact to preserve posterior hip stability in the ambulatory patient.

The blood supply to this muscle is derived from the

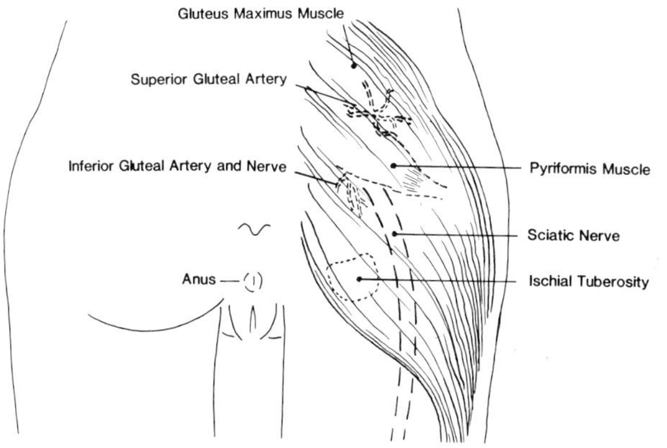

Figure 1 Anatomy of the gluteus maximus muscle. The inferior gluteal nerve also supplies the superior portion of the muscle. (Figures 1 to 4 are reproduced with permission from: Orgel MG, Kucan JO. A double-split gluteus maximus muscle flap for reconstruction of the rectal sphincter. Plast Reconstr Surg 1985; 75:62–66.)

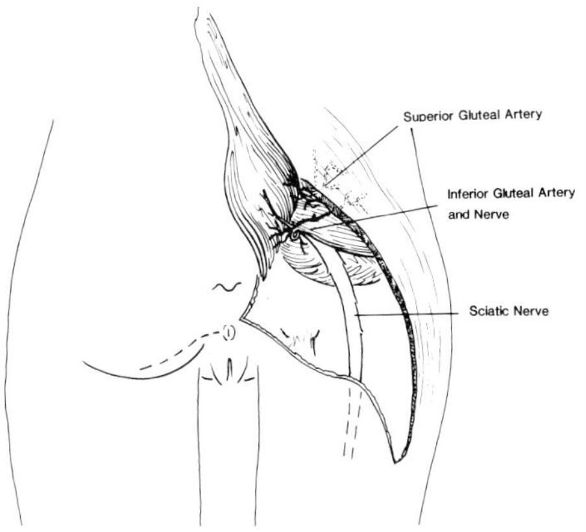

Figure 2 Incision lines and the raising of the inferior portion of the gluteus maximus muscle. Note proximity of sciatic nerve.

superior and inferior gluteal branches of the hypogastric artery that independently supply the superior and inferior halves of the muscle. However, the nerve supply to the muscle is singular and derives only from the inferior gluteal branch of the sciatic nerve. This nerve accompanies the inferior gluteal vascular pedicle and splits into superior and inferior branches near its origin to supply respective parts of the muscle.

SURGICAL TECHNIQUE

The patient is placed in a supine, flexed position on the operating table. Either gluteus maximus muscle may be chosen and a long incision is made on the selected side. It commences 2 cm from the anus, continues laterally just above the gluteal fold, and then extends in a gentle curve longitudinally over the femur (Fig. 2).

Skin flaps are elevated to visualize the total muscle in order to divide it accurately into superior and inferior halves. The muscle is then bluntly teased apart at this juncture, from origin to insertion, carefully preserving the nerve supply to the superior portion.

The inferior half of the gluteus maximus muscle is then detached from its insertions to the femur and the iliotibial tract and a generous strip of the fascia lata is retained for secure attachment of the muscle to the contralateral ischial tuberosity. This detached muscle half is then elevated from its bed and the underlying sciatic nerve should be kept in mind. The muscle should be mobilized until the inferior gluteal neurovascular bundle is visualized and carefully preserved.

The mobilized inferior half of the gluteus maximus muscle is then transposed posteriorly, and the extent of its second division is determined by positioning the muscle over the anus. Careful dissection then divides the muscle from this point to its distal insertion into two equal parts (Fig. 3). Few muscle fibers should be disrupted by this maneuver, and only small crossover vessels will be encountered. A mattress suture of nonabsorbable material should be placed at the apex of the second split to avoid further separation of the muscle when it is placed under tension around the anus.

A separate incision is then made on the contralateral buttock, from the ischial tuberosity to 2 cm from the anus (Figs. 2 and 4). The sacrotuberous ligament superficial to the ischial tuberosity is exposed for reinsertion of the gluteus muscle flap. Generous subcutaneous tunnels are then dissected anterior and posterior to the rectum to connect the medial portions of the buttock incisions. It is important to visualize the rectal wall on both sides at this point so that the reconstructed sphincter can function without the interposition of extraneous tissue. The split halves of the muscle flap are then threaded through the anterior and posterior tunnels, and the distal ends are sutured to themselves and to the periosteum and ligamentous tissue over the ischial tuberosity, with the retained

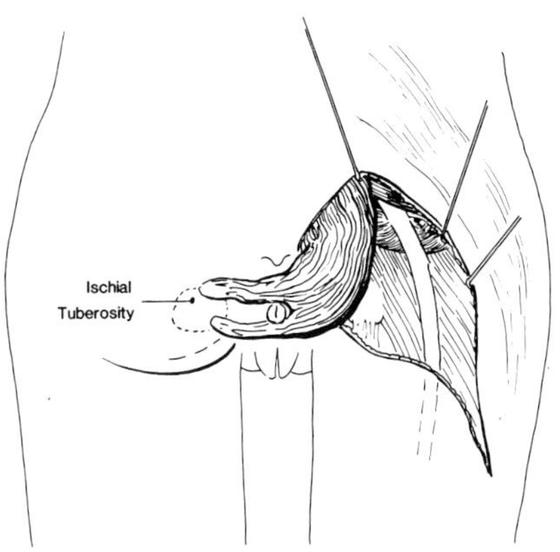

Figure 3 Further splitting of the inferior half of the gluteus maximus muscle. Muscle position over anus determines extent of muscle split.

fascia lata being used for a secure purchase (see Figs. 3 and 4). Correct tensioning of the muscle can be aided by accurately spaced superficial sutures in the distal muscle, placed prior to detachment of the muscle from its insertion. The muscle is then stretched to these measurements again when it is reinserted into the ischial tuberosity. The superior and inferior muscle halves are then reunited from the ischial tuberosity to the anus with nonabsorbable suture material. Only small bites of muscle are taken so that neurovascular function is preserved. It is important to "cinch up" the muscle to both sides of the rectum so that the anus is as tight as possible (rectal examination should admit only the small finger). We have not seen a reconstructed sphincter that was too tight. The opposite situation, however, was the rule until the importance of this step was realized.

The wounds are thoroughly irrigated, suction drains are placed bilaterally, and a layered closure of the skin flaps is performed. Colostomy diversion of the feces has not been utilized in our patients unless already in place. A low residue diet is used postoperatively until the wounds are well sealed. The patient is rolled to a standing position and ambulated the first postoperative day. Sitting and conscious contraction of the gluteus maximus muscles are avoided for a period of 3 weeks.

PATIENT SELECTION AND TIMING OF TREATMENT

Most of our patients have sustained trauma to the anal region that has caused significant disruption, or loss, of a portion of the external sphincter. Almost all of these patients have had one or more attempts at direct repair of the sphincter. We have not treated any patients who have had surgical ablation of the anal region for disease control, although this, theoretically, would be possible. However, as noted above, successful reconstruction of the anal sphincter depends upon an intact sensory nerve supply to the rectal ampulla. This point must be determined by history, physical examination, and possible neurologic workup prior to institution of therapy.

Rectal sphincter reconstruction with the double-split gluteus maximus muscle flap may be done at any time after scar maturation has occurred, to allow the determination of correct surgical planes. Our original report documents successful repair of the external anal sphincter mechanism up to 12 years after the traumatic event.

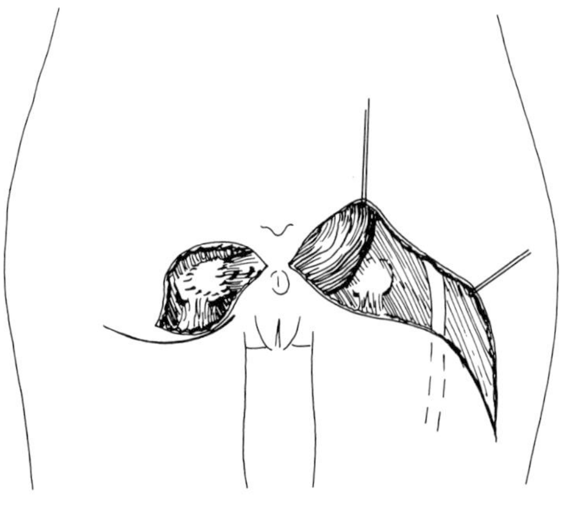

Figure 4 Attachment of muscle to the contralateral ischial tuberosity. Note fascial attachment to distal muscle and ischial tuberosity. Nonabsorbable suture reunites the muscle halves to form the sphincter.

SURGICAL PRINCIPLES

The successful use of the gluteus maximus muscle for rectal sphincter reconstruction involves careful analysis of the problem and correct selection of patients. The surgical approach is then based upon the following principles:

1. Preoperative bowel preparation is similar to that for any colonic or rectal surgery. Routine use of a diverting colostomy is not necessary.
2. Full exposure of the muscle for an accurate first division.
3. Careful preservation of the neurovascular supply to the inferior half, and the nerve supply to the superior half of the muscle.
4. Retention of a generous piece of fascia lata for strong reinsertion of the muscle.
5. Use of nonabsorbable suture material for insertion of the muscle to opposite ischial tuberosity and for reunification of the muscle portions around the anus.

It is most important to free the rectum from surrounding scar and subcutaneous tissues at the level of the anterior and posterior tunnels. It is then possible to suture the muscle halves accurately and securely up to the rectal wall. A lighted retractor or head lamp improves visualization for this critical step.

Both incisions should be drained at the time of wound closure. It had been our policy to drain only the donor wound until we saw, in two patients, the development of a small hematoma and subsequent infection on the reinsertion side. This problem has been solved subsequent to bilateral wound drainage. Prophylactic antibiotics have also been used just prior to surgery and for 24 to 48 hours postoperatively.

RESULTS

Patients who undergo rectal sphincter reconstruction with this unilateral gluteus maximus muscle flap have not experienced normal rectal sphincter function. However, all patients have developed the ability to control rectal contents by activating the reconstructed sphincter. Most patients have been able to return to their previous occupations and no longer require the use of absorbable padding in their underclothing. Episodes of diarrhea, however, may cause a temporary relapse to partial incontinence, because the reconstructed sphincter cannot sustain tonus as well as the normal sphincter.

Several patients have required a second operative procedure to tighten a lax, reconstructed sphincter after the development of infection secondary to hematoma on the side of reinsertion of the muscle flap. Suction drainage on both sides and the use of permanent suture material to construct the sphincter have decreased the incidence of these problems.

Although we have no experience with rectal sphincter reconstruction after surgical ablation of the anal region, the double-split gluteus maximus muscle flap may find further use for this purpose. If normal sensation is present in the retained segment, a "pull through" procedure could be used that would obviate the need for the full second split of the muscle. When the motor nerve supply to the rectal sphincter and contiguous, similarly innervated muscles has been destroyed, the gluteus maximus muscle, with its isolated neurovascular supply, may be the donor of choice for reconstitution of rectal continence.

Thanks are given to John O. Kucan, M.D., my former associate, with whom the idea for this reconstructive procedure was formulated.

SUGGESTED READING

BenHur N, Gilai A, Golan J, Sagher U, Issac M. Reconstruction of the anal sphincter by gracilis muscle transfer: the value of electromyography in the preoperative assessment and postoperative management of the patient. Br J Plast Surg 1980; 33:156–160.

Berek JS, Lagasse LD, Hacker NF, Leuchter RS. Levator ani transposition for anal incompetence secondary to sphincter damage. Obstet Gynecol 1982; 59:108–112.

Bruining HA, Bos KE, Colthoff EG, Tolhurst DE. Creation of an anal sphincter mechanism by bilateral proximally based gluteal muscle transposition. Plast Reconstr Surg 1981; 67:70–72.

Castro AF, Pittman RE. Repair of the incontinent sphincter. Dis Colon Rectum 1978; 21:183–187.

Hentz VR. Construction of a rectal sphincter using the origin of the gluteus maximus muscle. Plast Reconstr Surg 1982; 70:82–85.

Holschneider AM, Hecker WC. Reverse smooth muscle plasty: a new method of treating anorectal incontinence in infants with high anal and rectal atresia. J Pediatr Surg 1981; 16:917–920.

Orgel MG, Kucan JO. A double-split gluteus maximus muscle flap for reconstruction of the rectal sphincter. Plast Reconstr Surg 1985; 75:62–66.

Pickrell KL, Broadbent TR, Masters FW, Metzger JT. Construction of a rectal sphincter and restoration of anal continence by transplanting the gracilis muscle. Ann Surg 1952; 135:853–862.

GENITOURINARY STRUCTURES

HYPOSPADIAS

CHARLES E. HORTON, M.D., F.A.C.S.
MARTHA S. MATTHEWS, M.D.

Hypospadias is one of the most common urogenital anomalies and occurs in one out of every 300 infants. It is defined as a proximal malposition of the urethral meatus on the ventral surface of the penis. This is caused by an arrest in development of the male genitalia due to withdrawal of normal androgen stimulation. The abnormal meatus may be anywhere from proximal glans to perineum. It is associated with a deficiency of corpus spongiosum, Buck's fascia, and dartos fascia and is frequently associated with ventral curvature of the penis, know as chordee. Our approach to hypospadias is based on complete and accurate diagnosis, careful parental counseling, and a team approach to treatment that utilizes the expertise of plastic surgery and urologic surgical disciplines.

DIAGNOSIS AND PREOPERATIVE EVALUATION

Diagnosis of hypospadias should ideally be made in the newborn nursery, although repair is normally not undertaken until the penis is of adequate size. Circumcision is contraindicated in these infants, as the prepuce is an important source of tissue for later repair.

Initial evaluation of hypospadias categorizes the meatal position as glandular, distal, or proximal. In glandular hypospadias, the meatus is proximal to its normal position on the tip of the glans, yet entirely on the glans. Distal hypospadias occurs when the meatus is at, or just proximal to, the coronal sulcus. The term proximal hypospadias encompasses meatus from midshaft to perineum and can be further delineated into proximal shaft, scrotal, and perineal types.

Recognition of chordee is important for complete correction of the condition. Chordee is ventral curvature of the penis, caused by abnormal fibrous tissue that spans the gap between the proximally displaced meatus and the glans. This often becomes more prominent as the child grows and is most obvious with erection. Most children with hypospadias have chordee as well.

Initial evaluation of the infant with hypospadias includes a search for other abnormalities. A number of inherited syndromes are associated with hypospadias. Other congenital anomalies, particularly peculiar facies, skull, and hand abnormalities, should alert the clinician to possible syndromes. Marked proximal hypospadias, undescended testes, and penile-scrotal transposition indicate possible intersex abnormalities. Full evaluation of these children, including chromosomal studies, is mandatory prior to surgery.

Parental counseling is an important aspect of care. Parents are concerned about the prognosis for normal urologic and sexual function, permanent deformity, and the risk of future offspring being affected. We advise the parents that the repair is normally accomplished in one stage. We delay surgery until the child is old enough to cooperate with his care, at approximately 2 years of age. Repair is completed prior to entry into school. Parents of children with glandular hypospadias are advised that the deformity is principally cosmetic; yet significant psychological distress can result from being "different." We feel repair is indicated for this reason.

Although the majority of cases of hypospadias are idiopathic, there are some autosomal dominant and recessive conditions that are associated with hypospadias. Recognition of these syndromes is important for genetic counseling of the parents. It appears that the incidence of hypospadias in siblings of a child with idiopathic hypospadias is not increased.

As the child reaches the age for surgical intervention, a careful history is taken and a physical examination is again performed. This should include, if possible, observation of voiding and erection. Cystourethrography is done if there is suggestion of voiding difficulties. If kidney pathology is suspected, the patient should have ultrasound or intravenous pyelography. Cystoscopy is usually done at the time of repair, but may be done preoperatively. Intersex work-up, when indicated, should be complete. Routine laboratory work-up prior to surgery includes a complete blood count and urinalysis.

THE HOSPITAL EXPERIENCE

Hospitalization and surgery, particularly on such a psychologically sensitive area as the genitalia, are anxiety-laden experiences for parents and child. We make every attempt to minimize this, as a relaxed and cooperative child is much easier to treat. When possible, the child is admitted on the morning of surgery, thereby avoiding unnecessary and stressful preoperative hospitalization. All surgery is done at a pediatric hospital, which has preoperative teaching programs geared to children and parents. Parents are encouraged to room-in with the child and assist in his care. Access to the reconstructive team is important for the parents and is facilitated by the presence of a nurse clinical specialist.

In the postoperative period, every attempt is made to keep the child comfortable. Pain medication is available intravenously if needed. The patient is kept supine in Trendelenburg position for 48 hours to decrease edema. Small children often require leg restraints to prevent them from turning and a bed cradle is used to keep heavy blankets off the repair. Strict bedrest is maintained for about 5 days.

OPERATIVE TECHNIQUES

General

Some features are common to all hypospadias repairs. Meticulous, gentle technique is vital. All proposed incisions are marked prior to surgery. Fine instruments and sutures are used, as is magnification when necessary. Careful hemostasis is mandatory. When large tissue flaps are elevated, drains are used as well. We use either minivac or Penrose drains, which are removed on the first postoperative day.

Cystoscopy is done on virtually all patients. Utricular abnormalities, strictures, and diverticuli are noted. Artificial erection is done on all patients to check for chordee. A small butterfly catheter is placed into one of the corporal bodies. Both corporal bodies are compressed in the perineum and injectable saline is instilled through the catheter. This produces an erection that is reversible by releasing pressure on the corporal bodies; it can be repeated.

A stay stitch of 4–0 silk is placed in the dorsum of the glans at the beginning of the procedure. This is helpful during the case for traction and stabilization of the penis and, at the conclusion, it can be used to anchor the urethral stent.

Bladder drainage is employed for all patients. Those who have flip-flap repairs have a stent made of a No. 8 French Silastic tube and a No. 5 French feeding tube is run through the stent into the bladder. The smaller tube is removed about 5 days postoperatively and the child can void through the stent. Suprapubic tubes are used in conjunction with full-thickness grafts and preputial flaps. These repairs are also stented with a No. 8 French tube. Perineal urethrostomy is rarely done.

Antiobiotic prophylaxis with a parenteral cephalosporin is routine. The suture lines are kept clean with peroxide swabs. We use Bioocclusive (Ethicon) as a postoperative dressing. It adheres well, protects the wounds and also provides postoperative compression.

Specific Techniques

The procedure of choice for glandular hypospadias is the meatal advancement, or MAGPI, procedure (Fig. 1).

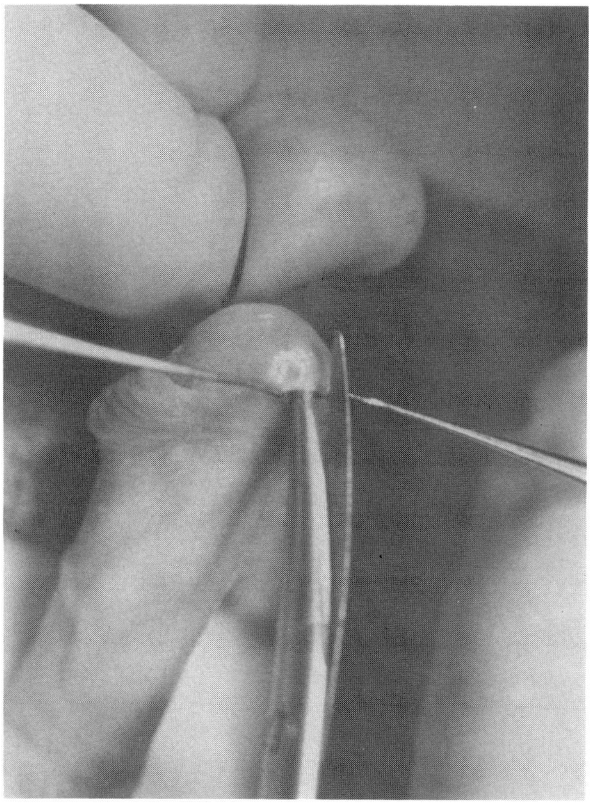

Figure 1 MAGPI procedure. Dorsal urethral wall incised longitudinally to glans tip.

The dorsal wall of the urethral groove is incised longitudinally to the glans tip. The incision is then closed transversely with 6–0 chromic suture. A circumcising incision is done and the ventral glans is freed from the corporal bodies in two wings on either side of the urethra. These wings are then reapproximated in the midline with 5–0 PDS (polydioxanone, Ethicon) deep sutures and 6–0 chromic skin sutures. This corrects the typical spatulate glandular deformity. The circumcision is then completed and the wound closed with 6–0 chromic suture. We do not routinely use urinary catheters in these patients.

Those patients with distal shaft hypospadias and *no chordee* are treated with a flip-flap urethral repair (Fig. 2). A flap is outlined on the ventral shaft skin, based on the existing meatus. The flap is slightly wider than the diameter of the meatus and long enough to reach the glans tip. This flap will be flipped up to become the ventral wall of the urethra. The dorsal wall is formed from the urethral groove from the meatus to the glans. The dorsal wall is marked and the skin is incised. The skin edges of what will become the dorsal urethral wall are elevated enough for suture to the flip-flap. The flap is elevated above Buck's fascia to the meatus and then turned up. It is sutured to the dorsal wall with a running subcuticular suture of 6–0 PDS. Care is taken to invert the epithelium into the neourethra. The anastomosis is then checked for leaks with dilute methylene blue. The glans wings are elevated and advanced to the midline, as described earlier. The new meatus is attached to the glans with 6–0 chromic suture. A subcoronal circumcision incision is completed, and the pre-

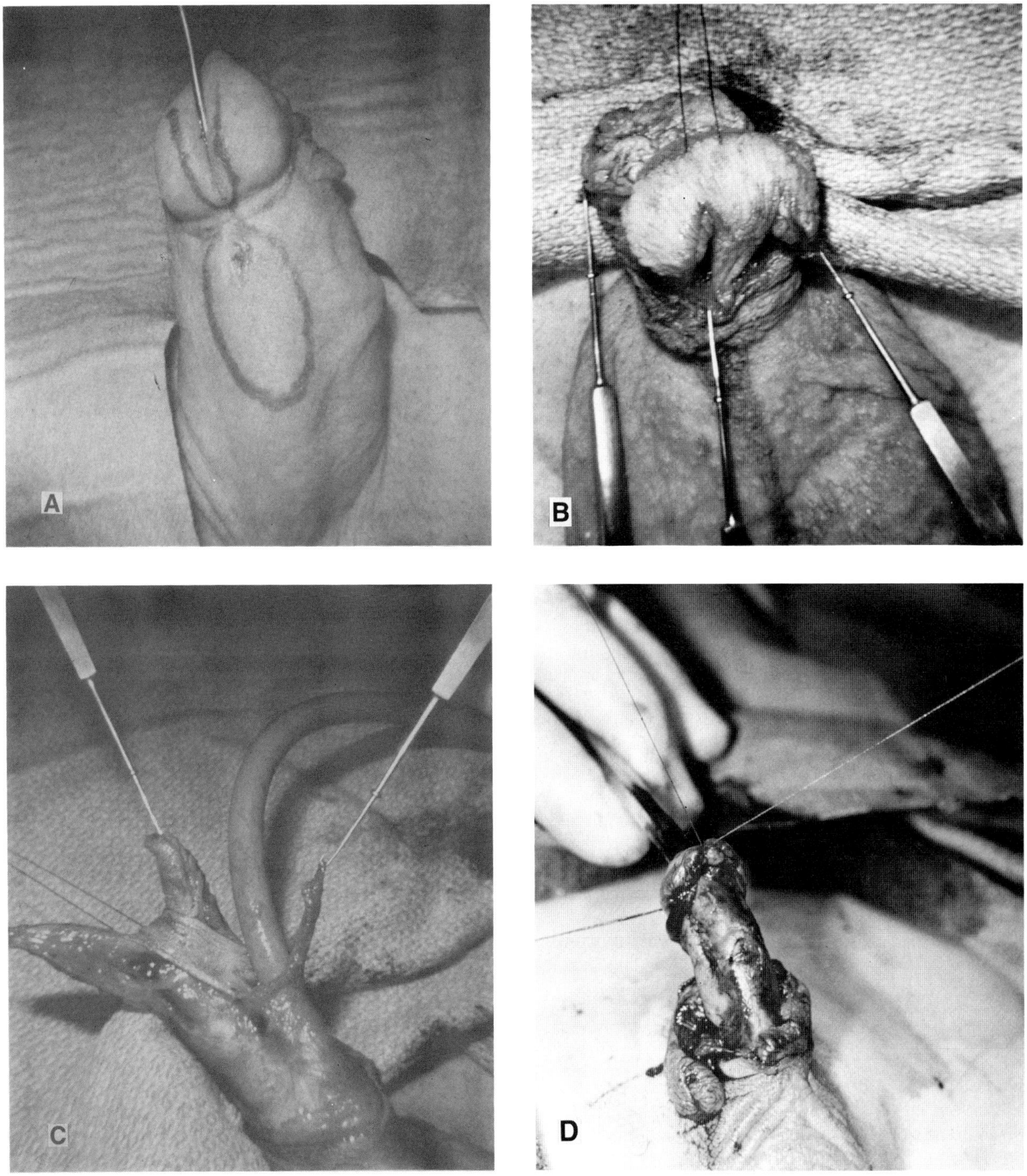

Figure 2 Flip-flap procedure. *A*, Flip-flap outlined on glans and shaft. *B*, Glans wings developed. *C*, Flip-flap elevated and sutured to V-flap of urethral groove. *D*, Glans wings reapproximated over completed neourethra.

puce is elevated. It is split dorsally, and the redundant skin is brought ventrally to close the shaft. The incisions are closed with 5–0 PDS subcuticular suture and 6–0 chromic skin suture. The repair is stented with a No. 8 French Silastic tube and the bladder is drained with a No. 5 French tube.

In the case of distal hypospadias *with chordee*, the flip-flap remains the same, but the treatment of the dorsal wall of the neourethra differs. The flip-flap is marked and elevated as previously described. The circumcision incision is made, and the penis is degloved above the level of Buck's fascia. A V-flap is marked on the glans with its base at the glans tip and its apex at the coronal sulcus. It is incised and the V is elevated from the glans. All chordee is excised between the old meatus and the glans and is checked with an artificial erection. The V-flap from the glans is advanced across the defect to the meatus. A slit is made in the dorsal wall of the meatus, and the tip of the V-flap is inset and sutured in place with 5–0 PDS. The flip-flap is then turned up and sutured to the limbs of the V-flap with 6–0 subcuticular PDS. The V-flap becomes the dorsal wall of the neourethra, and the flip-flap becomes the ventral wall. Glans wings are developed as before, preputial skin is redraped, and the wounds are closed.

In proximal hypospadias, the urethra can be reconstructed either with a full-thickness skin graft (Fig. 3) or an island preputial flap (Fig. 4). We do not have a strong preference for one over the other, but tend to use the full-thickness skin graft more often.

Both procedures begin with a subcoronal skin incision, as well as a midventral vertical incision from the coronal sulcus down to and around the meatus. The penis

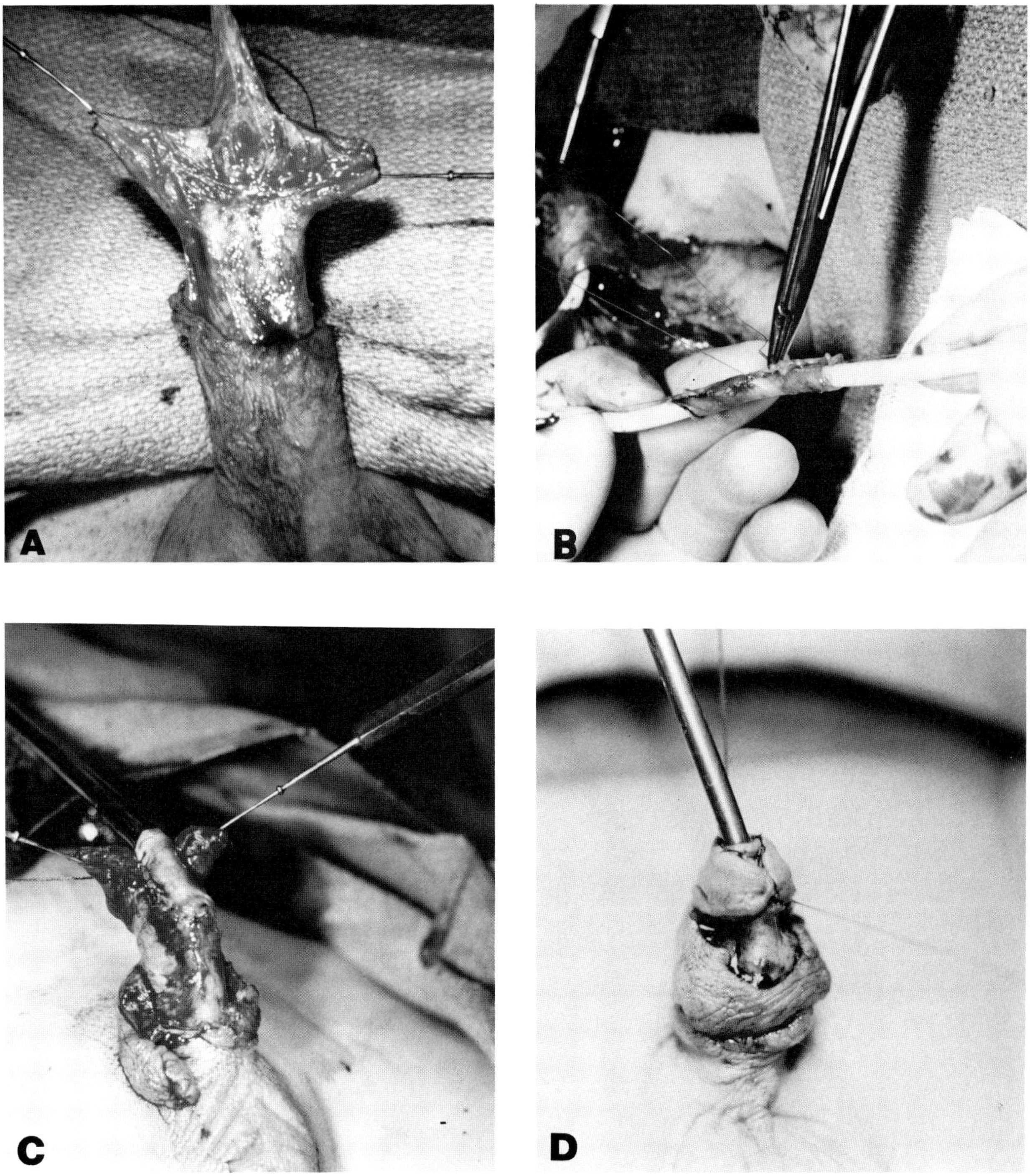

Figure 3 Full thickness graft. *A*, V-flap and glans wings developed. *B*, Full thickness graft tubed. *C*, Proximal anastomosis completed and distal end sewn to V-flap and glans. *D*, Glans wings closed.

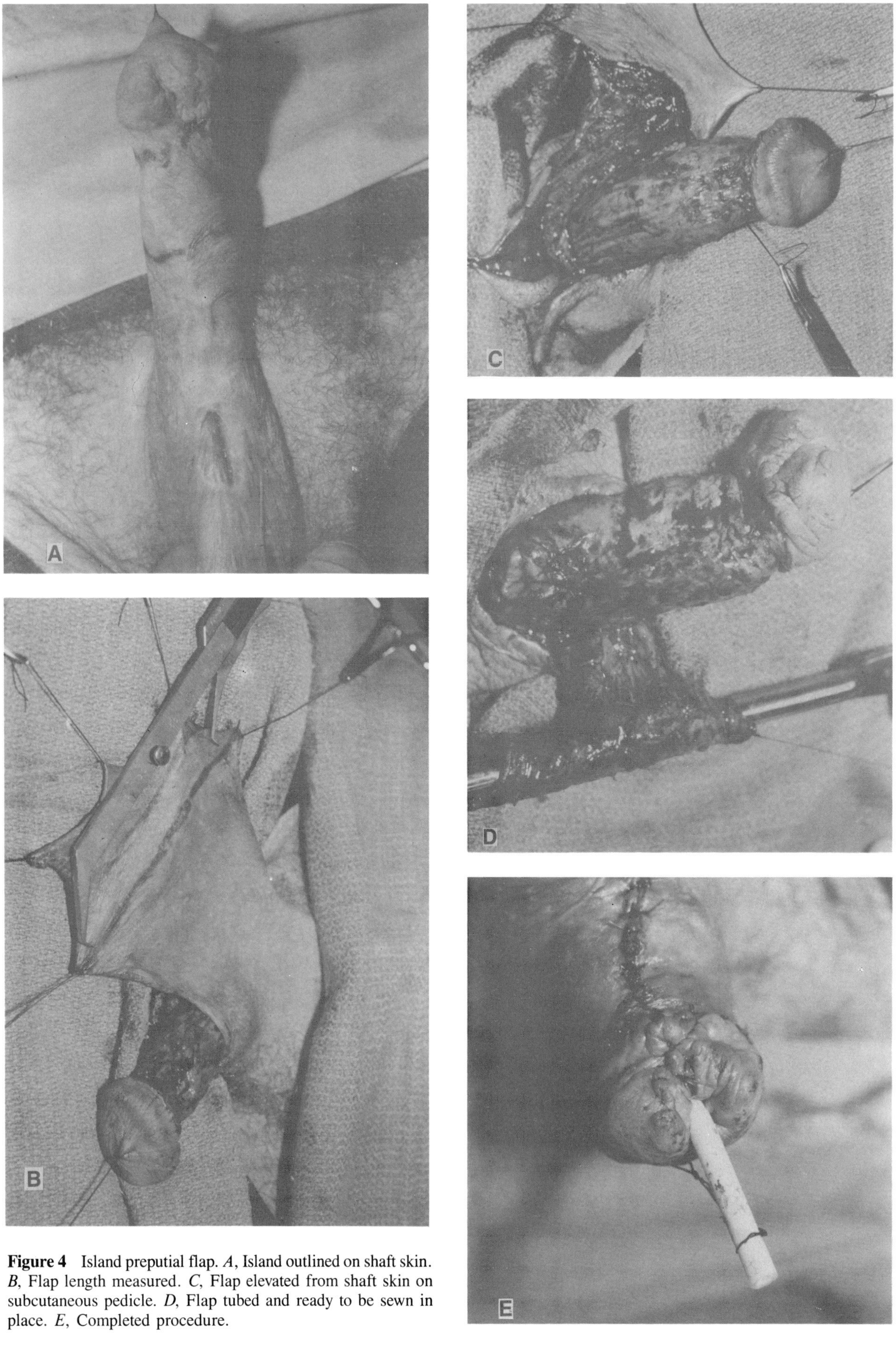

Figure 4 Island preputial flap. *A*, Island outlined on shaft skin. *B*, Flap length measured. *C*, Flap elevated from shaft skin on subcutaneous pedicle. *D*, Flap tubed and ready to be sewn in place. *E*, Completed procedure.

is then degloved above Buck's fascia. All chordee is resected, and artificial erection is done to check for residual chordee.

When a full-thickness graft is planned (see Fig. 3), the native meatus is freed slightly and a 2 to 3 mm vertical slit is made ventrally to accept a spatulated anastomosis. A V-flap is outlined on the glans and glans wings are developed. An appropriately sized ellipse of skin is then outlined on the prepuce of adequate length to span the defect after being tubed. The ellipse is excised as a full-thickness graft and trimmed to remove all subcutaneous fat. The graft is then tubed over an appropriately sized (corresponding to the normal proximal urethra) No. 12 French catheter with skin side facing in. It is sewn with running 6–0 PDS suture, with care taken to invert the skin into the lumen. The proximal and distal anastomoses are then constructed in a spatulate fashion using 6–0 PDS suture. The glans wings are closed over the neourethra, and the neomeatus is sewn to the glans with interrupted 6–0 chromic suture. The remaining preputial skin is divided down the midline (Byers), brought ventrally, and then redraped and closed with subcuticular 5–0 PDS and interrupted 6–0 chromic sutures. If there is inadequate preputial skin, the full-thickness graft can be harvested as an ellipse from the flank. The donor site is closed primarily with 5–0 Vicryl and 5–0 nylon suture.

The other option, when adequate preputial skin exists, is the island preputial flap. After the subcoronal and ventral incisions have been made, as described above, a rectangular flap is outlined on the distal dorsal skin of the portion of the prepuce that faces the glans. The long axis of the flap is oriented transversely. Its length equals the length of the defect and its width the circumference of the neourethra. The proximal edge of the flap is incised just through the epidermis. With the use of fine hooks for traction and fine pointed scissors, the dorsal penile skin is elevated from the dartos fascia and the subcutaneous tissue immediately beneath it. The blood supply for the distal skin paddle is provided by dorsal linear vessels, which can be dissected from the dorsal penile skin and used to transfer the preputial flap to the ventral side of the penis. The pedicle is dissected free for the width of the flap and is of sufficient length to allow rotation to the ventral surface of the penis. After the flap is elevated, it is tubed around a sound with 6–0 subcuticular PDS. All chordee is corrected. Proximal and distal anastomoses are spatulated and sewn with 6–0 chromic suture. As with the full-thickness graft, glans wings are developed and brought ventrally, and the remaining skin is redraped and closed. If vascularity of the flap is questionable, this can be checked with fluorescein. If the flap does appear devascularized, it can be used as a full-thickness graft. The pedicle must not be twisted as the flap is transferred to the ventral surface of the penis.

Both the full-thickness graft and the preputial flap are stented for 10 days. Urinary diversion is by suprapubic tube. A voiding trial is done on the tenth day. If there is no fistula, the suprapubic tube is left clamped and the child is discharged. The suprapubic tube is removed in the office.

SUGGESTED READING

Barakat AV, Seikaly MG, Der Kaloustian VM, et al. Urogenital abnormalities in genetic disease. J Urol 1986; 136(4):778–785.

Blair VP, Byers LT. Hypospadius and epispadius. J Urol 1938; 40:814.

Duckett JW. MAGPI (meatoplasty and planoplasty): a procedure for subcoronal hypospadias. Urol Clin North Am 1981; 8(3):513–519.

Horton CE Jr, Horton CE. Complications of hypospadius surgery. Clin Plast Surg 1988; 15(3):371–380.

Sadove RC, Horton CE, McRoberts JW. The new era of hypospadius surgery. Clin Plast Surg 1988; 15(3):341–354.

Vorstman B, et al. Current hypospadias techniques. Ann Plast Surg 18(2):164–173.

PHALLOPLASTY

DONALD R. LAUB, M.D., F.A.C.S.
DONALD R. LAUB Jr., M.S.
VINCENT R. HENTZ, M.D.

What greater damage to body image is there than absence or loss of the penis? Greater losses do exist, but the deficit of penis loss and the technical complexity of its restoration support the first statement.

The challenge of the reconstructive genitourinary surgeon in the 1980s is the formation of a penis with:

1. Sensitivity.
2. The ability to stand to urinate.
3. A passable to good appearance.
4. Ability for intromission in sexual intercourse.

Gilbert has enunciated these criteria on several occasions.

The techniques for achieving the construction of a penis are evolving rapidly. The techniques for gender dysphoria and for traumatic amputation are similar in principle and can be discussed together.

The professionals who have worked in the field of gender dysphoria for a number of years have become familiar with this disease entity. Most workers have come to the belief that the gender dysphoric patient carries a discrepancy that is as valid an indication for surgery as that in the intersex patient. The lack of wholeness of the gender dysphoric patient lies in the difference between the gender of body and mind.

The surgeon adjusts the anatomy of the body after legal, economic, social sexual, and psychological adjustments are complete in the gender of choice. The task of the social scientist is to determine the true gender and whether the particular patient is appropriate for surgery.

Workers approach the patients with principles of rehabilitation in mind: that interdisciplinary talent is needed; that patients must enter society as workers; and that self-help is superior to help from others. The surgeons change the body to fit what has been determined to be the real, or true, or best gender. As Edgerton has said: "We deal with gender confirmation surgery, not sex-change surgery."

With this philosophy, the Harry Benjamin International Gender Dysphoria Association (HBIGDA) was born as a professional association in 1978, so that the disciplines could interchange information and, most importantly, set down professional guidelines to help define the appropriate patients for surgery. The HBIGDA guidelines for gender confirmation surgery have begun to be accepted by the legal profession, third party insurance payers, the medical professions, and in the malpractice "arena." The guidelines contain prerequisite criteria for the diagnosis of gender dysphoria. Two social scientists, one with Ph.D. or equivalent, must participate in the diagnosis. One of these must have known the patient over a 6-month period. The patient must have had feelings of being in the wrong body or demonstrated discomfort in the gender role for at least 2 years, must be free of psychosis, and must desire to rid him or herself of the genitalia. The criteria for surgery are: (1) recommendation in writing by two behavioral scientists, one of whom has been in a therapeutic relationship with the patient for 6 months and (2) successful cross-living test over a 1-year period with legal, social, psychological, and sexual success accomplished during this period. Before any gender surgical rearrangement is performed, there is appropriate monitoring and documenting of other medical conditions, as well as the effects of hormones upon the liver and other organ systems.*

Presented here is a menu of surgery options in the interest of perspectives (Table 1). Our own choices are emphasized, as might be expected. "Post Modern" Phalloplasty, called Plan A, is preferred as the top of the line. Plan A, meets most of the criteria of Gilbert and consists of the Chinese forearm flap for sensibility and the neourethra the standard midline abdominal flap for shaft bulk, a split-thickness skin graft for shaft surfacing, and a baculum for mechanical support during intromission (Fig. 1).

TABLE 1 Post Modern Phalloplasty

Experience	
Standard abdominal tubes	180
Post modern phalloplasties	6
Traumatic loss (tree shredder)	1
F→M gender dysphoria	5
Morbidity	
Flap loss, total or partial	0
Venous occlusion ("take back")	1
Abscess, perineum	1
Fistula, urinary	2
Poor nerve regrowth (not fully assessed)	2

* The "Guidelines" may be obtained from the Harry Benjamin Gender Dysphoria Association Inc, Judy Von Maasdam, Executive Director, 900 Welch Road 20, Palo Alto, CA 95304.

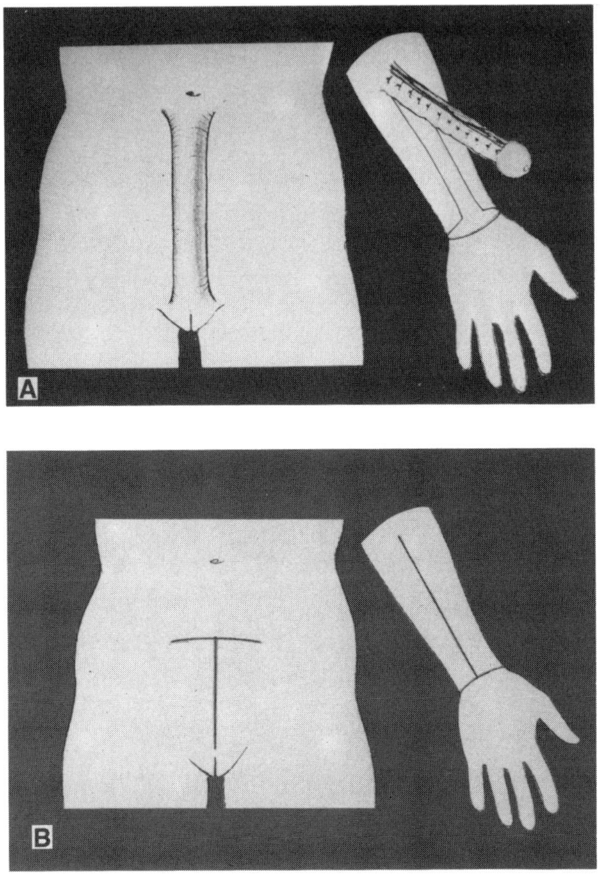

Figure 1 *A,* Diagram of the tissues used for the Post Modern Phalloplasty: a midline abdominal bipedicle flap for shaft bulk surfaced with split-thickness skin graft and the radial forearm flap for the neourethra and sensibility. *B,* Diagram of residual defects.

A definite alternate plan is metaoidioplasty (available only for gender dysphoric patients), which utilizes local existing tissue of the female external genitalia to fashion male external genitalia (Plan B).

Another alternative is the midline abdominal flap that uses devices rather than surgery to achieve function (Plan C) (Fig. 2).

In the Post Modern Phalloplasty, the ingredients are:

1. Sensitivity: lateral antebrachial cutaneous nerve from Chinese flap.
2. Urethra: glabrous skin from forearm—Chinese flap—smooth external appearance—split-thickness skin graft from hip.
3. Appearance: smooth surface from split-thickness skin graft, and bulk from subcutaneous tissue of midline abdominal flap.
4. Intromission: radial artery tumescence or baculum insertion.

More specifically, the standard midline abdominal tube pedicle flap is a fasciocutaneous flap based on the superficial external pudendal artery (SEPA) and not on

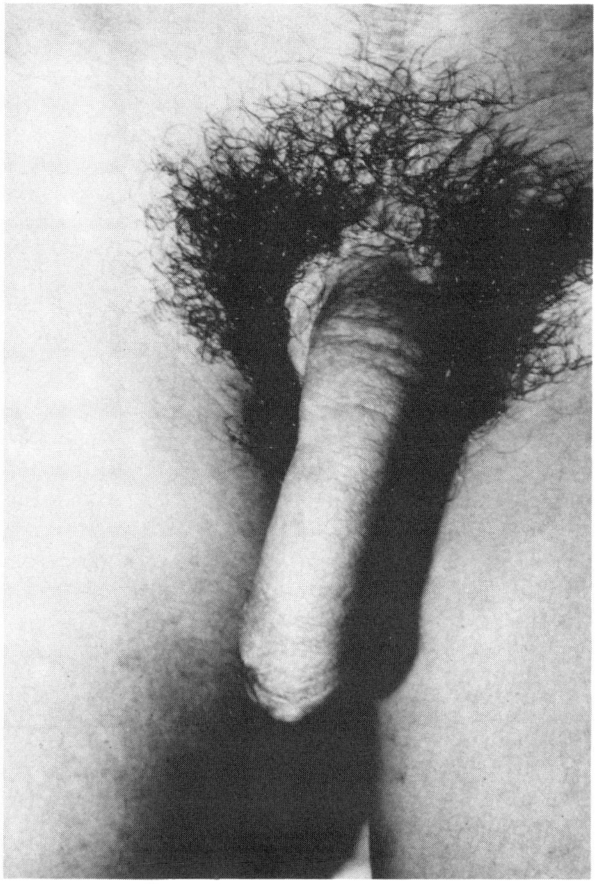

Figure 2 Example of the standard phalloplasty (not post modern) using midline lower abdominal inside-out pedicle flap, covered with a skin graft, placed on the external surface on Scarpa's fascia. Devices such as baculum and urinary assist device are necessary for function.

the superficial inferior epigastric artery. This flap is tubed inside-out and covered with a thick split-thickness skin graft for improved appearance. The resultant internal tunnel consists of abdominal skin. This phalloplasty is a two-stage procedure with a bipedicle tube formed in stage one.

The Chinese or radial forearm flap is based on the radial artery itself, which is then anastomosed to the deep inferior epigastric artery (DIEA) or the femoral artery itself. The lateral antebrachial cutaneous nerve of the flap is connected to the internal pudendal nerve (of Gilbert) for erotic cerebral connections. This flap is tissue-conservative in that it utilizes only a 3 cm by 2 cm strip of skin that can be closed as a linear scar. Preflap placement of tissue expanders into the forearm is usually helpful to obtain the best possible donor site scar. This flap is not associated with significant postoperative arm or hand morbidity.

The technical aspects, and the anatomic or physiologic reasons for these details, are as follows. Over the last 19 years, 195 phalloplasties have been performed using the midline abdominal inside-out SEPA-based fasciocutaneous flap (Plan C). Each surgical experience advances the technique in a small way. At the present time, only six combined or "Post Modern" Phalluses (Plan A) have been produced. The complications have been dealt with successfully by alteration of technique in subsequent cases. Forty metaoidioplasties (Plan B) have been performed, and none of them has completely brought the urinary stream to the tip of the glans. Bouman, as the first stage of phalloplasty, uses quite similar flaps (labia minora and anterior vagina) to form a neourethra just ventral to the clitoris. He quite correctly points out the embryologic homology of labia minora and male urethra pars fixa. He also notes that the result of his first stage is accepted as definitive therapy by some patients. However, in the brilliant surgery described by Eicher, the clitorispenoid, the patient does urinate from the neopenis, albeit with a more posteriorally placed penis than the metaoidioplasty. It is offered at the University of Mannheim, West Germany.

STAGE-ONE: ABDOMINAL SEPA FLAP

Two incisions are made in the anterior lower abdominal skin near the midline in the parasagittal position, from the level of the superior cleft of the labia majora, for 15 cm in a superior direction. The thickness of the abdominal wall is considered when determining the distance between these incisions. Some patients have more subcutaneous fatty tissue than others, and there is more subcutaneous fatty tissue in the mons veneris than in the concave configuration of the subcutaneous tissue in the infraumbilical hollow. The usual lower abdominal collection of fat that occurs in the female is familiar to those surgeons who perform suction-assisted lipoplasty procedures for body contouring. Typically, the pinch test is helpful in this determination. The incisions in any patient diverge from 5 to 10 cm apart in order to achieve uniform thickness of the penile shaft. If the free flap is planned as the second procedure, the penis is made more slim than usual because more tissue will be added at stage two. The subcutaneous tissue is undermined just subjacent to Scarpa's subcutaneous layer, and a bipedicle flap is tubed inside-out, with Scarpa's fascia and its great blood supply placed as the external surface of the tube (except near the seam or the suture line). One must beware because Scarpa's may easily close the entire tube under tension thereby creating a tourniquet effect and fatal ischemia. The abdominal skin forms an internal tunnel. The superficial inferior epigastric artery is sacrificed because it enters this tissue in a surprisingly superior position. The superficial external pudendal artery (SEPA) nourishes the flap with a fasciocutaneous circulation (documented recently by Patil, Dias, and Thatte). Some writers see no need to delay the flap; however, we do. The SEPA enters the tissue 2 cm superior to the most inferior incision. It must be gently pushed downward, yet be allowed to enter the tube without excessive tension. A thick (e.g., 18/1,000 inch) split-thickness skin graft is placed on the smooth external surface of the bipedicle flap on Scarpa's fascia. The skin graft is held in place with mild pressure of Davis and Geck black polyurethane foam prep ''sponges,'' sculptured and sutured in place around the tube flap. This gentle pressure is necessary. Without it, multiple seromas occur.

The flap donor site is closed with tension, using retention sutures and wide undermining. The foam sponges are removed at 1 week postoperatively. Both topical antibiotic solution and exposure to the air are used postoperatively to prevent infection over the ensuing 10 days.

STAGE TWO

Twelve weeks or more later, stage two is performed. It consists of parts or all of: (1) release of the upper end of the bipedicle flap, that forms the glans penis, and microsurgical transfer of forearm tissue, and (2) hysterectomy, bilateral salpingo-oophorectomy suction lipectomy, vaginectomy, and urethroplasty.

Patients who have not elected the microsurgical procedure utilize instead the baculum, which is placed in the skin tunnel on a p.r.n. basis for intercourse, and also use the urinary assist device in order to stand to urinate (Fig. 3).† Other patients have requested the microsurgery

† Baculum and Urinary Assist Device (UAD) may be obtained Precision Ocular Prosthetics. Tom Schulz, Anaplastologist, 39 Birch Street, Redwood City, CA.

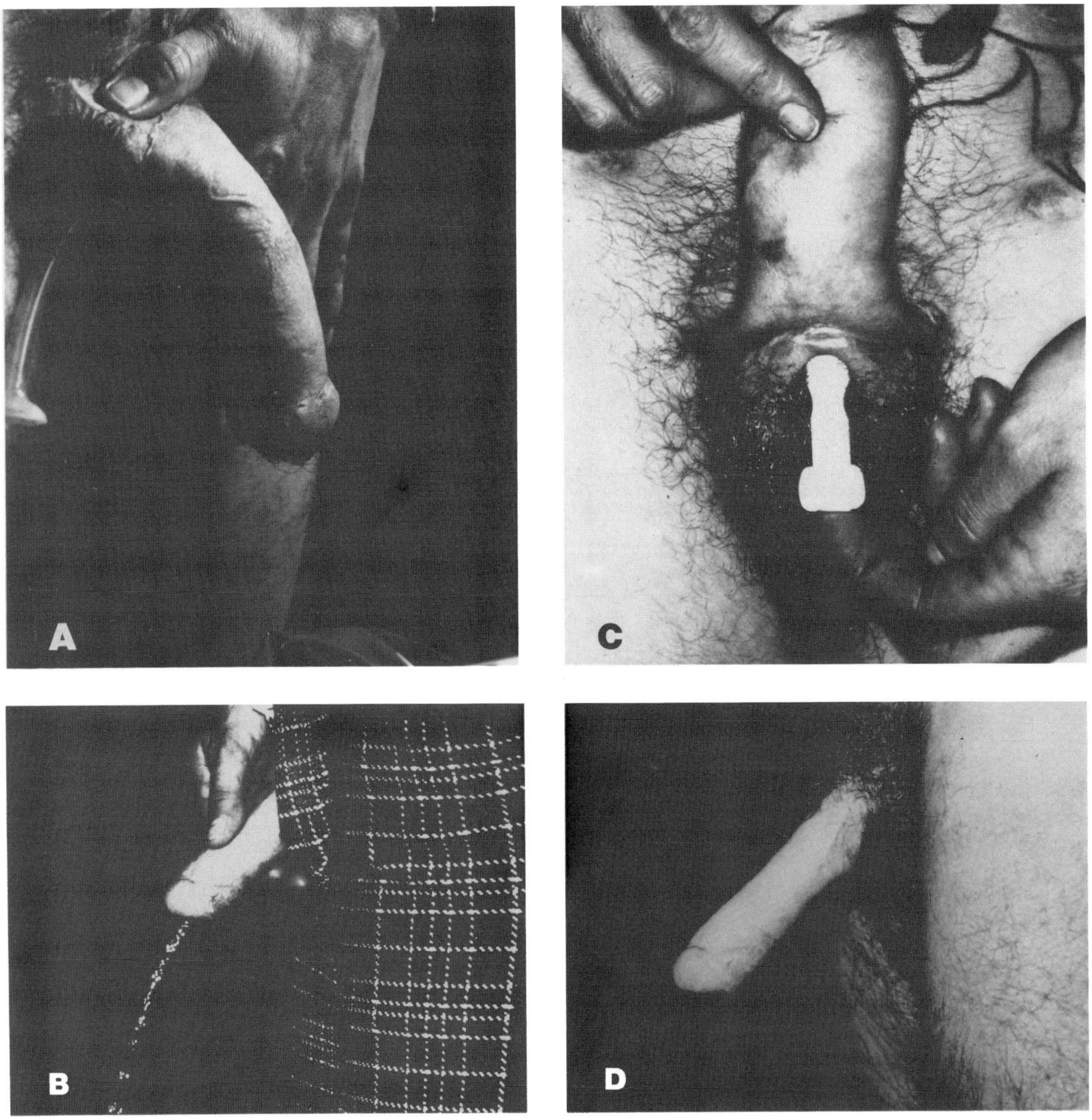

Figure 3 Illustrates the devices. The urinary assist device *A*, is used to conduct the urine from a cup held under the existing or female urinary meatus into the tunnel inside the flap. Urine exits orthostatically *B*, through the meatus at the neoglans. The baculum *C* or stiffener *D*, (os penis) is used on a p.r.n. basis. It transmits motion and feeling to the more erotic areas of the genitalia.

as a third or later stage after completion of much of the above surgery. The lateral antebrachial cutaneous nerve of the forearm (LACN) ends in the nicely sensitive area on the palmar side of the distal wrist (Fig. 4). This tissue is used to form a sensitive glans penis. The proximal end of LACN (formerly just distal to the elbow) is anastomosed to the erotic deep pudendal nerve (of Gilbert) as it exists from beneath the pubic bone to become one of the two dorsal nerves of the penis (or clitoris). The fascicular repair is performed under magnification. The donor site of the forearm is closed primarily, either with a tight skin closure (with occasional use of a small skin graft, subsequently excised) or, preferably, after the forearm has been prepared with a tissue expander so that it closes easily in a tension-free linear scar. A 3 cm-wide strip, 15 to 20 cm long, preferably glabrous in nature, is used for the urethroplasty. It is an important point that the donor site is inexpensive in that no deforming skin graft remains on the forearm. The arterial supply to the hand is uninterrupted via the ulnar artery. A vein graft could possibly reconstitute the radial artery but we have not used it. Very little anesthesia results in the forearm and hand because almost all the skin supplied by the LACN is removed.

The neoglans and urethroplasty skin are elevated without destroying the five to eight perforators from the radial artery (Fig. 5). The level of the branching of brachial artery into radial and ulnar dictates the length of the radial artery leash beyond the flap itself. Venae comitantes may not be as usable as the large superficial veins. The flap includes a subcutaneous fascial layer. A 30 mm-wide strip of skin theoretically equates to a French 30 tube (1 mm of circumference equals one French unit), but with suturing, French 24 caliber is expected.

A multiperforated Jackson Pratt round soft silicone drain is used as a stent over which the forearm skin is surgically tubed, while still on the forearm and, attached to the local vascular system. Fine absorbable sutures are used to adhere dermis to dermis (not epidermis). The fascia becomes the external surface of the tube.

The tourniquet is released; the tube flap is revascularized, and the vessels are then severed and transferred to the lower abdomen. The DIEA and veins have been traced to the femoral bulb and adequate leash length is obtained. The inguinal ligament is loosened to help prevent kinking of the vessels at this level.

The anastomosis is end-to-end, but occasionally end-to-side when the femoral artery and the saphenous vein at the bulb area are used.

The forearm flap tissue is placed on and into the new dorsal surface of the penis, which has been opened and debulked. The tube is routed down to the perineum by traversing through the base of the bipedicle flap at the level of the pubic symphysis. A comfortably wide tunnel is easily made through the midline of the base of the neopenis without any interruption of blood supply. The forearm flap urethroplasty tunnel is brought into the perineum to anastomose with the truncated urethral meatus of the male or the neomeatus of the female, usually already extended up to the level of the clitoris by a flap of the anterior wall of the vagina.

The deep pudendal nerves exit parasagittally at the root of the penis (or clitoris) on the posterior aspect of the pubic symphysis. One of these two nerves is selected for an interfascicular repair to the LACN, using microscope magnification.

In this way, the end organs of the neoglans penis (the distal palmar forearm skin) are able to transmit via LACN and deep pudendal nerve to the erotic centers of the brain, thus approximating a natural reflex.

The complete connection of the two portions of the urethra in the perineum may judiciously be postponed to help avoid complications. A temporary fistula allows good hygiene to be carried out during healing, using the Jackson Pratt stent for irrigation. A perineal urethrostomy allows better drainage and less bladder spasm than suprapubic diversion.

The existing glans from stage one is augmented with the inset of potentially very sensitive skin of the distal forearm.

A split graft may be necessary to resurface the dorsum of the penis over the new urethra—a stent or tie-over dressing with compressible foam is useful.

Postoperative management includes: (1) bedrest and restriction from hip flexion for 48 hours, (2) no anticoagulation and no aspirin, (3) drains to suction reservoirs, (4) elastic compression on the neopenis for 6 weeks to prevent edema. (Significant interruption of lymphatics occurs with the reconstruction, and the compression prevents edema as well as shortening and thickening of the penis), (5) irrigation of the neourethral skin with topical antibiotic solution, and (6) closure of the fistula at 3 weeks or more.

The advantages of the procedure are:

1. Function is achieved (Fig. 6).
2. The glans and the urethra are erotically sensible.
3. Ability to stand to urinate is achieved.

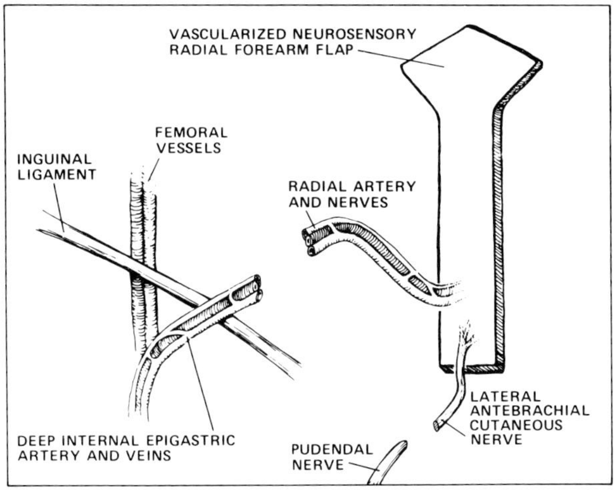

Figure 4 The nerve, artery, and vein hookups involved in the microsurgery.

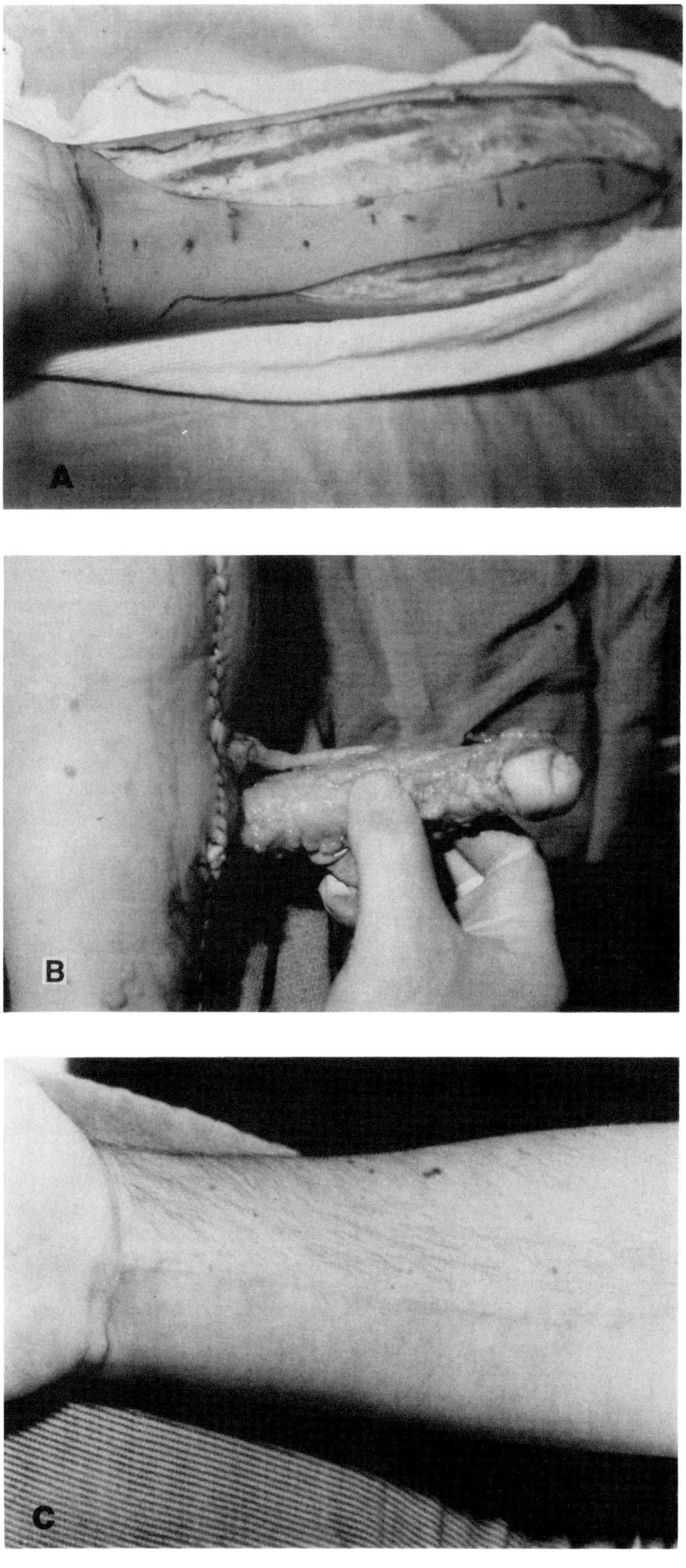

Figure 5 The radial forearm flap: *A,* Skin 25 or 30 mm by 20 cm. *B,* It is tubed in place on the forearm prior to transfer, and *C,* Resultant scar after primary closure. Tissue expanders are helpful.

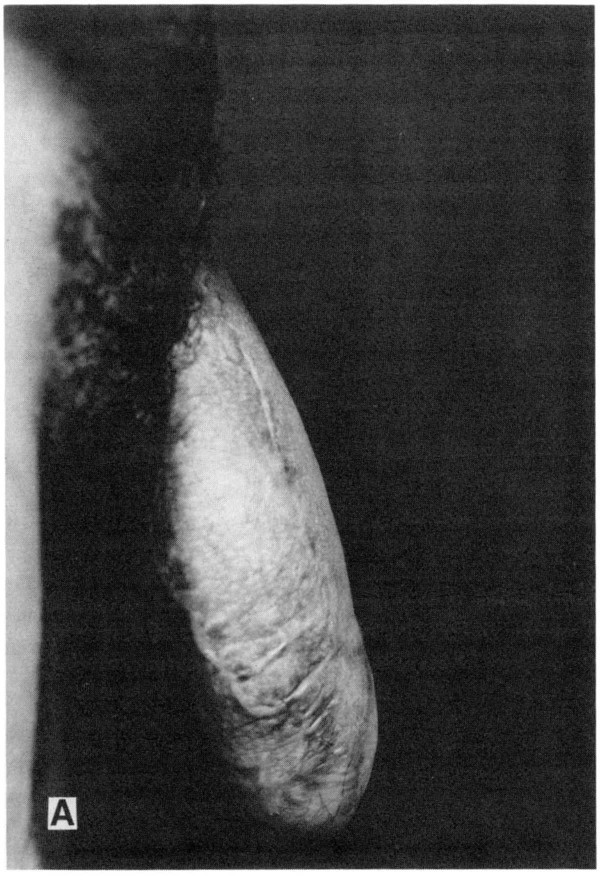

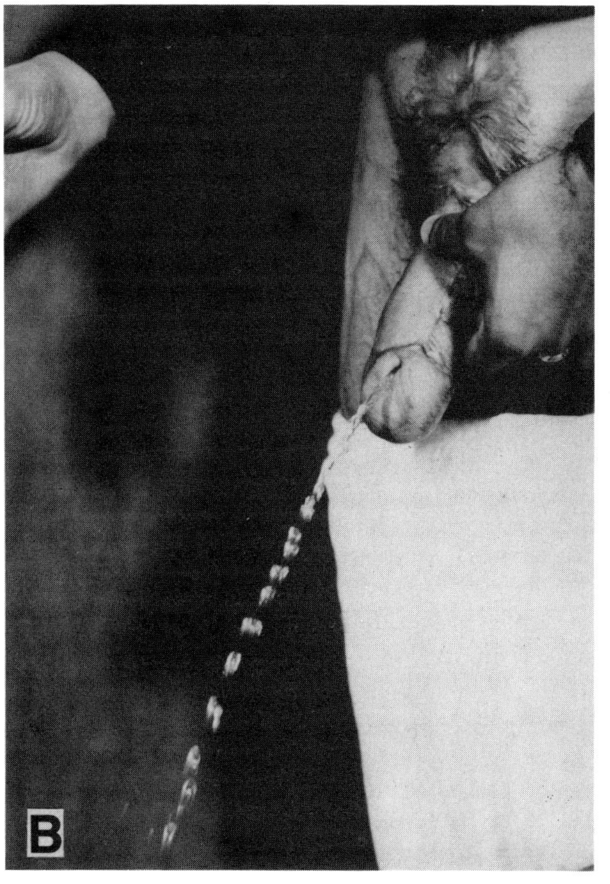

Figure 6 *A* and *B*, Results of a post-traumatic reconstruction.

4. The donor sites are not excessively expensive.
5. All of the patient's individual needs can be taken into consideration.

The disadvantages are:

1. There are two or more stages involved.
2. There is a skin graft donor site scar.

Techniques of phalloplasty are evolving in several centers. Consensus will be achieved with exchange of new information in the years ahead. The achievement of the dreams of the reconstructive surgeon requires that we first do dream. We are well on our way to beginning to solve the tissue deficit of no penis.

SUGGESTED READING

Bouman FG. The first step in phalloplasty in female transsexuals (letter). Plast Reconstr Surg 1987; 79:662–664.

Chang T-S, Hwang WY. Forearm flap in one-stage reconstruction of the penis. Plast Reconstr Surg 1984; 74:251–258.

Dubin BT, Sato RI, Laub DR. Results of phalloplasty. Plast Recon Surg 1979; 64:163–170.

Edgerton MT. The role of surgery in the treatment of transexualism. Ann Plast Surg 1984; 13:473–481.

Gilbert DA, Horton CE, Terzis JK, Devine CJ Jr, Winslow BH, Devine PC. New concepts in phallic reconstruction. Ann Plast Surg 1987; 128–136.

Hoopes JE. Surgical construction of the male external genitalia. Clin Plast Surg 1974; 1(2):325–334.

Patil UA, Dias AD, Thatte RL. Anatomic basis of the SEPA flap. Brit J Plast Surg 1987; 40:342–347.

VAGINAL RECONSTRUCTION

GORDON R. TOBIN, M.D.

Reconstruction is done for total or partial vaginal absence in two clinical settings: congenital agenesis; and excision during pelvic exenteration or abdominoperineal resection for pelvic cancer.

RECONSTRUCTIVE OPTIONS

Skin Grafts

Vaginal reconstruction with a skin-grafted perineal pouch was introduced by Abbe and popularized by McIndoe. This technique is the current procedure of choice for reconstruction of congenital absence, and is also used to restore lining if flap reconstructions suffer partial loss. Skin grafts do not provide a satisfactory vaginal reconstruction for pelvic exenteration defects because of the resultant inadequate bed.

Gracilis Myocutaneous Flaps

Vaginal reconstruction with bilateral gracilis myocutaneous flaps was introduced by McCraw and coworkers. This method provided the first highly satisfactory reconstruction for cancer resection defects, and it showed that myocutaneous flaps are vastly superior to all previously used donor tissues for reconstruction of these defects. However, gracilis flaps have a substantially higher incidence of flap failure than do rectus abdominis flaps. Therefore, I reserve the gracilis reconstruction for exenteration patients in whom the rectus abdominis unit is not available.

Rectus Abdominis Myocutaneous Flaps

Since its introduction, the distally based rectus abdominis myocutaneous flap vaginal reconstruction has proved to be the most satisfactory method for pelvic exenteration or abdominoperineal resection defects. It cannot be used when its inferior epigastric vascular pedicle has been interrupted by previous abdominal incision or by resection during the cancer resection. Its use for reconstruction of agenesis would provide a vagina of excellent quality, but would introduce an unnecessary abdominal scar.

Gluteal-Thigh Fasciocutaneous Flaps

Vaginal reconstruction can be done with bilateral gluteal-thigh fasciocutaneous flaps from the posterior thigh, as introduced by Hurwitz and co-workers. This method of vaginal reconstruction has not had nearly as extensive clinical application and evaluation as rectus abdominis or gracilis myocutaneous reconstructions, but experience to date shows it to be a satisfactory method that can be used as backup when neither myocutaneous flap technique can be used.

Skin Flaps

Vaginal reconstruction with local skin flaps, such as the method described by Williams, provides vaginal pouches that extend along the perineal surface rather than enter the pelvis. This method should be considered when reconstruction was not done at the time of resection and redissection of the pelvis poses substantial risks.

Bowel Segments

Both ileal and sigmoid colon segments have been transposed on mesenteric vascular pedicles for vaginal replacement. Because of a fragile lining and excessive secretions, ileal segment use has been abandoned. Sigmoid colon epithelium is more durable and less secretory, and a sigmoid colon segment can provide a vaginal reconstruction, although skin grafts for congenital defects and myocutaneous flaps for acquired defects are preferred.

Nonoperative Dilation

A technique of progressive dilation of the pelvic floor with graded prosthetic dilators to create a vaginal pouch has been described by Frank and analyzed by Broadbent and Wolf. This technique is an acceptable alternative for reconstruction of the congenitally absent vagina in selected cases where the patient is willing to pursue the process of gradual dilation. Moreover, it does not preclude subsequent surgical reconstruction if the nonoperative approach gives an unsatisfactory result.

PREFERRED APPROACH FOR CONGENITAL DEFECTS

The procedure preferred for vaginal agenesis is the Abbe-McIndoe procedure of lining a surgically created perineal pouch with skin grafts. Although postoperative management of skin-grafted pouches is more difficult than that of myocutaneous flap pouches, scars are not left on the abdomen or thighs, as they are when flap reconstructions are done. Alternatively, the limited experience with progressive dilation shows promise. Also, if a preexisting midline abdominal scar were present, the advantages of a rectus abdominis reconstruction could be provided without creating a new scar.

Patient Selection

Vaginal reconstruction with skin-grafted perineal pouches is done for natural and assigned phenotypic females with absent or incomplete vaginas. The most commonly presenting patient is a female with vaginal agenesis (Rokitansky-Kuster-Hauser syndrome). Other candidates include assigned females with male genotypes and testicular feminization syndrome, females with adrenogenital syndrome, females with gonadal dysgenesis (Turner's syndrome), and true or pseudohermaphrodites with female phenotypes. Rarely, this procedure is required for females born to mothers who take androgens or who have androgenic-producing tumors, and for males assigned a female gender in the neonatal period because of phallic amputation or true microphallus. The guiding principle throughout this diverse set of gender disorders is the provision of a capability for normal sexual activity to adult women, irrespective of original gonadal status or genotype. The work-up includes a history and physical examination, karyotyping, an intravenous pyelogram for detection of commonly associated urinary tract anomalies, and, frequently, a laparoscopy for evaluation of the internal genitalia. Hormonal assays are done where there are abnormalities of adrenocortical synthetic pathways. In the rare, complex, intersex patient, gonadal biopsy may be required. In testicular feminization patients, gonads predisposed to subsequent malignancies are removed. When needed, hormonal supplementation or psychiatric support is provided.

Timing of Surgery

Reconstructions of these patients is best done just prior to marriage and commencement of regular sexual activity, which helps maintain luminal diameter, or when the patient is strongly motivated to have the procedure and to participate diligently in the postoperative care regimen of stenting and luminal diameter monitoring.

Principles and Technique

The principle of the Abbe-McIndoe vaginal reconstruction is surgical dissection of a connective tissue pouch in the perineum, which is then lined with a skin graft. A complete mechanical and antibiotic bowel preparation is done preoperatively. The procedure is initiated by a transverse incision through the apex of any vaginal depression, or midway between the urethral orifice and rectum. An oversized pouch is made by meticulous dissection in the plane between the rectum and bladder to just below the pouch of Douglas, or into a closed vaginal remnant and hematocolpos, if present. Following complete hemostasis, a split-thickness skin graft having the surface area of the pouch is harvested, draped over a stent with its epithelial surface facing inward, sutured along its lateral margins, and placed in the pouch. Graft immobilization is facilitated by closure of the perineum over the stent, which is taken down at the first dressing change in 7 to 10 days. Prophylactic antibiotics are usually given for the first 4 to 7 days. The vaginal lumen is stented for 6 months to lessen contraction. Regular intercourse is allowed after 6 weeks of graft maturation and encouraged when appropriate. Pouch dimensions are calibrated regularly to insure adequacy.

Tricks and Traps

Accurate dissection of the vaginal pouch is facilitated by placement of a Foley catheter in the urethra and a gloved finger in the rectum to protect these structures from entry. Hemostasis of the dissected pouch should be absolute. Although medial thigh or lower abdominal skin graft donor sites are used by some authors, I prefer the central buttocks region, which will be hidden by panties and swimsuit bottoms. Although many rigid and flexible stents have been used, I prefer the commercially available Heyer-Schulte stent, with a foam core covered by a silicone elastomer envelope, that can be collapsed during placement and reexpanded in the pouch. Postoperatively, the Foley catheter is replaced by a suprapubic bladder catheter, and defecation is delayed by opiates and a low-residue diet.

Outcome

Series of vaginal agenesis reconstructions with skin grafts report a success rate of over 90 percent. If the graft fails to take, regrafting salvages most reconstructions.

PREFERRED APPROACH FOR RECONSTRUCTION OF VAGINAL RESECTIONS

Vaginal reconstruction for pelvic exenteration defects is best done with myocutaneous flaps. Myocutaneous flaps not only provide high-quality vaginal lining and a functional vagina, but they also obliterate pelvic dead space and bring a well-vascularized muscle pedicle into the pelvic wound, which is usually irradiated and contaminated by the resection. Gracilis myocutaneous flaps originally provided the preferred technique, but, since introduction of the rectus abdominis reconstruction, I prefer this latter method because of the greater reliability of the rectus abdominis flap, the need for only a single flap, and a more rapid surgical procedure.

Patient Selection

Vaginal reconstruction is done for all female patients who undergo pelvic exenteration, even if resumption of sexual activity is not intended, because of the ability of myocutaneous flaps to fill pelvic dead space and revascularize the irradiated wound, thereby lessening the incidence of perineal herniation, pelvic infection, and chronically open perineal wounds.

Timing

Reconstruction is done simultaneously with the exenteration or abdominoperineal resection. If vaginal reconstruction was not done at the time of exenteration and the patient subsequently desires a vagina, a decision must be made whether to reenter the pelvis and dissect a site for placement of a myocutaneous vagina or to construct a perineal surface pouch with local flaps, such as described by Williams.

Principles and Technique

The principle of myocutaneous vaginal reconstruction is the transfer into the pelvic defect of a well-vascularized muscle pedicle that carries a myocutaneous paddle fashioned into a vagina. Gracilis reconstructions require bilateral flaps joined into a pouch with the skin paddles facing the lumen. The larger skin paddle carried by the distally based rectus abdominis muscle pedicle provides a vagina from a single myocutaneous paddle, inversely tubed as illustrated. The cutaneous paddle is designed as a 12 to 15 cm-wide vertical ellipse centered over the superior one-half of the muscle and extending from the costal margin to just below the umbilicus (Fig. 1). When inversely tubed, this paddle provides a vaginal diameter of approximately 4 cm. Following incision of the skin-fascial paddle, the muscle is transected at the cephalic apex of the paddle, and the superior epigastric vessels are divided. The flap is elevated by sequential division of the segmental vessels and nerves that enter the lateral muscle border until the paddle reaches the perineal defect. The inferior epigastric vascular pedicle is carefully protected during dissection. Following pedicle mobilization, the flap is transposed to the groin region, and the skin paddle is inversely tubed to form the vaginal pouch while the urinary conduit and colostomy are simultaneously constructed (Figs. 2 and 3). The flap is passed into the pelvis through the midline peritoneal incision distal to the posterior rectus sheath termination at the linea arcuata (semicircular lines of Douglas), and the open end of the pouch is inset into the perineal defect. The abdominal wall donor site is reconstructed by joining the anterior and posterior rectus sheaths along the entire vertical midline incision (Fig. 4). Rectus fascial closure of the donor site, and over the site of pedicle passage into the pelvis, prevents subsequent incisional hernia. The cutaneous paddle donor defect is closed in a linear fashion in continuity with the laparotomy incision by direct approximation of the elliptical margins (Fig. 5).

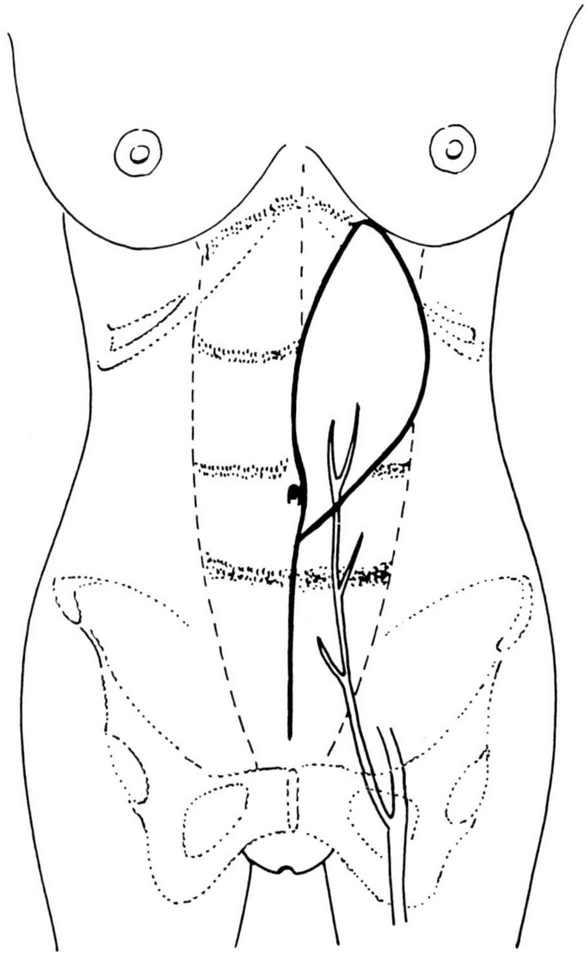

Figure 1 The cutaneous paddle design of rectus abdominis flaps for vaginal reconstruction shows the paddle's relationship to the muscle, vascular pedicle, laparotomy incision, and surface landmarks.

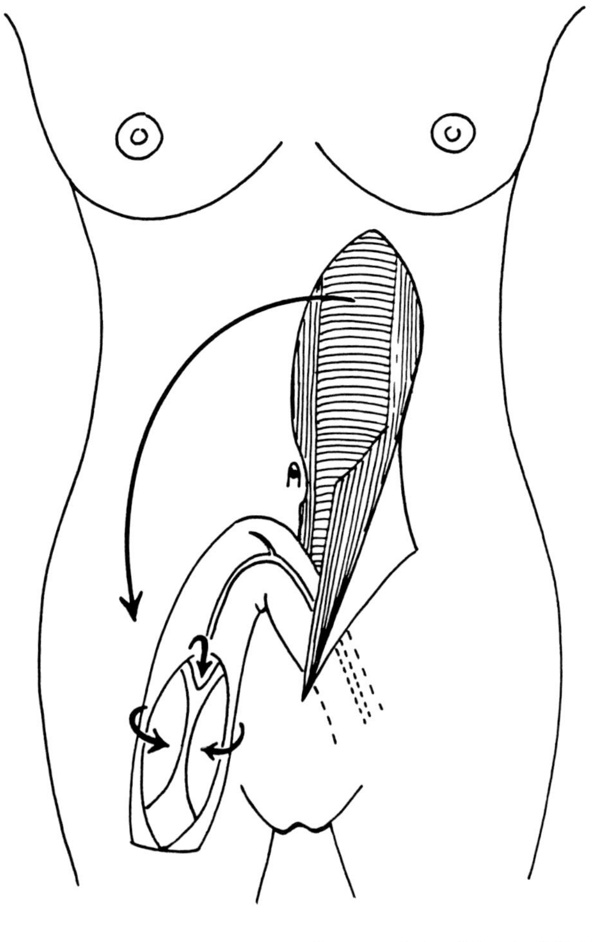

Figure 2 Transposition of the flap out of the abdominal field for formation of the vaginal pouch allows simultaneous urinary conduit and colostomy construction.

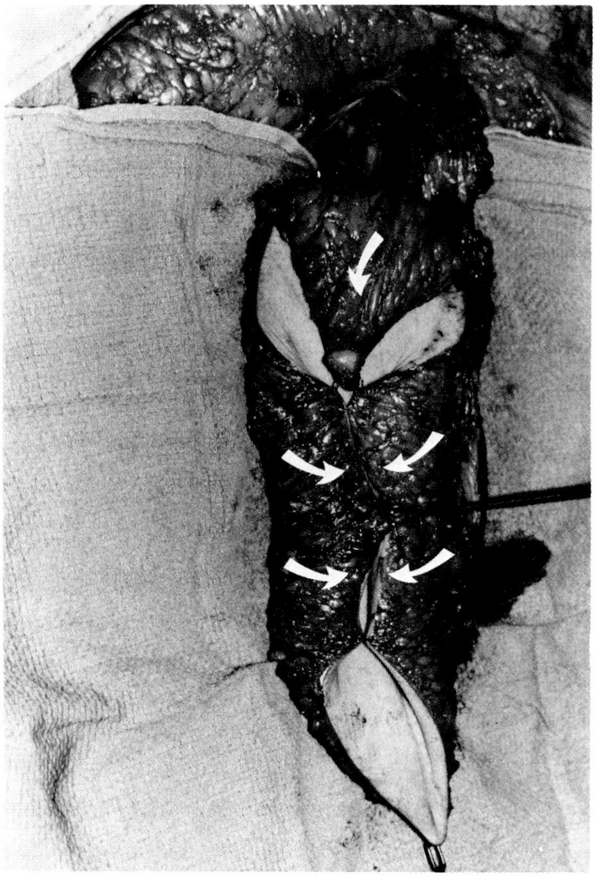

Figure 3 Inverse tubing (arrows) of the skin paddle creates a vaginal pouch.

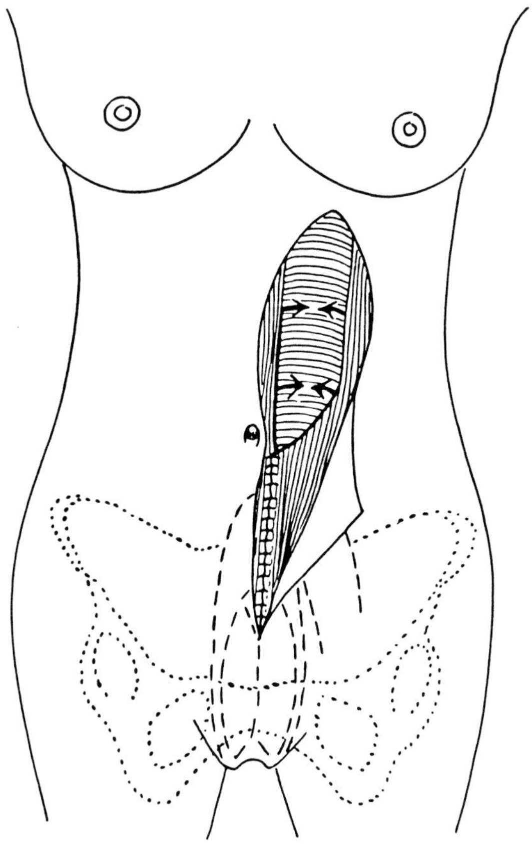

Figure 4 Following flap inset and stomal placement, abdominal wall integrity is restored by direct closure of the anterior rectus fascia distally, and its remnants proximally (arrows). The posterior rectus sheath beneath the fascial donor site also prevents hernia.

Tricks and Traps

One must be sure that the inferior epigastric vascular pedicle is not divided during the pelvic cancer resection. If this occurs, the contralateral rectus abdominis flap is used. If both pedicles must be resected, a gracilis reconstruction is done. Closure of the epigastric anterior rectus fascial donor site is facilitated by leaving 1 cm of anterior rectus fascia along the linea alba and 2 cm of anterior rectus fascia and muscle laterally. These fascial remnants are closed one to another.

Outcome

Distally based rectus abdominis myocutaneous flaps provide a vaginal replacement of exceptional quality (Fig. 6) and have been successful in all patients to date. An 8 percent incidence of partial paddle loss occurred that involved 2 to 3 cm of the flap tip. This was easily resolved by excision of the unperfused tissue and revision by primary closure, without the need for second flaps. In gracilis myocutaneous vaginal reconstructions, a 21 percent incidence of flap loss has been reported. However, most gracilis flap paddle losses can be skin-grafted or allowed to re-epithelialize, and second flaps are not usually required.

BENEFIT-RISK ANALYSIS

Vaginal reconstruction for agenesis provides the capability for sexual intercourse at minimal risk. The principle risks are rectal or urethral injury during pouch dissection, graft loss, and postoperative pouch constriction; all of which can be minimized by measures discussed above.

The benefits of myocutaneous vaginal reconstruction are restoration of sexual function and improved wound healing of the perineal defect. Perineal herniation, pelvic infection, and chronic perineal wounds are minimized or eliminated. Compared with these benefits, risks are minimal. The principle risk is flap loss, which occurs in the incidence described above and can be corrected in virtually all cases. Donor site complications are a potential risk that has not been observed to date.

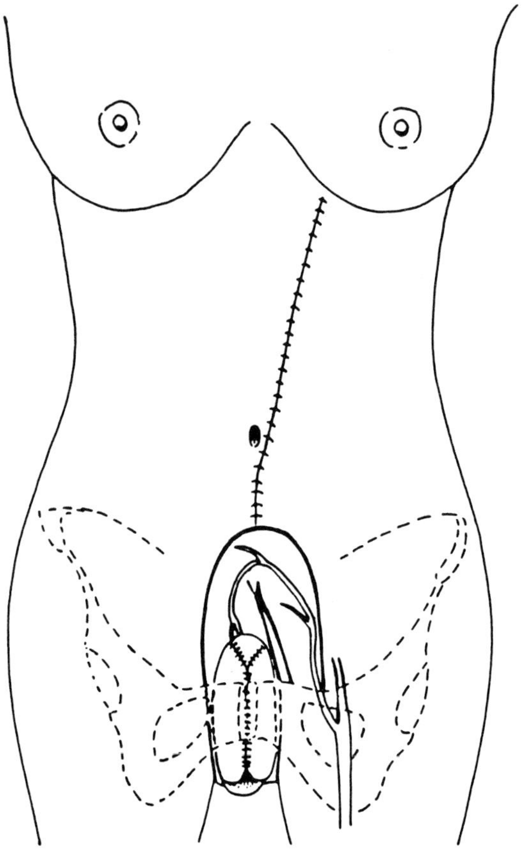

Figure 5 The cutaneous donor site is closed directly, in continuity with the laparotomy incision.

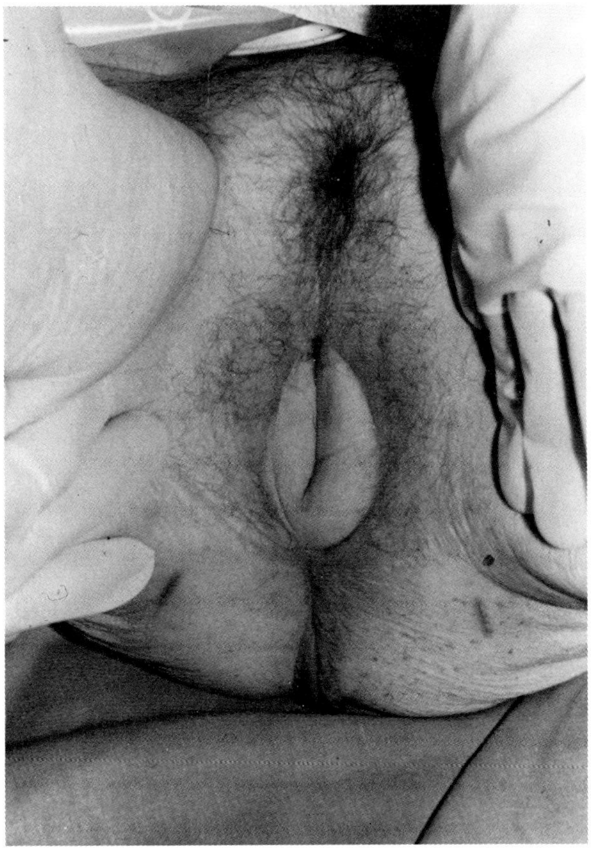

Figure 6 A rectus abdominis myocutaneous flap provides the most reliable and satisfactory vaginal reconstruction currently available.

SUGGESTED READING

Abbe R. New method of creating a vagina in a case of congenital absence. Med Rec 1898; 54:836–838.

Broadbent TR, Wolf RM. Congenital absence of the vagina: reconstruction without operation. Br J Plast Surg 1977; 30:118–122.

Hurwitz DJ, Zweibel PC. Gluteal thigh flap repair of chronic perineal wounds. Am J Surg 1985; 150:386–391.

McCraw JB, Massey FM, Shanklin KD, Horton CE. Vaginal reconstruction of gracilis myocutaneous flaps. Plast Reconstr Surg 1976; 58:176–183.

McIndoe A. Treatment of congenital absence and obliterative conditions of the vagina. Br J Plast Surg 1950; 2:254–267.

Pratt JH. Vaginal atresia corrected by use of small and large bowel. Clin Obstet Gynecol 1972; 15:639–649.

Tobin GR, Day TG. Vaginal and pelvic reconstruction with distally based rectus abdominis myocutaneous flaps. Plast Reconstr Surg 1988; 81:62–70.

Williams EA. Congenital absence of vagina: a simple operation for its relief. J Obstet Gynecol Br Commow 1964; 71:511–516.

EXSTROPHY

CALVIN R. PETERS, M.D.

The incidence of exstrophy of the urinary bladder reportedly varies from one per 25,000 to one per 50,000 live births, with a 2:1 ratio of males to females. Embryologically, it is a direct result of delayed perforation of the cloacal membrane. The occurrence in offspring of parents with this anomaly has recently been found to be approximately one per 70 live births, thus indicating a higher than previously assumed inheritance.

Prenatal sonography recently has been found to be helpful in establishing a diagnosis of bladder exstrophy prior to birth. Exstrophic bladders at term often have an irregular shape and are generally smaller than normal and, therefore, easily may be overlooked during sonography. The finding of exstrophy can be confirmed by repetition of the examination or by checking fetal bladder filling after intravenous administration of diuretics to the mother.

The primary objectives of the surgical management of bladder exstrophy are to provide a secure abdominal wall closure, to obtain urinary continence with preservation of renal function, and to reconstruct cosmetically acceptable and functional genitalia.

In the male with bladder exstrophy, the goal of surgical reconstruction of the genitalia is the achievement of a straight penis with an urethra capable of transporting urine and semen. Successful genital surgery implies a satisfactory cosmetic result, with the penis angulated downward in the standing position, a straight penis of adequate length at erection to allow sexual intercourse, and preservation of fertility potential.

The female patient usually has an unnatural appearance of her vulva and pubic hair (escutcheon). The vaginal orifice is commonly stenotic, causing dyspareunia when intercourse is attempted. Surgical correction of the introitus is usually easy, but should not be undertaken until the woman is ready for intercourse, as it may allow a prolapsing cervix to emerge from the vagina.

METHODS OF TREATMENT

The complications of treatment have provided controversy regarding the most suitable approach to rehabilitation. Treatment has varied among many different approaches: closure of the bladder with and without ileal osteotomy; internal diversion with and without antireflux anastomosis; one-stage functional closure; antirefluxing ureterosigmoidostomy; external diversion by ileal conduit; staged functional closure and colon conduit; and subsequent undiverted cystoplasty or colocolostomy. The multiplicity of these approaches attests to the fact that no one procedure is ideally suited to all patients with classic exstrophy.

Functional primary bladder closure and bladder neck-reconstruction achieve the most desirable cosmetic and functional restoration of the urinary tract. The technique provides a secure abdominal wall closure and urinary continence and can be achieved with minimal morbidity. Selection has been a definite factor in success. Some patients with small or severely scarred bladders, as well as those with extensive ectopic bowel mucosa or penile duplication, are diverted. Hydroureteronephrosis is also considered a contraindication to primary closure. Small bladders may enlarge surprisingly after closure. A bladder capable of holding only 5 ml initially may sometimes gradually increase to a 50 ml capacity, then up to 250 ml, after bladder neck plasty.

Primary bladder closure, bladder neck reconstruction, and epispadias repair are performed as staged procedures in the surgical reconstruction of bladder exstrophy. Primary bladder closure should be performed within the first 72 hours of life, since, at this time, the pubic symphysis can be approximated without the need for bilateral osteotomies.

EXTERNAL APPEARANCE

Regardless of the type of surgical repair performed, these patients exhibit characteristic deformities upon reaching adolescence and adulthood. Women and men alike have absent escutcheons and mons veneris, with hairbearing skin located laterally in the inguinal crease. Often there is hypertrophic scarring of the lower abdominal wall with marked diastasis recti.

The mature female patient presents with an unnatural appearance of her external genitalia and pubic region. These women may be sexually active and, occasionally, even postpartum. Almost all have a bifid clitoris, with abnormally placed labia. The vaginal mucosa may be everted, which results in dryness and dyspareunia. Many complain of "riding breeches" deformity; a result of the pelvic diastasis.

Male patients, in contrast, usually present with ejaculatory fistulas. Classically, they exhibit dorsal penile fistulas. Because of previously performed urinary diversion, their major complaint is related to sexual activities. Many also have an associated short penis due to the diastasis of the pubis. Both men and women complain of absence of the escutcheon and the extension of hairbearing skin into the inguinal region.

PSYCHOLOGICAL FACTORS

Adolescents with exstrophy and genital abnormalities suffer great problems in psychosexual adjustment. Important adolescent developmental tasks include achievement of a stable sexual identity early in adolescence, while becoming comfortable with pubertal body changes.

Like many other chronic illnesses in adolescents, attention must be paid to the psychological impact of these deformities on normal developmental tasks. Maladaptive behavior is common in adolescents with congenital urinary problems. Delinquency, sexual promiscuity, lack of social skills, and a poor self-image are characteristic of such patients during adolescence and young adulthood.

In order to achieve a normal life expectancy for patients with exstrophy of the bladder, it is important to work diligently to ensure an improved psychological adjustment as well as a functional one.

SURGICAL TECHNIQUES

The male patient usually requires a single-stage closure of the dorsal penile shaft fistula (epispadias). The two corpora cavernosa are mobilized from the widened pelvic bones to gain additional penile length and compensate for the short penis that is characteristic of this anomay. Bilateral fan flaps, with hairbearing skin, are developed in the inguinal region. These are elevated and rotated to the midline to reconstruct the escutcheon.

The female patient frequently requires correction of

the bifid clitoris and ectopic labia. Most patients require excision of the unstable and esthetically displeasing scar tissue of the lower abdominal wall, in addition to repair of the diastasis recti and reconstruction of the escutcheon with bilateral fan flaps.

CONCLUSION

These relatively simple techniques invariably produce a satisfactory cosmetic and functional end result in what has been referred to as a devastating anomaly. They complete what has frequently been a long and difficult rehabilitation.

Great strides have been made in the last decade regarding the general management of exstrophy, but further advances are needed. Exstrophy has challenged the skill and ingenuity of urologists and plastic surgeons for generations and will continue to do so in the foreseeable future.

SUGGESTED READING

Farrow JA. Genital abnormalities and psychological problems. JAMA 1980; 243:433.
Jeffs RD. Complications of exstrophy surgery. Urol Clin North Am 1983; 10:509–518.
Lepor H, Jeffs RD. Primary bladder closure and bladder neck reconstruction in classical bladder exstrophy. J Urol 1983; 130:1142–1145.
Mirk P, Calisti A, Fileni A. Prenatal sonographic diagnosis of bladder exstrophy. J Ultrasound Med 1986; 5:291–293.
Peters CR, Dinner MI, Wacksman J. Escutcheon and external genitalia reconstruction following childhood correction of urinary bladder exstrophy. Ann Plast Surg 1981; 2:117–120.
Shapiro E, Lepor H, Jeffs RD. The inheritance of the exstrophy-epispadias complex. J Urol 1984; 132:308–310.

GENDER DYSPHORIA

JOHN G. KENNEY, M.D., F.A.C.S.

Cross-gender behavior, known as transsexualism, is a pediatric neuropsychiatric disorder affecting an individual's total concept of self. It is the most profound disorder of gender identity known. Approximately 10,000 patients in the United States, and over 50,000 patients worldwide, can be classified by the American Psychiatric Association Diagnostic and Statistical Manual of Medical Disorders* as suffering from transsexualism.

One's gender role in society is a summation of genetic, cultural, social, and psychological influences that begin in early childhood and mature through adolescence and adulthood. How people perceive themselves sexually, and project that image into their sexual role in society, is a much more complex phenomenon than simple genetic biologic sex.

Clinical transsexualism is a disorder whereby the patient lives in the role of his biologic gender opposite. It is the ultimate in body-image disturbance. Because of social intolerance and misunderstanding by health care professionals, these patients endure severe psychological hardships such as social isolation, ridicule, alienation, rejection, and desperation. Ongoing endocrine research seems to suggest abnormalities of the hypothalamus in the cyclic behavior of releasing hormones and their end-organ responses. These chemical abnormalities may play a significant role in the pathogenesis of transsexualism.

"Sexual reassignment" is probably a misnomer. These are psychologically complex patients who are convinced they *are* the opposite sex. They desire to have the fact that they are the opposite sex confirmed surgically and hormonally. The majority of transsexuals are normally intelligent and have no major mental illnesses. The surgical and psychiatric role is to restore sexual harmony to allow the patient to function normally in society. A true transsexual's biologic sexual organs are totally foreign to him or her. They are repulsive, a mistake of nature that does not belong. Hormonal and surgical therapy, in conjunction with continuing psychiatric counseling, complete an affirmation of their sexual identity.

Professional controversy concerning their transsexualism leaves many patients without access to reputable professional help. In the past, the ratio of male to female transsexuals seeking surgical treatment was approximately 4.5:1. However, over the past 5 years, the ratio has approached 1:1. With the evolution of new and improved surgical techniques, more patients are seeking operative treatment at an earlier age in conjunction with continuing psychiatric treatment.

PRINCIPLES OF PATIENT SELECTION

The multidisciplinary team approach is the most efficient means of adding objectivity to patient evaluation and treatment. In addition, this reduces diagnostic error that might follow examination by a single physician. Ideally, multidisciplinary evaluation and treatment teams of health care professionals would include a psychiatrist, a psychologist, an endocrinologist, an urologist, a gynecologist, and a plastic surgeon experienced in genitourinary reconstruction. Stringent patient selection criteria and evaluation allow for diagnostic accuracy, ethical objectivity, and long-term scientific follow-up. This allows surgical and psychological treatment programs to be evaluated objectively and scientifically.

Diagnostic criteria of transsexualism, as defined by the American Psychiatric Association, are as follows: (1) a sense of discomfort and inappropriateness about one's anatomic sex, (2) the wish to be rid of one's own genitalia

* Third edition (D.S.M. III, 7)

and to live as a member of the opposite sex, (3) a disturbance that has been continuous (not limited to periods of stress) for at least 2 years, (4) an absence of physical intersex or genetic abnormality, and (5) an absence of any mental disorder such as schizophrenia.

The psychiatrist's role in the diagnostic and treatment process of transsexualism is critical. If improper diagnostic criteria are used and a patient receives surgical treatment, a postoperative crisis may follow. Subgroups of gender disorders exist and these may complicate proper diagnosis. The spectrum between homosexuality, transvestism, and transsexualism may be very subtle. A true homosexual does not find his existing genitalia foreign. He will feel mutilated if castration and penectomy are performed. This is in sharp contrast to the expressions of relief and appreciation consistently reported by the true male transsexual after similar surgery.

Adult transsexual patients frequently give a history of psychosexual conflicts that began during early childhood. The male transsexual is manifested by extensive and pervasive femininity as a boy. This is usually confirmed by parental and sibling interviews. A disturbed parent-child relationship is also frequently reported. Despite peer ridicule, family pressure, and prolonged psychiatric counseling and testing, cross-gender feelings intensify and progress into adulthood, manifesting themselves in true male transsexualism.

PREOPERATIVE EVALUATION

Preoperatively, there are numerous psychological and social issues that must be addressed by each patient individually. The expectations of surgical outcome must be reasonable. Psychiatric guidance and support play an important role pre- and postoperatively. Prior to any surgical treatment, the patient needs to be involved in an active psychiatric therapeutic program for at least 1 to 2 years. During psychiatric therapy, various issues are addressed. These include: (1) the patient's gender identity in relationship to parent-child interaction during infancy, childhood, and adolescence; (2) the internal motivational patterns for surgery; (3) the social ramifications of living in the gender of conviction, as well as ways of informing family members, friends, and associates at the work place, and (4) legal name change on birth certificate, driver's license, and all other legal documents. In addition, the patient must fully explore the ramifications of permanently losing fertility postoperatively. During this trial period, the patient needs to begin a full-time cross-living lifestyle both socially and at the workplace. This real life test of gender confirmation is the most important single requirement for patient selection and preparation for surgery. Also during this period, hormonal therapy is begun, as well as electrolysis when necessary.

The psychiatrist's role is critical throughout the stages of treatment. Psychiatric treatment needs to be intensified during the perioperative period. The psychological stresses of staged surgery have a tremendous impact on the patient's emotional equilibrium.

Even when diagnostic prerequisites have been filled, certain patients do not make suitable operative candidates. Patients who should not be considered for surgical therapy include: (1) those patients with emotional sexual ambiguity, i.e., patients who waver in their sexual role or have unrealistic expectations of surgery; (2) patients who cannot give meaningful and informed consent, i.e., patients less than 18 years of age; (3) patients with severe psychiatric disorders, who suffer from delusions or severe paranoia; (4) the patient who refuses presurgical psychotherapy; (5) the patient who exhibits antisocial behavior such as uncontrollable alcoholism or criminal behavior; (6) patients without support of significant others in their lives; and (7) the effeminate homosexual who wishes to escape the stigmata of homosexuality.

SURGICAL TECHNIQUES—MALE TO FEMALE

Surgical treatment deserves consideration in many patients who meet the DSM III criteria of male transsexualism. Long-term results and patient satisfaction are, in general, excellent, and no patient treated at the University of Virginia Medical Center has regretted surgical therapy. In addition, surgery becomes the only alternative for many patients when there is an absence of effective long-term nonsurgical treatment.

It is now possible to create an esthetically acceptable functional vagina for the male transsexual patient. Initial hormone treatment leads to moderate breast development and the deposition of fatty tissues over the lateral thigh and trochanteric area, thus creating a female body habitus. Surgical goals include: (1) creation of a vagina of adequate depth for satisfactory intercourse; (2) the ability to achieve and maintain orgasm; and (3) external genitalia acceptably female in appearance.

Various techniques are available for surgical vaginoplasty in male transsexual patients. Our preferred method is the penile skin fascial flap (Fig. 1). In this technique, the extensible skin of the male penile shaft is preserved as a pedicled skin and fascial flap. The pedicle is then shifted posteriorly to the appropriate operative site for the vaginal introitus. The flap is then inverted and the penile skin becomes the lining for the new vagina. The scrotal tissues are used to create the labia and the clitoral hood. Initially a Foley catheter is placed into the bladder to protect the urethra. An inverted V incision is made above the base of the phallus, and bilateral orchiectomy is then performed. The cord structures are divided at the level of the external inguinal ring, which is then closed. The inverted V allows for a 5 cm posterior displacement of the penile flap into a normal vaginal position. The penile skin and subcutaneous fascia is then dissected off the corpora cavernosa. The skin (and subcutaneous fascia) is left attached to its blood supply, which enters posteriorly through the perineal arteries in a posterolateral fashion. The glans penis is debulked internally and is left attached to the penile skin flap. The distal glans will then become the cervix during the latter portion of the procedure. The corpora cavernosa are ligated and removed.

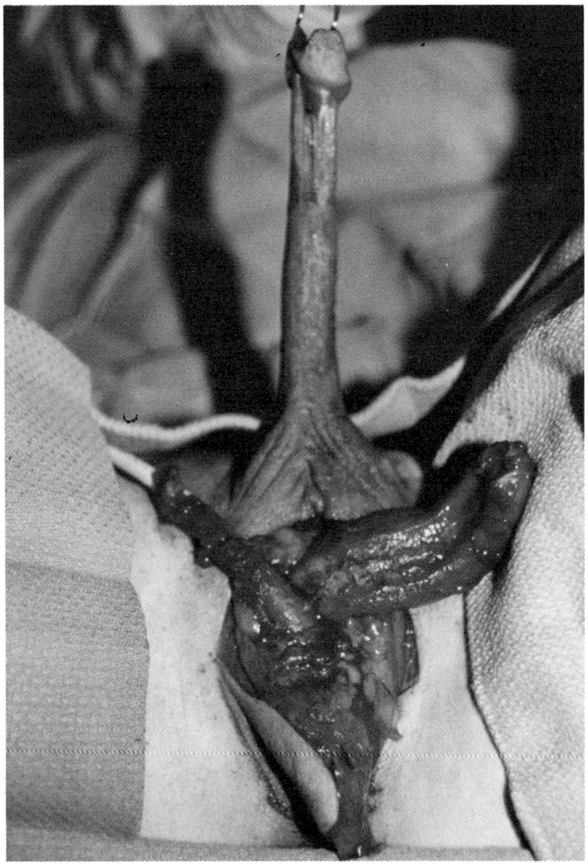

Figure 1 Intraoperative photographs demonstrate dissection of penile fasciocutaneous flap for vaginal reconstruction.

At this point, a cylindrical tissue expander is placed in the inverted penile skin fascial flap and expanded to the maximal level (Fig. 2). This allows direct observation of the flap venous drainage as well as its primary expansion, and thus allows for maximal tissue utilization for total reconstruction of the vagina. The tissue expander is then removed and replaced in the vaginal vault as a temporary stent at the end of the operative procedure. The operator's finger is then placed in the rectum and a cruciate incision is made in the posterior scrotum and perineum. The central tendon of the pelvic diaphragm is divided and a pocket dissected superiorly along the anterior wall of the rectum, just beneath the Denonvilliers' fascia on the posterior surface of the prostate. This is taken to the level of the pelvic peritoneum to gain adequate depth for the new vagina. It is important to stay just beneath the bladder neck during this dissection to avoid entrance into the rectum. In addition, the rectal sphincter must be carefully avoided. The pelvic levator muscles are divided laterally in dissection, proceeding laterally directly to the pelvic periosteum. This pocket should be approximately 14 to 16 cm in depth and as wide as the entire bony pelvis. Care must be taken during the dissection to avoid the obturator vessels and nerves as well as the pudendal artery and nerve. The penile flap is then inverted to make the lining of the vagina and is directly sutured to the apex of the dissected pocket, taking care not to enter or injure the rectum. Absorbable sutures attach the flap directly to the lateral periosteum of the pelvic wall. The tissue expander is then wrapped with petroleum gauze, reinserted, inflated with air, and placed as a stent. The lateral tabs of the expander are sutured to the introitus. The urethra is short-

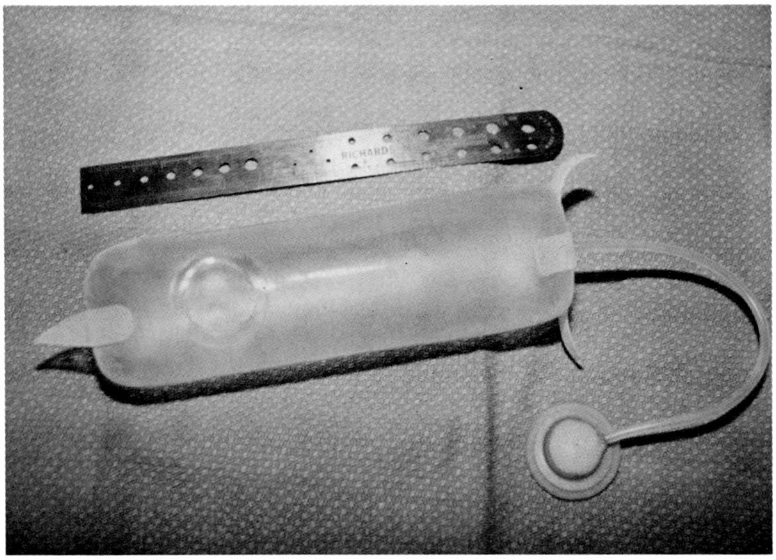

Figure 2 Custom-designed tissue expander is used for primary expansion of penile fasciocutaneous flap.

ened and a new position is selected, with the urethra base sewn directly and brought out through a cruciate incision in the anterior skin flap. The corpora are divided at an appropriate level and sutured together to recreate a sensate clitoris. The tissue expander stent is left in place for approximately 1 week, at which time the first dressing change is made (Fig. 3).

During the postoperative period, the patient remains at strict bedrest. Redundant scrotal tissues are left intact. In approximately one-half of the patients, a secondary procedure is required to transpose scrotal flaps to the area above the level of the urethral and clitoral hood in order to reconstruct the labia majora. In the remaining patients, this can be done during the primary procedure. There are many advantages to this technique. The penile pedicle skin flap of skin and fascia gives a pliable and noncontracting lining for the vagina. The patient is not required to use a vaginal form or stent for a prolonged period of time postoperatively. In addition, donor site scarring is minimal and covered by pubic hair. A large amount of sensation is retained to allow the patient to have satisfactory intercourse and achieve orgasm (Figs. 4 and 5). The only disadvantage to the penile flap method of reconstruction is the potential for flap necrosis, which is possible with any flap technique.

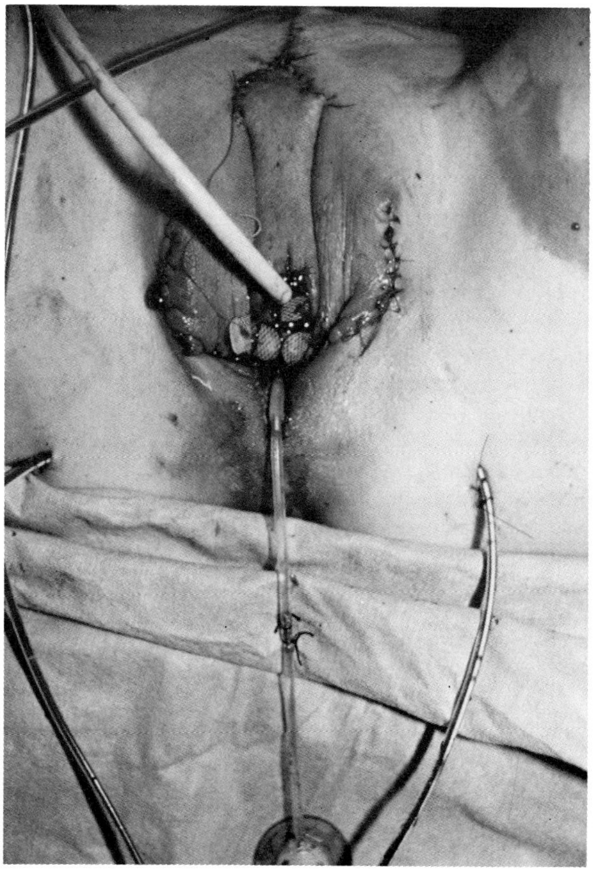

Figure 3 Completion of operative procedure, with tissue expander retained as a temporary stent.

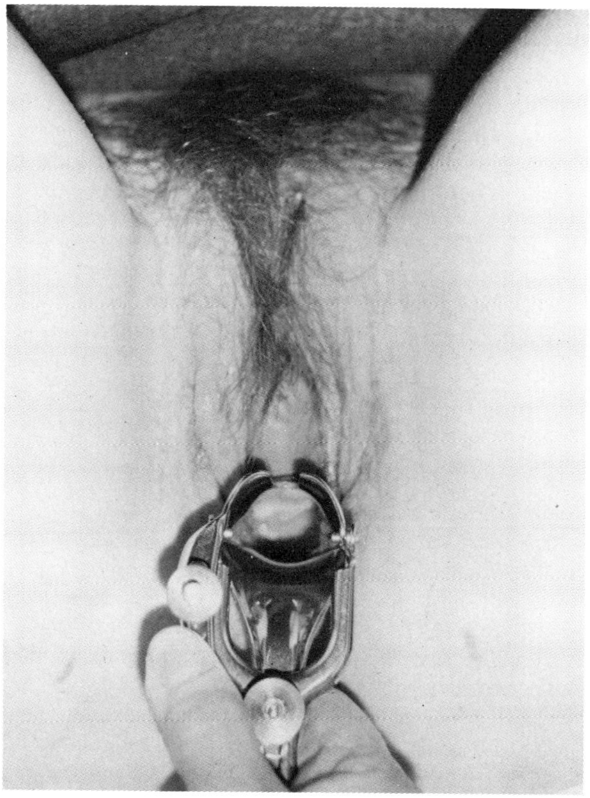

Figure 4 One-year postoperative speculum examination demonstrates a functional and esthetically acceptable vagina.

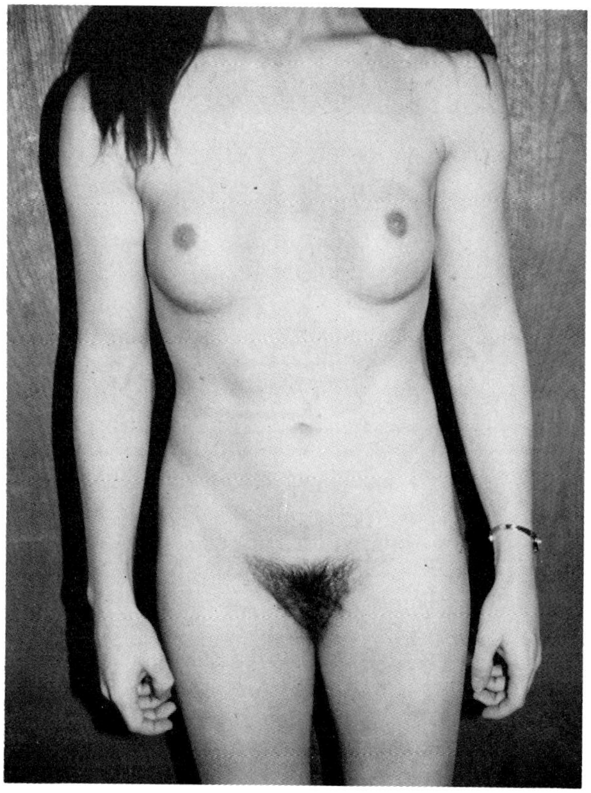

Figure 5 External escutcheon one year postoperatively.

There are various alternative techniques for reconstruction of the vagina. The first and simplest method is a modification of the McIndoe operation, originally used for congenital absence of the vagina. Modification of that operative technique utilizes a split-thickness skin graft from the thigh or a full-thickness free skin graft from the penile shaft to line the newly created vaginal pocket. In both methods, the scrotal skin is then used to reconstruct the labia. The free skin graft method is usually a one-stage procedure and demands meticulous attention to detail during the operative procedure to ensure full and complete healing of the graft. There is a tendency for a skin graft to contract secondarily when placed into the neovaginal pocket. This may produce a vagina of unacceptable depth and width. In addition, the skin-grafted patients are required to wear a vaginal conformer or dilator for at least 6 to 12 months postoperatively. Patient compliance is essential because when the free skin graft technique fails, a nonfunctional vaginal pocket results. The skin graft method is useful for patients who have undergone previous penectomy, either surgically or by self-mutilation. It is also a useful salvage technique for patients who have had an unsuccessful attempt at vaginal reconstruction with the penile flap technique, or in patients who experience partial flap necrosis.

Another method of vaginal reconstruction involves the use of paired gracilis muscle flaps with skin grafts placed over the gracilis muscles. This method is preferred to use of gracilis musculocutaneous flaps. The narrow width of the android pelvis can make such flaps too bulky for a functional vaginal lumen. The problem may be avoided by a preliminary suction lipectomy to the inner thighs prior to gracilis musculocutaneous flap transfer. Gracilis muscle flaps with skin grafts are seldom used unless there is prior mutilation, local tissue loss, or the need for additional blood supply in the area of vaginal reconstruction. This technique has been successful in patients who previously have received irradiation to the pelvic area.

Other methods have been proposed for reconstruction of the vagina in the transsexual patient. These include use of a short section of small bowel (ileum) or of the sigmoid colon for vaginal wall reconstruction. Such operations should only be used in the treatment of the patient who has experienced complications of a rectovaginal fistula after previous attempts at standard vaginal reconstruction. The segment of large bowel that forms the neovagina brings its own blood supply through branches of the superior and inferior hemorrhoidal vessels. When bowel is used for reconstruction of the vagina, the sigmoid is more satisfactory than a section of small bowel, because it does not produce troublesome mucous secretions in the neovagina and also allows the patient some degree of sensation in the vaginal lining. Reconstruction of the vagina from the sigmoid colon does entail the inherent risks and potential morbidity that accompany a major abdominal operation. In these cases, a temporary diverting colostomy should be considered. This is wise, especially in the patient who is being treated synchronously for a rectovaginal fistula. Rectovaginal fistulas also have been successfully treated by rotation of an inferiorly-based rectus abdominis flap between the neovagina and the rectum.

COMPLICATIONS

As with any major operative procedure, a variety of complications can occur. Most of these are directly related to surgical technique and can be avoided. However, some complications, such as infection and small hematoma, are unpredictable. Meticulous hemostasis throughout the operative procedure is essential in order to prevent hematoma formation. Partial tissue loss, or loss of a skin flap or skin graft, is a potential complication and occurs in approximately 10 percent of patients. These tissue losses generally respond to conservative treatment and, unless they are severe, do not compromise the overall vaginal reconstruction. The most serious complication is development of a fistula, either cystovaginal or rectovaginal. Rectovaginal fistulas generally occur from inadvertent direct dissection into the rectum, unbeknown to the operator during the operation, or following infection of the penile skin fascial flap. If the rectum is knowingly entered during the operative procedure, it should be repaired directly in anatomic layers. Communication between the neovagina and the rectum produces severe infection, scarring, troublesome drainage of feces into the neovagina, and even obliteration of the neovaginal vault, all of which lead to a totally unacceptable result for the patient. Mild to moderate introital stenosis occurs in approximately 10 percent of all patients. This is treated readily by nonoperative methods: repeated dilation and stent application for a period of 6 to 12 months postoperatively. When introital stenosis persists after that period of time, either a local Z-plasty flap transposition or application of a thick split-thickness skin graft to the area alleviates the problem. Direct suturing of the penile fascial flap to the internal pelvic periosteum and to the base of the bladder has eliminated foreshortening of the vaginal canal and problems with midvaginal stenosis.

Inadequate incision of periurethral erectile tissues can lead to severe dyspareunia, which can be very troublesome. Local steroid injections or secondary resection of periurethral erectile tissue, performed on an outpatient basis, ususally remedy this problem. Another potential complication that can be avoided by careful operative planning is malpositioning of the urethra. The urine stream should be directed downward rather than forward. In addition, placing multiple Z-plasties around the circumference of the urethrocutaneous junction eliminates urethral stenosis and problems with an altered urine stream during voiding.

ANCILLARY PROCEDURES

In addition to vaginal reconstruction of an esthetic and functional quality, many male transsexual patients require additional plastic surgery to maximize their functional feminine role in society. Hormonal treatment alone will produce adequate breast development in more than half of the patients. The rest usually request augmentation mammoplasty to recontour the chest wall. In addition, all patients require electrolysis and hormonal therapy during their course of therapy. Approximately half of the patients request rhinoplasty to produce a more esthetic female facial appearance. This can often be combined with contouring mentoplasty and a cosmetic cheiloplasty. Approximately one-quarter of patients request a laryngeal cartilage shave to improve the contour of the neck. Many older patients request foreheadplasty, blepharoplasty, and rhytidectomy to soften facial features and produce a more restful, pleasant appearance.

When the neuropsychiatric disorder known as transsexualism can be identified clearly during childhood, environmental modification may offer promising treatment. When discrete hormonal and releasing factor abnormalities can be accurately identified in the hypothalamus, it may be possible to modify them chemically to alter psychosexual behavior earlier in the history of the disorder and thereby allow the patient to deal comfortably with his original biologic sex. Until such breakthroughs occur, however, patients with transsexualism will still request surgical and hormonal treatment. These operations, at the minimum, bring the anatomic and psychological genders into harmony and provide a high degree of subjective patient relief. The overwhelming majority of patients treated by operative therapy give consistent reports of markedly improved self-image and personal satisfaction. At the University of Virginia Gender Identity Clinic, some patients have been followed for over 25 years. To date, there has been no patient in this series who regretted surgical treatment and this includes patients who experienced one or more major complications during reconstructive procedure. I have found transsexual patients to be consistently well-motivated, cooperative, and highly appreciative when reasonable surgical results are obtained.

SUGGESTED READING

American Psychiatric Association. Diagnostic and statistical manual of mental disorders. 3rd ed. Washington, D.C.: American Psychiatric Association, 1987.

Edgerton MT Jr, Langman MW, Schmidt JS, et al. Psychologic considerations of gender reassignment surgery. Clin Plast Surg 1982; 9:355–366.

McIndoe AH. The treatment of congenital absence and obliterative conditions of the vagina. Br J Plast Surg 1950; 2:254–267.

Mezer R, Kesseling UK. One-stage reconstruction of the vagina with penile skin as an island flap in male transsexuals. Plast Reconstr Surg 1980; 66:401–405.

Turner UG, Edlich R, Edgerton MT Jr. Male transsexualism—a review of genital surgical reconstruction. Am J Obstet Gynecol 1978; 132:119–133.

UPPER EXTREMITY

RADIOLOGIC EXAMINATION

LOUIS A. GILULA, M.D.
DAVID C. HARDY, M.D.

There are two major indications for preoperative radiologic examination of the upper extremity. The first is to identify the extent of a known soft tissue or bone abnormality. The second is to identify an underlying osseous abnormality prior to an operative procedure. This is especially important in our current medicolegal climate. In the absence of preoperative x-ray films, an unrelated osseous abnormality might later be mistaken as a consequence of the operative procedure. In our experience, it is not uncommon to find unsuspected underlying abnormalities (Fig. 1).

There are routine and specially tailored roentgenographic examinations available for various parts of the body to evaluate many individual problems. It is important that the referring physician conveys specific pertinent patient problems to the radiologist so that appropriate examinations and the best possible result may be obtained.

AVAILABLE RADIOLOGIC TECHNIQUES

Of the many different radiologic procedures available, we will briefly consider some of the different examinations available for each part of the upper extremity. These include:

1. Conventional ("routine") x-ray studies.
2. Detailed roentgenographic views for each anatomic site of question.
3. Fluoroscopically-directed spot views.
4. Nuclear medicine examination (bone scan).
5. Tomography.
6. Computed tomography.
7. Other specialty examinations, including:
   a. videotape or ciné
   b. arthrography
   c. angiography
   d. magnetic resonance imaging (MRI)
   e. ultrasound.

1. *Radiologic examinations.* Routine radiologic examinations are available for all parts of the body. In the upper extremity, the shoulder, arm, elbow, forearm, wrist, and hand have their own routine examinations, which may vary slightly between radiologic installations. The shoulder joint can be routinely examined in two views: (1) the anteroposterior (AP) position with the arm in internal rotation, and (2) the posterior oblique position of approximately 45 degrees, which profiles the glenohumeral joint and places the humeral head in external rotation (Fig. 2). When the humerus is in external rotation, the greater tuberosity is profiled. As these two views can be obtained without genohumeral joint motion, this examination can be obtained without potential injury to the patient that could be caused during positioning for x-ray studies. Numerous other views are available for the shoulder, depending on whether or not information is desired about the glenohumeral joint, acromion, clavicle, scapula, biceps tendon groove, glenoid labrum, acromioclavicular joint, etc. Additionally, pain can be referred from the neck into the shoulder. Therefore, the appropriate shoulder examination depends entirely on the specific problem and site of interest determined by the referring physician.

A routine arm examination is obtained in AP and lateral views and should include both the elbow and shoulder joints. For our routine elbow examination, we prefer an AP view with the elbow extended, and AP external rotation and lateral views (Fig. 3). The AP external rotation view is valuable to profile the radial head and the radioulnar articulation. The lateral view, as well as showing the bony structures, is valuable to define fluid or synovial thickening within the elbow joint, as indicated by abnormal displacement of either the anterior or posterior fatpads.

The forearm is routinely examined in both AP and lateral positions that include the elbow and wrist. The AP view of the entire forearm should be obtained with the hand in supine position and the forearm flat on the table. To obtain a lateral view of the forearm at right angles to the AP view, the wrist and elbow should be flat on the table (or x-ray film) with the elbow and shoulder at the same level above the floor.

A survey examination of the wrist should include four views. They are posteroanterior (PA) with the palm of the hand flat on the x-ray film, 45-degree oblique position (with the thumb elevated off the x-ray film), and PA ulnar deviation view (to profile the scaphoid more completely).

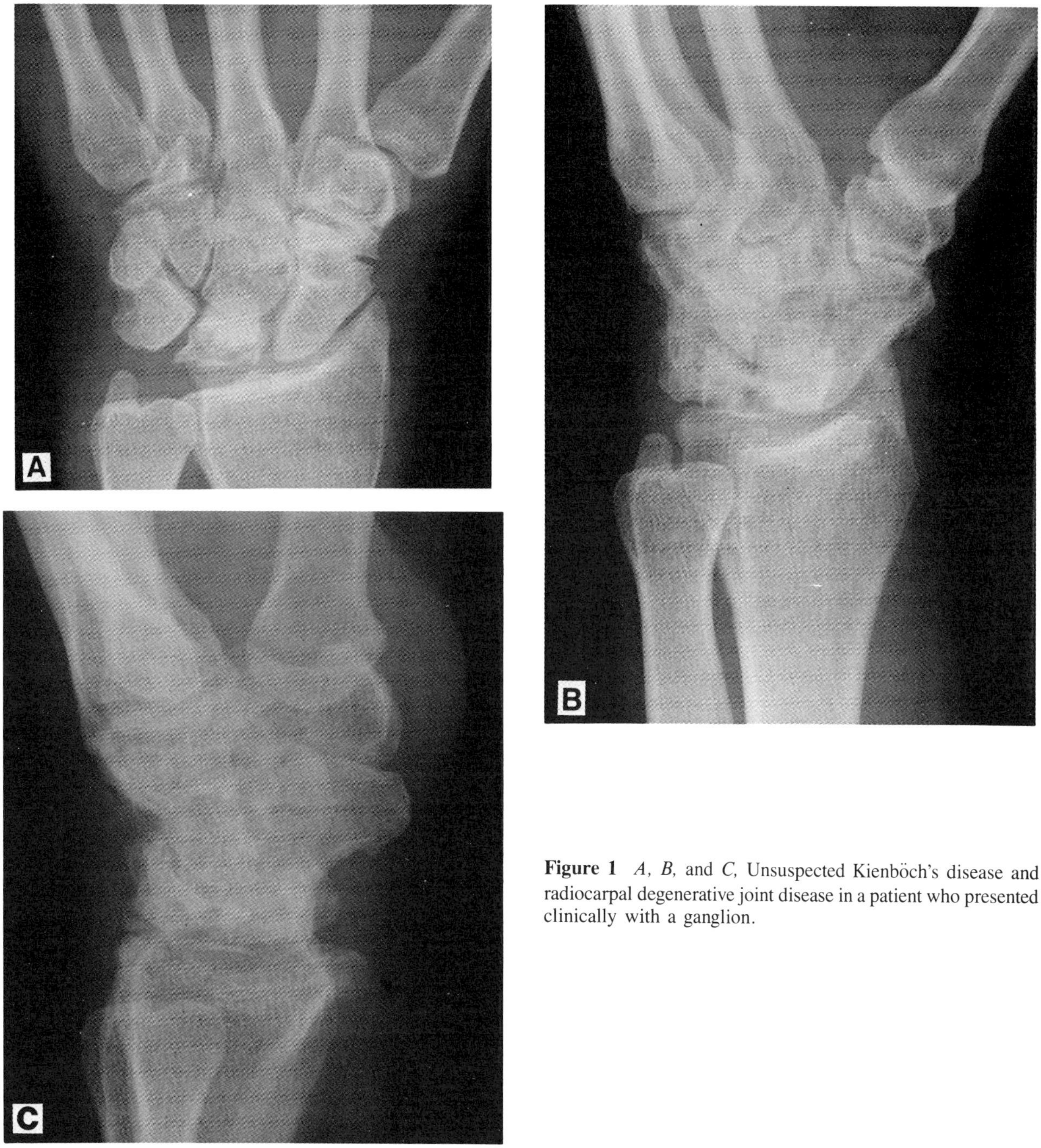

Figure 1 *A, B,* and *C,* Unsuspected Kienböch's disease and radiocarpal degenerative joint disease in a patient who presented clinically with a ganglion.

These three views should be obtained with the elbow, wrist, and shoulder in the same plane above the floor. The fourth routine view for the wrist should be obtained in the lateral position with the elbow at the patient's side. This combination of views provides a survey examination for the wrist and also displays the ulna in right angle positions (Fig. 4).

Routine examination of the hand includes PA, oblique, and lateral views. Fingers should be extended and not flexed on the oblique view, to prevent foreshortening of the phalanges. On the lateral view, the fingers should be separated to eliminate overlapping (Fig. 5). Such separation of the fingers allows ready evaluation of the dorsal and ventral aspects of all the phalanges. Failure to obtain routine lateral views of the hand and wrist can lead to failure to spot significant abnormalities. A detailed three-view examination of the fingers can be obtained in the PA, lateral, and oblique projections to include the entire area of interest.

2. *Detailed spot views.* For every site of anatomy within the upper extremity, as well as elsewhere in the body, coned down or detailed views, using routine radiologic examination, can be obtained to display specific sites of anatomic interest. For some sites, routine views are

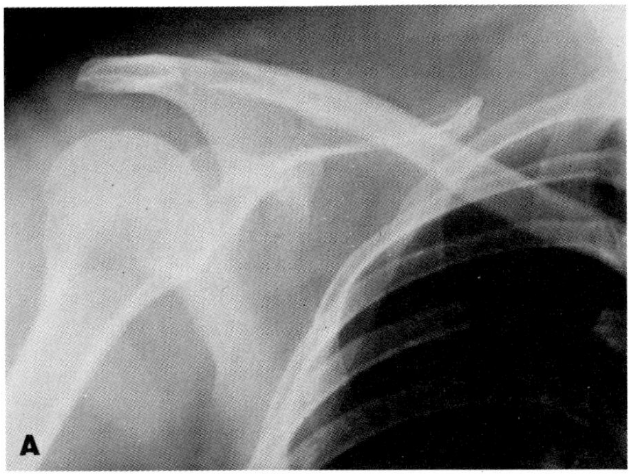

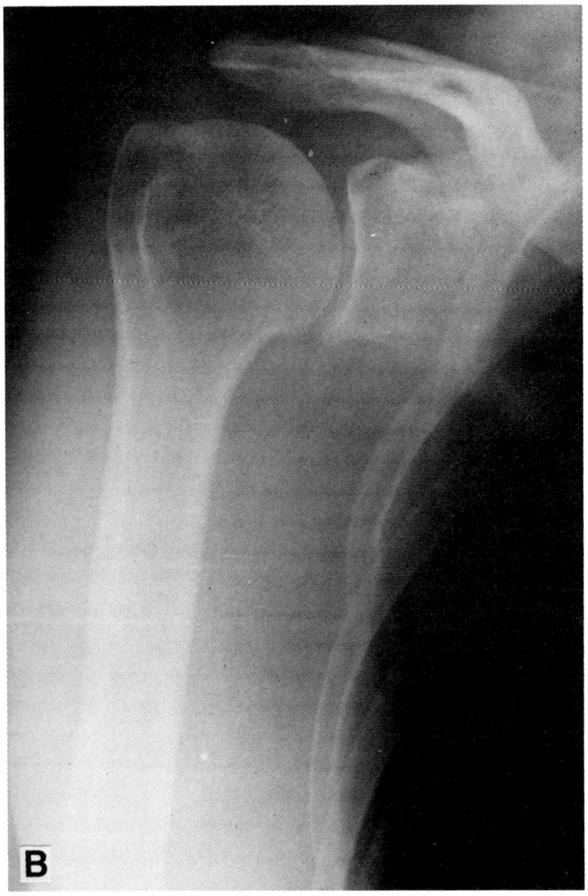

Figure 2 Routine radiologic examination of the shoulder in *A*, Anteroposterior (AP) and *B*, Posterior oblique positions.

available (Fig. 6). Work done in cooperation with a radiologist allows determination of other specific views designed for any localized area of question. One method of obtaining detailed views is to perform x-ray film exposures at multiple degrees of obliquity at small increments, i.e., 2 to 5 degrees tangent to an area of interest. This may enable profile of subtle bony abnormalities that are seen only when the abnormality is placed precisely tangent to the x-ray beam.

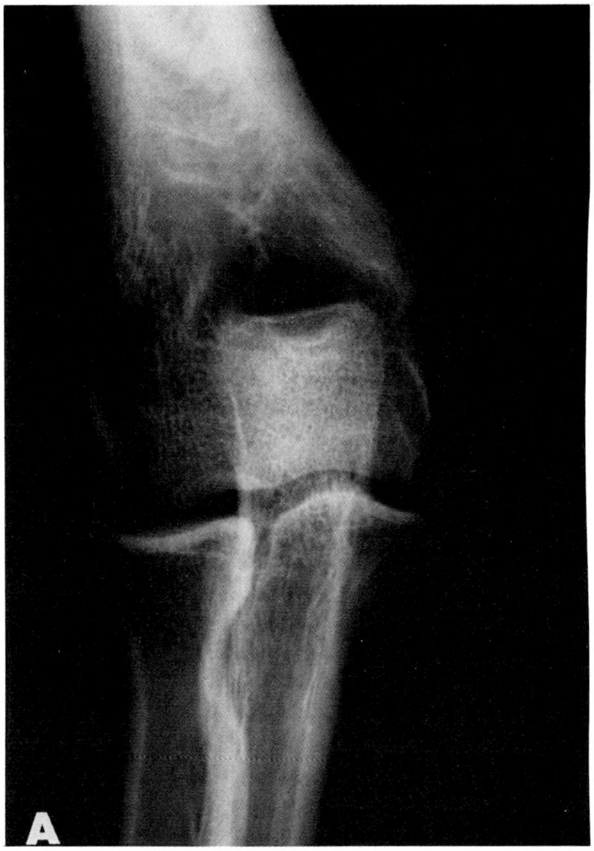

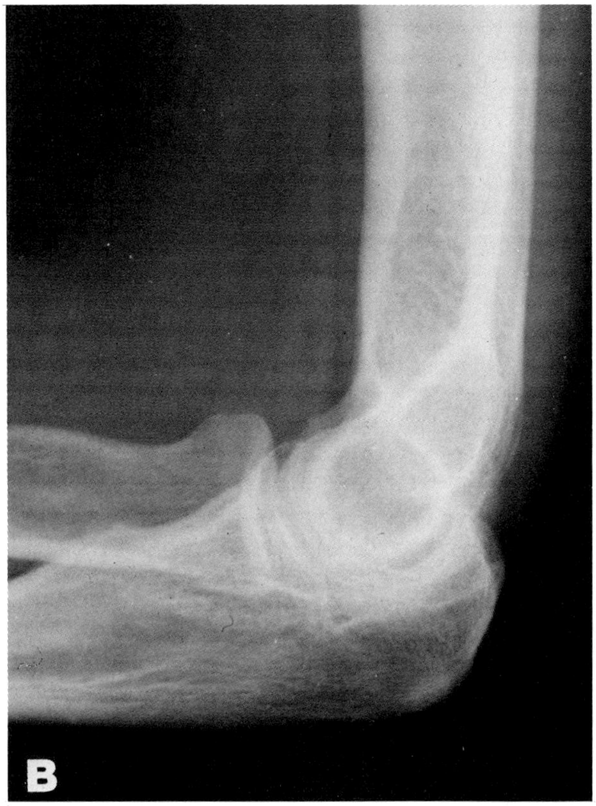

Figure 3 Routine radiologic examination of the elbow in *A*, AP, and B, Lateral views.

Figure continues on opposite page

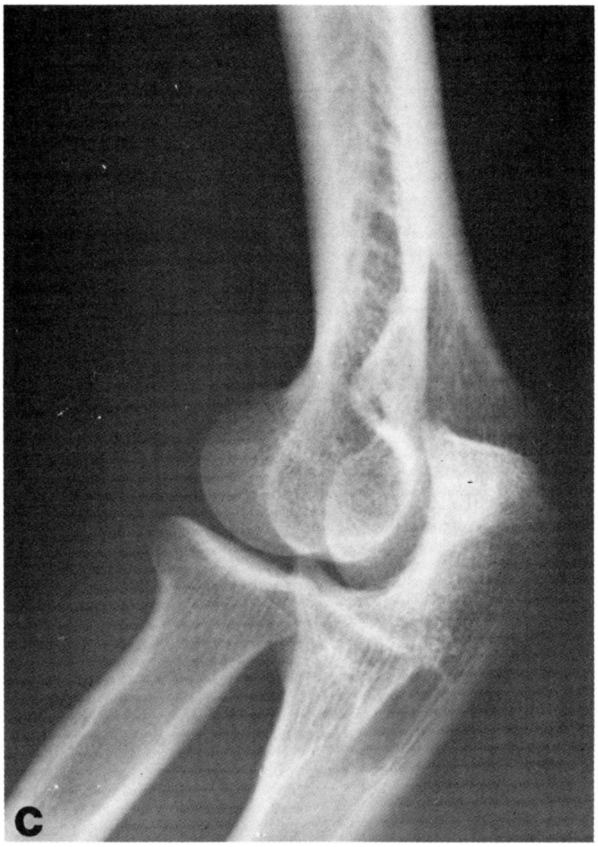

Figure 3 (continued) Routine radiologic examination of the elbow in *C*, AP external oblique view.

3. *Fluoroscopic spot views.* These are often most helpful when routine overhead obliques, as described in section 2, above, are not satisfactory. Fluoroscopic spot views may be particularly valuable in areas of complex bony anatomy, such as the wrist, where there is a desire to profile a joint or a specific cortical surface.

4. *Nuclear medicine examination.* A triple phase bone scan is performed by injecting a radioisotope, typically technetium^{99m} methylene diphosphonate. The radioisotope flow can be imaged immediately after injection to provide a map of upper extremity arterial filling, typically in the forearm and hand. The second phase image is performed at the end of the arterial flow and demonstrates soft tissues of the forearms and hand. The final phase is performed 2 to 4 hours later and comprises static images of radioisotope within bone. A detailed bone scan can also be performed to center at any portion of the body, including the elbow, shoulder, hand, or wrist. Detailed imaging of a specific joint, with comparison to the opposite side, produces finer resolution and greater detail than a bone scan that shows the entire body. Again, desires of the requesting physician must be transmitted to the radiologist, so that an appropriate study can be performed.

Generally speaking, the bone scan will be hot or abnormal in most patients by 3 days after a bone injury if it is going to become abnormal. It should be hot by 24 hours in 80 percent of people of all ages and 96 percent of persons under 65 years of age; by 3 days in 95 percent of persons of all ages and 100 percent of persons under 65 years of age; and by 1 week in 100 percent of people.

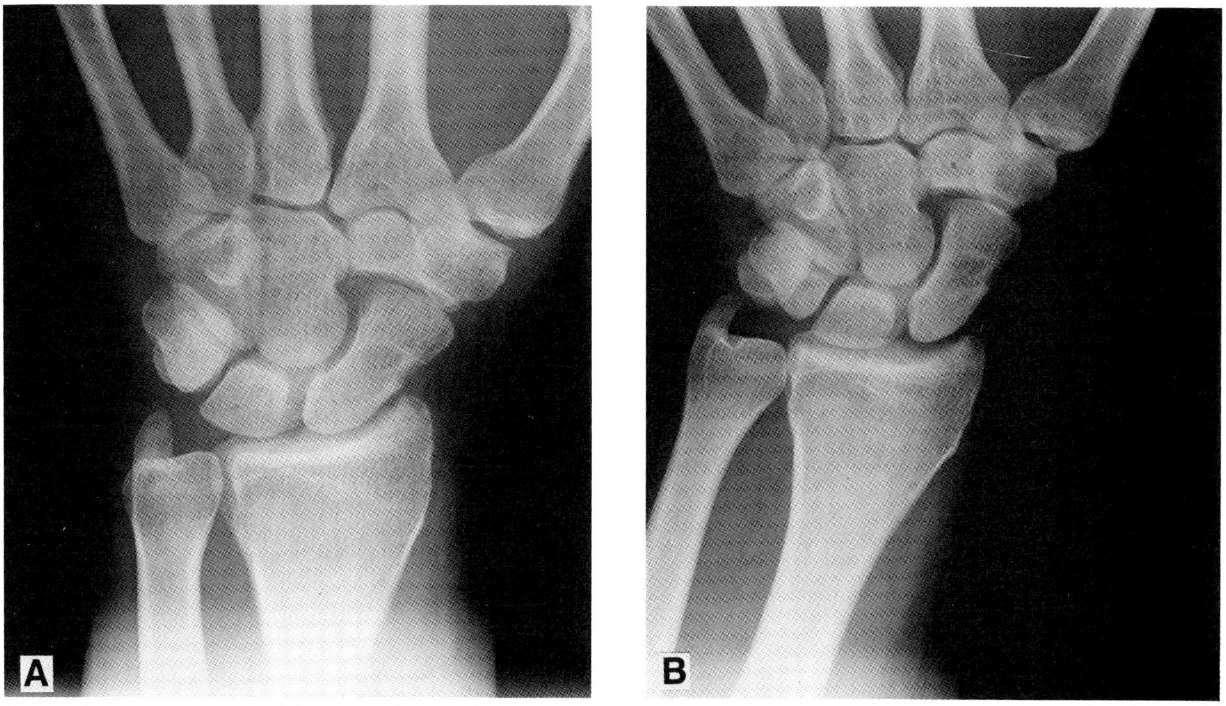

Figure 4 Routine wrist radiologic examination in *A*, Posteroanterior (PA), *B* (PA) ulnar deviated (scaphoid view).

Figure continues on following page

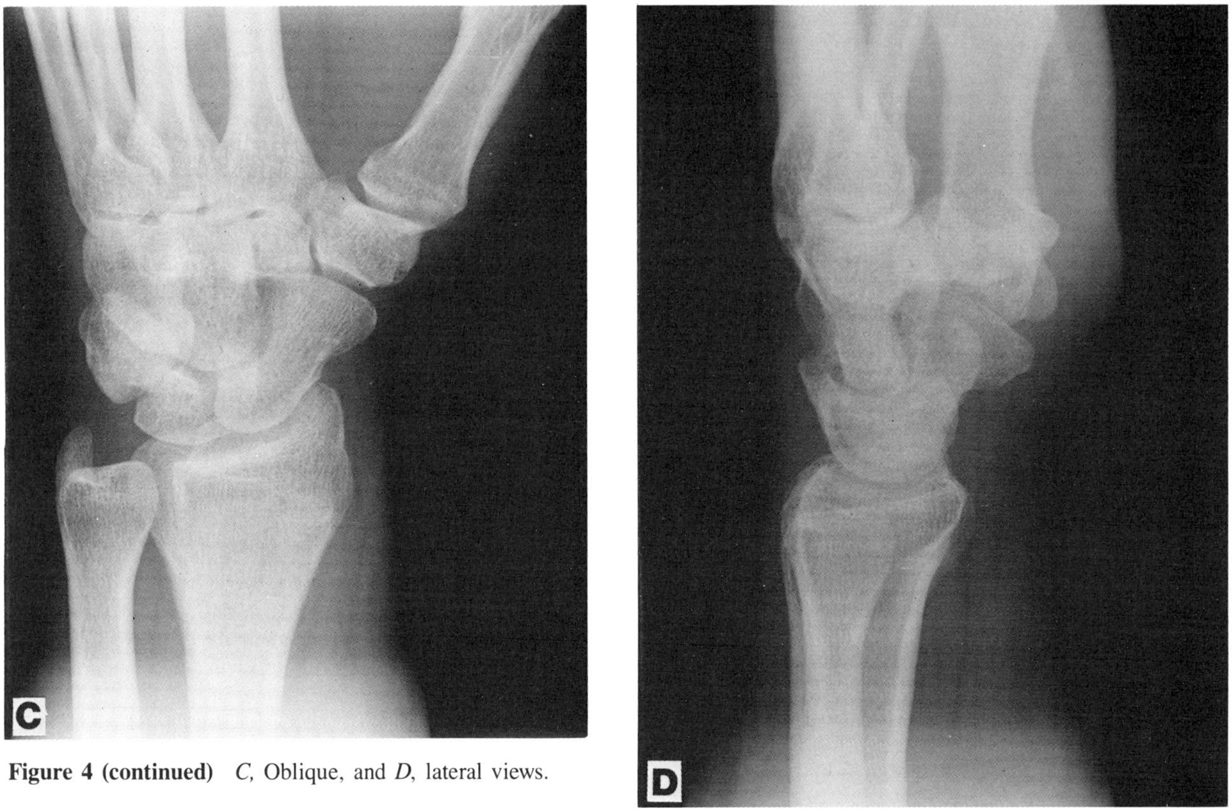

Figure 4 (continued) *C,* Oblique, and *D,* lateral views.

Practically speaking, the exception to scans becoming hot when there is an underlying bony abnormality, is when a patient can no longer form bone, or when a destructive process is present without bone formation, as encountered in some cases of multiple myeloma and occasional, very destructive metastases. Although it is not proven, there are some who feel that there may be increased tracer uptake early after an injury, due to ligamentous injury. However, chronic focal increased uptake probably represents osteochondral abnormality. In the face of a persistent focal hot spot, we believe it is worthwhile to obtain a sequential series of examinations until an abnormality is defined. This sequence may begin with routine x-ray studies, followed by detailed spots, fluoroscopic spots, precisely positioned tomograms, and, lastly, computed tomography or MR images to verify the cause of a focal area of bony abnormality. A hot area may be due to chondromalacia or a small osteochondral chip, and the aim of additional radiologic procedures is to identify some type of bony abnormality. Magnetic resonance imaging or arthrography may be necessary to demonstrate a cartilage abnormality. In the occasional patient, where no radiologically demonstrable abnormality can be found, surgical exploration may be indicated to find a focal cartilage or small osteochondral abnormality that may then be treated to relieve a patient's pain.

5. *Tomography (linear and pluridirectional).* Tomography is performed by moving the x-ray tube and film so as to provide images at different levels above the x-ray table. Depending on the area of involvement, variable thicknesses of tomographic sections may be obtained. In general, with small bony parts, narrow sections should be obtained to enable evaluation of a small osteochondral abnormality. When dealing with small bony parts, such as a metacarpal head or carpal bone, it is probably best to obtain 1 mm-thick sections with a fairly complex path of the x-ray tube through the area of interest. If only linear tomography is available, i.e., the path of the tomographic machine can only move in a linear fashion and not in a complex path, the bone surface of question should be placed so that the x-ray tube travels in a path at right angles to the cortex of interest. It is important that linear or pluridirectional tomography is performed so that the bone surface or joint of interest is placed in a position that allows the resulting tomographic sections to display the area of interest best.

6. *Computed tomography (CT).* This is now widely available and can display anatomic structures in a cross-sectional manner. The image is obtained by passing an x-ray beam through an anatomic site of interest, measuring the attenuation of the beam on the opposite side by digital detectors and then displaying the anatomy in a digital form, so that resulting images can be seen on a cathode ray tube or printed on x-ray film. The images can be reformatted into various planes by using the axial data, so that cross-sectional anatomy can be displayed, typically in sagittal or coronal planes, as well as other planes in some applications. Newly available software and hardware packages allow three-dimensional reconstruction of images.

CT can show bony structures well, and in sites with abundant fat, soft tissues can also be displayed clearly. Performance of the CT examination should be tailored to the

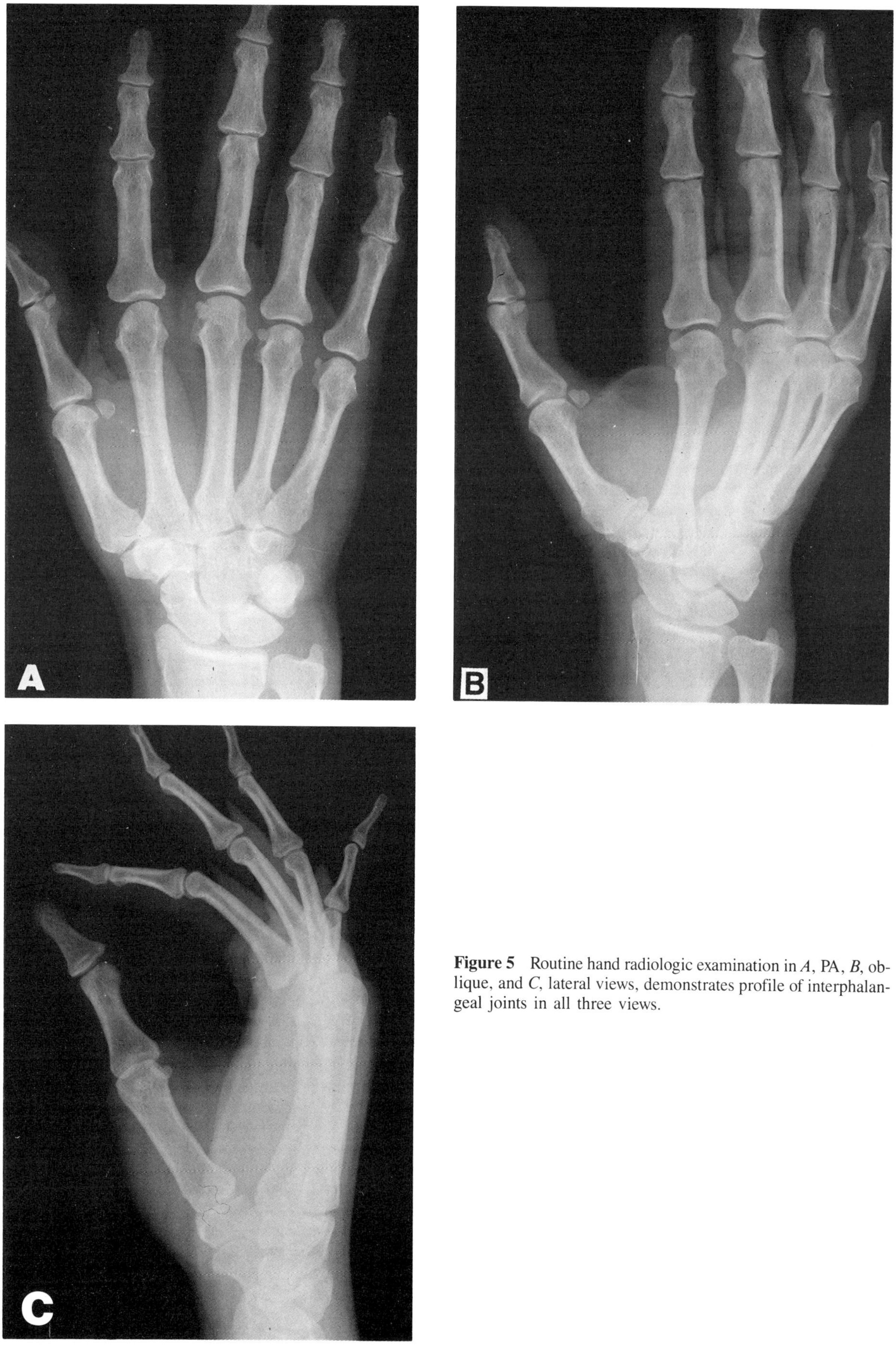

Figure 5 Routine hand radiologic examination in *A*, PA, *B*, oblique, and *C*, lateral views, demonstrates profile of interphalangeal joints in all three views.

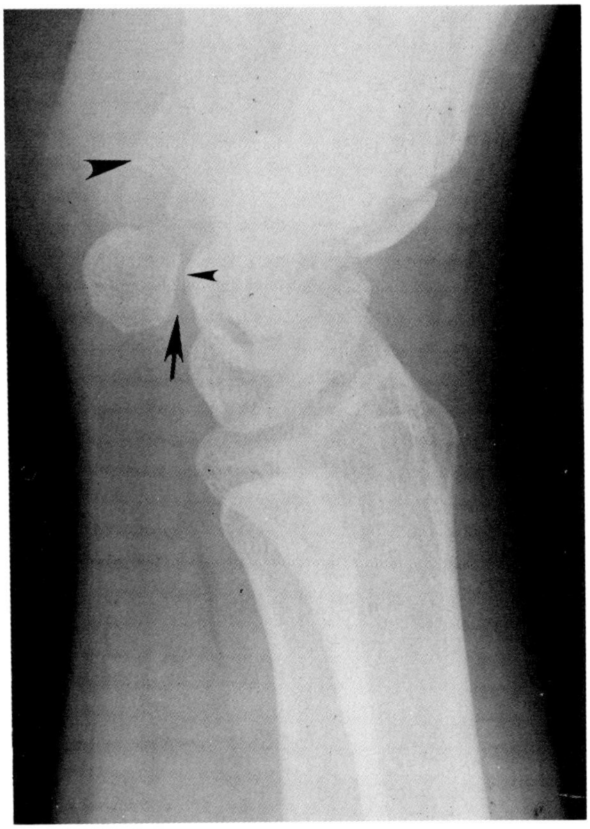

Figure 6 Off-lateral view of the wrist profiles the pisotriquetral joint (arrow), the tip of the hamate hook (large arrowhead), and the ventral surface of the triquetrum (small arrowhead).

specific question at hand, for example, in the wrist one could select coronal or transaxial approaches. When detailed anatomic information is desired about a small bony structure, or an area of complex anatomy, thin sections at close intervals (i.e., 2 mm-thick sections at 2 mm intervals) prove satisfactory. At other times, wider sections at overlapping intervals (i.e., 4 mm-thick sections at 2 mm) can be obtained. When information is desired about a large area of interest, for instance the extent of a large soft tissue or bony tumor, greater intervals may be obtained, i.e., 1 to 4 cm between sections. For best performance of three-dimensional reconstruction, thinner sections with very narrow intervals, i.e., 2 mm-thick at 2 mm or 1 mm intervals are optimal.

CT is best used when more precise bony detail is desired than is available with routine tomography, especially in sites where bony structures cannot be clearly separated by routine radiologic procedures. CT provides very clear definition of the cortex of rounded structures, as it displays the entire circumference of a rounded structure. Such information is not otherwise available even with multiple tangential oblique views. Computed tomography can be used to detect medullary involvement in the case with known cortical involvement. The low attenuation marrow fat is abnormal when it is replaced by higher attenuation soft tissue density.

A variety of other examinations can be used in specific instances. They include (a) videofluoroscopy or ciné, (b) arthrography, (c) angiography, (d) magnetic resonance imaging (MRI), and (e) ultrasound.

a. *Videofluoroscopy* of a joint can be performed when there is a desire to record motion—to watch for "popping" or some abnormal motion that cannot be clearly understood by physical examination alone. This can also provide a valuable way to record the abnormal motion. Ciné consists of rapid filming sequences with numerous exposed x-ray films. It requires significantly higher roentgen ray exposure, higher film cost, and is more time-consuming than videotape or fluoroscopy.

b. *Arthrography* can be used in the shoulder, elbow, wrist, and finger joints. It is used to demonstrate articular cartilage, ligament, and capsular abnormalities.

Shoulder. Shoulder arthrography is used to demonstrate rotator cuff tears, adhesive capsulitis, biceps tendon abnormalities, and a variety of capsular and intracapsular problems. Double contrast arthrography, using air and water soluble contrast agent, is preferred for the shoulder by many authors. Double contrast technique has the advantage of demonstrating the characteristics and size of a rotator cuff defect better than a positive contrast examination. Additionally, double contrast usually shows cartilage surfaces better than a single contrast examination. Currently, the best procedure available to demonstrate cartilage abnormalities of the glenoid labrum is computed tomography in combination with double contrast arthrography.

Elbow. Arthrography in the elbow may be used with or without tomography to look for intraarticular bodies that cannot be shown by routine radiologic examination, and can verify if bodies seen on routine examination are intraarticular or extraarticular. The cartilage surfaces can also be demonstrated with elbow arthrography. Either double contrast or single contrast studies may be used in various radiology departments.

Wrist. Wrist arthrography is usually done as a single contrast examination and can be performed by injection of one or all of the midcarpal, radiocarpal, or distal radioulnar joints. Most commonly, arthrography performed at the radiocarpal or midcarpal joints is used to look for tears of the triangular fibrocartilage and scapholunate and lunotriquetral ligaments. It may also be used to demonstrate tears along the radial or ulnar sides of the capsule. Contrast injection into the distal radioulnar joint can be used to demonstrate ulnar capsule defects, as well as tears at the proximal triangular fibrocartilage surface, if a defect has not already been identified by injection of the radiocarpal or midcarpal joints.

Finger joints. Arthrography of interphalangeal and metacarpophalangeal joints can be performed to document integrity of the articular capsule. An additional use of arthrography, using small amounts of contrast, is to verify intraarticular placement of medication, i.e., steroids.

c. *Angiography.* Arteriography is of value when definition of the arterial supply, or differentiation of normal from abnormal arterial anatomy, is required. In patients with questionable vascular insufficiency, arteriography may demonstrate evidence of vasculitis, vascular stenosis, or occlusion. Arteriography has been used to determine the vascularity of a bone or soft tissue mass, and also to demonstrate to better advantage the periphery and extent of a mass. However, contemporary computed tomography and magnetic images can usually evaluate soft tissue masses better than arteriography. Arteriography requires intraarterial needle and catheter placement and is more invasive than computed tomography and magnetic resonance imaging. Arteriography may be performed, if necessary, by injection of venous structures with digital subtraction techniques.

Another indication for arteriography is to demonstrate the arterial supply of skin and soft tissue flaps. It is of utmost importance to make certain the angiographer knows the exact reason for the arteriogram prior to the procedure, so that the desired angiographic information will be provided. Venography is used most commonly in the upper extremities when there is question of thrombophlebitis, old or new. Occasionally, venography is also performed to define the venous anatomy for venous procedures, or to define a vein source for harvest, or occasionally to create dialysis fistulas.

d. *Magnetic resonance imaging.* This relies on a strong magnetic field affecting orientation of various substances within the cell. Sophisticated digital recording of behavior of these particles is performed after the particles are lined up in the same direction as the magnetic field. The image is recorded as they return to their original pattern after the orientation of the magnetic field has been altered. Soft tissues can be imaged directly, and cortices of bones can be seen by contrast with the soft tissue structures within and outside the bone. MRI does not usually display calcifications or bone directly, unless the calcification or bone is large enough to be outlined by increased signal of adjacent soft tissues. Moving tissue that exits the section, such as blood, exhibits no signal, but is also visible by contrast with the signal in the surrounding soft tissues that outlines the vascular structures.

MRI shows soft tissue structures better than any other imaging technique, but it is more expensive than most other noninvasive imaging techniques. In general, when MRI is compared to CT, it may be stated that CT can show bony structures as well as MRI; however, if there is any soft tissue involvement, MRI generally will surpass CT. Therefore, if neoplasia or a process that involves bone is expected to involve soft tissue, or if a process involves soft tissues only, MRI would be the procedure of choice to determine the extent and exact anatomic area of involvement. A few patients may not be candidates for magnetic resonance imaging. Specifically, these are patients with ferromagnetic metallic vascular clips in the skull, patients with pacemakers, or those with some other apparatus that may be adversely affected by the magnetic field. A small group of patients who are claustrophobic, i.e., who cannot tolerate lying within a round cylinder, will not be able to tolerate either MRI or CT. Patients may have to lie on the examination table for a longer period of time for MRI to be successful than for CT. In the future, magnetic resonance imaging will produce still better images with the development of newer coils and faster imaging methods.

e. *Ultrasound.* In some institutions, ultrasound of musculoskeletal structures is routinely performed. Ultrasound can be used to look at certain structures, i.e., rotator cuff to see if it is intact, and to evaluate the status of various ligaments and tendons. It can also be used to see if a soft tissue mass is present and to determine the composition of the mass, i.e., whether or not it is cystic. The use of ultrasound is highly operator-dependent and is still in an evolving stage.

APPROACH TO UPPER EXTREMITY EVALUATION

In general, the first procedure to be obtained for the shoulder, arm, elbow, forearm, wrist, and hand is the standard examination as described above in section 1. This routine examination should be sufficient to identify unsuspected underlying osseous abnormalities prior to any other operative procedure (see Fig. 1).

To identify the extent and character of known bone or soft tissue abnormalities after a routine radiologic examination has been performed, the combination of bone scan with CT or MRI should be considered. The bone scan is valuable to show the extent of bony abnormality in the area of known pathology and also to detect other possible sites of bony abnormality. As described above, if MRI is available, it should be used if there is any question or possibility of soft tissue involvement. CT may be valuable to demonstrate complex bone anatomy or early signs of bony healing. CT will show calcifications where MRI will generally not show them unless they are large enough to create a large defect within the soft tissue structures. Such large calcifications should usually be identified on ordinary x-ray studies. CT is still of value to examine soft tissues if MRI is not available, especially where there are abundant fatty planes.

In the upper extremity, CT can be of definite value in the shoulder and about the elbow, wrist, and metacarpal areas, as there are fairly abundant fatty planes in these sites. In the arm and forearm, where there is relatively little fat and much more solid muscle, MRI is preferable; however, CT in these sites can sometimes be of value, especially when the opposite side is used for comparison. CT of the wrist, performed in the coronal fashion, provides an easy way to demonstrate the carpal bone anatomy in an easily understood manner. However, at times, CT should be performed with an axial orientation to demonstrate the distal radioulnar joint or a hook of the hamate fracture—in the exceptional case that a hook of hamate fracture cannot be shown by routine radiologic examination.

In patients with chronic, unexplained pain in the upper extremity, after we have done a routine radiologic examination, we prefer to use bone scan to see if there is support for an osteochondral abnormality, as suggested by a focal hot spot. Additional, detailed, oblique or tangential views of that specific hot spot are usually performed next, followed by an additional sequence of examinations as listed in section 4 under Nuclear medicine examinations.

In the face of a focal hot spot on bone scan, after routine radiologic examinations (see Section 4) have been performed, a decision may arise about the use of routine tomography or computed tomography. Such a decision depends on the area of interest. CT is preferred when fine bone detail is desired in an area of complex bony anatomy, such as that about the carpal bones and, sometimes, the elbow joint. If an answer is not evident, MRI may be considered to look for intraosseous abnormality, such as osteonecrosis. This may provide the earliest radiologic demonstration of an abnormal marrow space, after detection by bone scan.

For the painful wrist, a variety of combinations of these above procedures may be utilized, as described in an earlier work by Gilula et al.

SUGGESTED READING

Biondetti PR, Vannier MW, Gilula LA, Knapp R. Wrist: coronal and transaxial CT scanning. Radiology 1987; 163:149–151.

Freiberger RH, Kaye JJ. Arthrography. New York: Appleton-Century-Crofts, 1979.

Goldman AB. Double contrast shoulder arthrography. In: Weeks PM, ed. Acute bone and joint injuries of the hand and wrist. St. Louis: CV Mosby, 1981: 165.

Goldman AB. The wrist. In: Weeks PM, ed. Acute bone and joint injuries of the hand and wrist. St. Louis: CV Mosby, 1981:277.

Gilula LA, Destouet JM, Weeks PM, Young LV, Wray RC. Roentgenographic diagnosis of the painful wrist. Clin Orthop 1984; 187:52–64.

Hudson T. The elbow. In: Weeks PM, ed. Acute bone and joint injuries of the hand and wrist. St. Louis: CV Mosby, 1981:261.

Kaye J, Schneider R. Positive contrast shoulder arthrography. In: Weeks PM. Acute bone and joint injuries of the hand and wrist. St. Louis: CV Mosby, 1981:137.

Matin P. The appearance of bone scans following fractures, including immediate and long-term studies. J Nucl Med 1979; 20:1227.

Reinus WR, Conway WF, Totty WG, et al. Carpal avascular necrosis: MR imaging. Radiology 1986; 160:689–693.

ROLE OF PHYSICAL THERAPY

PAUL G. PIN, M.D.
PAUL M. WEEKS, M.D.

The purpose of hand physical therapy is to maximize the recovery of lost hand function and to minimize secondary dysfunction of structures not involved by the primary disease process. This is accomplished with techniques that modify wound healing so as to restore and/or maintain motion and strength. The largest group of patients who benefit from hand therapy are those who have suffered a work-related injury. Therapy is directed at complete rehabilitation of the patient, with return to previous occupation in a minimal amount of time. The hand therapist is frequently asked to see a patient prior to elective surgery. Such an encounter is educational for the patient and encourages active involvement postoperatively. The therapist's preoperative assessment establishes a functional baseline for the patient and allows an objective evaluation of the surgical outcome. Such prospective assessments also permit the hand surgeon quantitatively to compare the results of various treatment modalities. A final group of patients that benefits from hand therapy are those with inflammatory disorders, such as arthritis. Exacerbations in symptoms can frequently be managed without loss of motion by proper joint support using custom-made splints.

At the outset of therapy, each patient undergoes a complete assessment, which includes functional limitations, range of motion measurements, and documentation of strength and sensation. The assessment begins with a history of the mechanism of injury and of pertinent medical illnesses. Hand dominance and occupation are also recorded. Observations are made regarding skin color and texture, swelling, and the status of wounds and scars. Inquiry is made about the site and severity of pain, numbness, tenderness, and swelling. Sensibility is determined by pin-prick, static and moving two-point discrimination. Dellon's modified pick-up test, and by the Semmes-Weinstein aesthesiometer. Edema is quantified by circumferential digital measurements in both the injured and uninjured hands. Unless contraindicated, passive and active range of motion measurements are made of each joint in the extremity using an appropriately sized goniometer. Assessment of gross grip strength in the normal and injured hands is made with the Jaymar dynamometer on all five settings. Lateral key pinch is measured with a calibrated pinch gauge.

Data obtained from the assessment is conveyed to the referring physician and a therapeutic plan is formulated based on preexisting protocols modified for the individual patient. This plan is then discussed with the patient. Basic pathophysiology and natural history are described as is the expected outcome of treatment. Strong emphasis is placed on the central role the patient plays in determining the success or failure of therapy. Every effort is made to create an atmosphere where recovery and return to work are the primary goals.

Following the initial assessment, the actual treatment begins. Wound care is an integral part of the therapy of the postoperative and post-traumatic hand. Care consists of cleansing, minimal debridement, suture removal, and application of dressings. The patient receives instruction in wound management so that wound care can be continued at home. A practical knowledge of wound healing on the part of the therapist allows appropriate modification of exercise programs that might otherwise interfere with wound healing. Wound complications identified during therapy are called to the attention of the referring physician.

Exercise consists of a combination of active and passive range of motion, as well as resistive exercise. Through the adjunctive use of splints, select joints remain immobilized while others pass through the entire range of motion. Movement of injured tissues obviously causes some discomfort. Care must be taken to distinguish this sensation from the severe pain associated with destructive motion. Since individual pain tolerance is variable, exercise must be adjusted to the individual. The hypersensitive patient must be positively encouraged to tolerate the inherent discomfort of therapy, while the stoic must be constantly reminded that over-zealous manipulation of injured tissues is harmful. Particular caution is required in the presence of a sensory nerve deficit where there is no intrinsic feedback present to prevent inadvertent injury. Motion that causes persistent, significant pain in the post-exercise period may ultimately result in reflex sympathetic dystrophy. In responsible patients, written instructions and precautions can permit a home exercise program. Such programs are less disruptive to patients' daily activities and permit the patient more responsibility for rehabilitation.

Splinting constitutes the cornerstone of hand therapy. Static splinting in proper positions allows unimpeded healing while limiting secondary stiffness. Dynamic splinting helps favorably modify both developing and preexisting scar tissue and thus can be used to enhance motion. The development of thermoplastic materials for splint construction allows precise, custom fitting for each patient. As edema resolves and motion increases, poorly-fitting splints can be discarded in favor of new ones.

Edema accompanies every hand injury. Persistent edema prolongs the inflammatory phase of wound healing, thereby encouraging fibroblast proliferation and a resultant increase in scar formation. Since scar formation necessarily limits range of motion, all hand edema must be treated aggressively. The normal mechanism by which the hand rids itself of edema fluid is motion. Thus, edema control begins with passive and active motion. Edema ensues when hydrostatic and oncotic pressures are higher intravascularly than extravascularly. Extremity elevation reduces intravascular hydrostatic pressure and thus allows the elimination of edema fluid. Compression finger wraps and intermittent massage are useful in edema reduction.

Our Hand Center infrequently employs transcutaneous nerve stimulation. Generally, the effectiveness of these units appears attributable to a placebo effect rather than to a physiologic manipulation. Modalities such as ultrasonography, heat, paraffin and whirlpool (other than for debridement) are not used at our Hand Center.

Outlined below are basic strategies for hand care following common injuries and surgical procedures. Protocols are presented separately, though in the clinical setting, injuries frequently involve more than one structure, thus necessitating creative modification of these procedures.

Fractures

Therapy for hand fractures is determined by the presence or absence of articular involvement, the method of fixation and the bone fractured. Regardless of the exact fracture and method of fixation, hand therapy is directed at reducing edema, maintaining joint motion and tendon gliding without impairing bone healing. Nondisplaced fractures and fractures that are stable following reduction are usually treated by immobilization for 3 to 4 weeks. Depending on the injury, dorsal splinting may be used to keep the wrist in 30 degrees of extension, the metacarpophalangeal (MP) joints in 70 to 90 degrees of flexion and the interphalangeal (IP) joints in full extension. Immobilization of the IP joints is usually unnecessary in metacarpal fractures. Conversely, MP joint motion is usually possible in many phalangeal fractures. Likewise, uninjured fingers are not immobilized.

Internal fixation is required in unstable fractures and is almost always employed in fractures that have undergone open reduction. Internal fixation offers the distinct advantage of allowing early, active and passive motion. Depending on the rigidity of fixation, protective splinting in the position described above may be used between exercises. Internal fixation may be performed either percutaneously or openly. The latter procedure has the disadvantage of adding soft tissue trauma in addition to a wound. Occasionally, comminuted, intra-articular fractures are not amenable to fixation and reduction. Treatment consists of early active motion in the hope of developing a functional pseudoarthrosis.

Nerve Injuries

Repaired nerves do not tolerate tension in the early postoperative period. Primary neurorrhaphy frequently requires some joint flexion to minimize stress at the repair site. For these reasons, therapy for nerve repairs consists of strict immobilization for 1 week, followed by full active flexion. Extension is limited according to the amount of tension on the suture line at time of repair. Progressive extension is permitted at 4 weeks so that full extension is obtained by 6 to 8 weeks postoperatively.

In contrast, nerve grafting is performed with full digital extension and the repair sites are under no tension. Full active motion is, therefore, permitted at 1 week, though protective splinting is used for 3 to 4 weeks. A baseline sensory battery is obtained preoperatively and repeated at bimonthly intervals postoperatively until a plateau is reached. Mobilization is complemented by protective and dynamic splinting until 8 weeks when the protective splint is completely discarded. Dynamic splinting is continued until full range of motion is required.

Extensor Tendon Injuries

Repaired extensor tendon lacerations proximal to the MP joint are immobilized in extension for 4 weeks in a volar based wrist splint. The number of digits included in the splint depends on which tendons are lacerated. Digital immobilization is unnecessary if only the wrist extensors were injured. With extensor digitorum communis lacerations, the wrist is immobilized in 30 degrees of extension and the MP joints are immobilized in 70 degrees of flexion. Passive flexion and extension of the PIP and DIP joints are permitted; a static splint with the IP joints in extension is worn between exercises. At 4 weeks, light use of the hand and wrist is allowed and active flexion exercises are begun. At 5 weeks, dynamic flexion splinting and resistive exercises are initiated. Full use of the hand is allowed by 8 weeks.

Generally, the more distal a laceration to the extensor mechanism, the longer the required immobilization. This is because extensor tendon healing is slower as one proceeds distally. Furthermore, premature motion results in elongation of the extensor mechanism, which is particularly hard to treat. Though prolonged immobilization may lead to IP joints stiff in extension, this is much easier to treat than extensor lag.

Repaired extensor lacerations between the MP and PIP joints are treated by strict immobilization for 4 weeks, with the MP joint in 70 degrees of flexion and the IP joints in full extension. Repaired lacerations distal to the PIP joint are treated by strict immobilization in this position for 6 weeks. Following immobilization, active and passive exercises are begun and are supplemented by dynamic flexion splinting at 8 weeks.

Closed rupture of the terminal extensor tendon from the distal phalanx, results in an extensor lag (mallet finger). Untreated, DIP extension will be poor, and frequently a secondary hyperextension deformity (swanneck) of the PIP joint will develop. Since results of surgical repair of this injury are poor, proper hand therapy is essential to preserve digital function. A volar-based extension splint is used continuously for 6 weeks to immobilize the DIP joint. Hyperextension of the DIP joint consistently causes a stiff joint and should be avoided. The rest of the hand may be used in daily activities. At 6 weeks, gentle exercises and night splinting are employed. Gradual progression in use is allowed unless an extensor lag develops. In this situation, continuous splinting is restarted for at least 2 more weeks. In uncomplicated cases, full use is obtained by 10 to 12 weeks.

Flexor Tendon Injuries

The major dilemma in flexor tendon surgery is how to allow tendon healing without permitting the development of adhesions that will obstruct tendon gliding. This is accomplished by a combination of splinting and early motion. A dorsal splint is constructed during the first visit. The wrist is positioned in 30 degrees of flexion, the MP joints in 40 degrees of flexion and the IP joints in 10 to 20 degrees of flexion. Motion may begin as early as the first postoperative day and consists of *active* digital extension and *passive* digital flexion (Fig. 1). Numerous electromyographic studies have documented that active extension fails to activate flexor muscles, and thus adds

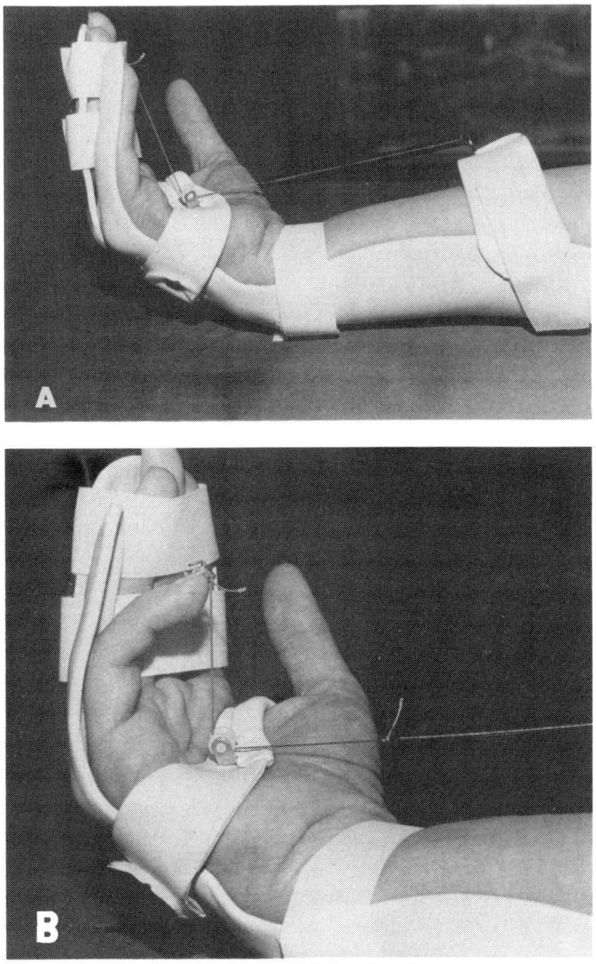

Figure 1 The dorsal splint used following flexor tendon repairs. Early motion consists of active extension (A) and passive flexion (B).

no additional tension to the repair site. Since the profundus tendons share a common muscle belly, active flexion of "uninvolved" digits is disallowed. If desired, rubberband traction consisting of an elastic extending from the nail to a splint wrist strap can substitute for passive flexion. It is critically important when using this method that the PIP joint be fully extended, less a flexion contracture develop.

At 3 weeks, gentle active flexion is begun. A hand-based protective splint is substituted to prevent sudden extension. At 5 weeks, resistive exercises are initiated and dynamic flexion splinting is pursued. Scar massage and edema management proceed as with any injury. Full use is permitted by 12 weeks.

When the tendon bed is scarred, the pulley system destroyed, or the tendon itself is inadequate, staged repair is performed. This sequence begins with the placement of a silastic tendon rod. The objective of hand therapy is to maximize passive MP and IP joint motion while a pseudosheath forms around the rod. Ideally, passive motion should be excellent prior to rod placement. Passive range of motion exercises are begun on the first postoperative day. Between exercises, a trapper splint is worn continuously to keep joints supple. When passive motion is limited, dynamic flexion and extension splints are used as needed.

Usually by 2 to 3 months after placement of the silastic rod, the tissues have softened sufficiently to allow the rod to be replaced by a tendon graft. When there is persistent edema, scarring, or poor passive motion, grafting is deferred until these problems are solved either by time, further hand therapy, or surgery. Unlike a repaired tendon, a tendon graft has no intrinsic blood supply and it must, therefore, adhere to the surrounding tissue. Like any skin graft, this neovascularization depends on strict immobilization. Flexor tendon grafts inserted after rod removal are continuously immobilized for 4 weeks, at which time active flexion and extension exercises are begun. Resistive exercises, dynamic flexion splinting and passive extension splinting are initiated, if needed, at 5 to 6 weeks. Dynamic extension splinting is added 1 week later. Full use of the hand is anticipated by 10 to 12 weeks after grafting.

Tenolysis

Tendon surgery in general and flexor tendon surgery in particular, frequently result in a loss of active range of motion from tendon adhesions. This is especially true after tendon grafting. Tendon gliding can be improved by tenolysis, but tenolysis is delayed at least 6 months after grafting. Ideally, full passive flexion should be present prior to tenolysis. Frequently, however, stiff joints develop synchronously with tendon adhesions. Joint stiffness not amenable to preoperative dynamic splinting is commonly treated at the time of tenolysis by capsulotomy.

Following tenolysis, gentle, hourly active range of motion exercises must begin on the first postoperative day. Pain and edema are managed aggressively as they are precursors of recurrent stiffness. Resistive exercises and dynamic splinting are added at 1 week, and full use is allowed by 4 to 6 weeks.

Stiff Joints

Joint stiffness results from the scarring of structures either intrinsic or extrinsic to the joint. Intrinsic elements include joint capsule, collateral ligaments, and the volar plate. The extrinsic group consists of the flexor and extensor tendons, digital fascia, and skin. Prevention of stiffness is based on continued motion when possible and on proper positioning when immobilization is mandatory.

Because of their eccentric location, the MP joint collateral ligaments are taut in flexion and lax in extension. Therefore, to prevent ligamentous shortening, the MP joints should be immobilized in 70 to 80 degrees of flexion. In contrast, the length of the true collateral ligaments of the interphalangeal joints is unaffected by flexion and extension. Yet the ligaments dorsal and volar to the true collateral ligaments are affected by joint position. The dorsal ligaments are taut in flexion and lax in extension. The volar collateral ligaments are taut in extension but lax in flexion. These joints are immobilized in extension, as joints that are stiff in extension are more successfully treated than those stiff in flexion.

Some stiffness invariably results following even proper immobilization. This stiffness can almost always be successfully treated by hand therapy. Such therapy consists of passive and active exercises in conjunction with dynamic and static splinting. Passive motion should be monitored to prevent pain and edema from excessive tissue trauma. The end point of therapy should be a return of normal motion.

Joint stiffness associated with tendon and ligamentous injuries or with intra-articular fractures frequently requires operative capsulotomy to restore joint motion. In these cases, therapy should begin as soon as possible postoperatively. Delay in therapy inevitably leads to recurrent stiffness. Active and passive motion exercises are instituted to maintain motion. Static and dynamic splinting are useful to prevent relapse, and the type of splint used is determined by the preoperative deformity.

CONCLUSION

Hand therapy has a central role in the successful management of hand patients. Early motion, supplemented by proper splinting, edema control, and wound care, is the basis for therapy. Though broad guidelines can be established to aid in managing particular conditions, hand therapy must be individualized for each patient. The therapist must consider pain tolerance, wound status, severity of injury, and patient motivation in making these modifications. Working together, the surgeon, the therapist and the patient can hope to attain the best possible result for the patient.

SUGGESTED READING

Doyle JR. Extensor tendons—acute injuries. In: Green DP, ed. Operative hand surgery. St. Louis: CV Mosby, 1978:1441.

Fess E. The effects of Jaymar dynamometer handle position and test protocol on normal grip strength. Proceedings American Society of Hand Therapist. J Hand Surg 1982; 7:308–310.

Lister GD, Kleinert GE, Kutz JE, et al. Primary flexor tendon repair followed by immediate controlled immobilization. J Hand Surg 1977; 2:441–451.

Szabo R, Gelberman R, Williamson R, et al. Vibratory sensory testing in acute peripheral nerve compression. J Hand Surg 1984; 9A:104–109.

THE BURNED UPPER EXTREMITY

ROGER E. SALISBURY, M.D., F.A.C.S.

The complications of healed burns of the upper extremity that require surgical intervention have become more common and more complex in the past 20 years. Improved resuscitation from burn shock, early diagnosis and treatment of inhalation injury, and prevention of infection through the use of topical chemotherapeutic agents have all markedly increased survival. Thus, many patients who previously died are now surviving and seeking an improved quality of life. These patients are apt to have major problems with function and cosmesis in other parts of the body. The determination of surgical priorities becomes as important as the execution of the task.

The burn surgeon should ask himself some basic questions—What? Who? When?—as he develops a treatment plan.

What? All the patient's deformities are carefully documented from head to foot. No attempt is yet made to rate them in importance. But a complete examination is extremely important. A two-column page is set up. The catalogued deformities are placed one under the other in the lefthand column. In the righthand column, potential surgical solutions are listed, again without preference regarding the deformity.

Who? The presence of an anatomic abnormality is not the indication for an operation. The patient is now counseled in depth on the deformities, surgical solutions, and complications. He helps determine what is important to him. What does he think his major problems are? What does he want corrected first? Many factors determine possibilities of correction. The patient's background and personal history are important and relevant. Disturbing numbers of individuals who get burned have known personality disorders and prior psychiatric histories. Drug addicts, alcoholics, and arsonists are regularly admitted to our burn units. Because postoperative compliance and commitment to a splinting and therapy program are essential to success, these individuals are screened very carefully. Otherwise, the surgery merely amounts to a technical exercise. Age has to be a consideration in patient selection. A serious burn contracture of the little finger of a dominant hand in a machinist might warrant correction, whereas a nursing home resident would not be a candidate for the same procedure. Injury to the dominant versus nondominant hand is significant. The correction of limitations in the dominant hand gives a degree of independence that boosts morale, and allows therapy and the performance of daily activities. The presence of systemic disease may make the risk of some procedures unacceptable, whether they are functional or cosmetic.

Speed in reconstruction can be achieved by grouping procedures and using a team of surgeons. For instance, multiple corrective procedures can be done on the face and upper extremity by two teams working simultaneously, thus decreasing the number of hospitalizations and anesthetics.

The questions "what?" and "who?" are best applied after careful consideration of each tissue of the upper extremity and hand—skin, muscle and tendon, bones, nerves, and blood vessels. The patient's preburn occupation is highly significant. Is the surgeon attempting to restore power, fine movement, or both, and is it realistic even to consider the return of this patient to his former occupation? Sometimes, it is very obvious that the patient is going to need the help of the Office for Vocational Rehabilitation and Job Retraining, regardless of any surgical magic. A quick arrival at this conclusion saves the patient time and money and protects him from needless or incorrect surgery and later disappointment.

When the elbow or shoulder is also involved, I always release contractures of these areas before I approach the hand—or else do it simultaneously. This is because good extremity range of motion is needed to perform hand therapy effectively, especially when a work simulator program is involved.

When to perform surgery is a confusing question. Some think that time should elapse to allow scar to mature. This is a concept frequently not applicable to severe burns. When hypertrophic scarring and contractures occur, secondary deformities in unburned tissue may result, such as ankylosis, or dislocation of joints, or tendon adhesions. Although it is true that many burn scars or skin grafts improve with time, scarring far too often becomes progressively worse in spite of compression garments and aggressive splinting. A deformity that does not respond to splinting and therapy should be operated on before secondary deformities occur.

AXILLARY CONTRACTURES

For axillary contractures, I prefer flap reconstruction when possible, as recurrence is less frequent than with a skin graft. When only the anterior and midaxilla have been involved with the contracture, the posterior axilla can be mobilized as an advancement flap. Once a release is done, the flap is advanced into position. The trick is to hold the arm in an adducted position postoperatively so that the flap tip is not put on stretch or tension. Because the flap has bulk soft tissue, no significant shortening or recontracture will occur. Three weeks postoperatively, when the skin is healed, one can gradually begin extension or abduction of the arm. For longstanding contractures, unburned tissue that is shortened may have to be incised to get true overcorrection. The deficit may be too large for flap coverage. Sheets of thick, split-thickness skin grafts are laid in transversely so that suture lines and scars run against the contracting forces. Postoperatively, real problems occur with maintenance of correction if the patient will not wear an airplane splint, or modification of one. Recontracture is then likely since shortening of the graft will occur.

ELBOW CONTRACTURES

Correction of elbow contractures do not present the same postoperative problem as the axilla because the elbow hangs at the side and the normal weight of the extremity discourages recontracture. A posterior extension splint, worn all the time, allows hand function and ensures no recurrence. For the severe elbow contracture, I am always prepared to do step cut lengthening of the biceps tendon to achieve full correction. Although it seems redundant to warn about the brachial artery and the median nerve, their position is often distorted and they may be shortened. Under the tourniquet, with the artery and nerve lost in a scar field, one can imagine how easily a surgeon could injure one of these structures by cutting transversely across the scar. When in doubt, I extend my incision proximally and distally, after first identifying these structures in normal tissue. When this maneuver is not feasible, the tourniquet should be deflated to allow palpation of the brachial pulse, and identification of vessels along the epineurium, assists in nerve dissection. When a complete dissection does not yield a full release, it is sometimes possible to achieve the last 15 to 20 degrees of extension over time with a good therapy and splinting program. This is not a panacea for inadequate surgery, but normal exercise gradually allows some stretching in shortened tissues.

THE HAND

For operations on the hand, I let the quantity and quality of pathology guide my plan. For instance, when the patient has extensive total body injuries, I group compatible procedures and do them during one anesthesia. Each case is weighed on its merits and clichés of treatment are avoided. For instance, it is usually considered inadvisable to operate on both hands at the same time because of the patient's inability to eat and attend to personal toilet without help. Recently, however, we cared for a cardiologist with severe, healed-burn complications of the face and upper extremities. He could not do catheterizations because of the tight dorsal scar contractures over both hands. To save a busy professional time lost from work, a team excised the scarred dorsal skin, resurfaced both hands with thick, split-thickness skin grafts, and also reconstructed his eyelids and nostrils during the same anesthesia. During his week in the hospital postoperatively, we provided him with all of the help that he needed. There were no complications and healing was uneventful. If one calculates the cost of a few extra days in the hospital because both hands were bandaged, versus the cost of multiple admissions and anesthetics, it is obvious that much time and money were saved. Because of our experienced team and careful selection of patients, we have not found that the grouping of procedures during one anesthetic has caused increased complications such as infection.

Once the hand has been assessed for pathology and surgical needs, my preference is to start with skin and soft-tissue releases. The most common dorsal problem is an inadequate amount of skin, with extension contractures or inability to make a full fist because of skin tightness. When the quality of the skin is good but there is not enough of it, incisional release down to paratenon, and skin grafting, should restore a normal range of motion. The key in preoperative examination is to determine whether the maximum tightness is in the wrist, dorsum of hand, or fingers. Attempts at passive flexion will reveal the site. When multiple sites are identified, I start the release proximally. For example, once the wrist contracture is opened transversely, the overlying skin and soft tissue are reflected off underlying paratenon proximally and distally. Sometimes this maneuver, by freeing adhesions and releasing contracting forces, allows the skin to slide distally, and some metacarpophalangeal release will occur. Far more frequently, a separate incision is required over the metacarpophalangeal joints in order to yield full flexion. Simple incisional release of the fingers has not been found as efficacious, and excision of the scarred skin down to paratenon is usually necessary. Once a full passive release is achieved, overcorrection is maintained by placing the wrist and metacarpophalangeal joints in full flexion and the interphalangeal joints in neutral. I like to pin the joints with fine K wires to hold them in the desired overcorrected position. Thus, I am sure to insert adequate skin grafts. This point is important because, when unrestricted activity begins, some graft shortening will inevitably occur and there will still be enough skin to allow full range of motion. Pinning of the joints also protects the patient for 7 days postoperatively. Fingers can slip out of position in a soft dressing. When dorsal skin in unstable, of poor quality, or where there is a history of repetitive ulceration, full excision and replacement with thick grafts is indicated.

Volar releases for flexion contractures present a very real hazard when shortening and displacement of neurovascular bundles have occurred. For chronic contractures, there often is displacement of the bundles. Transverse incisions must be done under optical magnification since fibrous scar bands and shortened neurovascular bundles are difficult to differentiate under the tourniquet. I do not attempt to extend contracted fingers fully with a tourniquet inflated. Vessels can be stretched into spasm and gangrene of the fingers may result. Instead, the soft-tissue release is completed first and the shortened volar plate and collateral ligaments often need to be incised. The tourniquet is then deflated. Fingers are extended until blanching occurs. They are dropped back a few degrees into flexion until color returns, then pinned in that position and skin-grafted. It may be impossible to achieve a full release and the patient must be forewarned.

For release of the first web space, extreme care must be taken not to injure the ulnar digital nerve of the thumb or the radial digital nerve of the index finger. It is my practice, when the contracture requires a deep dissection (such as release of the adductor), to identify these nerves. Once the release is completed and full abduction achieved, I check for opposition. A common error is to overlook tightness and shortening of the carpometacarpal and/or metacarpophalangeal joints of the thumb. When the first web space is grafted, and the thumb immobilized for 2 weeks, an already stiff thumb gets worse. After release of the first web space, passive opposition is attempted. When there is tightness of either the carpometacarpal or the metacarpophalangeal joint, capsulotomy is done.

Dorsal hooding, unless severe, is rarely a functioning problem, but often a cosmetic one. When the sides of the fingers are unburned, I prefer to use a combination of local flaps and skin grafts. When there is scarring on the sides of the fingers, I use only incision and grafting because the vascularity of the flaps is too tenuous. The key to successful correction is longitudinal incision of the hood, proximally back up the intrinsic canal. Postoperatively, the danger of recontracture can be decreased if discrete pressure is applied to the spaces. This can be accomplished by placing cotton in tube gauze, inserting it in each web and then applying a Jobst glove.

The choices of syndactyly procedures are many but most use local flaps and grafts. My preference is Bevin's hourglass procedure, which gives a very normal-appearing web. The most serious complication to avoid is inadvertent devascularization of the fingers, intraoperatively or postoperatively. Intraoperatively, I always use optical magnification and assume the neurovascular bundles to be displaced from their normal position. Unlike a congenital syndactyly, where there is good soft tissue, the sides of the fingers are often severely scarred internally as well as externally. Both sides of a finger should not be done at the same time since the postoperative compression dressing may cause ischemia of the finger. Thus, alternate fingers are done 1 month apart.

Joint deformities are multiple, but the most common are hyperextension of the metacarpophalangeal joints and hyperflexion of the proximal interphalangeal joints (PIP). The hyperextension is usually due to inadequate dorsal skin and lack of splinting. The PIP hyperflexion is usually due to destruction of the extensor mechanism and unopposed pull of the flexors. I prefer the capsulotomy or capsulectomy procedures described by Curtis to correct the metacarpophalangeal joint deformity. Each joint should be explored through individual, longitudinal incisions rather than through a single, transverse one. If a transverse one is used, and the extended joints are flexed after capsulectomy, there will be a coverage problem. Exposed, released joints provide no bed for skin grafts. Individual, longitudinal incisions can always be closed. During the Curtis release, I am particularly careful to recreate the volar plate pouch. Otherwise, when the fingers are flexed, dislocation may result because the base of the proximal phalanx cannot slide volarly in a normal fashion. I always pin the joints in maximum flexion so that capsular structures heal in the lengthened position. Management of the PIP joints varies depending on the degree of pathology. When there is poor dorsal skin, severe hyperflexion, and total destruction of the extensor mechanism, arthrodesis in a functional position is desirable. Tendon grafts are not successful in this type of finger, and arthrodesis is a predictable, safe procedure. I leave the K wires in situ for 5 to 6 weeks because of the poor blood supply that invariably delays wound healing. When dorsal skin is good and there is a boutonnière deformity with good tendon remnant present, I have enjoyed success with Elliot's repair. The PIP joint should always be pinned, in neutral, to protect the repaired and advanced central slip. Passive positioning of the MP and DIP joints is started within 7 days to prevent stiffening. Vigorous therapy is needed after the pin is removed to prevent joint fixation in neutral.

The rapid recovery of patients treated with the continuous passive motion machine has been very impressive. There is no doubt that if the patient wears it, fingers become mobile more quickly. The machine is an excellent policeman. Specifically, we push our patients to attend a minimum of three therapy sessions per week and guide them through a very aggressive program. It is always questionable what they actively and voluntarily do on returning home. However, it seems to be psychologically pleasing and acceptable to most patients to let a machine do part of the work for them, and increased gains have been noted.

TISSUE EXPANDERS

One of the newer techniques deserves special mention. The use of tissue expanders is still experimental and complication rates as high as 40 percent have been reported nationally. Although the indications and levels of their utilization are still being sought, the future is very exciting. I find them useful for the removal of scars from the forearm and upper arm. It is safest to make the entire incision for insertion of an implant in normal skin with a normal blood supply. When the incision has been made partially in scar, we have had wounds open 5 to 6 weeks after surgery when expansion was started because of poor healing. Once expansion is completed, we wait several weeks before surgery, thus allowing the skin to remain stretched. This makes it easier to manipulate the skin and soft tissue intraoperatively for closure of defects.

FREE FLAP PROCEDURES

The use of free flaps, or composite grafts, is sporadically mentioned in upper extremity burn reconstruction. Many patients resent or refuse this surgery because of donor site morbidity. As one patient told me, "I have enough bad scars on my body, I don't want more." The state of the art is now so refined that, in good microsurgery centers, the complication rate is very low and the potential benefits very appealing. In selected cases, much more can be accomplished than with any other reconstruction technique. For example, the toe-to-hand transfer is ideal for individuals who have lost thumbs if there are recipient vessels. If the patient can be persuaded, it is far superior to other choices, such as first web space widening, or iliac bone graft and random pattern flaps for thumb lengthening. Other types of free flaps can be useful when there has been extensive tissue loss (such as in electrical injuries). I do not recommend a particular flap but urge careful patient selection since these patients have frequently sustained significant emotional, as well as physical, trauma. The flap is indicated if a simpler procedure cannot produce as good a result. Complications must be clearly outlined because these patients are frequently leery of any procedures that have significant morbidity and chance of failure.

SUGGESTED READING

Bevin AG. The hourglass procedure. In: Salisbury RE, Bevin AG, eds. Atlas of reconstructive burn surgery. Philadelphia: WB Saunders 1981: 180.

Curtis RM. Capsulectomy of the interphalangeal joints of the fingers. J Bone Joint Surg 1954; 36:1219–1234.

Elliott RA. Boutonnière deformity. In: Cramer LM, Chase RA, eds. Symposium on the hand. St. Louis: CV Mosby, 1971:42.

DUPUYTREN'S DISEASE

ROBERT M. McFARLANE, M.D., M.Sc., F.R.C.S.(C), F.A.C.S.

In order to treat Dupuytren's disease intelligently within our present state of knowledge, the surgeon should subscribe to one of two theories. The majority view is that Dupuytren's disease is a fibromatosis and that the disease process will continue unless it is completely removed. Another view is that the joint contractures are the result of biomechanical stresses upon the fascia. If the fascia is divided or interrupted by partial excision, these stresses can be overcome and contracture prevented. I believe that the disease is a fibromatosis and the operations described here are designed to remove disease and potentially diseased fascia.

Treatment is designed primarily to correct flexion contractures at the metacarpophalangeal and proximal interphalangeal joints. It is easy to correct contracture at the metacarpophalangeal joint, but difficult to correct joint contracture more distally. As a result, the operation is relatively easy in the palm and difficult in the finger. The terms introduced by Hueston best describe what operation is performed upon the fascia. A regional fasciectomy means that only the obviously diseased fascia is removed. An extensive fasciectomy means that the obviously diseased as well as the surrounding normal fascia are removed. In the palm, I suggest a regional fasciectomy and in the finger, an extensive fasciectomy.

THE STANDARD OPERATION

A common operation for Dupuytren's disease is one in which an attempt is made to correct a contracture of a single ray. Let us assume that the ring finger is involved with contracture at the metacarpophalangeal joint and the proximal interphalangeal joint. I suggest a midline longitudinal incision that begins in the proximal palm and ends just beyond the distal crease of the finger. The skin and subcutaneous tissue are then reflected to either side to expose the diseased fascia. In the proximal palm, the diseased fascia is deep not only to the skin but to a good thickness of subcutaneous fibrofatty tissue. This tissue can be left on the skin to assure its vascularity. However, as one proceeds distally, this fibrofatty tissue disappears so that in the distal palm and proximal segment of the finger the diseased fascia is intimately adherent to the overlying dermis. The skin and fascia can, however, be separated by sharp dissection, and loupe magnification helps to find this plane of dissection. In the palm, the skin is reflected each way until the normal-appearing fascia of the adjacent rays is exposed. In the finger, the skin is usually dissected back to the midlateral line.

If the metacarpophalangeal joint is severely contracted, the dissection is facilitated by incision of the diseased fascia in the proximal palm. This permits extension at the metacarpophalangeal joint so that the diseased tissues are more readily seen.

The dissection begins by exposing each neurovascular bundle. This is best done by finding the neurovascular bundle at the level of the distal crease of the finger where it is quite superficial. Each bundle is exposed by a combination of sharp and blunt dissection. It is best to keep the artery and nerve together. It is easy to see the nerve, but sometimes difficult to see the artery because it contains little or no blood. Again, loupe magnification is extremely helpful. It is necessary to divide volar branches of both the nerve and the artery during this exposure. The branches of the artery should be coagulated with a bipolar unit while staying about 2 mm away from the main vessel. As one proceeds proximally to the level of the metacarpophalangeal joint, the neurovascular bundle disappears deep to the transverse fibers of the palmar aponeurosis. It is not necessary to expose the neurovascular bundle more proximally because the diseased fascia is always superficial to the nerves and vessels proximal to this level.

With both neurovascular bundles safely exposed, one can perform a block excision of the fascia. Again, starting distally, the fascia is excised from between the neurovascular bundles from the level of the distal joint proximally. At the proximal third of the middle phalanx the fascia is firmly adherent to the tendon sheath and must be removed by sharp dissection. No great harm comes from opening the tendon sheath at this level, although one tries not to do so. Over the proximal phalanx, the fascia is not adherent to the tendon sheath so is readily removed. At the level of the metacarpophalangeal joint, the fascia is adherent on either side to the septa of Lejueu and Juvara. These septa are not involved in the disease process but they must be incised in order to remove the pretendinous cord of the palmar aponeurosis.

When the diseased tissue from between the neurovascular bundles has been removed, the diseased and potentially diseased fascia, on either side of the neurovascular bundles and deep to the neurovascular bundles, are removed. Again, this tissue is best removed from distal to proximal. On one or other side there may be diseased tissue that extends distal to the distal crease of the finger, attached to the side of the distal phalanx. As one proceeds proximally, there may be a considerable amount of diseased tissue deep to the neurovascular bundle at the level of the proximal interphalangeal joint. This tissue terminates proximally by attachment to the side of the base of the proximal phalanx, to an intrinsic tendon, or passes to the adjacent finger within the diseased natatory ligament.

All of the diseased tissue has now been removed from between the neurovascular bundles, on either side, and deep to them. The contracture at the metacarpophalangeal joint is invariably corrected and the proximal interphalangeal joint should be fully extended as well. If the latter joint is still flexed, the surgeon must decide what further steps to take. In an older patient, i.e., over 60 years of age, I would accept as much as 45 degrees of residual flexion at the proximal interphalangeal joint. In a younger patient, i.e., less than 45 years of age, I would attempt to improve upon even 30 degrees of residual flexion contracture. Between these ages one must rely upon an individual evaluation of the patient. Postoperative therapy might improve upon a residual flexion contracture, but, more realistically, good postoperative therapy will maintain the correction gained at operation. If further surgical steps are considered, the first one would be to incise the flexor tendon sheath. Sometimes this alone permits extension at the joint. A second step could be the release of the checkrein ligaments of the volar plate, as described by Watson, although I prefer to excise the junction of the accessory collateral ligament to the volar plate, as described by Curtis. Both procedures are extra-articular procedures, and in the patient with Dupuytren's disease it is best to stop short of actual opening of the proximal interphalangeal joint in an attempt to overcome the residual contracture.

Closure of this midline longitudinal incision must be interrupted by Z-plasties in order to prevent postoperative scar contracture. Three Z-plasties are designed; one at the level of the proximal interphalangeal joint, another at the proximal crease of the finger, and a third at the distal crease of the palm. The limbs of these Z-plasties are about 1 cm long.

Postoperatively, the hand is immobilized with slight flexion at the wrist to relax the palmar skin, and slight flexion at the metacarpophalangeal joint to relax the proximal interphalangeal joint. The next day, or shortly thereafter, a thermoplastic splint is made, and the patient is seen frequently by the hand therapist. Emphasis is placed upon gaining full extension at the proximal interphalangeal joint, but also upon regaining flexion of all of the fingers by periodic removal of the splint. Ideally, the splint would be worn for varying periods of time for about 3 months but, in practice, patients lose interest in gaining the last few degrees of extension at the proximal interphalangeal joint and discard their splints within 6 to 8 weeks. It is more important for patients to regain full flexion of the fingers than to gain full extension of the involved finger. Almost always they regain full extension at the metacarpophalangeal joint.

MORE EXTENSIVE DISEASE

When there is more than one ray involved in the palm, and more than one finger contracted, although the principle of the operation is the same the operation in the palm is somewhat different. Let us assume that the fourth and fifth rays are diseased with contracture at the metacarpophalangeal joint and proximal interphalangeal joints of the little and ring fingers.

A transverse incision is made within the distal crease of the palm to extend from the ulnar border of the hand to the line of the middle finger ray. Skin flaps are raised proximally and distally. The proximal flap is easily dissected from the diseased fascia, and its viability is assured by a good thickness of fibrofatty tissue. It is doubtful that the more proximal fibers of the palmar aponeursis need be removed even though they are diseased, but this incision permits exposure of the palmar aponeurosis to the distal edge of the transverse carpal ligament. The distal flap is more difficult to develop because the pretendinous cords attach to the skin between the distal crease of the palm and the proximal creases of the fingers. However, with sharp dissection and magnification, a plane can be developed. This distal dissection is also difficult because there is a lot of fibrofatty tissue in the web spaces between the diseased pretendinous cords. Within this fibrofatty tissue lie the neurovascular bundles. The bundles within each web space, i.e., those that pass to adjacent sides of the fingers, must be exposed in the course of dissection. This dissection can be difficult if there is severe metacarpophalangeal joint contracture. However, this contracture can be overcome by simple incision of the diseased fascia, thereby making the dissection easier and safer. In this area, there are large branches from the metacarpal arteries that nourish the fat pads and pass to the dorsum of the hand. These arteries must be cauterized so that they do not cause trouble from postoperative bleeding.

The diseased fascia in the finger is exposed, as before, through a midline longitudinal incision. If the dissection in the distal palm and proximal finger is particularly difficult, then it is prudent to extend the longitudinal incision proximally to meet the transverse incision in the palm. This provides excellent exposure in this very difficult area of the distal palm. After the neurovascular bundles are exposed in each finger a block excision of the diseased fascia is performed as described above. The finger wounds are closed with Z-plasties, but the transverse wound in the palm is left open to heal by second intention. The principle of leaving the palm open is that the skin at the palm has become foreshortened by prolonged metacarpophalangeal joint contracture. If the skin is allowed to heal by second intention, it gradually stretches to its previous length. This seems to be true, because the resulting scars are linear and scarcely noticeable. The value of the open palm method is that a palmar hematoma cannot occur, postoperative pain and swelling are minimal, and both flexion and extension are readily regained. Postoperative splinting is, however, essential to maintain metacarpophalangeal joint extension during healing of the palmar wound and to maintain the extension gained at the proximal interphalangeal joint.

MODIFICATIONS OF THIS SCHEME

Both the palmar and digital components of these operations can be modified, depending upon the surgeon's goals. In the palm, especially in young people, an extensive fasciectomy might be performed in which the entire palmar aponeurosis is removed. This is an operation that should be reserved for the young person with extensive disease.

In the finger, a regional fasciectomy is indicated in the older patient. Nevertheless, the incision should extend at least to the distal crease of the finger in order to remove the tissue that contracts the proximal interphalangeal joint and is attached to the tendon sheath and periosteum of the middle phalanx.

Thumb web contracture is very common and can usually be treated by a regional fasciectomy, i.e., simple removal of the diseased tissue.

THE TREATMENT OF RECURRENT DISEASE

Persistent contracture at the proximal interphalangeal joint is the most difficult problem associated with the treatment of Dupuytren's disease. We have no solution to this problem other than to remove the diseased fascia that is causing proximal interphalangeal contracture. Some of the residual contracture is due to foreshortening of the joint structures, which is not readily amenable to treatment in the older age group, and some may be due to attenuation of the extensor mechanism. Recurrent contracture is a different matter. It is usually due to inadequate excision, comparable to the inadequate excision of a neoplasm. However, it may also be due to a biologic phenomenon known as severe Dupuytren's diathesis, in which it is almost impossible to prevent the reappearance of the disease by any surgical procedure. Hueston described the patient with a severe diathesis as a young person (under the age of 40) with extensive and aggressive disease in both hands, with knuckle pads, and possibly plantar and/or penile fibromatosis. This patient usually has a strong family history of Dupuytren's disease. This picture is not often seen, but variations in which the diathesis is less severely expressed are not uncommon. When a patient requires operation for a recurrent contracture, one should consider what Hueston describes as a dermofasciectomy as the operation of choice. In this operation, the overlying skin as well as the diseased fascia is excised. The defect is covered by a full-thickness skin graft. Hueston admits that his observations are empirical but says that excision of the skin avoids further recurrence and that the use of a full-thickness graft is more effective than a split-thickness graft.

A final comment concerns a persistent, severe, and annoying contracture at the proximal interphalangeal joint of the little finger. This is a common sequela of an otherwise successful operation for Dupuytren's disease. In the past, these patients have been offered an amputation of the finger or fusion of the proximal interphalangeal joint in a better position. Joint replacement is an improvement on either of these operations. By a generous excision of the head of the proximal phalanx, the little finger can be shortened enough to overcome the flexion contracture without the need to remove either scar or diseased tissue from the finger. The patient will retain some 40 to 60 degrees of movement within a better range.

SUGGESTED READING

Colville J. Dupuytren's contracture. The role of fasciotomy. Hand 1983; 15:162–166.

Gonzales RI. Dupuytren's contracture of the fingers. A simplified approach to the surgical treatment. Cal Med 1971; 115:25–28.

Hueston JT. Dermofasciectomy for Dupuytren's disease. Bull Hosp Jt Dis 1984; 44:224–231.

Hueston JT. Dupuytren's contracture. In: Flynn JE, ed. Hand surgery. 3rd ed. Baltimore: Williams & Wilkins, 1982:79.

King EW, Exeter NH, Boss DM, Watson HK. Treatment of Dupuytren's contracture by extensive fasciectomy through multiple Y-V-plasty incision. J Hand Surg 1979; 4:234.

McCash CR. The open technique in Dupuytren's contracture. Br J Plast Surg 1964; 17:271–280.

McFarlane RM. Dupuytren's contracture. In: Green DP, ed. Operative hand surgery. 2nd ed. New York: Churchill Livingstone, 1988:553–589.

GANGLIONS AND OTHER BENIGN TUMORS OF THE HAND

DAVID J. SMITH Jr., M.D.

Ganglions and other benign tumors of the hand are among the most frequently encountered surgical lesions. Large, deep soft tissue hand tumors, exclusive of ganglions, lipomas, and giant cell tumors, are frequently malignant. About 95 percent of the remaining masses are included in the following categories: (1) reactive lesions, (2) mucoid or degenerative cysts, (3) giant cell tumors of tendon sheath, (4) epidermoid inclusion cysts, (5) pyogenic granulomas, (6) foreign body reactions, and (7) fungal infections. A review of these lesions, plus those of other soft tissues such as nerve and blood vessel, would be encyclopedic. Their treatment does not differ from that in any other part of the body; however, their clinical presentation may be unique. For example, epidermal inclusion cysts and lipomas may be more symptomatic in the hand because, as they enlarge, they may distort or compress adjacent structures. This emphasizes the importance of meticulous dissection and loupe magnification in their removal. Some of the lesions more distinctive to the hand are described in the following section.

Ganglions are the most common tumors of the hand and wrist and represent 50 to 70 percent of all soft tissue masses in this area. The dorsal carpal ganglion is the most common. Conservative measures have been uniformly unsuccessful in management; however,if the ganglion has been present for only a short time, i.e., a matter of weeks, the patient is usually asked to wait for about 3 to 6 months because some spontaneously resolve. When this fails, the patient is scheduled for surgery. Loupe magnification is used, and the procedure is done under tourniquet with an axillary block, which is preferred to Bier block because it allows for the tourniquet to be released and hemostasis obtained. After ganglion removal, the presence of a hematoma is particularly troublesome for the patient because it immediately raises the question of ganglion recurrence. Nearly 95 percent of dorsal carpal ganglions arise from the scapholunate ligament; therefore, a transverse incision should be placed so that the ganglion can be removed and the scapholunate ligament visualized. Usually the ganglions project distally, and lie over the capitate. Once the ganglion has been identified, the cyst wall should not be skeletonized. If a small remnant of fibrous tissue is left on the cyst, clamps or pickups can be used to control the cyst during dissection without puncturing the cyst wall. As the ganglion is dissected, the base of the capitate may be mistaken for the origin of the cyst; however, it is the scapholunate ligament, not the scaphocapitate ligament, that is the most frequent site of origin. When the ganglion is left attached only to the wrist joint capsule, usually by dissection between the extensor pollicis longus and extensor digitorum communis tendons, the capsule should be opened to expose the base of the ganglion. A rectangular flap of capsule can be created to allow a good view of both the base and scapholunate area. The ganglion is then shaved off the scapholunate ligament, taking care not to damage the ligament, since this might lead to scapholunate dissociation. After the ganglion has been excised, the base is cauterized with bipolar cautery, the tourniquet released, and hemostasis obtained. Closure of the wrist capsule is usually attempted using 4–0 Vicryl sutures. If this is not possible, a retinacular flap is developed to close the defect, or it can be left open. A plaster splint, which holds the wrist in a neutral or slightly flexed position with the digits free, is applied to prevent dorsal tightness. The splint is worn for 10 to 14 days, at which time motion, without lifting or resistive activity, is begun. The sutures are removed at 3 weeks, and full activity, including strengthening, should return 6 to 12 weeks postoperatively.

Treatment of volar carpal ganglions parallels that of dorsal carpal ganglions with a few exceptions. Lister has emphasized that treatment of the ganglions should not involve sacrifice of the radial artery. If necessary, a rim of cyst wall should be left attached to the artery to ensure arterial continuity. If there is great concern about radial artery identification, extremity exsanguination should not be complete, thereby making it easier to visualize the blood-containing artery. If necessary, on both dorsal and volar ganglions, the cyst should be opened and dissected from inside rather than risk damage to surrounding structures by dissection in a firmly scarred area. Most volar carpal ganglions arise from the scaphotrapezoidal joint. Frequently, a preoperative diagnosis of flexor carpi radialis tendinitis will mask, or be associated with, a volar carpal ganglion. In such cases, the skin incision is designed longitudinally so that it can be carried over the thenar crease as this allows for thenar musculature elevation in order to expose the ganglion. More frequently, however, dissection and exposure of the ganglion proceeds between the flexor carpi radialis and abductor pollicis longus tendons to the wrist joint capsule and then to the scaphotrapezoidal joint. The wrist is splinted in 15 to 20 degrees of extension for 2 weeks to prevent capsule tightness.

The third most common ganglion is the volar retinacular ganglion, which most frequently originates between the first and second annular pulleys or from the proximal annular pulley. A transverse incision may be used if the size is small, but often a curved or angular incision is necessary for adequate exposure. Once the digital neurovascular bundles have been protected, the cyst is identified and traced to the tendon sheath. Excision of the base, including a small portion of the pulley, assures complete removal. The dressing should be simple and light to allow for early mobilization.

The so-called mucous cyst must be recognized as a ganglion cyst of the distal interphalangeal (DIP) joint, often associated with Heberden's nodes and an arthritic DIP joint. Adequate treatment must address both the cyst and the arthritic osteophytes of the joint. Usually, a gently-curved incision is made that extends proximal to the DIP joint. When the skin lying directly over the cyst is thin and attenuated, it should be excised with the cyst. This is most easily done by carrying the incision distal as an ellipse around the attenuated skin. The cyst usually lies to one side of the extensor tendon, between the eponychium and dorsal distal joint crease. During dissection, care must be taken not to disrupt the insertion of the extensor tendon or injure the nail matrix. The cyst (and overlying skin) is mobilized, traced to the joint, and then excised with joint capsule. The opposite side of the tendon should also be explored for occult ganglions, osteophytes, or hypertrophied synovial tissue. A synovectomy of the joint is completed, if necessary, and all osteophytes removed with a fine rongeur. Essentially all soft tissue between the collateral ligament and the lateral aspect of the extensor tendon is removed. If skin has been excised, primary closure can usually be achieved by rotation of the curved incision distally; otherwise, a full-thickness graft is used. Early postoperative motion is allowed with primary closure but, if a graft is used, motion is restricted until the graft is stable. Ganglions of the proximal interphalangeal joint are also relatively common and are handled similarly to those of the DIP joint, although skin closure is not a problem.

Although ganglions present in other places in the hand, they are rare and will not be discussed. It must be remembered that conditions such as de Quervain's disease, carpal tunnel syndrome, and Guyon's canal compression can all be caused by ganglions, and these should be searched for at the time of operation. Although rare, intraosseous ganglions are increasingly recognized as a source of wrist pain. Another benign condition often confused with the dorsal wrist ganglion, is the carpometacarpal boss, an osteoarthritic spur at the base of the second and/or third carpometacarpal joints. Nearly one-third of such cases have a ganglion associated with them. The area is surgically approached through a gently-curved transverse incision over the mass. The extensor digitorum communis and extensor indicis proprius tendons are usually retracted ulnarward. The mass is exposed either ulnar to the extensor carpi radialis brevis or between this tendon and the extensor carpi radialis longus. When a ganglion is present, it is removed as previously described. The osteoarthritic spurs and adjacent joint that form the metacarpal boss are exposed subperiosteally via a longitudinal incision in the second and/or third carpometacarpal area. A small osteotome removes the tissue until normal cartilage is identified on both sides of all four joints. The most common problem is inadequate removal of tissue; therefore, the area should be carefully palpated through the skin to assure that all prominent areas have been removed. All soft tissue should be anatomically approximated, and periosteum, joint capsule, and adjacent tendons restored to their appropriate position with a 4–0 Vicryl suture. A plaster splint, including the digits, is applied and worn for 2 to 3 weeks before postoperative rehabilitation begins.

Giant cell tumor of the tendon sheath is actually a misnomer. It is most correctly called a "localized pigmented villonodular tenovaginosynovitis" or localized nodulartenosynovitis. It is the second most common tumor mass in the hand. While it is felt to be of reactive synovial origin, its etiology is poorly understood. The tissue usually has a distinctive brownish stain and it is mandatory that all such stained tissue be removed. Color varies depending upon the amount of hemosiderin, the number of histiocytes, and the amount of collagen present. These tumors spread along the planes of least resistance with varying degrees of encapsulation. Removal involves careful dissection around multiple structures, especially nerve tissue. At times, partial excision of the tendon sheath is necessary, or the collateral ligament of an adjacent joint should be taken down to remove the tissue in its entirety. Ligament reconstruction is then necessary.

Juvenile aponeurotic fibroma is an uncommon benign tumor that occurs mostly in the hands and wrists of children under 20 years of age. This lesion emphasizes the confusion and therapeutic dilemmas caused by the fibrous and neoplastic tumors in this area. Juvenile aponeurotic fibroma and nodular fasciitis are the most confusing diagnostically because they appear malignant histologically but are usually self-limited reactive lesions clinically. Desmoids, although histologically less a cause for concern, behave much more insidiously and aggressively. These lesions emphasize that a close working relationship between surgeon and pathologist is mandatory. Juvenile aponeurotic fibroma involves the wrist and hand in over 50 percent of cases. The lesion is usually painless, although surrounding fat and skeletal muscle may be invaded by the tumor, and there may be areas of dense collagenous tissue. No instance of metastases has been reported; therefore, treatment should be conservative, and consist of local excision even if the tumor seems to invade tendons and neurovascular bundles, so that these vital structures are not sacrificed. Excisions can be repeated as necessary.

Awareness of the extensor digitorum brevis manus muscle (EDBM), first described in the nineteenth century, has clinical relevance because it may be confused with such common masses as ganglions. Clinical symptoms are usually similar, and consist of a dorsal hand swelling and some discomfort and pain, aggravated by continued use or heavy work. The EDBM is fusiform-shaped, parallel to the extensor tendons and freely mobile. Failure to transilluminate separates it diagnostically from a ganglion. The term EDBM is almost generic and describes several anatomic variations. The most common origins are the dorsal carpal ligaments or joint capsule and the dorsum of the carpal bones; the most common insertions are the extensor digitorum communis tendon and, less frequently, the extensor indicis proprius. Regardless of the anatomy, excision of the muscle is the only treatment that consistently relieves pain. Other than pain, there is probably no reason for exploration or excision.

Vascular tumors, particularly hemangiomas and lymphangiomas, are discussed elsewhere; however, the glomus tumor of the hand is of particular interest. In 1812, Wood first described glomus tumors as "painful subcutaneous nodules" characterized by intermittent severe pain, susceptibility to temperature changes, long duration, small size, and firm consistency. It was not until 1934, however, that Popoff described its normal anatomy and correlated it with temperature regulation. The normal glomus is an end-organ that is an arteriovenous anastomosis without an intermediary capillary bed. While it is distributed widely over the body in the stratum reticulum, the deepest layer of the corium, it is found most frequently beneath nails and with less frequency on the ventral surface of fingertips. Most patients have a classic triad of symptoms—pain, tenderness, and temperature sensitivity. Pain is usually the first manifestation of the lesion. Complete removal of the tumor results in nearly 100 percent cure. All procedures are done with tourniquet assistance and loupe magnification. Although usually localized to the distal portion of the digit, axillary block anesthesia is preferred. When the lesion is entirely subungual, the nail is removed. Usually one, but occasionally two, vertical incisions are necessary to expose the tumor. It can usually be shelled out in its entirety with the residual bed generously curetted to bleeding cancellous bone before closure with interrupted 7–0 catgut sutures. The nail is then replaced and a light, nonadherent dressing applied. New nail growth will take about four months. When the lesion is partially subungual and at the periphery of the nail, the latter need not be removed. A longitudinal incision adjacent to the nail fold allows complete removal. When the lesion is entirely separate from the nail, careful preoperative marking is necessary. The tumor appears light brown with the limb exsanguinated, but with tourniquet release shows a dark reddish color and swells. This may make localization easier if uncertainty exists.

Although nerve tumors of the hand and wrist are rare, two deserve mention. The neurolemmoma, or schwannoma, is the more common of the two benign tumors. It is usually located along the course of a peripheral nerve but rarely has associated sensory or motor abnormalities. Clinically, it may be confused with a ganglion, lipoma, or lymph node. It is usually solitary, presenting either on the side of a nerve trunk or completely intraneural with fasciculi spreading out over the tumor. Treatment is complete surgical removal using loupe magnification. Surgical enucleation is usually accomplished by dissection between fasciculi, then shelling out the tumor. Because recurrence is rare, and malignant degeneration has not been reported, normal surrounding nerve should not be damaged or excised. A light dressing that allows immediate motion is applied.

On the other hand, the neurofibroma is interwoven with the functioning nerve fascicles. Neurofibromas, frequently recognized in von Recklinghausen's disease, may be large and soft, with a reported rate of malignant degeneration of 15 to 30 percent. Despite this, excision is usually indicated only if the tumor changes its biologic behavior or becomes symptomatic. Solitary lesions are less prone to malignant degeneration. Complete removal without nerve damage is difficult, if not impossible. If the lesion is peripheral and cutaneous, complete excision with possible reconstruction may be warranted. On the other hand, removal from a major nerve trunk may not be justified. A compromise may be intraneural dissection using the operating microscope. This limits fascicular loss or damage and maximizes tumor excision. In any case, the clinical result must justify any nerve excision.

Although common, ganglions and other benign tumors of the hand and wrist can present frustrating problems. Careful preoperative identification and diagnosis, coupled with meticulous dissection aided by loupe magnification and tourniquet control, should improve success rates and decrease recurrences.

SUGGESTED READING

Lister GD, Smith RR. Ideas and innovations—protection of the radial artery in the resection of adherent ganglions of the wrist. Plast Reconstr Surg 1978; 61(1):127–129.

McFarland GB Jr. Soft tissue tumors. Part 1. In: Baird P, Green MD, eds. Operative hand surgery. New York: Churchill Livingstone, 1982:1654.

Moore JR, Weiland AJ, Curtis RM. Localized nodular tenosynovitis: experience with 115 cases. J Hand Surg 1984; 9A-3:412–417.

Popoff NW. The digital vascular system. With reference to the state of glomus in inflammation, arteriosclerotic gangrene, diabetic gangrene, thromboangiitis obliterans, and supernumerary digits in man. Arch Pathol Lab Med 1934; 18:295–330.

Wood W. On painful subcutaneous tubercle. Edinburgh Med J 1812; 8:283.

VASCULAR PROBLEMS IN THE HAND

RONALD M. ZUKER, M.D., F.R.C.S. (C), F.A.C.S.
PATRICIA E. BURROWS, M.D., F.R.C.P. (C)

The hand, an end vascular organ, is particularly susceptible to alterations in blood flow because collateral circulation does not develop readily.The complex anatomy of the hand allows for only mild degrees of vascular distortion before function is comprised. Problems associated with excessive vascularity include cardiac failure, excessive growth or both. Diminished vascularity may lead to pain, inability to combat infection, and, of course, ischemic tissue death.

In this chapter, we provide a clinical approach to vascular problems in the hand rather than an exhaustive description of all clinical variations and therapeutic modalities.

CONGENITAL VASCULAR LESIONS

Vascular problems may be congenital or acquired. Congenital lesions generally involve excessive blood flow or growth; acquired lesions usually produce deficient blood flow. The relatively recent classification of congenital vascular anomalies by Mulliken et al into hemangiomas and vascular malformations has been of great assistance in the organization of a realistic approach to management.

Hemangiomas

Hemangiomas in the hand, as elsewhere, grow rapidly during the first 9 months of life and then involute over the subsequent 5 to 7 years. The end result usually is so good that early intervention would only increase morbidity. As the hand is easily traumatized, small areas of ulceration may develop. The ulcers are managed with frequent cleansing, topical antibiotics, and immobilization, especially when they occur around mobile joints or web spaces. Surgical intervention should be avoided despite parental wishes until involution is complete. The vast majority of patients with hemangiomas require no surgery. Minor contouring procedures may be helpful to reduce the excessive residual fibrofatty tissue.

Vascular Malformations

Vascular malformations are congenital anomalies or dysplasias of the blood and lymphatic vascular channels, generally believed to result from a regional insult that leads to an arrest in the development of the vascular bed. Although many classifications and a vast terminology exist in the published literature, vascular malformations are classified most simply and practically according to the morphology of the channel anomalies (Table 1). Combinations of channel abnormalities frequently co-exist. While histologic assessment of vascular malformations provides useful information, they are probably most accurately classified in vivo according to their angiographic features.

TABLE 1 Classification of Vascular Malformations

Arterial dysplasia
Arteriovenous malformations
High-flow
Low-flow
Small vessel (capillary, venular)
Capillary-venous
Venous
Lymphatic
Hemolymphatic dysplasia

CLINICAL PRESENTATION

Vascular malformations are almost always congenital lesions and, according to Mulliken and associates, differ from hemangiomas by their absence of growth by endothelial cell proliferation and absence of involution by endothelial cell drop-out. Typically, they are present at birth and enlarge in proportion to the growth of the child. However, they may undergo periods of rapid transformation and either increase in volume with opening of arteriovenous shunts, or decrease in volume associated with channel thrombosis. The external appearance of the lesion and its physiologic effects and symptoms are related to the type and location of the channel abnormalities present and to the presence or absence of involvement of adjacent tissue structures.

ARTERIOVENOUS FISTULAS

Arteriovenous fistulas consist of direct connections between arteries and veins. Large communications result in the presence of a pulsatile mass with a thrill and bruit, prominent arterial pulsations, and dilated tortuous veins, both proximal and distal to the fistula. Large fistulas may be associated with an increase in circulating blood volume and tachycardia. The most common cardiac manifestations of the shunt are tachycardia, cardiomegaly, and dyspnea on exertion. Infants and young children with large shunts may present with overt congestive heart failure and failure to thrive (Fig. 1). The bradycardia reaction, or Branham's sign, describes the decrease in heart rate that occurs when the flow through the fistula is prevented by the application of local pressure or a tourniquet.

Increased skin temperature and sweating are frequently present over the site of the fistula, but, peripherally, tissue temperature may be abnormally low.

Tissue ischemia distal to the arteriovenous fistula is a frequent complication. Although a "steal" effect from run-off of blood from the major artery may contribute, the ischemia probably is predominantly due to the resulting elevation in distal venous pressure, which leads to vascular stasis. The tissues around and distal to an arteriovenous fistula are usually perfused by collateral vessels. Secondary effects of the fistula include distal cyanosis, ischemic pallor, edema, atrophic skin changes (hyperkeratosis, ulceration), and tissue atrophy. Pain is frequently present and may be secondary to edema and venous congestion when it is associated with dependency of the affected extremity, or it may be caused by the mass effect of the lesion itself, or involvement of nerves or muscle. Dysfunction of the hand is also relatively common and my be caused by the same mechanisms. All of these symptoms may be relieved by successful obliteration of the fistula. This may be accomplished surgically if access to the fistula itself is possible, or else by the intravascular embolization techniques.

ARTERIOVENOUS MALFORMATIONS

Arteriovenous malformations are complex lesions that consist of nidus, a dysplastic vascular network, feeding arteries and draining veins. The lesion may be focal, but more often infiltrates surrounding tissues and may be quite extensive, involving most of the hand and, frequently, the forearm and arm. The effects of the lesion depend on the size and rapidity of flow through the arteriovenous connections and on the extensiveness of the lesion. Lower flow lesions produce symptoms related to local mass effect and venous distension. Higher flow arteriovenous malformations, fortunately uncommon, exert systemic effects similar to large arteriovenous fistulas. Local symptoms of warmth, pain, and paresthesia, as well as limb overgrowth and deformity, are also common. Initial elastic compression may improve symptoms temporarily, while surgery is reserved for significant complications as is discussed later.

SMALL VESSEL MALFORMATION

This category includes abnormal networks that consist of arteriolar, capillary, or venular channels and combinations thereof. Those limited to the dermal layer (port wine stains) mainly produce cosmetic effects. However, they are frequently a superficial marker that indicates associated vascular malformations or dysplasias in the deep tissues. Intramuscular small vessel malformations (Fig. 2) are characterized by local pain on exertion, which resolves when the activity is terminated. Small vessel malformations are low-flow lesions and associated with little, if any, enlargement of the adjacent arteries and veins. Usually, treatment is unnecessary. However, where exertional pain is a major feature, custom-made compression gloves are often effective. Esthetically, the surface staining may be improved by laser electrocautery or cryosurgery. Surgical excision with resurfacing should be reserved for the rare situation where the lesion becomes heaped up and verrucous.

CAPILLARY-VENOUS MALFORMATIONS

These are low-flow vascular malformations that consist of ectatic sinusoidal spaces, which fill through tiny connections with slightly enlarged feeding arteries and drain into regional veins, which are often also dysplastic. They present as purple or blue nonpulsatile masses, which may be localized or diffuse (Fig. 3). They do not have systemic effects, but produce deformity, pain, and decreased function. Some regression may occur with

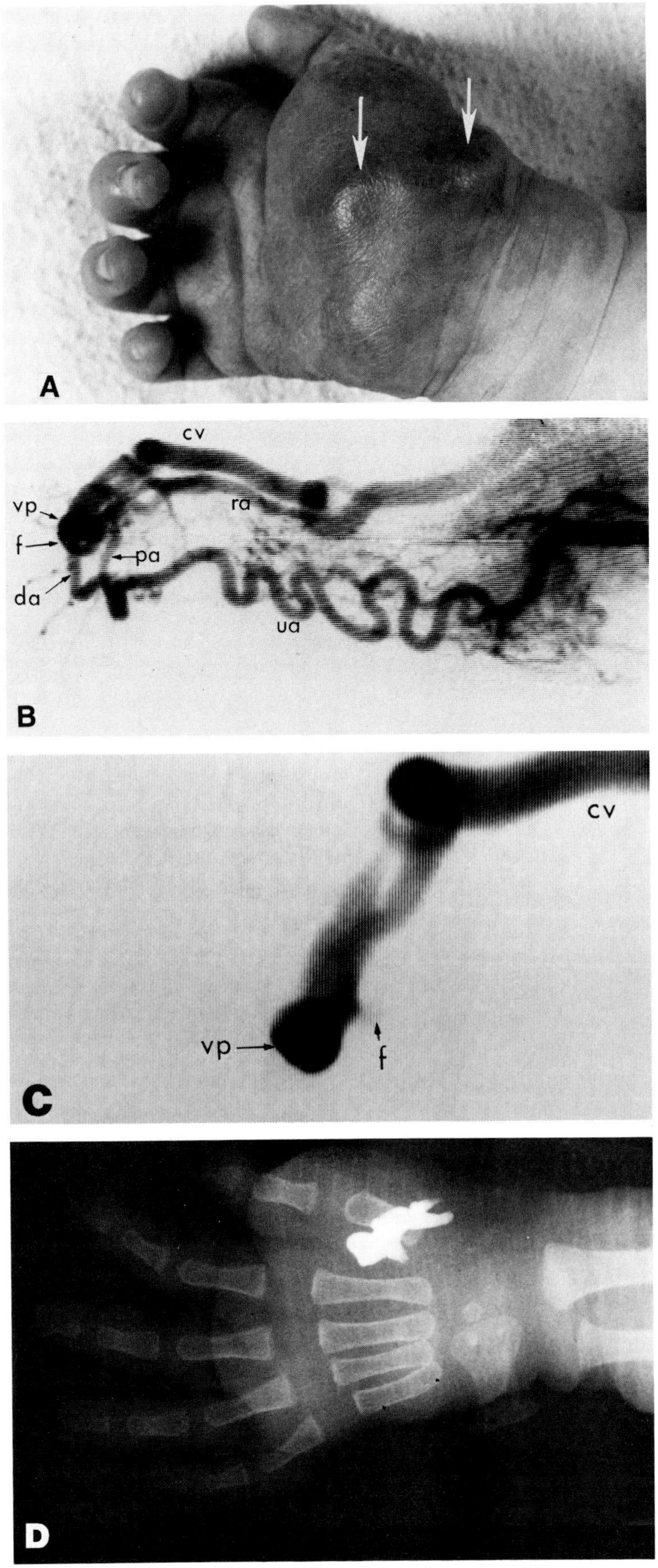

Figure 1 Diffuse vascular malformation of the right upper extremity with a palmar arteriovenous fistula, associated with congestive cardiac failure. Particle embolization of multiple arteriovenous malformations in the newborn period produced significant improvement in cardiac function, but there was still evidence of cardiac overload. The infant initially had a flail wrist with little movement of the fingers. After occlusion of the distal radial artery with isobutyl-2 cyanoacrylate (IBCA) during an attempt to occlude the fistula at 3 months, the flow diminished and neuromuscular function improved. The child still appeared to have local pain and poor function of the thumb. Further improvement in hand function and decrease in cardiac size occurred after transvenous percutaneous embolization of the fistula. *A*, Right hand at 9 months of age shows port wine discoloration, diffuse mass at thenar emminence, and dilated superficial draining veins (arrows). *B*, Brachial (transfemoral) digital subtraction arteriography at 9 months of age shows a diffuse small vessel malformation at the elbow, a tortuous, dilated ulnar artery, occlusion of the proximal radial artery and a fistula between the distal palmar arch and a tributary of the cephalic vein. *C*, Digital subtraction angiogram after percutaneous cannulation of the venous pouch opacified the venous pouch, fistula, and cephalic vein. *D*, Roentgenogram of the hand after injection of radiopaque IBCA. After application of a pressure dressing for 1 week, the thrill and bruit disappeared completely. (cv = cephalic vein; da = distal palmar arcade; f = fistula; pa = proximal palmar arcade; ra = radial artery; ua = ulnar artery; vp = venous pouch).

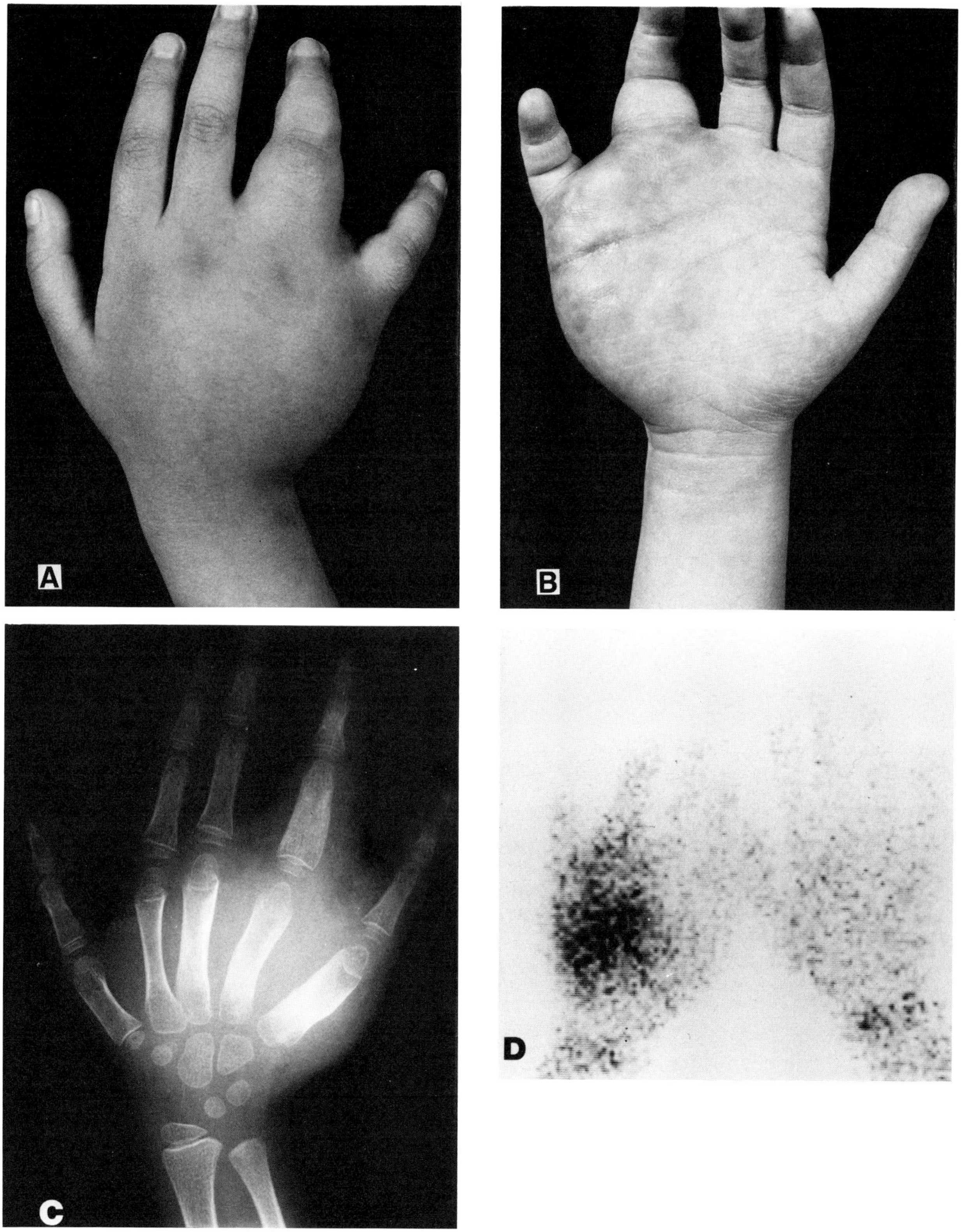

Figure 2 Small vessel malformation of the right hand in a 3-year-old girl is shown. The hand appeared normal until it was injured in a car door at 1 year of age. She demonstrated muscular dysfunction and complained of pain. Treatment consisted of continuous use of a compression glove, which produced some improvement in the swelling. *A* and *B*, Clinical appearance of the dorsum and palm of the hand. Note the diffuse mass effect with spreading of the digits, discoloration of the palm, and prominent veins over the middle phalanx of the dorsum of the ring finger. *C*, X-ray film of the hand shows soft tissue overgrowth, osseous deformity, and osseous hypertrophy (cortical thickening). *D*, Blood pool image from a 99m technetium pyrophosphate bone scan shows increased activity in the areas of the soft tissue mass.

Figure continues on following page

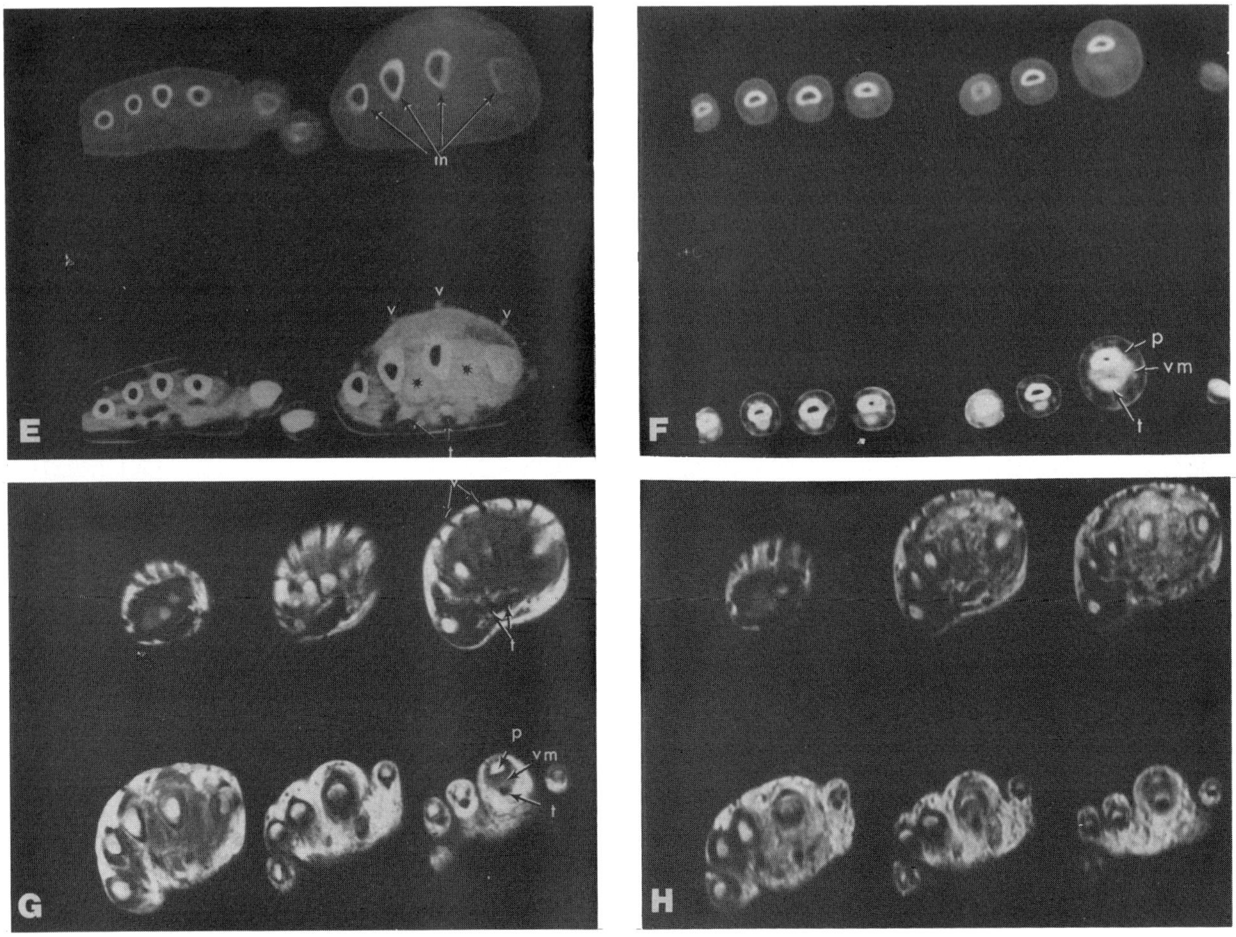

Figure 2 (continued) *E*, Contrast-enhanced axial computed tomographic (CT) images through the metacarpal bones (m), palms down, at bone (above) and soft tissue (below) window settings show diffuse enlargement and enhancement of the intrinsic hand muscles (*) as well as dorsal subcutaneous tissues. The scan includes the head of the fifth metacarpal. The other metacarpals have normal marrow fat density, which indicates absence of involvement. Note the prominent veins (v) over the dorsum of the left hand and in the palm (arrows). *F*, Contrast-enhanced axial CT images of both hands, at the level of the proximal phalanges, palms down, show the involvement of the ring finger with abnormal vascular tissue between the phalanx and the tendon and its attachments. *G* and *H*, T-1 (*G*) and T-2 (*H*) weighted axial magnetic resonance images of the right hand, palm down, from wrist (above left) to proximal fingers (lower right). In *G*, the subcutaneous fat and bone marrow are white, and blood vessels are black. The diffuse muscular enlargement shows up well. In *H*, the curvilinear dark ares within the masses represent vascular channels. (m = metacarpal; p = phalanx; t = tendon; v = veins; vm = vascular malformation).

spontaneous thrombosis. The masses typically distend with exertion, dependency, and obstruction to venous drainage.

VENOUS MALFORMATIONS

The term venous malformations applies to localized varices, pouches, or tangles of systemic veins, as well as to sinusoidal spaces that have no angiographically-demonstrable connection with adjacent arteries and small or non-demonstrable connections with regional systemic veins. They characteristically produce bluish discoloration and focal or diffuse masses which, like capillary venous malformations, distend with dependency and obstruction to proximal venous flow.

The symptoms in both capillary-venous malformations and venous malformations may be improved with local elastic compression. Surgery is rarely indicated but major contour irregularities may be excised. In some localized cases, percutaneous injection of sclerosing agents may be effective.

LYMPHATIC MALFORMATIONS

These lesions have been classified according to the size of the space (Table 2). Although they may present as localized, spongy or cyst-like soft tissue masses, they are frequently diffuse lesions that produce generalized expansion of the extremity. They are frequently associated with dysplasia of blood vessels (hemolymphangioma or

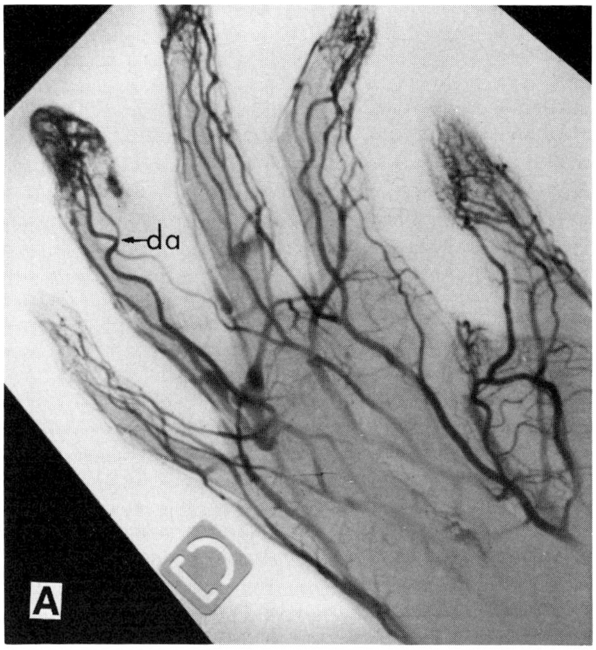

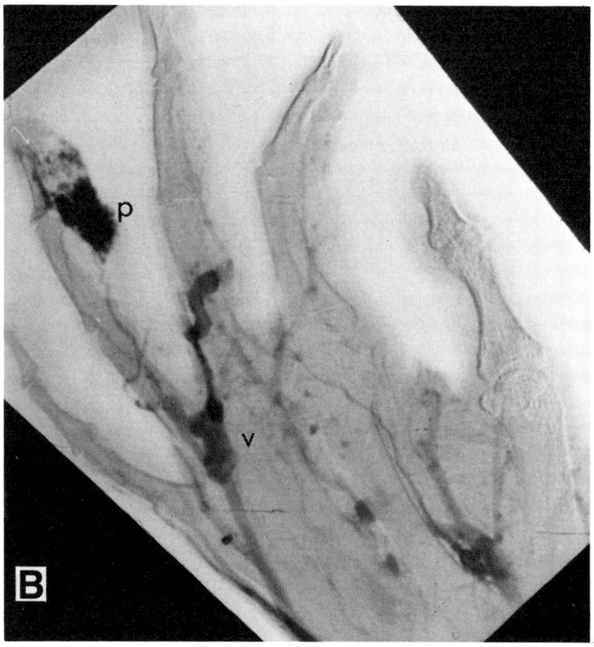

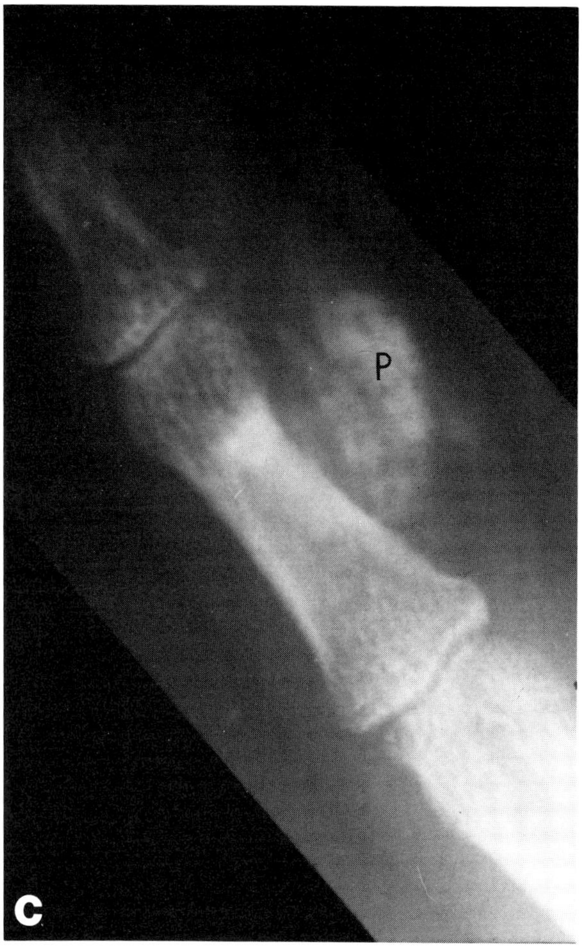

Figure 3 Localized capillary-venous and venous malformation in a young journalist, who complained of bluish distention and pain of the soft tissues of the distal ring finger (aggravated with typing). The venous pouch became completely flat within 5 weeks after percutaneous injection with alcohol. Late arterial (*A*) and phases of (*B*) a right brachial arteriogram shows mild enlargement of the digital arteries in the ring finger, prominent subungual vessels, opacification of focal sinusoidal spaces, and dysplastic draining veins. *C*, X-ray film of the index finger after injection of the sinusoidal pouch with 100 percent sterile ethanol, opacified with metrizamide powder. (Courtesy of Dr Pierre Lasjaunias, Hopital Bicêtre, Université de Paris, France). (da = digital artery; p = venous pouch; v = venous varix).

hemolymphatic dysplasia). The associated vascular malformations are usually venous or capillary-venous in nature, but may also include arteriovenous connections. The spaces in lymphatic malformations may also contain blood due to hemorrhage via communication with adjacent systemic veins, without the presence of an associated hemovascular malformation. They are subject to painful episodes of rapid enlargement, which are generally attributed to hemorrhage, thrombosis, or inflammation. Spontaneous regression may occur, but is usually partial.

DIAGNOSTIC APPROACH TO VASCULAR MALFORMATIONS

Most vascular malformations can be diagnosed and the nature of the underlying channel abnormality can often be predicted by a careful history and physical examination. As discussed above, vascular malformations are nearly always congenital and, typically, they enlarge in proportion to the growth of the child. They may show periods of rapid expansion, especially at puberty, during

TABLE 2 Lymphatic Abnormalities

Classification	
Lymphangioma:	Capillary or simplex
	Circumscripta
	Cavernous
Cystic hygroma	
Lymphedema	
Lymphangiectasia	

From: Williams HB. Embryology and classification of lymphatic abnormalities. In: Williams HB, ed. Symposium on vascular malformations and melanotic lesions. St. Louis: CV Mosby 1983; 175.

menses or pregnancy, or following trauma, and may show partial regression with thrombosis.

However, the history of rapid enlargement during the first year of life followed by slow regression, which is typical of hemangiomas, is not a feature of vascular malformations. A history of rapid enlargement of the lesion during periods of hormonal change may indicate a lesion with increased potential for evolution, such as recurrence or progression following partial removal.

Discoloration may indicate a superficial location of the lesion, or may simply reflect distended regional veins that are draining a deeper lesion. High-flow lesions can be predicted by the presence of increased pulse pressure, thrill, and bruits.

IMAGING OF VASCULAR MALFORMATIONS

Although angiography is the most precise modality to demonstrate vascular malformations, it should probably be reserved for use in patients who are being considered for intervention, or for patients in whom the diagnosis is unclear. Noninvasive imaging modalities (see Fig. 2) are excellent to define the extent and, therefore, resectability of vascular malformations.

PLAIN RADIOGRAPHIC FEATURES

Radiographic findings include soft tissue deformities, bony changes, and soft tissue calcifications, usually phleboliths. Bony changes are frequent, and include sclerosis, cortical thickening, modelling abnormalities, and increase in size. Less commonly, the affected extremity or digits may be shorter due to premature fusion of the epiphyseal plates. Coarsening of the medullary trabecular pattern indicates a high probability of bone marrow involvement. Joint space narrowing or destruction may result from hemarthrosis. Scintigraphic bony scanning is useful in two ways. Firstly, the flow and blood pool phases help to distinguish lymphatic from hemovascular malformations by the presence of accumulation of activity in the latter. Delayed images demonstrate increased activity in bone in the presence of cortical thickening. Tagged red blood cell imaging is probably a more reliable way of distinguishing vascular malformations from avascular lesions, and is useful in showing the extent of the vascular abnormality.

COMPUTED TOMOGRAPHY AND MAGNETIC RESONANCE IMAGING

Axial computed tomographic imaging, performed with and without intravenous contrast administration, is useful to demonstrate the extent of the vascular malformation, the involvement of structures such as muscle, neural sheaths, tendons, and bone, and helps to differentiate between pure lymphatic and hemolymphatic dysplasias. In the presence of tissue enlargement, cross-sectional imaging is useful to differentiate between tissue infiltration with the vascular malformation, tissue hypertrophy, and increased fat content that is frequently present in diffuse vascular malformations of the extremities. Magnetic resonance imaging is a superb modality for demonstrating the integrity or involvement of soft tissue structures.

ANGIOGRAPHY

The purpose of angiography is to demonstrate the nature and extent of the vascular malformation, and to map out precisely the angioarchitecture of the nidus, its arterial supply, and its venous drainage, prior to intervention. It also provides information about the vascular supply to the normal tissues.

Angiographic features of high-flow lesions, such as arteriovenous fistulas (see Fig. 1) and arteriovenous malformations, include enlargement and tortuosity of the feeding arteries, the presence of abnormal vessels supplying the nidus, rapid flow through the fistula or nidus (network), and rapid filling of dilated veins. Vascular malformations frequently include other signs of vascular dysplasia, such as aneurysms of the feeding vessels within the nidus, or of the draining veins.

Capillary-venous malformations show filling of the sinusoidal spaces by tiny branches of slightly dilated regional arteries. This opacification occurs earlier than that of the normal regional veins. The draining veins often also appear abnormal, with areas of dilatation.

Venous malformations typically do no fill from the arterial injection, or fill at the same rate as the systemic veins. Those sequestered from the normal arterial tree may require opacification by direct percutaneous puncture and injection with contrast material

EMBOLIZATION TECHNIQUES

In recent years, embolization techniques have been refined due to improvements in catheters and materials. The techniques involve deposition of occlusive material via a catheter, ideally into the nidus or fistula. Occlusion of only proximal vessels is as ineffective as surgical ligation.

There are basically two approaches to embolotherapy: presurgical devascularization of a lesion prior to excision, and primary embolization without surgery. The latter should be reserved for patients with isolated arteriovenous fistulas, or for complications of inoperable lesions.

Techniques include occlusion of larger arteriovenous communications with detachable balloons, wire coils, or polymerizing liquid agents (isobutyl-2 cyanoacrylate) (see Fig. 1) and flow-directed occlusion of the nidus of the arteriovenous malformation with liquid agents or calibrated particles (polyvinyl alcohol foam). These agents are usually delivered through a catheter, but, in peripheral lesions, access may be more readily obtained by direct puncture of the nidus (see Fig. 1 and 3) or feeding artery. Localized low-flow (venous) malformations may respond to percutaneous injection (under fluoroscopic control) of sclerosing agents such as opacified 100 percent sterile alcohol (see Fig. 3C).

Partial embolization of high-flow lesions will be followed by recurrence, but may offer some temporary symptomatic relief. Specific indications include congestive heart failure, bleeding, pain, and decreased function.

SURGICAL EXCISION

Gelberman and Goltner have published a review of their own experience with surgical excision of vascular malformations as well as that reported in the literature. They found that only 12 of 28 attempts at excision of vascular malformations involving the hand were successful; 16 had persistent or increased symptoms and 3 procedures were followed by gangrene of a digit. They also reviewed the results of 28 amputations performed in 18 patients. Nine of 19 finger or ray amputations were curative, while the others resulted in persistent or worse symptoms with proximal proliferation of the mass. Simple ligation was curative in only one case. Proximal vessel ligation is not only ineffective but contraindicated, as it leads to the reperfusion of the arteriovenous malformation via the collaterals that previously perfused the healthy tissues, thereby increasing tissue ischemia and making future excision or embolization more difficult.

Gelberman and Goltner concluded that the likelihood of success from surgical treatment was related to the localized or diffuse nature of the lesion. Diffuse digital masses with involvement of the palm and adjacent digits, and those lesions with bony involvement, respond poorly, with a high recurrence rate and persistent worsening of symptoms. Localized lesions, with single feeding vessels without bony involvement, respond best to excision. The authors stressed that single-channel continuity must be maintained to prevent gangrene, and they recommended the use of a vein graft if necessary. They suggested that, in the presence of osseous involvement or decreased distal flow, amputation of a digit or ray and excision of any adjacent mass is the procedure of choice. Patients with diffuse masses should undergo surgery only as a last resort.

The onset of significant complications requires surgical intervention. This occurs in the arteriovenous fistula and arteriovenous malformation groups. Such complications consist of intractable pain, progressive ischemic ulceration, compartment syndrome from intralesional bleeding, and development of an overgrown, weighty, functionless extremity, particularly with high-flow systemic symptoms. Prior to surgery, as much information as possible regarding the lesion should be obtained through the imaging techniques outlined above. Embolotherapy for presurgical devascularization facilitates the dissection enormously. As noted earlier, proximal vessel ligation is of no benefit and, in fact, may worsen the situation. As complete an excision as possible, particularly in relatively localized lesions, provides the best chance at success. Vascular reconstruction that utilizes microvascular surgical techniques may be necessary after excision of the lesion. Clearly, preservation of function with careful attention to joints, tendon complexes, and nerves is of foremost importance.

Should this prove unsuccessful or vascular shunting create a life-threatening situation in a weighty, functionless limb or distal part, then amputation of the limb or affected part may be the only route.

ACQUIRED VASCULAR LESIONS

The etiology of acquired vascular problems in the hand may be local, systemic, or on a vasospastic basis. Within the hand, vascular injuries, arterial thrombosis, aneurysm formation, and vascular tumors may occur. Systemic emboli or generalized systemic disease also may cause hand problems. Lastly, vasospastic conditions (Raynaud's) are commonly seen in the hand.

Acquired Local Vascular Problems

Vascular Injuries

Vascular injuries may take many forms. Local trauma, whether sharp, blunt, or avulsive, may disrupt flow and compromise distal perfusion. Reconstruction is then indicated and may take the form of direct vessel repair or vein grafting, utilizing microvasular techniques. The question as to whether a transected single digital artery should or should not be repaired when its mate is uninjured is the topic of an ongoing clinical research project in our unit. Preliminary results indicate a marginal advantage to repair.

Intra-arterial injection injuries, either iatrogenic or as seen in drug addicts, pose major problems. Burning pain onsets immediately with interruption of blood flow; blanching and later cyanosis follow. Thrombolytics and direct mechanical flushing are effective in the early stages, followed by systemic anticoagulation and vasodilators. In drug addicts, the presentation is often late and, despite the above measures, little can be done to prevent gangrene and eventual amputation of affected tissue.

Aneurysm Formation

An aneurysm may form at the site of arterial trauma whether the latter is of an external penetrating type or caused by blunt injury. True aneurysms involve intimal, muscular, and adventitial layers, whereas pseudo or false aneurysms involve intimal and fibrous tissue only. The clinical presentation is that of a painful, pulsatile mass, often in an area of recent trauma (Fig. 4A). Distal digital pain or ischemia may result from emboli that originate in the aneurysm. The Allen's test gives useful information regarding the flow in both the involved and noninvolved vessel. The treatment is surgical and consists of complete resection, and arterial reconstruction with a vein graft (Fig. 4B).

Vascular Tumors

Acquired vascular tumors in the hand are uncommon. The majority are benign, have a specific clinical picture, and are readily resectable. The glomus tumor is the most common in this group. Its prominent feature is localized pain, often exquisite. The lesion is usually found in the nailbed, and a bluish or reddish discoloration. When present in the digital pulp, a painful mass is often palpable. The treatment is surgical excision, which is curative. Nailbed reconstruction is important if a nail deformity is to be avoided.

Another acquired vascular tumor in the hand, often seen in children, is the pyogenic granuloma. This elevated, pedunculated, red lesion is often crusted and bleeds easily when traumatized. Treatment is surgical excision with cauterization of base.

Other vascular tumors such as pericytoma, angiosarcoma, and Kaposi's sarcoma are very rare in the hand.

Acquired Systemic Vascular Problems

Systemic Emboli

Systemic emboli often originate from the heart or great vessels as a result of arrhythmias, infarction, or vascular disease. In the absence of cardiac disease, the thoracic outlet should be carefully evaluated, as this may also be a source of emboli. With compression of the subclavian artery, thrombi can form on the vessel wall and produce showers of microemboli with resultant ischemic hand symptoms. The effects of such emboli range from sudden limb ischemia due to large emboli to distal digital pain and ischemia caused by small embolic showers. Treatment should be directed at the cause, with a careful evaluation of other areas for the effects of such emboli. When impending gangrene results from a large embolus, surgical embolectomy should be undertaken immediately.

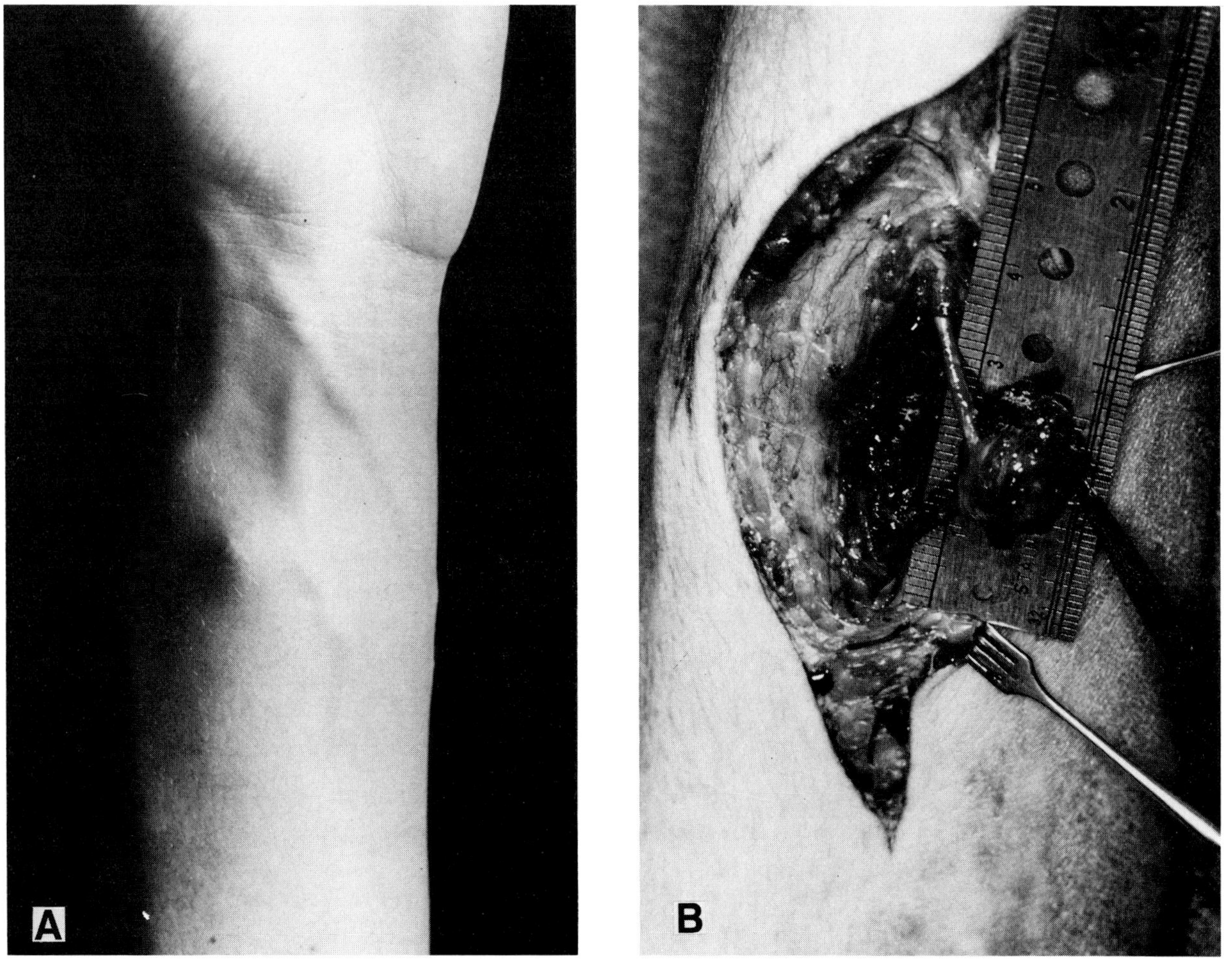

Figure 4 *A*, Photograph of acquired traumatic aneurysm of radial artery in distal forearm. *B*, The aneurysm is exposed for resection.

Systemic Disease Processes

The generalized systemic diseases most commonly associated with vascular hand problems are scleroderma, Thromboangiitis obliterans (Buerger's disease), and polyarteritis. The course of these conditions and the vascular component is highly variable. Although medical management is the mainstay of therapy, large vessel involvement occasionally occurs in scleroderma. Angiography may demonstrate localized areas suitable for microsurgical vein graft reconstruction.

Vasospastic Conditions

Raynaud's phenomenon consists of episodic digital blanching and numbness, precipitated by cold exposure or emotional stress and followed by digital rubor and paresthesia as the circulation returns. The pathophysiology is vascular spasm, which has a host of known causes both local and systemic. Where no cause is found after a thorough investigation and years of symptoms, the condition is known as primary Raynaud's or Raynaud's disease. Secondary Raynaud's consists of vascular spasm as a result of such local conditions as repetitive trauma, as in pneumatic hammer disease, localized arterial disease such as thromboangiitis obliterans and thoracic outlet compression, and systemic disease such as the collagen vascular diseases, particularly scleroderma.

A thorough search for organic disease as the basis of the vasospasm is mandatory. Treatment should be directed at correction of any underlying abnormality or disease and removal or minimizing of any precipitating stimulus. Conservative measures are probably most effective. Nonconstrictive warm clothing should be worn in an effort to avoid reflex vasoconstriction. Effective gloves are of critical importance in cool weather as are warm socks. The use of tobacco should be discouraged as this often induces vasoconstriction and precipitates an attack.

Specific control of the vasospasm through drug therapy is still evolving. Only those patients with severe symptoms or tissue necrosis should be considered. In addition to the adrenergic blocking agents (guanethidine, methyldopa, reserpine, phenoxybenzamine) much of the current activity revolves around prostaglandin E_1 and I_2, the slow calcium-channel antagonists (nifedipine and verapamil), the serotonin antagonist (ketanserin), and angiotensin-converting enzyme inhibitor (captopril). Topical 2 percent nitroglycerin ointment may provide temporary relief, although systemic absorption and cardiac ischemia upon withdrawal has been reported.

The surgical management of Raynaud's phenomenon by sympathectomy has been disappointing. Sympathetic ganglia resection is all too often followed by the return of autonomous vascular tone and symptomatology, as well as uncomfortably dry hands due to pseudomotor denervation.

SUGGESTED READING

Burrows PE, Mulliken JB, Fellows KE, Strand RD. Childhood hemangiomas and vascular malformations: angiographic differentiation. AJR 1983; 141:483-488.

Dowd PM. The treatment of Raynaud's phenomenon. Br J Dermatol 1986; 114:527-533.

Gelberman RH, Goltner JL. Congenital arteriovenous fistulas of the hand. J Hand Surg 1978; 3:451-454.

Liu P, Daneman A, Stringer DA, Smith CR. Computed tomography of hemangiomas and related soft tissue lesions in children. J Can Assoc Radiol 1986; 37:248-255.

Moore JR, Weiland AJ. Embolotherapy in the treatment of congenital arteriovenous malformations of the hand: a case report. J Hand Surg 1985; 10A: 135-139.

Mulliken JB, Glowacki J. Hemangiomas and vascular malformations in infants and children: a classification based on endothelial characteristics. Plast Reconstr Surg 1982; 69:412-420.

Williams HB. Embryology and classification of lymphatic abnormalities. In: Williams HB, ed. Symposium on vascular malformations and melanotic lesions. St. Louis: CV Mosby, 1983; 175.

Wisnicki JL. Hemangiomas and vascular malformations. Ann Plast Surg 1984; 12:41-59.

OCCUPATIONAL HAND DYSFUNCTION

MORTON L. KASDAN, M.D., F.A.C.S.

This chapter covers my approach to acute hand injuries and cumulative trauma disorders. In either situation, the goal of the treating surgeon is to restore the injured worker to a condition that would allow a return to his or her previous occupation. Too often one loses sight of the ultimate goal. Despite the tremendous costs of hand injuries, not enough is being done to cut these expenses by returning the patient to work. The price of medical care may represent only a fraction of the total cost. When the off-work disability payments and final workman's compensation settlement for an impairment of function are considered, the result is a serious economic problem. Multiple elaborate surgical procedures that do not result in a return to gainful employment accomplish very little for the patient or his employer.

When the acute hand injury is managed, every effort should be made to make the first operation the only one. Try to keep in mind the ultimate goal; that is, the return of the injured employee to his or her job. Each day the patient is off work, it becomes more difficult to rehabilitate him. A similar situation would be a child on sick leave from school. Each day it becomes harder to return the student to school. The same thing is true of adult workers.

They become progressively more fearful of returning to the work place.

The decision to return a patient to regular duty at work can be a tough call. The surgeon must keep in mind that there may be a reward for not getting well. Subjective complaints must be thoroughly and fairly evaluated. The final determination should be based on as much objective data as possible.

A good starting point for the hand surgeon is familiarity with the plant or factory where the patient was injured. This can be accomplished by an on-site inspection, or by reviewing a video tape of the exact hand function. It is possible, on occasion, to obtain a very accurate description from an articulate patient or supervisor at the place of employment. In any event, the surgeon must have a clear understanding of what is expected from the patient at his or her job. It helps to know if the patient has any secondary occupations or hobbies that require specialized hand function. The best rehabilitation for the injured worker is a return to work as soon as possible, but this does not necessarily mean he or she has to do the exact preinjury job; a light duty position may be available. Although one wants to believe the patient, it is important not to accept a statement that "they don't have light duty where I work." It does not take long to telephone the employer and find out what is available. This call can provide much information about the patient. For example, does he or she have a good (or bad) work record? Have there been multiple other injuries with lost time and disability settlements? It helps to know if the patient is "street wise" to worker's compensation suits. The person who pays the bill has a right to know what is going on with the employee.

The patient also has the right to know the diagnosis of his or her problem and the plans for treatment. The patient should be informed of the alternative methods of treatment and told what to expect with emphasis upon rehabilitation and return to work.

It is usually possible to give the patient any one particular function; it is often impossible to give a seriously injured hand a multitude of functions. I repeatedly stress to patients that I cannot make them well, that I can try to give them the potential to make themselves well, but that I cannot do it for them. Eighty percent of the final result will be the patient's participation in his or her own recovery and rehabilitation. I let patients know from the start my plans to return them to some form of work. The response to this dialogue gives good insight as to the patient's motivation.

CUMULATIVE TRAUMA DISORDERS

Three important consultants in the evaluation of a cumulative trauma disorder are the neurologist, the radiologist, and the clinical psychologist. The neurologist who works with me has saved the day on several occasions. He has picked up cases of systemic neurologic disorders. Carpal tunnel syndrome is the most common occupational peripheral nervous system disease; however, pain, numbness, and tingling in the classic median nerve distribution can also be caused by central lesions in the brain or lesions proximal to the carpal tunnel. The diagnosis is not necessarily carpal tunnel syndrome. Therefore, a neurologic consultation is usually scheduled for patients with symptoms of peripheral neuropathy. Recently, a patient who was to have surgery for carpal tunnel symptoms was seen for a second opinion. The neurologist found Charcot-Marie-Tooth Disease.

Choice of the right neurologist may be difficult. There are helpful tips one can use to select the right consultant. First, one should be sure that he or she tests the asymptomatic extremity. If both sides are symptomatic and tested, did the neurologist test an asymptomatic nerve, i.e., ulnar or peroneal? Second, was the patient so unhappy with the examination that he or she refused to be retested in a couple of months? In other words, the neurologist should be thorough and gentle.

The radiologist should have a special interest in the upper extremity. A quick check of his or her library for hand radiology books and *The Journal of Hand Surgery* provides excellent information. If the radiologist takes a history and examines the patient, he or she is the right consultant.

The clinical psychologist must be experienced in the evaluation of pain. It is a good idea to interview several psychologists and check their references. Is the psychologist a member of the State Board of Psychology and is he or she licensed? Is the specialist registered with the National Register or Health Service Providers in Psychology? One must be sure the psychologist is qualified to give the assessment instruments.

ACUTE HAND INJURIES

The only acute trauma to be discussed here is the high pressure injection injury. Most injuries can occur either at home, during hobby, or at work. The one injury that is usually found only at work is the high pressure injection injury. This is a surgical emergency and should never be underestimated. Thin hydrocarbons are especially dangerous. It is almost impossible to decompress and explore too much (Figs. 1, 2, and 3). The extent of soft tissue dissection by the fluid is amazing. One should be especially alert for systemic effects of the solution, and, if possible, try to find out the toxicology.

DISCUSSION

The doctor should use common sense, and if he does not feel the patient wants to get better, i.e., does not want to work, then he or she may be better off without an operation. The injured worker may be better motivated by a different surgeon. The physician should get to know his or her patients by letting them talk. Be careful with patients who blame all their troubles on the supervisor or company. They may blame their surgeon next. No case, especially a cumulative trauma disorder, should be taken over without a review of the medical records. If the patient does not listen when the doctor talks, the latter may be the wrong doctor for the case.

There should be good objective evidence of pathology before one institutes invasive therapy. For example, I do not operate for carpal tunnel syndrome without neurologic

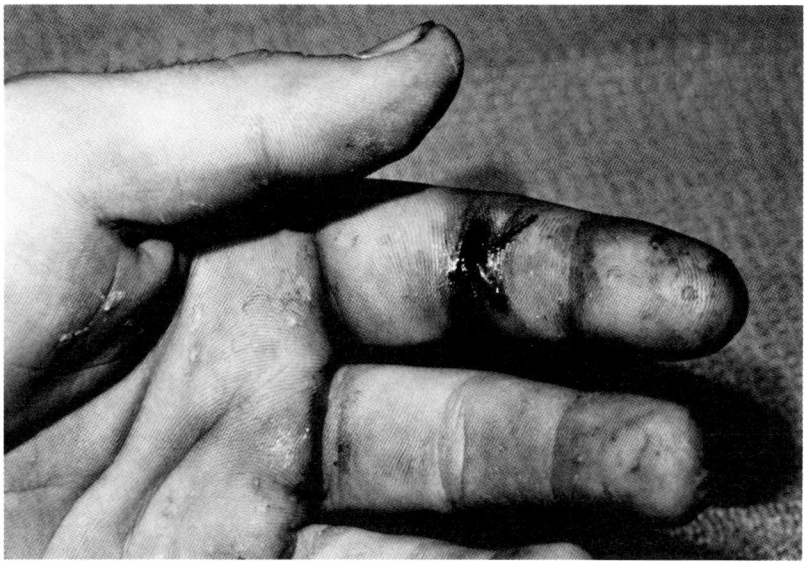

Figure 1 The patient was a 25-year-old male who was checking a high-pressure paint sprayer with his finger in front of the nozzle. The high-pressure spray gun developed 4,160 pounds of pressure.

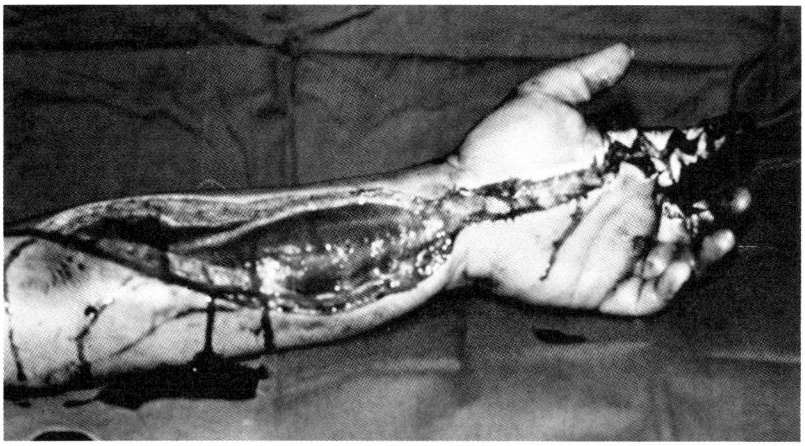

Figure 2 Extensive extravasation of an unknown paint thinner extended up to the proximal forearm. This required amputation of the left index finger, as well as decompression of the hand and forearm.

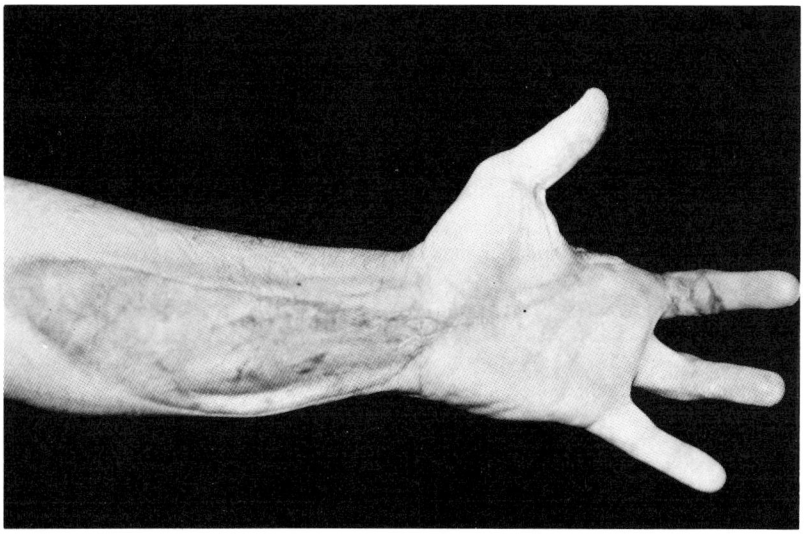

Figure 3 The appearance of the patient almost 9 months later.

testing. The worker with secondary gain in mind (time off work, disability settlement, or litigation) may know all the subjective responses to convince the inexperienced surgeon to operate.

One should do what is necessary; not what is possible. The surgeon who tries for the perfect result may have a "successful" operation and a psychologically crippled patient. It should be explained to both the patient and employer that perfection in the real world is not possible. There should be no operation if one does not feel the patient can be improved.

SUGGESTED READING

Chaplin E, Kasdan M, Corwin H. Occupational neurology and the hand, differential diagnosis. Hand Clinics 1986; 2(3):513–524.

Harter B, Harter K. High-pressure injection injuries. Hand Clin 1986; 2(3):547–552.

Johnson R. Psychological evaluation of patients with industrial hand injuries. Hand Clin 1986; 2(3):567–575.

Kelsey J, Pastides H, Kreiger N, et al. Upper extremity disorders: a survey of their frequency and cost in the United States. St. Louis: CV Mosby, 1980:2.

Wayne P. Radiology of the occupationally injured hand. Hand Clin 1986; 2(3):467–506.

NERVE COMPRESSION SYNDROMES

SUSAN E. MACKINNON, M.D., F.R.C.S. (C), F.A.C.S.

Chronic nerve compression, or entrapment neuropathy, is a common clinical problem managed by the plastic surgeon. Carpal tunnel was first described in 1854. It is now a well-recognized compression syndrome and by far the most frequently diagnosed. Compression of the ulnar nerve in the cubital tunnel was first described in 1878 and is the second most frequently diagnosed syndrome. Other nerve entrapments more recently described are, of course, less well-recognized. With increased clinical awareness, symptoms related to nerve compression are recognized earlier and at more anatomic sites. However, entrapment of the radial sensory nerve in the forearm is still frequently misdiagnosed as de Quervain's disease, and, while diabetics with diminished sensation in the hand are frequently diagnosed as having carpal tunnel syndrome, the same patient with numbness in the foot is rarely considered as having tarsal tunnel syndrome.

The treatment of a compressed nerve is relatively simple and involves decompression of the nerve at the anatomic point of compression. Many aspects of this problem are not so simply dealt with. Establishment of the clinical diagnosis of the less common compression neuropathies is difficult. Evaluation of patients with complaints referable to multiple entrapments, or entrapment neuropathies that present with pain rather than motor or sensory loss, is equally challenging. An understanding of the subtleties of the surgical anatomy can be critical in determining improvement of symptoms. The role of internal neurolysis remains highly controversial. Iatrogenic, superimposed nerve injury from inadequate or careless surgical decompression is a topic in itself and may be a source of litigation.

Considerable material is available that summarizes in detail all aspects of entrapment of neuropathy. This chapter highlights the author's personal approach to this very common problem.

PATHOGENESIS

It is important to review the pathogenesis of chronic nerve compression, since the pathology of this entity is reflected by the patient's symptoms and clinical findings. The histopathology of chronic nerve compression presents a broad spectrum, which progresses from no histological findings to severe Wallerian degeneration (Fig. 1). Initially, the patient's symptoms are in response to periodic ischemia, secondary to transient compromise of local blood flow. The earliest histologic change will be breakdown in the blood-nerve barrier, with resulting subperineurial edema. Eventually, connective changes will be seen, with thickening of both the external and internal epineurium. When nerve fiber changes are finally noted, they initially involve only the peripheral fibers of the peripheral fascicles of the nerve. The fascicles in the center of the nerve, or those fascicles away from direct pressure, appear normal. The large, myelinated fibers demonstrate segmental demyelination; the unmyelinated fibers degenerate and then demonstrate evidence of regeneration. Eventually, diffuse fiber changes are seen throughout the entire nerve, and Wallerian degeneration (which, by definition, relates only to myelinated nerve fibers) will be present. Both connective tissue and nerve fiber pathology increase directly with the amount and duration of compression.

CLINICAL IMPLICATIONS

Clinical Diagnosis

The surgeon should attempt to grade, or stage, the degree of compression neuropathy and should expect patients to demonstrate both symptomatology and clinical signs across a wide spectrum of severity. In the early stages of nerve compression, symptoms may only be elicited when provocative tests are used to render the nerve locally ischemic by manipulation of the extremity (e.g., wrist flexion for median nerve compression at the wrist; elbow

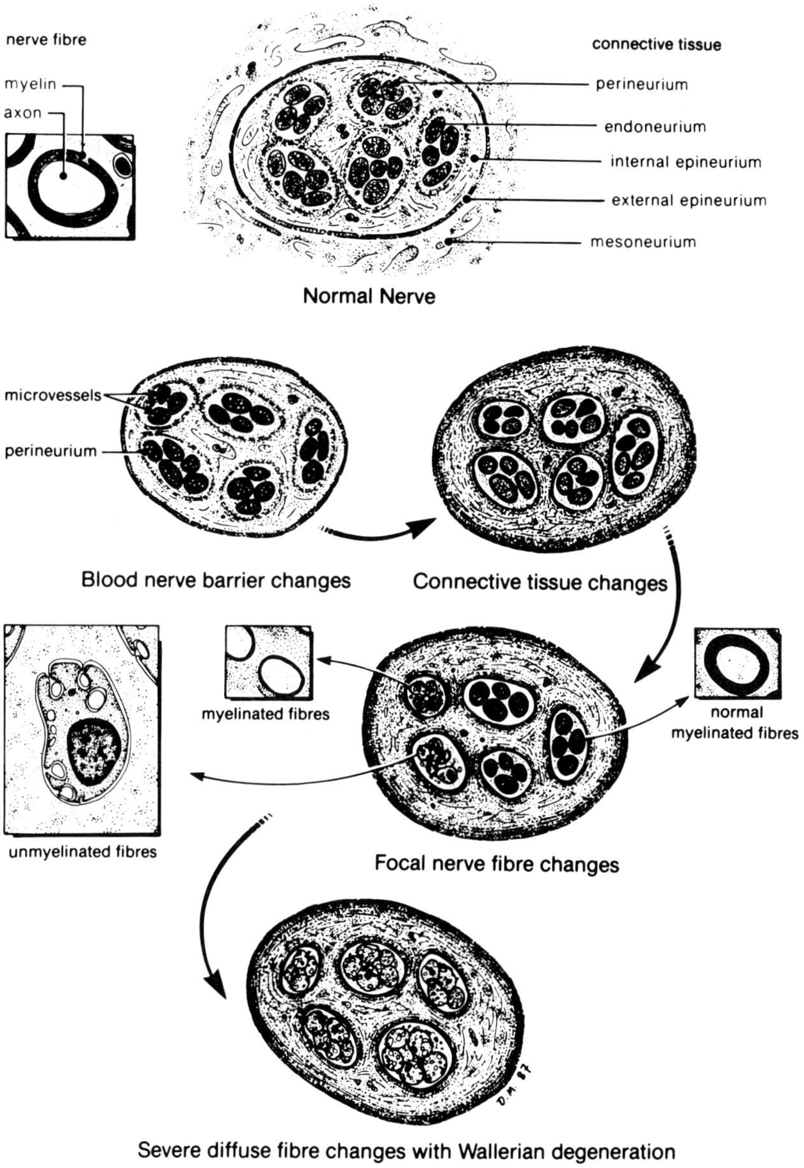

Figure 1 Schemata of histopathology of chronic nerve compression. The initial changes occur at the level of the blood nerve barrier. This is followed by connective tissue changes and then focal nerve fiber changes. The large myelinated fibers undergo segmental demyelination. The small, unmyelinated fibers demonstrate evidence of degeneration and regeneration with the presence of a new population of very small, unmyelinated fibers. Thus, a bimodal rather than unimodal population of unmyelinated nerve fibers is noted. With progression of the compression, diffuse Wallerian degeneration is noted. (From MacKinnon SE, Dellon AL. Peripheral nerve surgery. New York: Thieme-Stratton, 1988.)

flexion for ulnar nerve compression at the elbow or local pressure over the nerve). Persistent paresthesia is related to more chronic alternations in blood flow produced by intraneural fibrosis. Muscle wasting and loss of two-point discrimination are present only if there is advanced nerve compression with actual loss of nerve fibers, as occurs with Wallerian degeneration. The finding of Tinel's sign in chronic nerve compression should suggest a more severe degree of compression, with nerve fiber damage and attempts at regeneration.

Initially, only the nerve fibers in peripheral fascicles of the nerve are affected. Adjacent fascicles may be entirely normal. This would account for the frequent paradox of the patient who presents with marked symptomatology but normal electrodiagnostic findings. The abnormal histologic findings in the fascicles which demonstrate nerve fiber pathology, would account for the patient's symptoms, while the normal, large, myelinated fibers in the unaffected fascicles would account for the normal electrodiagnostic studies.

At this stage, when there is a variable fascicular pathology, the clinician should expect the patient to demonstrate other than classic or complete nerve palsies on physical examination. Patients with median nerve compression in the carpal tunnel often have varying sensory findings from digit to digit. Patients with anterior or posterior interosseous nerve entrapment may demonstrate marked variability in muscle weakness from muscle to muscle. Such a partial nerve palsy should not imply minimal nerve palsy, as those fascicles to the affected muscles or sensory receptors will demonstrate very severe fiber pathology. The patient should be investigated and treated as aggressively as if all units supplied by that nerve were affected.

Provocative Pressure Test

The clinical diagnosis of various entrapment neuropathies has been well-described. In general, the clinician anticipates the patient's symptoms, and signs will vary depending on the stage of chronic nerve compression. In every instance, however, he should be able to elicit or reproduce symptoms by some local provocative test. In my experience, chronically compressed nerves have a reduced threshold to mechanical stimulation compared to normal nerves, and are locally susceptible to direct mechanical stimulation. Direct pressure over the nerve quickly reproduces the patient's symptoms. The local *provocative pressure test* applies to all entrapped nerves. The examining physician exerts pressure with two or three digits, or the thumb, directly over the nerve in question, just proximal to the area of compression. This maneuver will reproduce the patient's symptoms if the nerve is compressed (Fig. 2). The pressure provocative test is performed on the contralateral extremity as a control test. Other provocative tests are specific to individual nerves (Table 1).

Electrodiagnostic Testing

For reasons outlined above, while an abnormal electrodiagnostic test is supportive of the diagnosis, findings will be entirely normal in many patients with chronic nerve compression. In a study that correlated a patient population, carefully staged for nerve compression, with electrodiagnostic testing, a 20 percent incidence of false-negative electrodiagnostic tests was noted in all staging categories for nerve compression.

Surgical Treatment

Following surgical release, immediate symptomatic improvement observed in some patients after peripheral nerve decompression, must be attributed to alterations in neural blood flow. More gradual improvement in recovery of sensation, muscle strength, and bulk is probably related to actual neural regeneration. Evaluation of the progressive pathology seen with chronic nerve compression leads us to speculate that internal neurolysis does not play a role in early nerve compression, when symptoms are due to compromise of local blood flow, with subsequent neural ischemia. At a later stage, when there are marked connective tissue changes, with thickening of the interfascicular epineurium and nerve fiber changes, neuro-

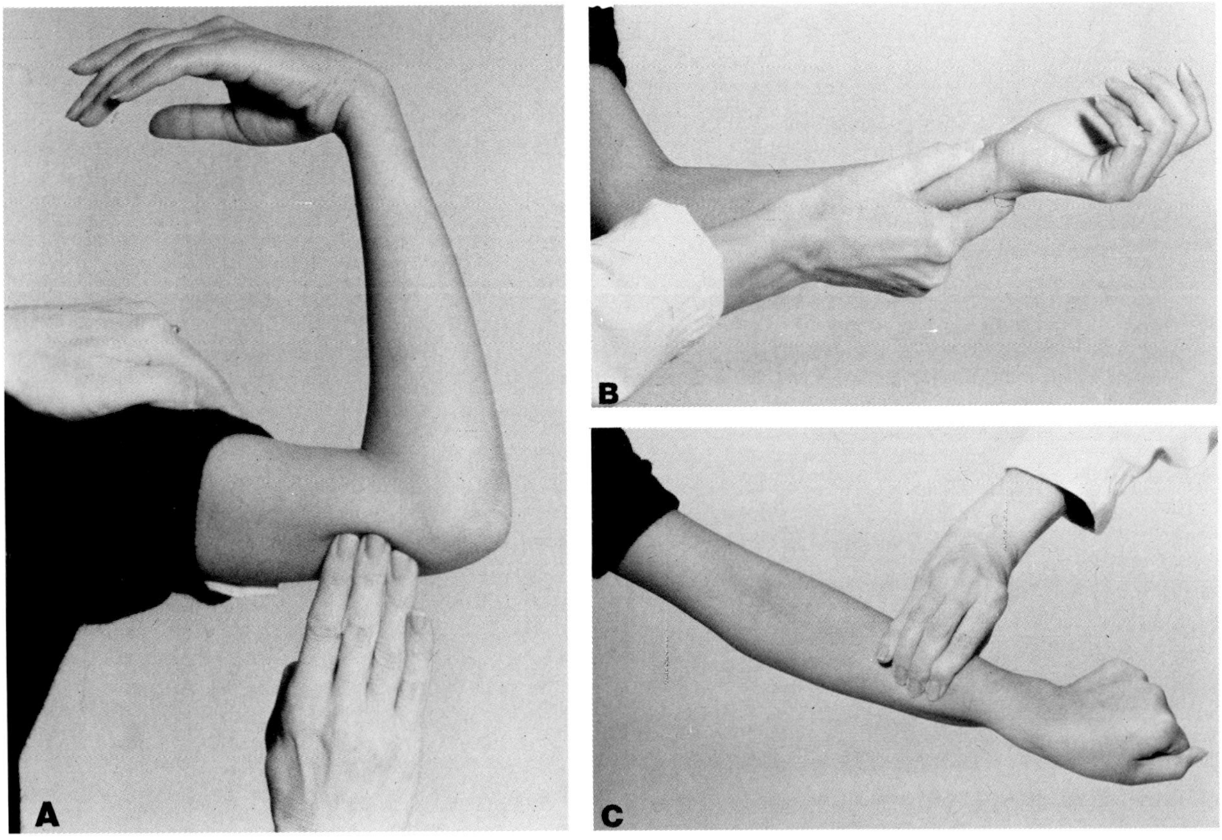

Figure 2 Direct mechanical pressure over an entrapped nerve will reproduce or provoke the patient's symptoms. *A*, Elbow flexion and direct pressure just proximal to the cubital tunnel will provoke cubital tunnel symptoms. *B*, Direct pressure over the median nerve, just proximal to the carpal tunnel, will reproduce the carpal tunnel patient's symptoms. *C*, Similarly, in those patients with entrapment of the radial sensory nerve, pressure over the nerve and forearm pronation with wrist ulnar flexion will reproduce symptoms.

TABLE 1 Provocative Tests for Nerve Entrapment

Nerve	*Entrapment Site*	*Provocative Test*
Median	Carpal Tunnel	Pressure proximal to carpal tunnel Phalen's test, reverse Phalen's (hyper-extension wrist)
Median	Proximal Forearm	Pressure over proximal forearm resisted-elbow flexion -pronation -finger flexion
Ulnar	Guyon's Canal	Pressure proximal to Guyon's canal
Ulnar	Cubital Tunnel	Pressure proximal to cubital tunnel elbow flexion
Radial (posterior interosseous)	Arcade of Frohse	Pressure over supinator resisted supination, resisted long finger and wrist extension (ECRB)
Radial (sensory)	Forearm	Pressure over junction of brachioradialis/extensor carpi radialis tendon forearm pronation
Posterior Tibial	Leg (tarsal tunnel)	Pressure at flexor retinaculum
Peroneal	Leg (fibular head)	Pressure at fibular head

lysis may theoretically proceed along the surgical plane provided by this interfascicular fibrosis, with resultant decompression of individual fascicles and a decrease in endoneurial fluid pressure. At the end stage of nerve compression, there would potentially be a point at which nerve fiber pathology would be so severe that little if any recovery could be expected.

Experimental studies have demonstrated that with mild to moderate nerve compression, internal neurolysis confers no benefit over simple decompression, while with severe nerve compression associated with Wallerian degeneration, significant improvement in nerve function is noted following internal neurolysis. The only prospective clinical study that addressed this problem did not document any quantitative motor tests pre- or postoperatively. The only sensory test quantitated was vibratory threshold.

Neurolysis is a graded procedure, that extends from external epineurotomy—to external neurolysis—to internal neurolysis. The procedure stops once a normal fascicular pattern is seen. The importance of the mesoneurium in facilitating gliding and movement of the nerve in a longitudinal direction has recently been emphasized, and this should lead us to encourage early movement of the nerve in its tissue bed following decompression or neurolysis.

I feel neurolysis should only be considered if the patient has constant sensory deficit and evidence of nerve fiber loss (motor atrophy or abnormal two-point discrimination), and suggest that neurolysis should only be done by those trained in microneurosurgical technique. Otherwise, certainly more harm than good will be performed.

Closed Nerve Injuries

It is apparent that the degree of chronic nerve compression varies with the amount of compressive force and the length of time it is applied. The patient with a closed nerve injury is treated expectantly unless the nerve is located at a specific anatomic site known to be susceptible to nerve entrapment. In these instances, the nerve should be decompressed so that nerve recovery progresses without the superimposed effect of nerve compression. It is generally accepted that a patient who presents with an acute carpal tunnel syndrome, with sensory and motor loss following a traumatic injury to the hand or forearm, should be considered for urgent decompression. Unfortunately, other nerves involved in identical clinical situations in known areas of anatomic entrapment are not treated in the same fashion. The patient who demonstrates a complete peroneal nerve palsy following a crush injury to the lower extremity, demonstrates the same pathology as the one who presents with an acute carpal tunnel following a crush injury to the upper extremity. In both instances, the nerve should be decompressed at the site of the anatomic point of nerve compression. When the nerve deficit is not localized to a known anatomic area of nerve compression, it is treated conservatively, with frequent clinical examination and electrodiagnostic follow-up.

Staging Nerve Compression

The correlation of the pathophysiology of nerve compression and the clinical signs and symptoms of nerve compression is now possible, based on the work reviewed in the foregoing sections. Stages of nerve compression can, and should be, described. In the *minimal* degree of nerve compression, the patient's symptoms are variable, and the physical findings may be limited to positive provocative tests, such as a positive pressure provocative test and a positive Phalen's sign in the carpal tunnel syndrome. Treatment is by nonoperative measures, such as treatment of any underlying medical disorder, alteration of daily or work activities, and splinting. In the *moderate* degree of nerve compression, the symptoms are still variable; the signs may now include diminished vibratory perception and measurable muscle weakness, and the treatment is still directed first at nonoperative measures. If the patient's symptoms are sufficiently severe in this stage, even though they may still be intermittent, and/or if the patient either is unwilling to continue splinting or does not wish a nonoperative management, then the treatment is directed to surgical decompression of the nerve—at which time it is usually found that there is minimal intraneural fibrosis, and an internal neurolysis is not included. In the *severe* degree of nerve compression, the symptoms are now persistent, the signs include either muscle wasting and/or abnormal two-point discrimination, and the treatment is now decompression of the nerve with an internal neurolysis.

SPECIFIC NERVE ENTRAPMENTS

It is worthwhile to highlight problems, in both diagnosis and treatment, specific to common nerve entrapments.

Median Nerve in the Carpal Tunnel

Patients are usually given a conservative course of treatment that includes vitamin B_6 treatment and night wrist-splinting. The wrist is splinted in a neutral position, as any movement of the wrist from the neutral position increases the pressures within the carpal tunnel. Injury to the palmar cutaneous branch of the median nerve is avoided by making the incision 5 to 6 mm ulnar to the thenar crease in line with the fourth digit. If only simple decompression is required, the incision does not cross the wrist crease. If a neurolysis is required, the wrist crease is crossed in a zigzag fashion. In every instance, the distal antebrachial fascia is decompressed. In those patients who demonstrate carpal tunnel syndrome following a forearm injury, significant thickening of the antebrachial fascia is anticipated. Particular attention is paid to decompression at this level. In patients who demonstrate muscle weakness, the motor fascicles should be explored, and careful attention paid to the distal anatomic course of the motor fascicle as it enters the thenar mass. Frequently, (56 percent incidence) the motor branch enters the thenar muscles through a separate fibrous tunnel. In patients whose persistent sensory symptoms demonstrate signs of loss of nerve fiber function (muscle wasting or abnormal two-point discrimination) a graded microneurosurgical neurolysis is carried out until good fascicular pattern is demonstrated (Fig. 3). Simultaneous, bilateral carpal tunnel release is not recommended. Early movement of finger flexors is encouraged in the postoperative period to allow the tendons to glide past the nerve. Splinting of the thumb in a well-opposed position helps to reconstitute the arch or the palm.

Median Nerve Proximal Forearm

The median nerve may be compressed at multiple levels in the proximal forearm by the lacertus fibrosis, or fibrous arches from the superficialis or pronator teres. Thus, a longitudinal incision to allow decompression along its entire length is suggested (Fig. 4). Tests of forced resistance to contraction of these muscles reproduce symptoms or elicit pain. Pressure over the median nerve in the forearm elicits symptoms. Compression of the median nerve in the proximal forearm is always suspected when the patient fails to respond to a carpal tunnel release, and is also suspected in patients with carpal tunnel syndrome who have assembly line type jobs that require repetitive pronation or finger flexion activities. Patients who present with anterior interosseous nerve palsy may demonstrate compression of the median nerve proximal to the anterior interosseous (AIN). Because the AIN is "relatively" tethered at take-off from the median nerve, it responds more significantly to the proximal median nerve compression much like Upton and McComas' "double crush" phenomenon.

Ulnar Nerve—Guyon's Canal

Occasionally the ulnar nerve is entrapped in Guyon's canal. A myriad of causes have been reported for this entity. Chronic, repetitive, or acute trauma to the hypothenar eminence, space-occupying lesions within Guyon's canal, or local fractures form the majority of the etiological factors. Careful examination of the function of the dorsal cutaneous ulnar, digital cutaneous branches, hypothenar muscles, and interosseous and adductor muscle function help to localize the area of compression precisely. In 20 percent of the normal population, a fibrous band exists at the origin of the flexor brevis muscle. The motor

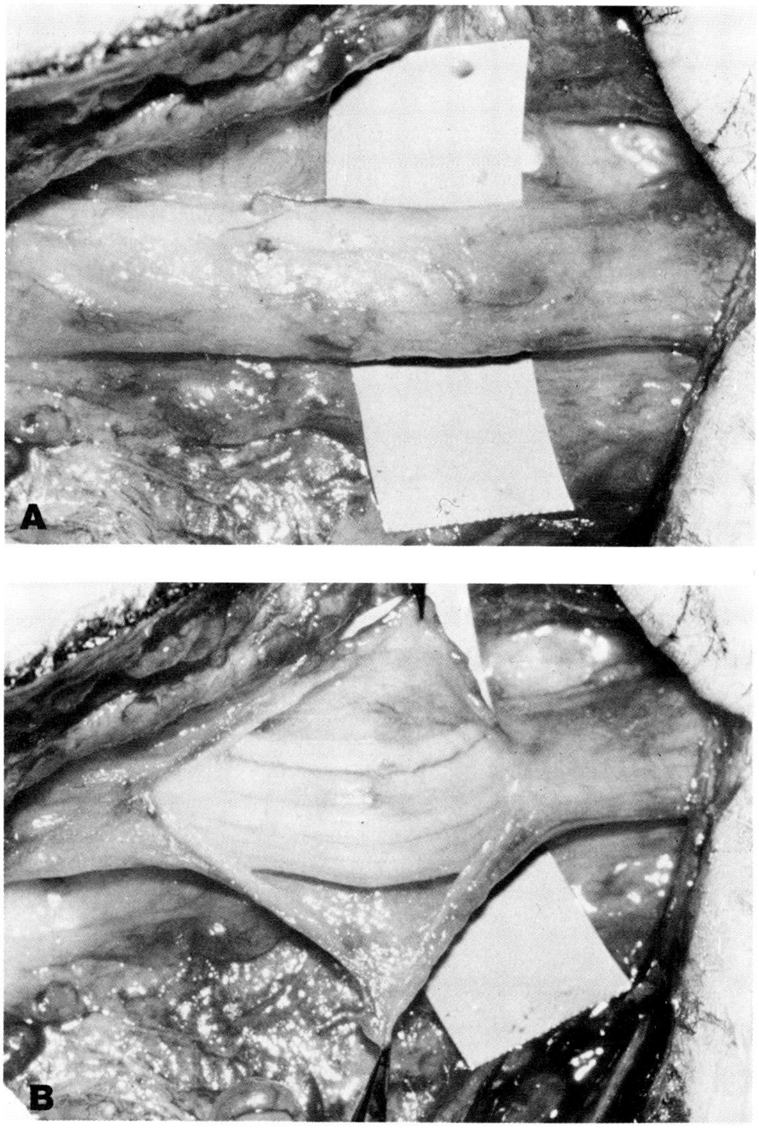

Figure 3 *A*, The median nerve of a patient with persistent sensory numbness in the distribution of the median nerve and thenar atrophy. Note the thickened epineurium. *B*, Using microneurosurgical dissection and loupe magnification, the external epineurium is opened (epineurotomy), thereby exposing a normal fascicular pattern. The external epineurium will be excised. Care is taken not to violate the perineurium, which is a site of the blood-nerve barrier.

branch of the ulnar nerve courses directly under this fibrous band and is, thus, anatomically predisposed to nerve entrapment at this level. Urgent decompression of the motor branch at this level is warranted in patients who present with intrinsic muscle weakness following closed injury to the hypothenar region of the hand.

Ulnar Nerve Cubital Tunnel

Subclinical ulnar neuropathy is a common clinical problem. Sensory symptoms in the ulnar one and half digits of the hand are better tolerated than sensory abnormalities in the median nerve distribution, as the patient must use the median nerve digits for precision sensory grip and tactilegnosis. Thus, patients who present with ulnar neuropathy frequently present at a later stage than those with carpal tunnel. Initial conservative treatment consists of demonstrating to the patient that elbow flexion will aggravate his or her symptoms. The patient is taught to recognize activities in his or her lifestyle that require such elbow flexion posture. Splints that prevent the patient from assuming a flexed elbow position at night are recommended.

Patients can unfortunately develop ulnar neuropathy following unrelated operative procedures. These patients often demonstrate an anatomic predisposition to ulnar compression neuropathy, such as a subluxating ulnar nerve or a wide carrying angle at the elbow. Intraoperative positioning of the arm in supination rather than pronation ensures that inappropriate direct pressure is not placed on the ulnar nerve during operative procedures, and in some cases prevents the development of such nerve injury.

Surgical treatment involves transposition of the ulnar nerve to an anterior position so that flexion does not result in decreased blood flow and ischemia to the nerve. Care must be taken not to damage the medial antebrachial cutaneous nerve as it courses across the operative site. I prefer a submuscular transposition but more important than the type of transposition is to ensure that there is no

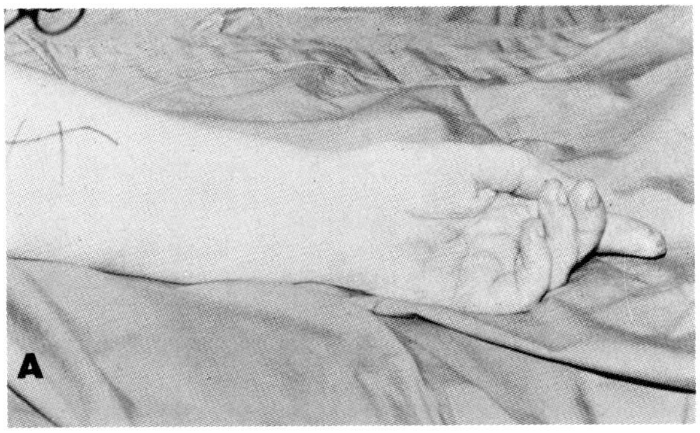

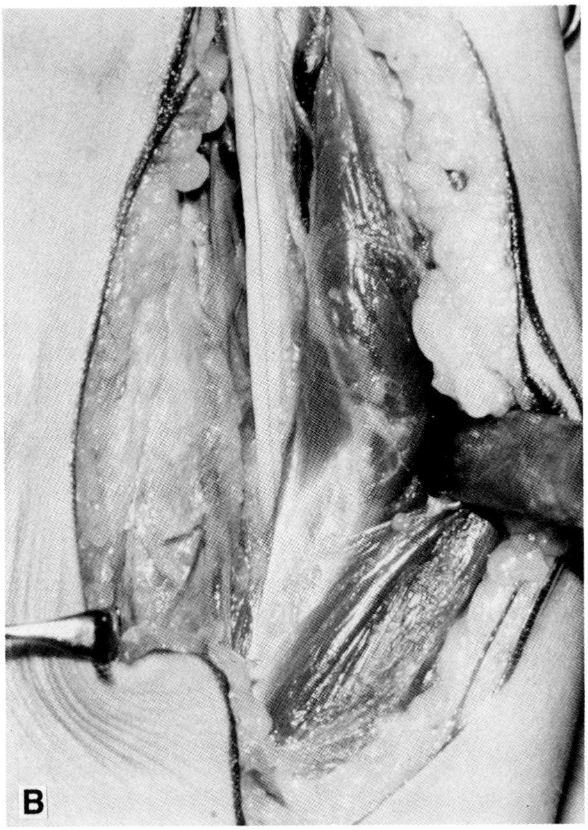

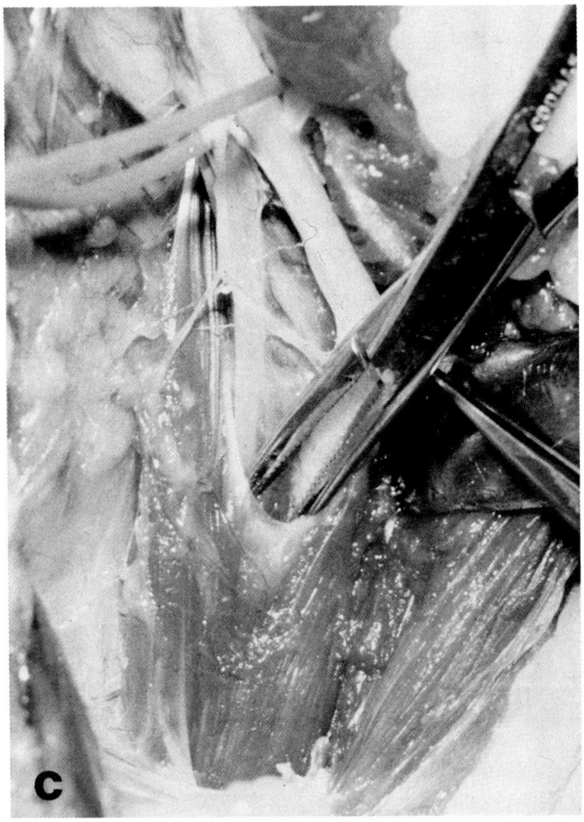

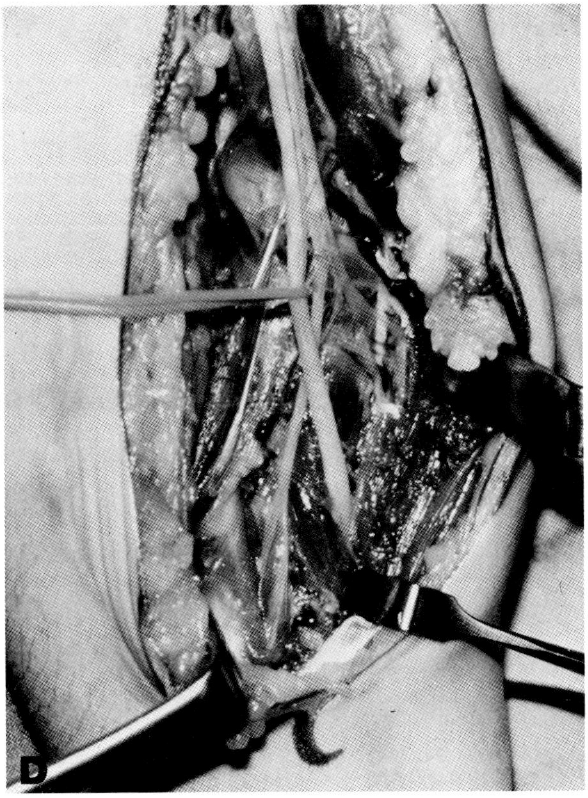

Figure 4 *A,* This patient, with compression of the anterior interosseous nerve, had previously been suspected of having a rupture of the flexor profundus of the index finger. Previous exploration of the digit had demonstrated an intact tendon. *B,* Through a longitudinal incision in the forearm, the median nerve was explored. The tendinous edge to the superficial head of the pronator teres is noted. *C,* Further dissection demonstrated a separate fibrous edge to the superficialis. *D,* The median nerve (vessel loop) and anterior interosseous nerve were decompressed along their length.

tension or kinking of the nerve at the proximal and distal transition points of the transposition. While the medial intermuscular septum will not affect the ulnar nerve in its anatomic position, it will kink the nerve in its new transposed location. Similarly, distal fascial tissue between the ulna and the two heads of the flexor carpi ulnaris will kink the nerve in the transposed position, and care must be taken to release or excise this distally as well.

Radial Nerve Arcade of Frohse

The anatomic structures important in decompression of this nerve have been well-described. The exposure between the brachioradialis and the extensor carpi radialis longus offers excellent decompression of the posterior interosseous nerve. The posterior cutaneous nerve of the forearm lies directly between these two muscles and serves as an anatomic landmark. Care must be taken, however, not to injure this nerve. I now suggest decompression of the radial nerve through a second, separate, proximal incision between the brachioradialis and the brachialis in order to release connective tissue bands that may compress the radial nerve at the radial head.

I have not found release of the posterior interosseous nerve particularly helpful for the relief of pain in those patients with pain that mimics tennis elbow, in the region of the Arcade of Frohse.

Superficial Sensory Branch Radial Nerve

In 1932, Wartenberg described entrapment of the radial sensory nerve in the forearm. The radial sensory nerve becomes entrapped between the tendons of the brachioradialis muscle and the extensor carpi radialis longus. The incidence of this nerve entrapment is more common than is recognized and is frequently misdiagnosed as de Quervain's disease (Table 2).

TABLE 2 Comparison Between De Quervain's and Wartenberg's Syndrome

	de Quervain's	*Wartenberg's*
Pain in dorsal radial wrist area	+	+
Positive Finklestein sign	+	+
Tenderness over 1st extensor compartment	+	−
Tinel's sign (junction BR and ECRL tendon)	−	+
Exacerbation of symptoms with forearm pronation or pressure over BR/ECRL junction	−	+
Abnormal sensibility testing radial sensory nerve distribution	−	+

Patients with de Quervain's disease have normal sensation in the territory of the radial sensory nerve. Those with entrapment of this nerve demonstrate a positive Finklestein sign, complain of pain over the dorsoradial aspect of the wrist, and, importantly, demonstrate abnormal sensory findings in the distribution of this nerve. Treatment does not involve release of the first extensor compartment, but rather release of the radial nerve between the brachioradialis tendon and extensor carpi radialis longus tendon in the mid forearm. In five patients who did not respond to release and neurolysis, the radial nerve was excised and transferred proximally into the brachialradialis muscle. In two other patients, the brachioradialis tendon was excised in order to completely decompress the nerve.

Lower Extremity

The common entrapment points in the lower extremity involve the peroneal nerve at the fibular head and the posterior tibial nerve in the tarsal tunnel. Early decompression of the peroneal nerve at the fibular head is recommended in those patients who, following traumatic injuries to the lower extremity, demonstrate loss of dorsiflexion of the ankle. Patients with symptoms of posterior tibial nerve entrapment require decompression. Surgical decompression of the tarsal tunnel historically involved release of the flexor retinaculum (lancinate ligament). The incomplete nature of this decompression has recently been reported. The flexor retinaculum is analogous to the antebrachial fascia in the arm. The anatomic tunnels that correspond to the carpal tunnel (medial plantar nerve) and Guyons' canal (lateral plantar nerve) are well distal to the flexor retinaculum under the abductor hallucis muscle itself. Adequate decompression requires decompression of these distal tunnels and resection of the interfascicular septum.

Diabetic Neuropathy

There appears to be a susceptibility to chronic nerve compression associated with diabetes. While this is well recognized for the carpal tunnel, it is not recognized for nerve entrapment at other sites. In particular, decompression of the tarsal tunnel in patients with diabetic neuropathy, may improve the sensibility in the foot so as to prevent catastrophic sequelae. Prior to diagnosis of "stocking and glove" anesthesia and a surgically "untreatable" neuropathy, care must be taken to rule out multiple superimposed "treatable" compression neuropathies. This is valid in both the upper (carpal tunnel, cubital tunnel, radial sensory compression) and the lower (posterior tibial, peroneal, sural compression) extremities. Unfortunately, at the present time, both surgeons and internists who care for diabetics, while aware of their patients' susceptibility to carpal tunnel, do not extrapolate this susceptibility to other nerves at other levels of anatomic entrapment.

Brachial Plexus Compression

Patients presenting with multiple nerve compressions in both upper extremities should be considered for brachial plexus nerve compression (otherwise known as thoracic outlet syndrome). Pressure over the trunks of the plexus between the scalene muscles will reproduce symptoms as will elevation of the arms above the head with superimposed pressure over the plexus. Vibratory threshold measurements (vibrogram) will be abnormal. Consideration will be given to proximal decompression of the plexus (scalenectomy, neurolysis plexus and first rib resection).

SUGGESTED READING

Dawson DM, Hallett M, Millender LH. Entrapment neuropathies. Toronto: Little, Brown, 1983.

Dellon AL, MacKinnon SE. Injury to the medial antebrachial cutaneous nerve during cubital tunnel surgery. J Hand Surg 1985; 10B:33–36.

Dellon AL, MacKinnon SE. Radial sensory nerve entrapment. J Hand Surg 1986; 11A:199–205.

Hall HC, MacKinnon SE, Gilbert R. The posterior interosseous nerve. Plast Reconstr Surg 1984; 74:435–437.

MacKinnon SE, Dellon AL. Peripheral nerve surgery. New York: Thieme-Stratton, 1988.

MacKinnon SE, Dellon AL, Hudson AR, Hunter DA. Chronic human nerve compression—a histological assessment. Neuropathol Appl Neurobiol 1987; 12:547–565.

MacKinnon SE, Dellon AL, Hudson AR, Hunter DA. Histopathology of chronic compression of the superficial radial nerve in the forearm. J Hand Surg 1986; 11A:206–210.

Spindler HA, Dellon AL. Nerve conduction studies and sensibility testing in carpal tunnel syndrome. J Hand Surg 1982; 7A:260–263.

Spinner M. Injuries to the major branches of peripheral nerves of the forearm. 2nd ed. Philadelphia: WB Saunders, 1978.

Upton ARM, McComas AJ. The double crush syndrome in nerve entrapment syndromes. Lancet 1973; 2:359–362.

INTERRUPTION OF NERVE FUNCTION

A. LEE DELLON, M.D.

The exciting neuroscience research of the past decade has provided a foundation for the unification of diverse approaches to the diagnosis and treatment of the clinical problems of peripheral nerve management. It is the purpose of this chapter to provide the conceptual framework within which surgeons trained in microneurovascular techniques can approach the end of this century and enter the twenty-first century with a new optimism about the peripheral nerve. As our understanding of the clinical spectrum of neural dysfunction increases, the surgeon who treats these problems must be prepared to deal with interruption of nerve function at all levels: *reversing* this interruption of nerve function in order to restore sensory and motor function, while intentionally *creating* interruption of nerve function in order to disrupt painful sensory input and the dysfunctional motor output of spasticity and asymmetry.

In the third quarter of this century, the questions asked were: Could a nerve regenerate if repaired? How should the nerve be repaired? When should the nerve be repaired? How should a gap in the nerve be treated? Through the anatomic studies of Sunderland, the pursuit of tension-free nerve reconstruction techniques by Milessi, and quantitative clinical assessment of sensory function by Moberg, the basis was provided to answer these questions. The following axioms summarize what I believe is the consensus among those doing a significant amount of peripheral nerve surgery today:

1. Preoperative and postoperative clinical assessment should be as quantitative as possible, recording at least the following: degree of muscle wasting and pinch and grip strength for the motor system and the presence or absence of protective sensation and innervation density (e.g., moving and static two-point discrimination) and, if possible, measurements of threshold, (e.g., vibrometer or nylon monofilaments) for the sensory system.
2. Whenever a tension-free nerve repair can be done, it should.
3. Whenever a nerve repair cannot be done without tension, an interposition, interfascicular nerve graft should be done.
4. Whenever the clinical condition permits, a primary nerve repair should be done.
5. Whenever the intraneural topography of the peripheral nerve permits, a grouped fascicular repair should be done; when the function of the fascicles is primarily mixed sensory and motor, without well-defined groups of fascicles, an epineurial repair should be done.

CORRECTION OF COMPLETE INTERRUPTION OF NERVE FUNCTION

The underlying assumption of the surgical approach to restoration of nerve function in the past decade has been that through increased magnification and decreased suture and needle size, the wisdom and technical experience of the surgeon could correctly align fascicles to permit maximization of neural regeneration. Implicit in this approach were the assumptions, supported by good experimental and clinical evidence, that provision of a tension-free environment would minimize scar tissue at the nerve repair sites and that proper fascicular alignment would minimize misdirected axons and minimize suture line neuroma formation. Unfortunately, however, the results of applying these now accepted, if not traditional, approaches to nerve repair (including grafting), still yield far from excellent results. It is clear that improved clinical results will not come from further refinements in microneurosurgical technique.

It is likely that future improvements will come through a greater understanding of the neurobiology of the tissues with which we must deal. The results of research into what is best termed neurotrop(h)ism provide a basis for the unifying approach to interruption of nerve function, outlined below. In summary, the controversy between Weiss and Cajal over contact guidance versus neurotrop(h)ism has been decided in favor of both. With contact guidance, a regenerating axon sprout grows preferentially along the components of basement membrane, i.e., laminin and type IV collagen. In both rats and primates, under the influence of some distal factor (and it is not clear whether this is released from the distal nerve or distal Schwann cell, or is circulating, or is derived from the target muscle or sensory end-organs), the proximal nerve regeneration can be guided appropriately. With this guidance, the proximal nerve can select a distal intact nerve versus a distal nerve segment; a distal nerve segment versus a distal motor or tendon segment; a correct sensory versus motor distal choice; and it appears that even a correct choice between appropriate distal nerve territories can be made. The critical factor is that the proximal nerve segment must have an opportunity to experience or come under the influence of the distal segment. It follows then that attempts to align specific fascicles precisely and intimately may, in fact, provide some detriment to neurotrop(h)ism; too much technical meddling may interfere with the basic neurobiologic potential.

Recently, it has been demonstrated that contact guidance also influences the orientation of axonal elongagation. In the isolated chamber model of nerve regeneration, axons elongate through the environment guided by the fibrin orientation: in a linear direction when fibrin strands are oriented in a linear fashion; in a random direction when a classic random dot pattern of matrix is present. The technical extension of this concept in neurobiology is to attempt to restore nerve function by permitting neural regeneration to occur through some form of nerve tube. The nerve tube technique already has been successfully demonstrated in lower mammals, as well as baboons and monkeys, by use of autogenous conduits, such as vein, mesothelial-lined pseudosheaths, nonabsorbable and bioabsorbable nerve tubes.

The ideal technique to correct a complete interruption of nerve function is a technique that permits the restoration of axonal continuity that existed prior to the nerve injury. If neurotrop(h)ism is sufficiently capable of inducing this to happen, then the ideal surgical approach is to provide the appropriate environment, such as a nerve tube filled with the appropriate material to permit neurotrop(h)ism to occur. The use of a nerve tube eliminates the need for a nerve graft donor site, with its morbidity of scar, area of sensory loss, and potential for pain. There is the secondary benefit that placement of proximal and distal nerve ends within a nerve tube minimizes loss of axons through any extrafascicular routing, or neuroma formation at the nerve repair site—which has been a problem with the traditional approaches to nerve repair, whether they are perineurial, epineurial or graft techniques (Table 1).

TABLE 1 Correction of Complete Interruption of Nerve Function

Traditional Treatment Terminology	*Nerve Deficit*	*Future Treatment Approach*
Nerve repair	None	Nerve tube
Nerve graft	Any size	Nerve tube
Neuroma	Any size	Nerve tube

Another situation that is most appropriately viewed in terms of an interruption of nerve function, where a nerve deficit exists, is the problem of a painful neuroma. By definition, these are so-called end-bulb neuromas and not neuromas in-continuity. In the latter case, there may be some nerve function that has not been interrupted and the clinical problem is to determine which fibers, if any, through the in-continuity neuroma are intact and have not had interruption of nerve function. Intraoperative nerve conduction recordings can determine which fascicles that remain in-continuity are appropriate to leave in-continuity and maintain function, and which fascicles have had sufficient disruption of nerve function that they should be resected. Once this is determined, the problem of a neuroma in-continuity can be converted, after the neuromatous fascicles are resected, into the same problem as the end-bulb neuroma.

What is the best technique to prevent recurrent neuroma formation? Primate experimental work has made it clear that classic neuroma formation can be altered by altering the microenvironment of the sensory nerve. The most successful way to do this, as confirmed clinically, is to implant the sensory nerve into a muscle. The nerve should be implanted loosely into a muscle that has minimal excursion (Fig. 1). The ideal approach to the treatment of the neuroma is the same as the ideal treatment to prevent neuroma formation, i.e., to direct the axons back to their prior destination. When a distal source for these proximal nerves exists, i.e., if the distal nerve is still present, then the ideal treatment is to restore nerve function through a nerve tube (Fig. 2).

If a nerve tube is to be the technique by which surgeons of the future repair nerves, reconstruct nerve deficits, and restore continuity when a painful neuroma is present, it is appropriate to ask, "What is a nerve tube?" A nerve tube may be any type of physical device that provides a framework for the nerve to grow from one place to another. An autogenous nerve graft is, in fact, a form of nerve tube. The most commonly used nerve tube has been one made out of a silicone elastomer. Through a Silastic tube, a nerve will regenerate no more than 15 mm in a rat. Yet it has been observed that the same rat sciatic nerve, left in its own natural milieu, will generate a mean of 2.4 cm, with an upper range limit of four cm. This suggests that there is something about the Silastic tube that inhibits neural regeneration. The Silastic tube probably is immunogenic and, since it is not bioabsorbable, can give rise to chronic peripheral nerve compression.

A nerve tube made of a bioabsorbable material has obvious advantages. Collagen tubes have been used as

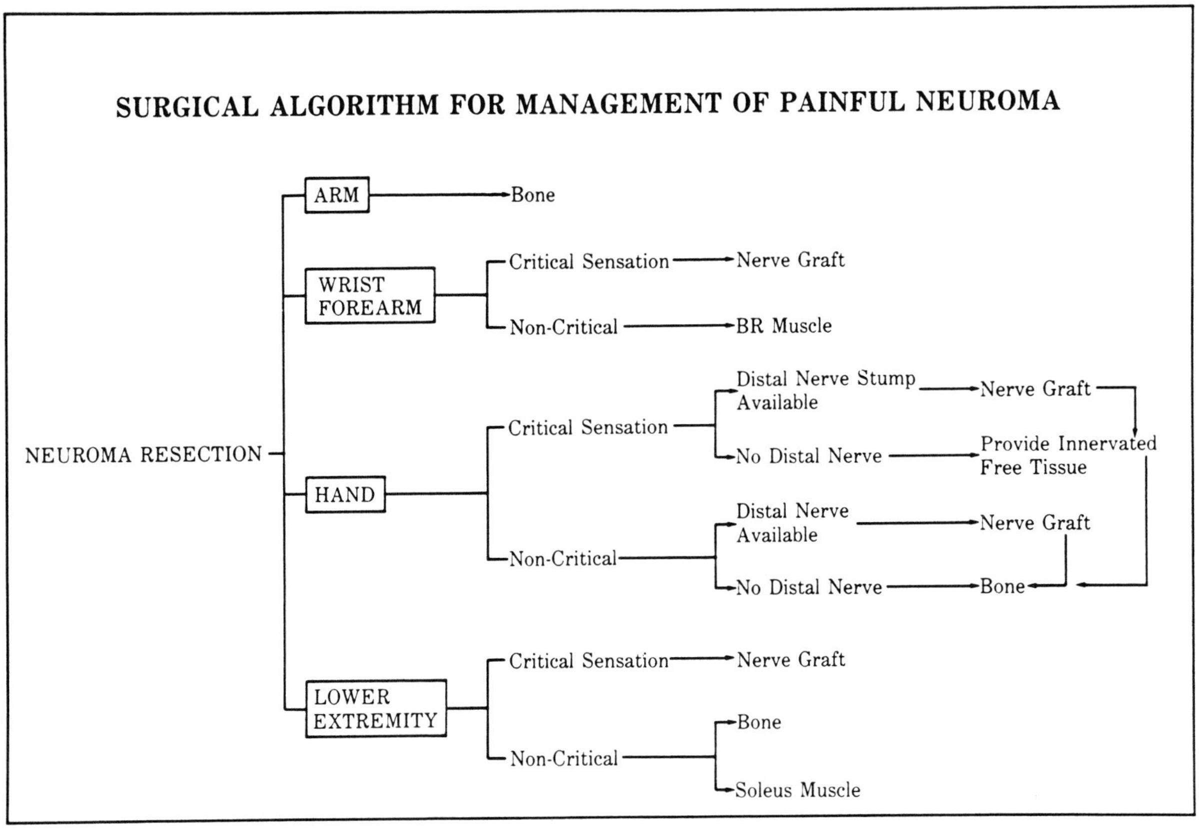

Figure 1 Algorithm for management of the painful neuroma. If a distal "runoff" for the regenerating axons exists, the first approach to management is correction of the complete interruption of nerve function by (traditionally) a nerve graft of a bioabsorbable nerve tube, if possible. (With permission from Mackinnon SE, Dellon AL. Algorithm for management of painful neuroma. Contemp Orthop 1986; 13:15–23.)

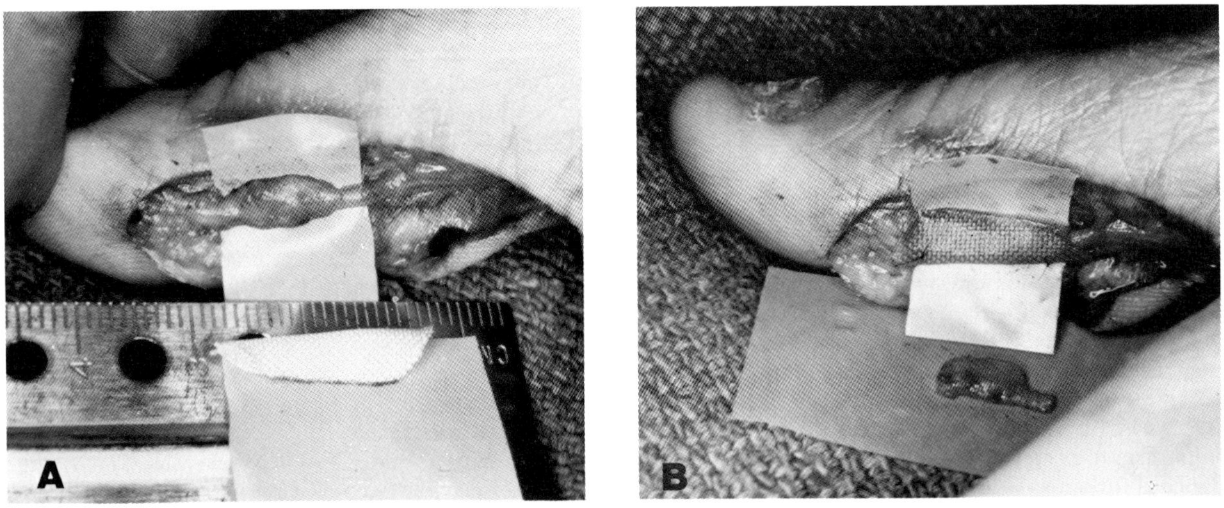

Figure 2 Patient with a neuroma of the ulnar digital nerve to the thumb with pain that prevented work. After neuroma resection, the nerve deficit is reconstructed, correcting the complete interruption of nerve function, with a bioabsorbable (polyglycolic acid; Davis & Geck) nerve tube. (From Mackinnon SE, O'Brien JP, Dellon AL, et al. An assessment of the effects of different treatment strategies, including internal neurolysis, on a chronically compressed rat sciatic nerve. Plast Reconstr Surg 1988; 81:251–256.)

nerve tubes and have demonstrated neural regeneration across gaps of less than 15 mm in rodents. Collagen, however, is immunogenic. It is of theoretical interest that collagen is present in basement membranes and may possibly help neural regeneration by means of contact guidance. However, current collagen conduits are Type I collagen, unlike the collagen Type IV that is present in the basal lamina. The substance "laminin" is also found in the basement membrane and has been shown to permit neural regeneration along specific pathways. Although it may be possible to include such large molecules as laminin and collagen within nerve tubes, or fabricate them into the nerve tubes themselves, the problems of their immunoreactivity must first be resolved before they can be utilized in patients.

A nerve tube to restore interrupted function across a small nerve deficit probably need not contain a factor such as laminin to enhance regeneration. Unless the nerve deficit to be reconstructed is significantly large, an increase in the rate of neural regeneration across a few centimeters would not have any real benefit over a nerve tube without such capacity. There should be no need for such nerve tube enhancement, especially if the nerve defect were located quite distally; for example, in the hand or finger where the distance from the nerve defect to the end-organ is small.

A bioabsorbable nerve tube that is not immunogenic would appear to be the ideal nerve tube. It has been demonstrated that the use of a polyglycolic acid nerve tube, with tensile strength that remains for 28 days and which is resorbed over a period of 90 days, can permit neural regeneration across a 3-cm gap in the ulnar nerve at the level of the elbow in the monkey. This regeneration has been shown to produce results equivalent to that of a sural nerve interposition interfascicular graft in terms of conduction velocity and amplitude, nerve fiber diameter, and nerve fiber density. Futhermore, this study has demonstrated recovery, by electrodiagnostic testing, of the abductor digiti minimi and the first dorsal interosseous muscle 1 year after the nerve tube procedure. There would be little, if any, expectation that a human ulnar nerve, treated by either nerve repair or nerve graft in the upper arm, would result in reinnervation of the intrinsic muscles of the hand (Table 2 and Fig. 3).

TABLE 2 Morphology of the Distal Ulnar Nerve Following Reconstruction of a 3 cm Gap by Sural Nerve Grafting or Polyglycolic Acid Nerve Tube

	Normal	*Sural Nerve Graft*	*Polyglycolic Acid Nerve Tube*
Mean fiber diameter (μ)	6.9 ± 2.7	4.1 ± 1.8*	3.0 ±0.4*
Fiber density (Fibers/mm²)	14,320	16,172	12,925

* p<.05

CORRECTION OF INCOMPLETE INTERRUPTION OF NERVE FUNCTION

When nerve function has been partially interrupted, nerve compression or a partial division of the nerve that has resulted in an in-continuity neuroma may be the cause. The approach to the in-continuity neuroma must be a careful preoperative assessment of sensory-motor function in the distribution of the nerve. At the time of surgery with prior consent of the patient, some sensations and motor functions that are present, but significantly abnormal, may be sacrificed willingly by interruption of nerve function in order to correct the incomplete interruption of nerve function in the hope of restoring better ultimate neural function. This restoration of nerve function may be done with a nerve tube, after an intraoperative intraneural neurolysis to separate each fascicle, then by intraoperative electrodiagnostic testing to determine the electrical function through each of these fascicles. The anatomic basis for this approach is the dissections by Sunderland and by Jabaley, Wallace, and Heckler. The electrophysiologic basis is the intraoperative dissections and recordings of Kline and Terzis. These confirmed the fascicular pattern of the peripheral nerve over a significant length, so that intraneural dissection (with awareness of the surgeon that interfascicular plexus can occur) may be carried out with safety. The computer assisted signal-averaging equipment now available makes measurement of the amplitudes of the fascicles more reliable. The surgeon must work with an experienced electrodiagnostic technician, or other physician, and with equipment that is familiar so that, when no electrical recording is obtained, the surgeon has confidence that it is because there are no axons across the nerve being tested and not a technical problem with the diagnostic equipment. It helps if an adjacent normal nerve can be stimulated and recorded to give a control. The current guideline is that no electrical recording suggests complete lack of axonal integrity across the segment tested, and the area should be resected. A recording of an electrical signal across the segment is not by itself considered sufficient to permit the nerve in question to remain. A small number of fascicles with appropriate myelination can cause the signal to be conducted with little alteration in the latency. The amplitude of the recorded action potential is the critical parameter. An amplitude of less than 25 to 50 percent of normal is considered insufficient to restore the appropriate innervation density to the target end-organs and, with appropriate clinical considerations, an amplitude of this modest size is considered an indication to resect the fascicle and reconstruct the nerve defect. An amplitude of 50 percent or greater of normal is considered indicative of a sufficient number of nerve fibers to permit restoration of good nerve function, and aneurolysis alone is done (Table 3).

The usual cause for a nerve to have partial interruption of nerve function, without a history of direct trauma, is chronic nerve compression. In addition to the common isolated chronic nerve compressions from idiopathic or repetitive trauma (work), there are systemic

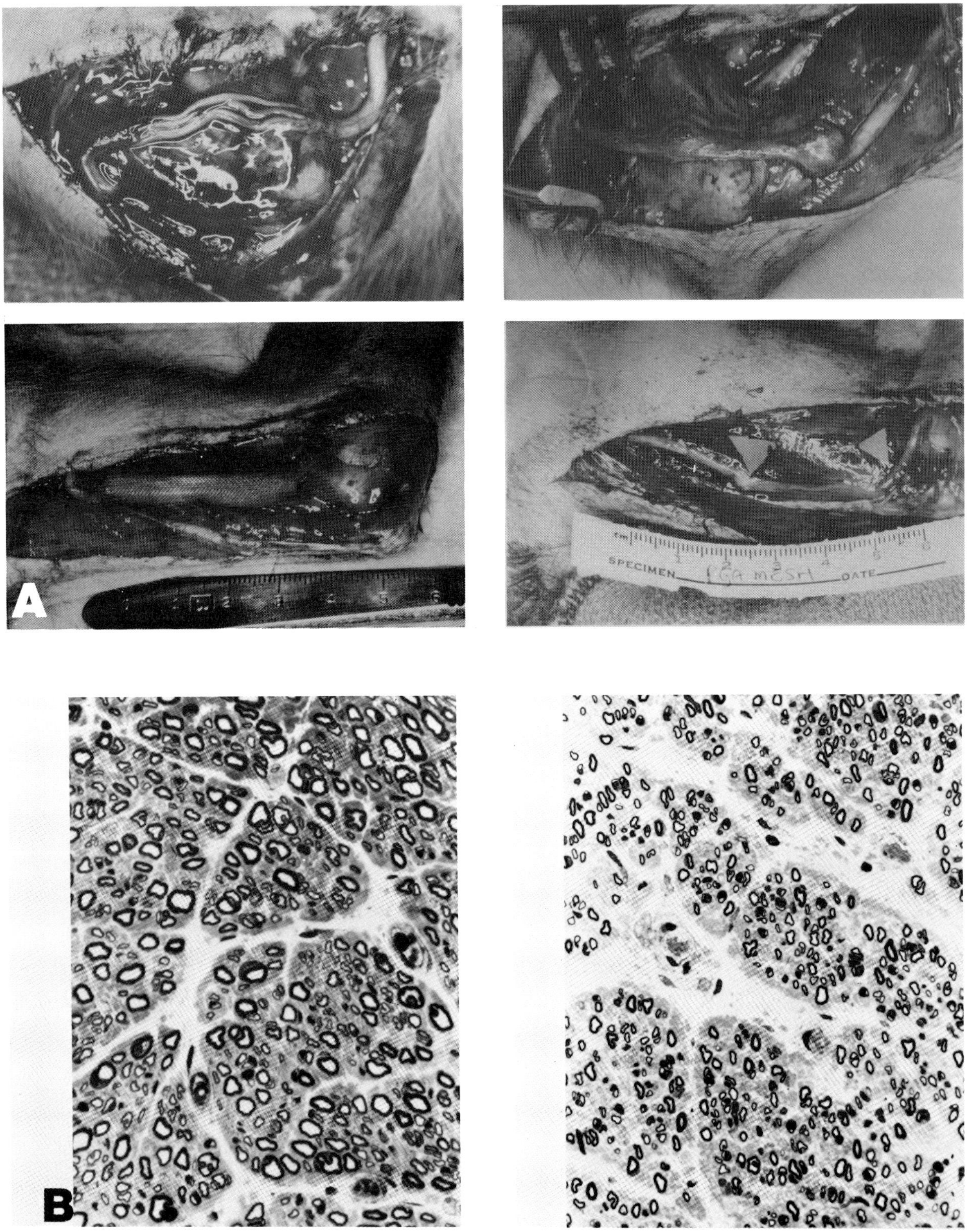

Figure 3 *A,* Correction of complete interruption of nerve function by nerve graft and nerve tube. At left, the monkey ulnar nerve at elbow at time of 3 cm neural deficit corrected by sural nerve interposition interfascicular nerve graft (*top*) and a polyglycolic acid mesh rolled into a tube (*bottom*) as a nerve tube. At right, one year postoperatively, note neuromas at proximal and distal nerve repair sites of the nerve graft (*top*), while the nerve tube has been absorbed, leaving a regenerated nerve in its place (*bottom*). *B,* Photomicrographs of ulnar nerve distal to sural nerve graft (*left*) and polyglycolic acid nerve tube (*right*) demonstrate regeneration of myelinated fibers (see Table 2 for morphometric analysis.)

TABLE 3 Correction of Partial Interruption of Nerve Function

Traditional Treatment Terminology	*Nerve Deficit*	*Future Treatment Approach*
Neurolysis	None	Internal neurolysis
	(Neuroma in-continuity)	Intraoperative nerve recording Possible nerve tube
Metabolic control only	None (metabolic neuropathy)	Internal neurolysis plus metabolic control
Nerve decompression	None (chronic nerve compression)	
	Moderate	External decompression
	Severe	Internal neurolysis

problems known to be associated with peripheral neuropathy and predispose to nerve compression, such as diabetes, alcoholism, thyroid dysfunction, vasculitis associated with collagen vascular disease, and amyloidosis. The most common of these is diabetic neuropathy, which is present in 25 percent of diabetics at the time they are diagnosed and the prevalence of which increases with the duration of the diabetes. While the surgeon cannot correct a metabolic neuropathy, he can treat the areas of compression of these susceptible nerves at known anatomic areas of tightness. The treatment for chronic nerve compression is neurolysis: this consists of a so-called external neurolysis or decompression of the nerve from factors compressing it from without, such as the deep transverse carpal ligament in the carpal tunnel syndrome, Osborne's band in the cubital tunnel and flexor retinaculum over the tarsal tunnel. For the appropriate case (with a severe degree of compression and muscle wasting and/or abdominal two-point discriminations and/or persistent sensory change), a microsurgical internal neurolysis may be added to the traditional nerve release. A study that used the models for chronic nerve compression in the primate median nerve was carried out in the primate and demonstrated that a microsurgical internal neurolysis could be performed in the presence of a moderate degree of chronic nerve compression without causing increased scarring when compared with an external decompression alone. Another study that used the model for chronic nerve compression in the rat sciatic nerve, was done in the presence of a severe degree of chronic nerve compression and showed that a microsurgical internal neurolysis gave better results in restoring the compressed nerve to normal (by morphometric assessment) than an external decompression of the nerve alone.

There may now be cause for optimism when a partial interruption of nerve function is due to a metabolic neuropathy, such as diabetes. Although the metabolic neuropathies have been generally considered to be progressive and irreversible, the concept of the double crush phenomenon has been extended to this problem area. The double crush hypothesis stated that a single site of nerve crush or compression, which by itself may not constitute sufficient constraint upon axoplasmic flow to cause neural dysfunction, may summate with a second nerve crush or site of compression, which by itself may not have been sufficient to cause nerve dysfunction, to create nerve dysfunction sufficient to produce symptoms. In the case of a metabolic neuropathy, the underlying axonal dysfunction may be considered as the first of the double crush insults. Any normally tight anatomic area, such as the carpal or cubital tunnel, may be the second crush site.

The metabolic neuropathy of diabetes has as its pathophysiologic correlate an edematous nerve: since there is no blood–nerve barrier to the elevated glucose in the blood, the increased intraneural polyhydrol metabolites cause water to come into the nerve. Additionally, although the mechanism is not clear, there is decreased axoplasmic flow in the diabetic nerve. Any normal area of anatomic narrowing creates a site for a further decrease in axoplasmic flow. A recent study that used streptozocin induced diabetes as a model, combined with the chronic nerve compression model already described, demonstrated that the sciatic nerve in the diabetic is more susceptible to chronic nerve compression than the banded nerve in the nondiabetic. In the metabolic neuropathies, there has been traditionally described a stocking or glove distribution pattern of sensory loss. A similar pattern could be mimicked by multiple peripheral nerve compressions. In essence, the susceptible nerves in the extremity would each be compressed, thereby resulting in the appearance of a diffuse sensory and motor loss. With the description of sites for the radial sensory nerve, and for the lateral sural and lateral cutaneous nerve of the calf to be entrapped, the potential for such multiple peripheral nerve entrapments was realized. The clinical application of these basic science research developments has been an attempt to treat symptomatic diabetic neuropathy by internal neurolysis of multiple peripheral nerve entrapments. The results of this approach have recently been reported. That study demonstrated that in 84 nerves in 33 patients, good to excellent sensory and motor results were achieved in more than 80 percent of the patients. These results held regardless of whether the patient was a Type I or Type II diabetic, or whether it was the upper or lower extremity that was operated upon. They also held whether the end result assessment technique was the subjective opinion of the surgeon, or the hard clinical measurements of vibratory perception, moving two-point discrimination, pinch and grip strength, muscle wasting, or the more objective results of the pre- and postoperative electrodiagnostic testing (Fig. 4).

CREATION OF INTERRUPTION OF NERVE FUNCTION

There are indications for deliberate interruption of nerve function. In the sensory sphere of the peripheral nervous system, the usual indication for deliberate interruption of nerve function is pain that arises from joints or skin. In the motor sphere of the peripheral nervous system, the most common indication would be spasticity, where overactivity of upper motor neurons creates muscle hyperactivity or contractions that interfere with function, or where a motor paralysis has permitted the antagonist muscle to be overactive, thereby creating a significant imbalance or asymmetry (Table 4).

The problem of joint pain may arise either from trauma or from one of the many varieties of arthritis. A common problem is persistent pain following a fall upon the outstretched hand where radiographically there is no evidence of fracture, despite nonoperative management in splints and anti-inflammatory medications. Similar pain may follow appropriate management of a fracture even though radiographically the joint surfaces appear appropriately aligned. In both circumstances, the pain may be shown to arise from joint afferents. The nerves that innervate the joint via the capsular structures may have been either damaged by tears in the ligament (as in sprains) or entrapped in callus of the healing fracture. Diagnostic nerve blocks of the appropriate nerves can demonstrate pain relief in the doctor's examining room. Frequently, there is increased range of motion as the pain is relieved. Whereas previous approaches to this problem have called for a total wrist denervation procedure, more recent anatomic studies have identified the terminal branch of the posterior interosseous nerve as innervating the dorsal wrist structures and the terminal branch of the anterior interosseous nerve as the innervator of the volar wrist structures. The block of the terminal branch of the interosseous nerve, when followed by relief of pain and increased hand function, permits a partial dorsal wrist denervation (Fig. 5). This can be done on an outpatient basis with local anesthesia proximal to the extensor retinaculum. The block of the terminal branch of the anterior interosseous nerve, when accompanied by relief of pain and increased wrist function, can suggest a partial volar wrist denervation procedure (Fig. 6). This is done through a carpal tunnel-style approach, with a more proximal extension into the distal forearm to allow division of the terminal

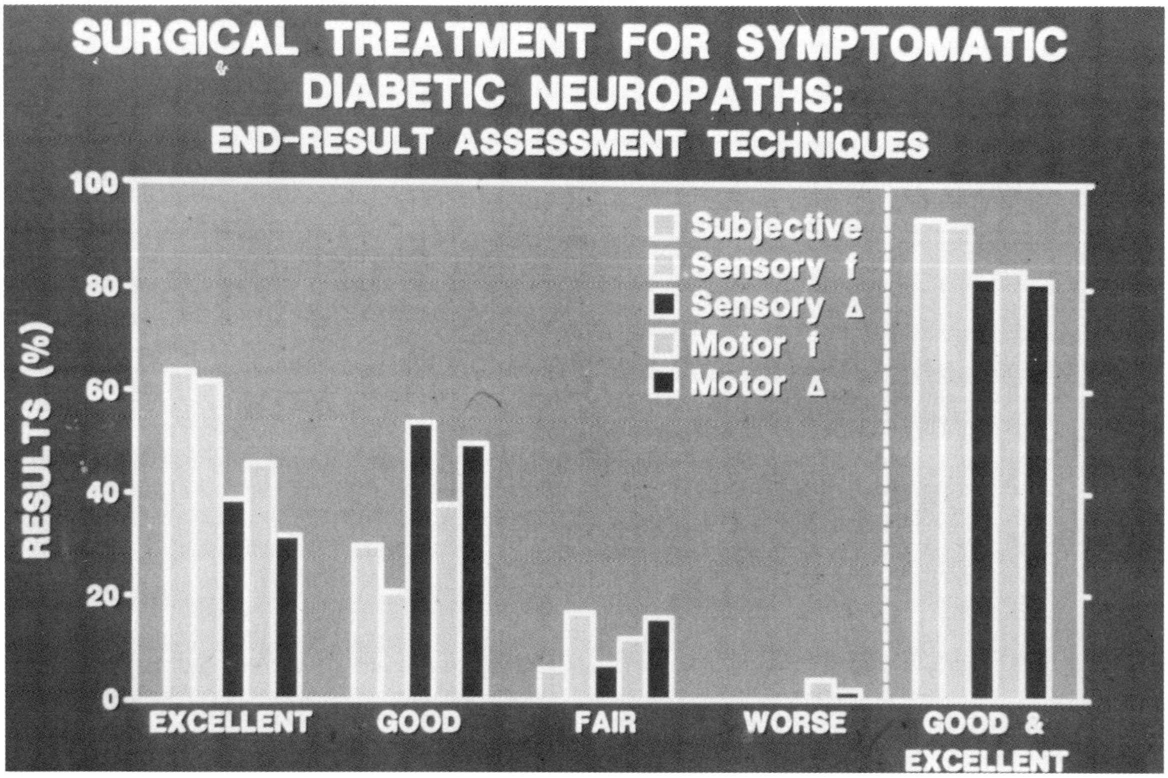

Figure 4 Treatment of symptomatic diabetic neuropathy by internal neurolysis. For Type I and Type II diabetes, the result of treating 84 nerves in 33 patients, with a mean follow-up of 17.2 years, was the achievement of more than 80 percent good to excellent results by any of the clinical criteria employed.

TABLE 4 Creation of Interruption of Nerve Function

Traditional Diagnosis	*Type of Neural Dysfunction*	*Future Treatment Approach*
Strained joint, arthritis	Sensory: Joint pain	Partial joint denervation
Painful neuroma	Skin pain	Diagnostic nerve block; follow algorithm for neuroma treatment
Cerebral palsy	Motor Spasticity	Tendon transfer, denervation
Facial palsy	Asymmetry	Cross-facial nerve graft, innervated free-muscle transfer

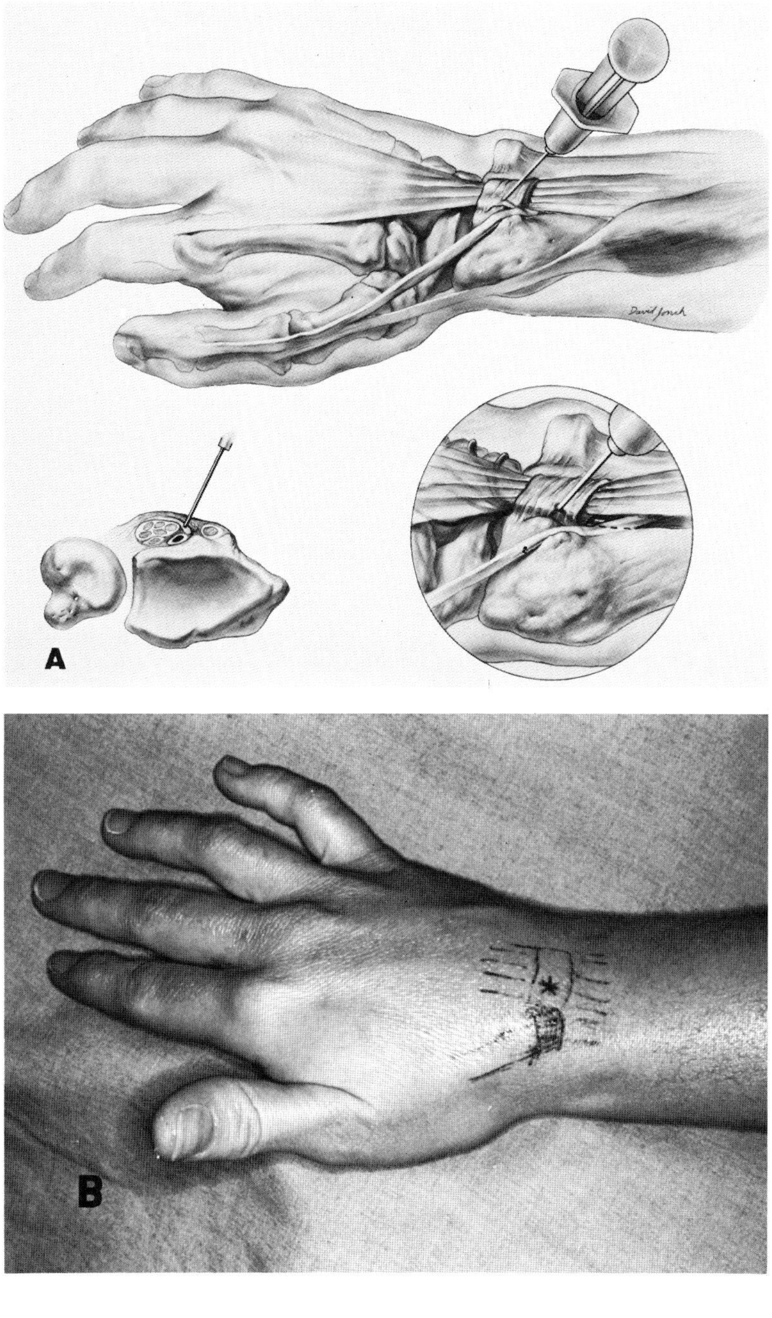

Figure 5 *A*, Deliberate interruption of nerve function to relieve pain by means of partial dorsal wrist denervation procedure. Terminal branch of posterior interosseous nerve is located on radial side of fourth dorsal extensor compartment (also noted by asterisk in 5B). Schema demonstrates technique for diagnostic nerve block, which can be placed proximal to extensor sheath to avoid also injecting the radial carpal joint. *B*, Skin markings show third and fourth dorsal compartments. Asterisk marks location of nerve branch at this level. The denervation is done 2 cm proximal to this. (With permission from Dellon AL. Partial dorsal wrist denervation. J Hand Surg 1985; 10A:527–533.)

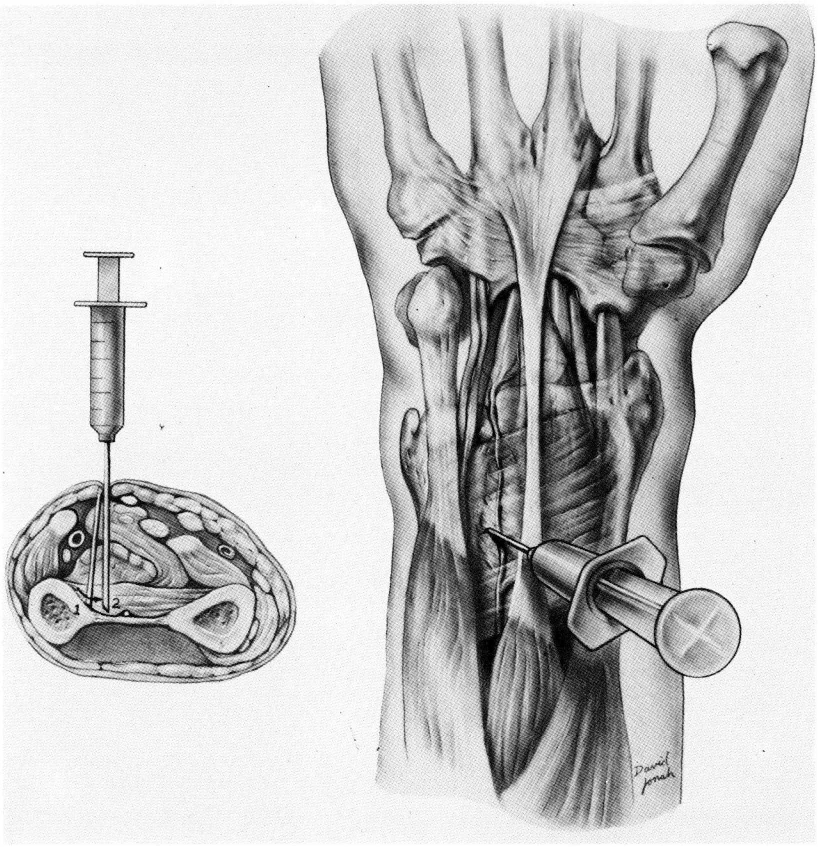

Figure 6 Deliberate interruption of nerve function to relieve pain by means of partial volar wrist denervation procedure. Terminal branch of anterior interosseous nerve located beneath pronator quadratus on interosseous membrane. Schema for diagnostic nerve block; first touching ulna, then repositioning needle to interosseous region. (With permission from Dellon AL, et al. Terminal branch of anterior interosseus nerve as a source of wrist pain. J Hand Surg 1984; 9B:316–322.)

branches as they transit from below the distal end of the pronator quadratus muscle into the volar wrist ligaments. For pain associated with degenerative or posttraumatic arthritis, where there is radiographic confirmation of the arthritis but sufficient range of motion remains for more aggressive joint procedures, such as joint replacement or partial fusion, not to be indicated, the partial wrist denervation procedures permit a conservative operative approach. This relieves pain, if so demonstrated by the preoperative block, while retaining range of motion. Although it is likely that in the future, if the arthritis progresses, additional surgery will be required, such a joint-sparing initial attempt may give the patient additional years of function. These approaches are not recommended for the carpal instability patterns.

The deliberate interruption of nerve function of pain of cutaneous origin is most commonly indicated for neuromas. In the section on correction of complete interruption of nerve function, this subject was discussed with regard to a neuroma of a peripheral nerve where there are sufficient distal neural structures to permit a nerve tube approach. When such distal neural structures are not available, or cannot be provided, review of the algorithm (see Fig. 1) suggests that the appropriate course of treatment is to resect the end-bulb neuroma and transfer the nerve to a site away from any target-derived neurotrop(h)ic stimuli, away from tension or traction provided by joint movement, and into a nonstimulating environment, such as an innervated muscle. Results of this approach have been gratifying, with greater than 80 percent success in relief of pain and improvement in hand function, even for the difficult neuromas over the dorsoradial aspect of the hand. Critical in this approach are preoperative diagnostic nerve blocks and the recognition that 75 percent of people have an overlap of the lateral antebrachial cutaneous nerve with the radial sensory nerve. Thus, many patients who have been treated for radial sensory neuromas in the past and who have had their treatment fail, may, in fact, have had an appropriate treatment for the radial sensory nerve itself, but pain persists because of a concomitant injury to the lateral antebrachial cutaneous nerve. Success has been possible in patients with work-related injuries. It has been poor in those with digital neuromas where no appropriate muscles for implantation exist in the hand. The muscles of the hand are of too small diameter and have too much excursion to permit successful use for muscle implantation. In these instances, the nerve is implanted into bone after neuroma resection.

Deliberate creation of interruption of nerve function has been thought to be desirable in cases of spasticity. The general setting is the patient with cerebral palsy, or other upper motor neuron type problems, where overactivity in a muscle either directly interferes with function or further limits hand function by creating joint contractures or dysfunctional positions. Although many individuals believe that such spastic muscles cannot be transferred to achieve any useful end, and, therefore the desirable course of action should be a nerve division or neurectomy (or the same effect can be obtained with a tenotomy), the alternative remains an option: removal of function of the spastic muscle by transfer into another desired area. It is a worthwhile approach to attempt to transfer the muscle, bearing in mind that such a transfer always can be reversed, thus in effect reversing to the interruption of nerve function situation. For example, the overactive pronator teres muscle can be rerouted in the opposite direction about the radius to make it a supinator (unpublished technique of Ivan Matev, M.D., Bulgaria). Similarly, the usually spastic flexor digitorum sublimis to the middle and ring fingers can be transferred through the interosseous membrane to add force to wrist extension. When this transfer has been placed into the extensor digitorum communis, the transfer has proved too strong, and has resulted in hyperextension at the metacarpophalangeal joints for these fingers. The concept is that, in an attempt to rebalance the spastic hand, the deliberate creation of an interruption of nerve function can be carried out by tendon transfer rather than by neurectomy itself, with the hope of achieving some additional increased function by rebalancing where extra force is needed.

An additional role for the deliberate creation of interruption of nerve function exists in the motor system where facial paralysis results in significant facial asymmetry. The current favored approach builds upon the ability to carry out an innervated neurovascular muscle transfer following cross-facial nerve grafting. The placement of the cross-facial nerve graft requires selective nerve division on the innervated side. This selected denervation of the facial nerve territories on the active side of the patient with facial paralysis, partially corrects the asymmetry. Once the transferred muscle has become reinnervated and has reached sufficient strength, the stage is set for additional operative procedures to rebalance the face further. Frequently, the smile is distorted with a downward or depressor function on the innervated side. In this case, a deliberate creation of interruption of nerve function is done to the marginal mandibular branch, in an attempt to weaken the depressor anguli oris group of muscles.

SUGGESTED READING

Dellon AL. Evaluation of sensibility and re-education of sensation in the hand. Baltimore: Williams & Wilkins, 1981.

Dellon AL. Optimism in diabetic neuropathy. Ann Plast Surg 1988; 20:103–105.

Dellon AL. Partial dorsal wrist denervation: resection of distal posterior interosseus nerve. J Hand Surg 1985; 10A:527–533.

Dellon AL, Mackinnon SE. An alternative to the classical nerve graft for the management of the short nerve gap. Plast Reconstr Surg 1988 (in press).

Dellon AL, Mackinnon SE. Segmentally innervated latissimus dorsi muscle: microsurgical transfer for facial reanimation. J Reconstr Microsurg 1985; 2(1):7–12.

Dellon AL, Mackinnon SE, Daneshvar A. Terminal branch of anterior interosseous nerve as a source of wrist pain. J Hand Surg 1984; 9B:316–322.

Mackinnon SE, O'Brien P, Dellon AL, et al. An assessment of the effects of different treatment strategies, including neurolysis, on a chronically suppressed rat sciatic nerve. Plast Reconstr Surg 1988; 81:251–256.

Mackinnon SE, Dellon AL. Results of treatment of recurrent dorsoradial wrist neuromas by neuroma resection and muscle implantation. Ann Plast Surg 1987; 19:54–61.

Mackinnon SE, Dellon AL. Surgery of the peripheral nerve. New York: Thieme, 1988.

Mackinnon SE, Dellon AL, Lundborg G, et al. A study of neurotropism in primate model. J Hand Surg 1986; 11A:888–894.

BRACHIAL PLEXUS INJURIES

JULIA K. TERZIS, M.D., Ph.D., F.R.C.S.(C)
HALLENE MARAGH, M.D.

The brachial plexus is formed by the anterior branches of the last four cervical spinal nerves (C5, C6, C7, C8) and the first thoracic spinal nerve (T1). The brachial plexus provides the motor and sensory innervation to the upper extremity—the shoulder, elbow, wrist, and hand. Injuries to the brachial plexus can be partial or complete and can be classified into those with shoulder sparing and those with hand sparing.

EVALUATION

At evaluation, the aim is to determine, as accurately as possible, the type and site of lesion of the brachial plexus. This is done by a meticulous clinical examination and specialized testing.

From identification of the mechanism of the injury, several factors help in determining the type and the severity of the injury.

1. The arm position indicates the type of neurologic deficits that might be expected. If the injury is sustained while the arm is in a classic upward position, the lower plexus is most affected; if the arm is pulled sidewards, the central plexus is maximally involved. If the mechanism of injury is such that the arm is in the abducted position, the upper plexus is affected.
2. Multiple levels of injury should always be considered. Identification of dislocation of the shoulder is important since, in addition to a supraclavicular injury, a dislocated shoulder can also result in an infraclavicular plexus injury. Distal fractures may also result in multi-level neural injury.
3. Associated vascular injuries suggest, more frequently than not, an infraclavicular type of brachial plexus injury. In such injuries, root avulsions are rarely encountered.
4. Pain is usually a symptom associated with an avulsion

lesion of the C8 and/or T1 root. Such pain is confined mainly to the hand and the patient usually describes it as being severe and noted immediately after the onset of the paralysis.

PHYSICAL EXAMINATION

All muscles that serve the upper extremity must be examined. A tabulation of muscle function, graded on a scale of zero to five by the manual muscle tests, is done and recorded on a convenient chart (Fig. 1). All the muscles of the upper extremity, including the shoulder girdle and the trapezius muscle, which is supplied by the spinal accessory nerve, are tested and exact records are kept. Sensibility assessment is done for each dermatome, the cervical and brachial plexi included. Testing includes pain and temperature appreciation, static two point and moving two point discrimination, constant touch, and vibration with a tuning fork at both 30 and 256 cycles per second.

Objective sensibility testing, which primarily addresses the sudomotor system, is carried out by the Ninhydrin sweat test in the palms. In addition, thermography of both palms is performed in an effort to measure the temperature changes that effects of nerve injuries cause on the skin of the palm. Tinel's sign is executed in a distoproximal fashion, with each of the major peripheral nerves tested separately. The presence of a proximal Tinel's sign in the neck usually indicates a proximal neuroma, and usually is a good prognostic sign. However, the absence of a Tinel's sign in the neck is an important clinical finding because it indicates total plexus avulsion, unless proven otherwise.

The eyes are examined to document evidence of Horner's syndrome, which includes ptosis, meiosis, and anhidrosis. The absence of Horner's sign is a good prog-

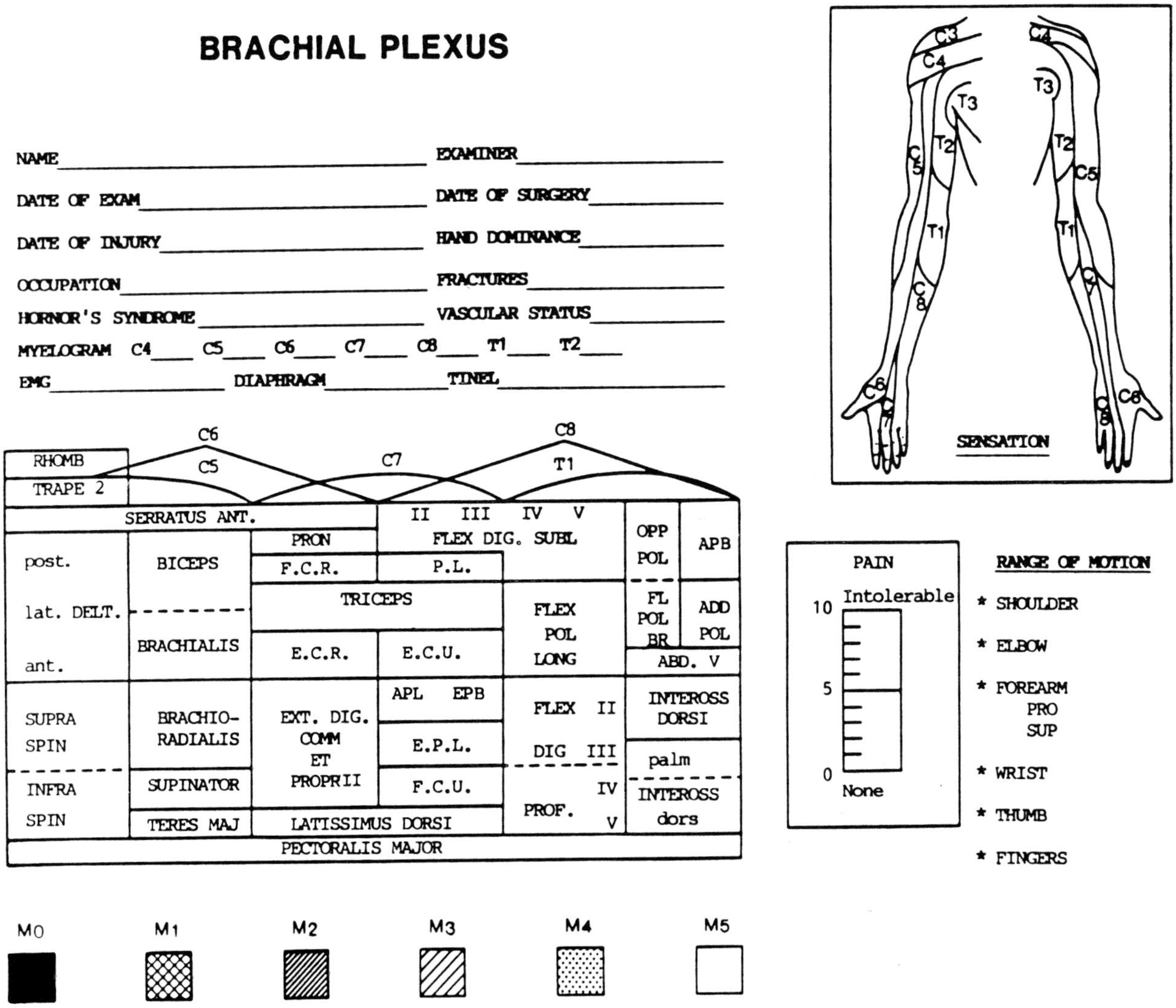

Figure 1 Chart used to tabulate and record results of manual muscle tests performed on all muscles of the upper extremity.

nostic feature, while its presence usually implies C8 and/or T1 avulsion from the spinal cord.

ELECTRODIAGNOSTIC EXAMINATION

These tests include conduction velocity studies, electromyography (EMG), and percutaneous invasive spinal nerve stimulation. The aim of conduction studies is to try to quantitate the number of axonal carrythroughs and the speed of axonal transmission. Preoperatively, motor conduction velocity permits one to determine the continuity of the involved nerve and the degree of the injury. Postoperatively, motor conduction velocity can be useful to ascertain the rate and maturity of the regeneration process.

The sensory conduction velocity permits the diagnosis of an avulsion injury in specific cases. From the clinical examination, one ascertains whether the patient can perceive along the median, ulnar, and radial nerve distribution. When the patient has no sensory perception in the hand but the distal sensory latencies are normal, this indicates that the roots are interrupted proximal to the sensory ganglion, which is a positive sign for avulsion injury.

EMG helps to predict the localization and extent of the lesion. However, the test has two limitations: (1) EMG predicts avulsion of a root only in the absence of other postganglionic lesions corresponding to the same root, and (2) needle EMG may show good electrogenesis although the mechanical function of the muscle may still be gravely compromised.

A powerful new preoperative electrodiagnostic test is the one introduced by Liberson in 1984. It involves the percutaneous introduction of stimulating needle electrodes down to the vertebral laminae. The patient is awake and is simply asked to identify the fingers with referred sensory perception. This procedure is repeated for all the spinal nerves that contribute to the brachial plexus. If, for example, the patient identifies the little finger, the integrity of C8 or T1, or both, is ascertained. If no referred sensation in the fingers is identified, probably all roots are involved. We have used this technique in our clinic for the past 4 years, and it has greatly increased our accuracy in the preoperative diagnosis of avulsion injuries in the adult patient.

Preoperative radiologic testing includes plain myelography, or metrizamide myelography combined with computerized tomography (CT) scan and polytomography. In an effort to increase the accuracy of the preoperative neurodiagnostic testing we are also trying magnetic resonance imaging (MRI). However, our experience with this new tool is limited at present.

When the patient has suffered a concomitant vascular injury and has had vascular reconstruction of the subclavian artery, preoperative arteriography is indicated.

PRINCIPLES IN MANAGEMENT

Management should be considered under nonoperative and operative methods. Nonoperative management includes prevention of trophic lesions, maintenance of joint mobility, frequent massage of the extremity to reduce edema, continuous range of motion exercises, and maintenance of muscle bulk by galvanic and/or faradic stimulation.

Electrotherapy is applied in our clinic in a completely different fashion, based on exact calibration of signals obtained by the involved muscles. Thus, denervated muscles must be stimulated by slow pulses of current (above 100 milliseconds) and with electrodes applied below and above the muscle (longitudinal stimulation).

Reinnervated muscles are stimulated by a brief pulse stimulator to excite nerves and muscles, as developed by Liberson 25 years ago and later modified for use in patients with brachial plexus paralysis. We use the brief pulse stimulator for three purposes: (1) to increase the strength of the innervated muscle, (2) to bombard the centers with musculocutaneous feedback stimuli and, therefore, contribute to restoration of both the muscle and sensory perceptions, and (3) to reduce pain.

Other measures include psychological support and patient retraining.

OPERATIVE MANAGEMENT

Operative repair of the brachial plexus may be achieved primarily or secondarily. Primary repair is indicated in situations where there are clean lacerations of the brachial plexus and the plexus is explored as an emergency procedure to repair a vascular injury. In such a case, end-to-end repair of the severed plexus structures can be achieved primarily. Emergency nerve grafting procedures are not indicated.

Secondary Repair

This is carried out with all other brachial plexus injuries, namely closed injuries, or in patients who had vascular reconstruction elsewhere and were referred to our clinic for microreconstruction of the brachial plexus.

Timing of the Repair

When the mechanism of injury is blunt trauma, it is advisable to wait for 3 weeks before proceeding with preoperative diagnostic electrical testing. If the paralysis persists, then exploration is scheduled anytime between 8 and 12 weeks. By this time, the neurapraxic component of the nerve lesion has been restored, and all appropriate studies to localize and assess the extent of the injury are completed.

TECHNIQUES OF REPAIR

Neurorrhaphy

This is one of several available techniques of repair and is an end-to-end epineurial coaptation without any tension. The existing gap should not exceed 2.0 to 3.0 cm.

When there is evidence of moderate tension in the repair, then one should proceed to a nerve grafting procedure. As a rule of thumb, any nerve stumps that cannot be held together with two 8.0 nylon sutures should be grafted.

Interposition Nerve Grafts

The technique of interfascicular nerve grafting of corresponding fascicular groups is rarely applicable to proximal repairs of the brachial plexus. Instead, sectoral coaptation formulates the basis of repair. The types of grafts used include the following: (1) nonvascularized nerve grafts (cutaneous nerve grafts and trunk graft with complete epineurial resection), and (2) vascularized nerve grafts (vascularized trunk or cutaneous grafts transferred by microvascular technique and pedicled vascularized grafts).

Our indications for vascularized nerve grafts are a scarred bed, long defects, and use as riders for nonvascularized nerve grafts. The vascularized grafts that have been introduced and popularized for brachial plexus reconstruction by Dr. Terzis include vascularized ulnar and saphenous nerves. The indications for vascularized sural nerves are limited in brachial plexus microreconstruction as this necessitates turning the patient to a prone position.

Vascularized ulnar nerve grafts are used in cases where the C8 and T1 nerve roots are avulsed. This should always be confirmed by exploration of the C8–T1 roots prior to harvesting the ulnar nerve.

Neurolysis

This is indicated in the case of a lesion in-continuity, where there is documented function distally along the distribution of the involved nerve. We perform neurolysis as a staged procedure. It commences with a longitudinal epineuriotomy and, if there is no evidence of decompression of fascicular bundles, then a step-like decompression is performed until the entrapped bundles are decompressed. We, therefore, proceed from external to internal structures of the nerve. The stages would be continued as external epineuriotomy, external epineuriectomy and, finally, interfascicular microneurolysis. When there is no functional preservation distally, and when the fascicles are scarred with loss of perineurial integrity, then we proceed with resection and repair by interposition nerve grafting.

Neurotization

This is the principle of transferring a donor nerve to a dissimilar, more important recipient nerve to achieve innervation. Such procedures have often transferred the distal spinal accessory nerve directly onto the suprascapular nerve and used cervical plexus motor donors to musculocutaneous nerve.

Direct Muscle Neurotization

In the situation where a motor nerve is avulsed from its muscular target tissue, an attempt to implant a motor nerve is made close to the motor point in order to restore a neuromuscular junction. This technique yields inferior results compared to the ones obtained through a proximal nerve-to-nerve coaptation.

PRIORITIES IN BRACHIAL PLEXUS RECONSTRUCTION

In this series the order of decreasing priorities is as follows:

1. Shoulder Stability. The aim is to reverse shoulder subluxation by reinnervation of supraspinatus and deltoid muscles.
2. Elbow Flexion. When the shoulder is stable, the next single most important muscle is the biceps. Thus, reconstruction of the musculocutaneous nerve is of critical importance because, in addition to restoration of elbow flexion, the patient gets some sensory perception on the dorsum of the hand.
3. Hand Sensibility. Reconstruction of the median nerve is a high priority in brachial plexus management as it restores protective sensibility to the hand and in many cases, an appreciable degree of finger flexion. When the injury is supraclavicular, the degree of motor return in the long finger flexors is limited to M3 grades.
4. Long Flexors. The aim is to restore a strong grasp in the hand. This is not usually achieved by primary nerve repair when there are high lesions. So it is usually accomplished by tendon transfers a combination of "banking nerve motors" and free muscle transfers.
5. Long Extensors. The aim is to achieve wrist and finger extension. Again, this is not usually accomplished by primary nerve repair in supraclavicular lesions but by secondary procedures that include tendon and free muscle transfers.
6. External Shoulder Rotation. This can be accomplished by reinnervation of infraspinatus and teres minor muscles, through the suprascapular and axillary nerves respectively.

The minimal goal is to provide an upper extremity that has a stable shoulder, elbow flexion, and median nerve sensibility. This ensures that the extremity can be used as a "helper" to the normal extremity.

OPERATIVE TECHNIQUES

The aim of the operative technique is to identify the site of the injury and expose the injured nerve proximal to and distal to the site of the injury, so that the microsurgical repair can be done between good proximal and good distal stumps.

The first step is exploration of the supraclavicular plexus. Important landmarks to the brachial plexus include identification of the phrenic nerve on the anterior surface of the scalenus anterior muscle, which is situated posterior to the sternocleidomastoid muscle. Once the phrenic nerve is identified and stimulated, the dissection then proceeds proximally to trace the phrenic nerve as it receives contributions from the C4 and C5 spinal nerves. The C5 spinal nerve is first identified by palpation, followed by exploration. Then in step fashion we proceed from C5 to identification of C6, which is situated inferoposteriorly.

The dissection continues from medial to lateral on the superior aspect of C5 to identify the upper trunk. The superior border of the upper trunk is followed further peripherally. Just above the clavicle the suprascapular nerve is identified as it exits at the level of the juncture of upper trunk and posterior cord.

The C7 spinal nerve is exposed by gentle lifting of the upper trunk and by palpation of the vertebral foramen inferior to C6. The middle trunk is easily visualized as a prolongation of C7. At the level of the clavicle, the middle trunk proceeds to join the posterior cord with a smaller contribution to the lateral cord. The C8 and T1 spinal nerves are located below the level of the clavicle and just above the subclavian artery. The safest approach to these roots is to dissect in a plane posterior to the plane of upper and middle trunks and proceed in a medial fashion by lifting gently both trunks anteriorly. Once these roots are identified, they are then traced to the site of entry into the spinal cord. Care should be taken to respect the apex of the pleura and the large vessels that are situated just below the lower trunk. Other landmarks during plexus dissection are the omohyoid muscle and the transverse cervical artery and vein.

Exploration of the Infraclavicular Plexus Dissection

To identify the extent of a brachial plexus lesion, it is usually necessary to explore the infraclavicular plexus. This is approached by separation of the pectoralis major muscle from the deltoid muscle, while identifying and preserving the cephalic vein. Next the pectoralis minor muscle insertion to the coracoid process is taken down to facilitate access to the infraclavicular plexus. We first identify the lateral cord and its contribution to the median nerve. Once this is done, we can then identify the contribution from the medial cord to the median nerve, and when we trace this contribution proximally, the medial cord and ulnar nerve are exposed. The medial cord then turns posterior to the subclavian artery and, by proximal and distal dissection, the medial cord can be traced right up to its contribution from the C8 and T1 roots. In some cases, when there is a lot of scarring in the area, this is difficult to accomplish and a clavicular osteotomy may have to be performed at this point. The posterior cord is usually approached by retraction of the lateral cord medially and exposure inferior of the posterior cord, which is situated posterior to the lateral cord and the subclavian artery. The radial nerve and axillary nerve are identified by tracing the posterior cord distally, as well as the upper and lower subscapular nerves. The lateral pectoral nerves exit the lateral cord at the level of the clavicle and shortly afterward enter the pectoralis major muscle about 2 or 3 cm below the interior clavicular border.

Intraoperative Electrophysiologic Stimulation Studies

Electrical stimulation of each structure is carried out by routine use of a direct current stimulator and stimulation with one-half, one, and two milliamps. The plexus is stimulated proximal to the site of injury and distal to the site of injury. Each spinal nerve, trunk, cord, and peripheral nerve is stimulated at the moment it is exposed, prior to further microsurgical manipulation. This is a very important point to understand and conform to as minor surgical assault to the nerve can cause neurapraxia, which, on subsequent electrical stimulation, will not yield a positive muscular response. If intraoperative decisions are to be based on electrical stimulation findings, one has to make certain that the nerve is undisturbed, warm, and dry of surrounding fluids prior to stimulation. For instance, it is very common initially to get positive distal contractions with stimulation of a specific nerve, yet 2 hours later the same nerve may be totally silent to the same stimulus.

The accurate interpretation of the results of intraoperative stimulation studies is a difficult task that should be taken seriously, because false interpretation can lead to loss of function or, conversely, an euphoric interpretation can lead to continued paralysis of the target tissue.

While the supraclavicular and infraclavicular plexi are explored, decisions are made as to the exact diagnosis of the neural injury. Roots are biopsied as necessary to identify nerve fibers versus ganglion cells versus scar tissue. Before a final intraoperative diagnosis is reached as to whether a root is avulsed or ruptured, all the preoperative clinical, electrical, and neuroradiologic findings are correlated with the intraoperative surgical findings of the injured neural tissue, as well as how the nerves feel to palpation and appear to inspection under magnification.

On the basis of our understanding of the cumulative findings, decisions are made toward microreconstruction.

In reconstruction, donor nerves are used to restore spinal nerves C5, C6, C7, and/or upper and middle trunks, and/or lateral and posterior cords. Ulnar nerve reconstruction has not been a priority in adults as intrinsic recovery has been universally poor. Thus, our priorities in microreconstruction of the adult brachial plexus include reconstruction of shoulder stability, elbow flexion, hand sensation, finger flexion, elbow extension, finger extension and abduction, and external rotation at the shoulder.

Our approach to the injured adult brachial plexus is illustrated in four clinical cases; chosen as representative examples of different types of injuries. An example of high velocity penetrating lesions that involved the upper trunk is shown in Figure 2. This type of lesion is amenable

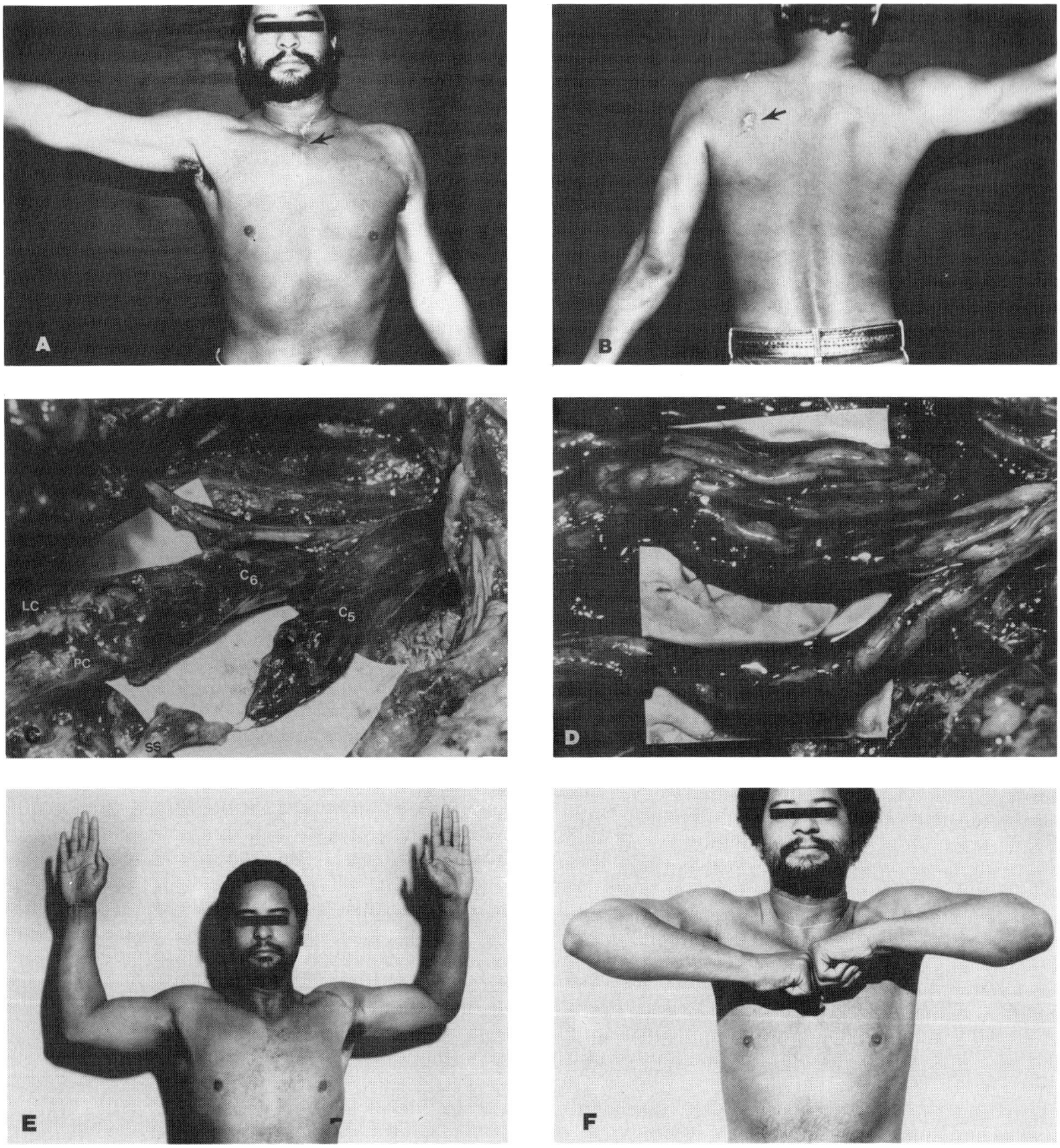

Figure 2 Example of upper trunk, high velocity penetrating lesion. A 26-year-old male had sustained a gunshot wound to the left supraclavicular plexus with transection of the suprascapular nerve and penetrating lesion to the upper trunk. The patient was initially explored by vascular surgeons and at 6 weeks the brachial plexus was explored. Microreconstruction was carried out by using nine interposition sural nerve grafts. *A*, Preoperative view of patient after the vascular exploration (note scar in the left neck and sternum [arrow]). Patient is unable to abduct shoulder, to externally rotate the humerus, or flex elbow. His triceps was preserved. *B*, Posterior view of patient preoperatively. Note exit wound of bullet over left scapular region (arrow). There is flatness of deltoid, supraspinatus and infraspinatus. Note bulk of triceps is preserved. *C*, Intraoperative findings upon exploration. Bullet tract had penetrated most of upper trunk, completely transected origin of suprascapular nerve from C5 spinal nerve and minimally injured the ipsilateral phrenic nerve. (P = phrenic, C5 = C5 spinal nerve, C6 = C6 spinal nerve, SS = suprascapular nerve, PC = posterior cord, LC = lateral cord). *D*, Situation following microreconstruction of the upper trunk with nine interposition sural nerve grafts. *E*, Postoperative view of patient at 2 years. His ability to abduct the shoulder is shown, as well as flexion of the elbow and external rotation of the humerus. *F*, Strong elbow flexion has returned, as well as near-normal abduction of the shoulder.

Figure continues on opposite page

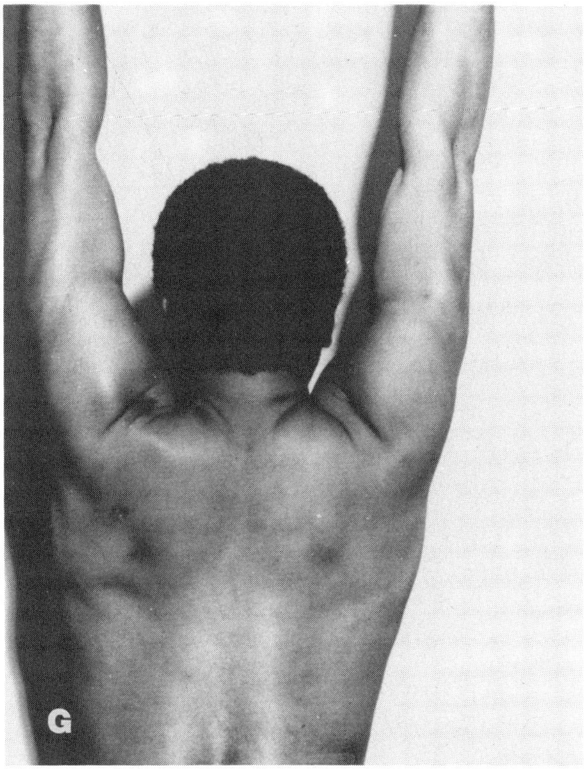

Figure 2 (continued) *G*, Complete elevation of the left upper extremity is shown. Note restoration of the muscle bulk of the deltoid, biceps, supra- and infraspinatus. The patient has returned to work as a longshoreman following extensive rehabilitation.

to microsurgical reconstruction, with favorable results. In this case, the patient resumed his previous work as a longshoreman.

An example of high velocity penetrating lesion that resulted in complete paralysis of the infraclavicular plexus, with associated vascular injury, is presented in Figure 3.

Traction lesions to the brachial plexus imply a longitudinal extent of injury to the involved plexus. In Figure 4, we present an example of severe traction lesion to the infraclavicular plexus, with associated vascular injury.

Figure 5 depicts a more common lesion, namely, severe supraclavicular traction lesion with three-root avulsion. Such lesions are common sequelae of motorcycle accidents and, up to recent years, carried a grave prognosis. The use of vascularized nerve grafts, as popularized by Dr. Terzis, and, specifically, the use of the vascularized ulnar nerve graft in cases of C8 and T1 avulsion has dramatically altered the prognosis in these devastating lesions.

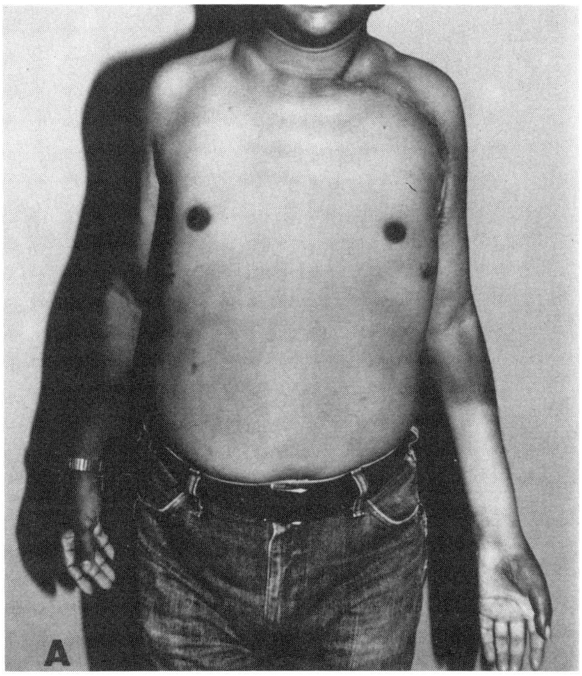

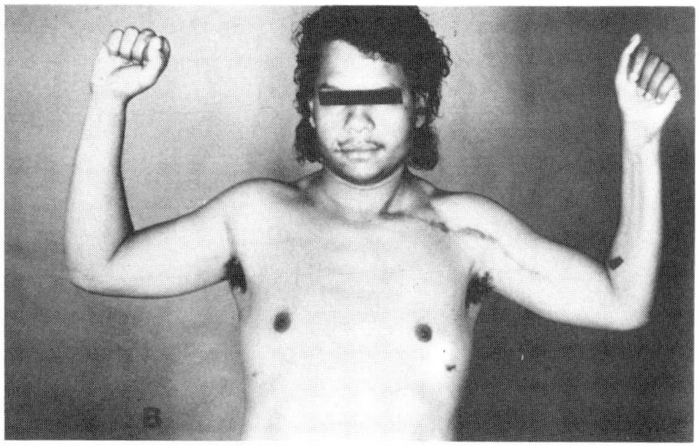

Figure 3 Example of complete infraclavicular brachial plexus palsy from high velocity penetrating lesion with associated vascular injury. A 24-year-old male sustained a gunshot wound in the left infraclavicular region with left subclavian artery transection and complete left infraclavicular brachial plexus paralysis. Two weeks after vascular repair of the subclavian artery, the brachial plexus was explored and the radial and median nerves were repaired by interposition sural nerve grafts. The ulnar nerve and musculocutaneous nerve were neurolysed. *A*, The patient, 6 weeks postoperatively, shows complete left upper extremity paralysis. Discoloration over distal forearm depicts usage of wrist splint. *B*, He is shown 3 years subsequent to microreconstruction of the left infraclavicular plexus. Note shoulder abductions, external rotation, elbow flexion, strong finger flexion, and excellent wrist extension.

Figure continues on following page

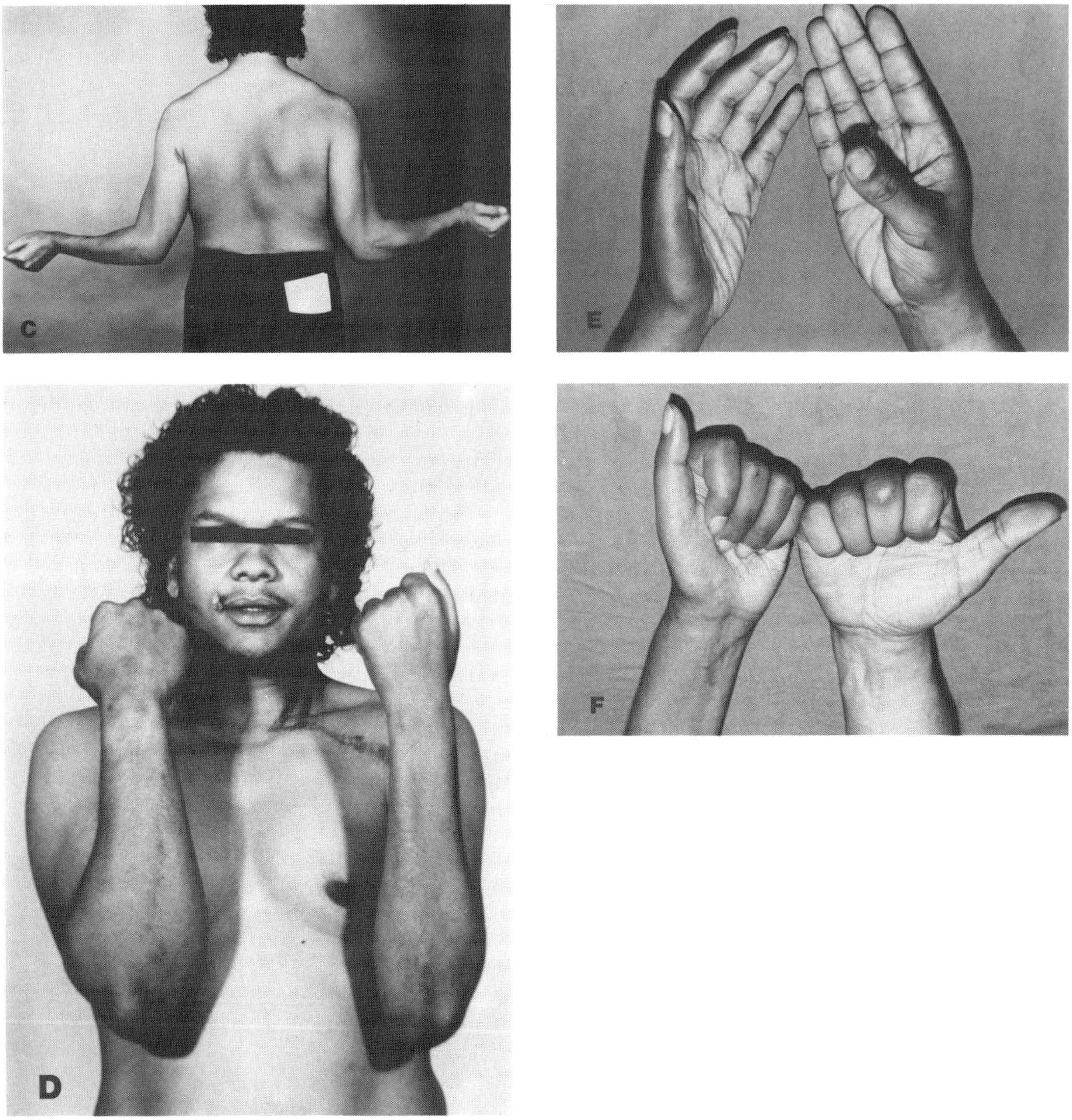

Figure 3 (continued) *C*, Posterior view of patient shows excellent external rotation and elbow flexion. Note return of brachioradials and wrist extensors and long finger flexors. *D*, He shows strong elbow and finger flexion. *E* and *F*, Some ulnar intrinsics have recovered. Also there is strong return of finger extension and flexion. Note inability to oppose thumb.

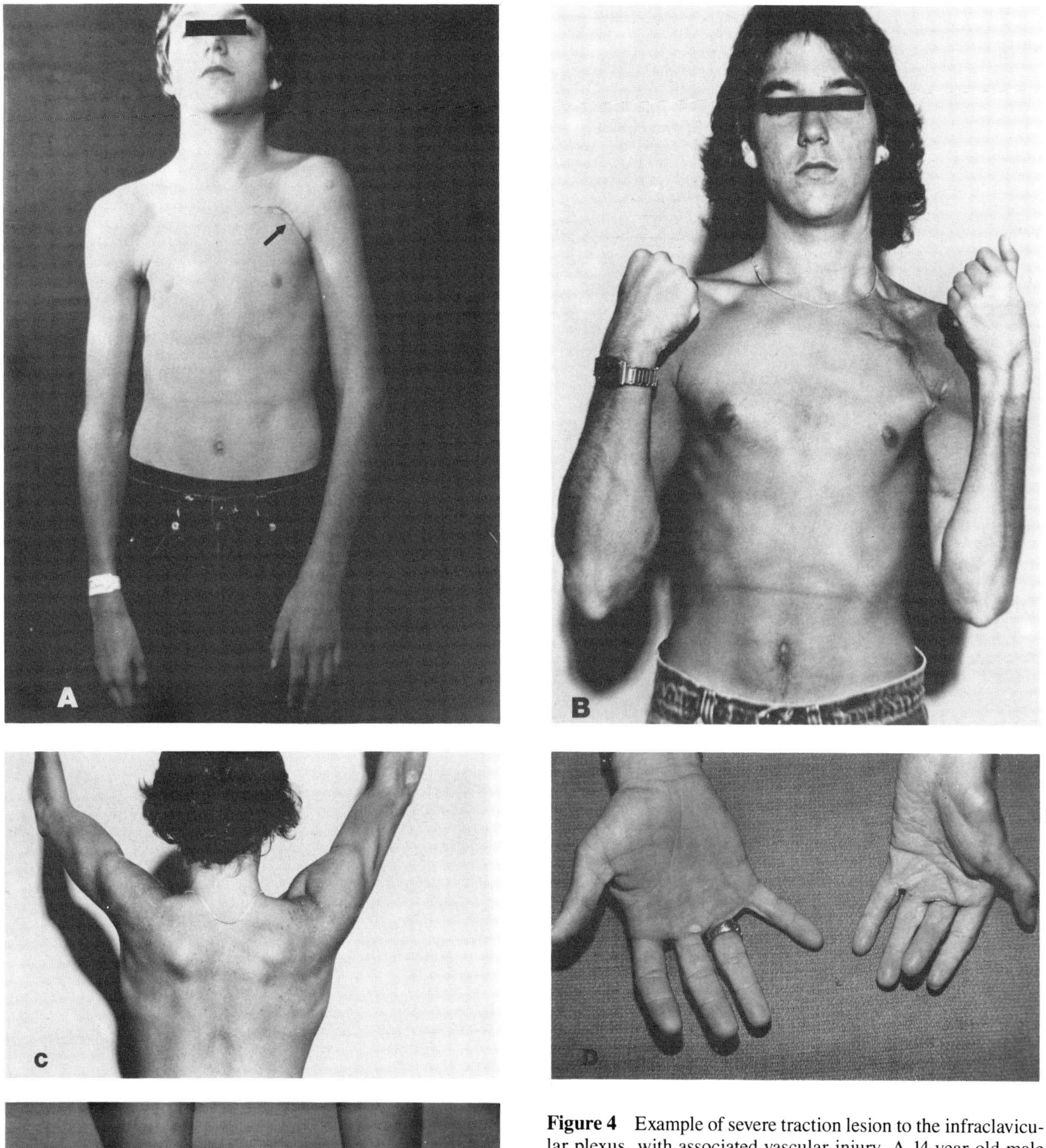

Figure 4 Example of severe traction lesion to the infraclavicular plexus, with associated vascular injury. A 14-year-old male sustained a motorcycle accident with a left total infraclavicular brachial plexus injury. At 3 months after the reconstruction of the subclavian artery with interposition vein graft, the brachial plexus was repaired by interposition sural nerve grafts to the musculocutaneous nerve, median, ulnar, radial, and axillary nerves. *A*, Preoperative presentation of the patient shows a completely paralyzed, left upper extremity with associated sudomotor paralysis, as depicted by mottled discoloration of the left hand. Note scar from previous vascular reconstruction (arrow). *B*, Postoperative view at 4 years reveals powerful elbow flexion, strong finger flexion, and good wrist control. *C*, Posterior view shows acceptable return of deltoid, excellent biceps, and adequate triceps. *D* and *E* are close-up views of the hands, showing finger extension and strong finger flexion. Patient has resumed his competitive wrestling career.

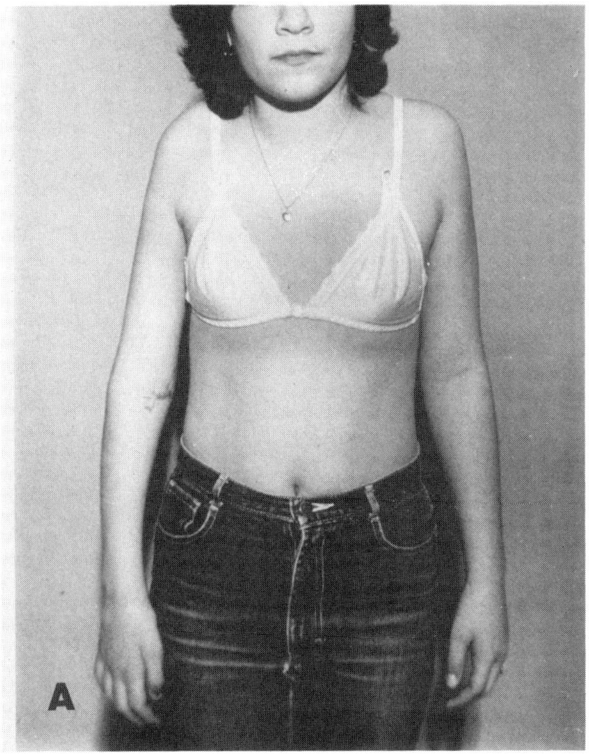

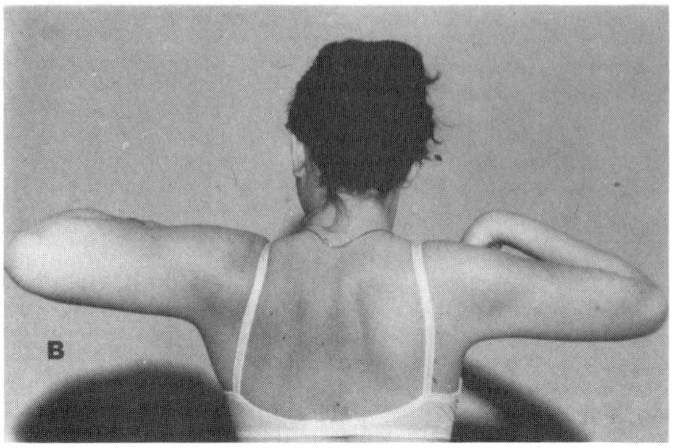

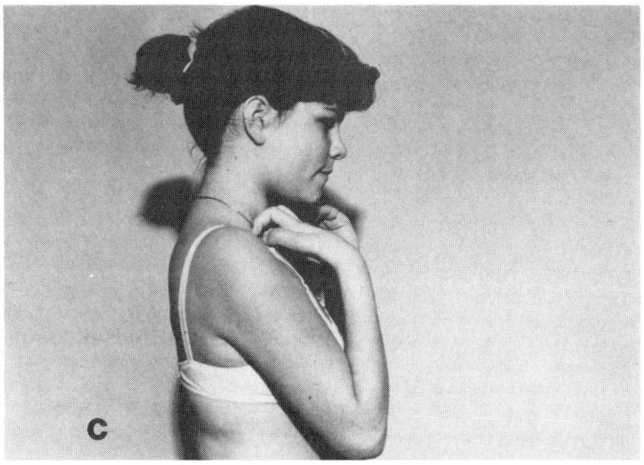

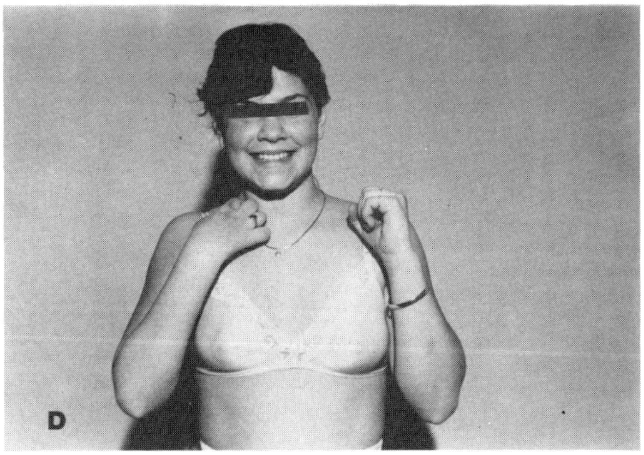

Figure 5 A severe high velocity supraclavicular traction lesion with avulsion of C7, C8, and T1 spinal nerves. A 14-year-old female had sustained a motorcycle accident in July, 1984, with a right total plexus injury with ruptures of C5 and C6 and avulsion of C7, C8, and T1 spinal nerves. The patient was referred to our clinic 10 months following her injury. At that time, the brachial plexus was repaired by microneurolysis of C5 spinal nerve and microreconstruction of the remaining plexus by the use of a vascularized ulnar nerve graft. *A*, Preoperative presentation of a total right brachial plexus paralysis, with no motor or sensory function at the shoulder, elbow, or hand. *B*, Postoperative posterior view at 2 years, following microreconstruction of the right brachial plexus. Note excellent return of shoulder functions, including abduction, elevation, and external rotation. *C*, Lateral view of patient shows strong elbow flexion. Finger flexion is minimal but increasing in strength with time. *D*, Anterior view of patient reveals strong elbow flexion and excellent shoulder function. Restoration of motor function is just beginning in the hand. However, she already has a respectable degree of sensory return in the right hand.

SUGGESTED READING

Terzis JK. Microreconstruction of nerve injuries. Philadelphia: WB Saunders, 1987.

MICROSURGICAL MUSCLE TRANSFER FOR UPPER EXTREMITY MOTORS

RALPH T. MANKTELOW, M.D., F.R.C.S.(C)

Microvascular techniques allow the transfer of tissues from one location to another and assure their viability. Muscle is one of the tissues that has been successfully transferred from many sites; survival of this tissue is reliable because of long predictable vascular pedicles and a vigorous blood supply. These muscles may be transferred as functioning units by a motor nerve repair in the recipient site.

Microneurovascular muscle transfer has been used successfully to reconstruct thenar, forearm flexor and extensor, upper arm flexor, and shoulder flexor musculature.

THERAPEUTIC ALTERNATIVES

There are many alternatives to microneurovascular muscle transfer for providing motor function, including tendon transfers, tenodeses, and fusions. If any of these procedures will provide adequate function, they are usually preferable to microvascular techniques. Tendon transfers, tenodeses, and fusions are usually reliable, relatively easy to carry out, and provide a useful functional return within a few months. Microneurovascular transfer, although reliable, is a tedious, long procedure that requires considerable attention to detail. The time for maximum functional return following such a transfer is 1 to 2 years.

PROCEDURE

Patient Selection

Patients who are suitable for this procedure are those who have sustained a total muscle loss of a functional group of muscles such as the long flexor musculature to the fingers. The most common causes of muscle deficiency are direct trauma and Volkmann's ischemic contracture. Other less common causes are long-standing nerve injury, electrical burns, gas gangrene, and posttumor resection.

After it has been determined that other simpler techniques will not provide an adequate solution to the patient's problem, the patient and the extremity are evaluated to assess their suitability. The extremity must have suitable anatomy so that a functioning muscle transfer is technically feasible. It also must have sufficient functional capability, such that the addition of a single functioning muscle will provide a significant improvement in the extremity's usefulness.

For example, a muscle transfer to the flexor aspect of the forearm requires a useful, undamaged motor nerve and adequate vasculature for microneurovascular anastomoses. Suitable skin cover must be present to enclose the muscle and to allow muscle-tendon gliding. The flexor tendons must be present and capable of gliding and the finger joints must be supple. In addition, there should be good sensibility and sufficient intrinsic function that balanced grip will be produced by activation of the flexor tendons in order for the hand to be useful. A mechanism for finger and thumb extension and wrist stabilization must be present.

Muscle Selection

The guidelines for muscle selection are as follows:

1. Suitable anatomy
   a) neurovascular anatomy that allows microneurovascular transfer
   b) gross anatomic fit, i.e., muscle length, location of neurovascular bundle, and tendon availability
2. Functional capability
   a) adequate strength
   b) range of muscle excursion
   c) stamina
3. Ability to be removed without leaving a significant functional or cosmetic defect in the donor site.

The location in the recipient bed of the motor nerve, vessels, and tendons to which the muscle will be attached can usually be determined by the surgeon's knowledge of the pathologic anatomy, examination of the arteriogram, and a functional assessment. However, the availability of a pure motor nerve to reinnervate the muscle may be difficult to assess except by direct exploration of the forearm and neurohistologic examination. If there is reasonable doubt, neurohistologic examination should be done either as a quick section assessment or as a preliminary diagnostic exploration prior to the planned muscle transplantation.

An understanding of the anatomy of the recipient bed allows the surgeon to match the anatomy of the various muscles that are available for transfer and to determine which one will provide the best fit.

The functional requirements of each muscle group are fairly well known. In the forearm, finger flexor tendon excursion is 7 to 8 cm, and finger extensor tendon excursion is 5 cm. As the muscle after transfer will likely have a slightly different tension than in its original site, it is necessary to select a muscle that has slightly more excursion than these amounts for transfers to the flexor and extensor surface. Strap muscles, such as the gracilis, latissimus dorsi, and tensor fascia lata, have an adequate range of excursion for finger flexion and extension. In addition, muscle strength is proportional to the cross-sectional area of the muscle's fibers. The gracilis, latissimus dorsi, tensor fascia lata, the rectus femoris, one-half of the gastrocnemius, the serratus anterior, and the pectoralis minor have all been used successfully for functioning muscle transfer.

For most muscle defects in the upper extremity, I

prefer the gracilis (Fig. 1). It is a relatively easy muscle to prepare, and it has a long and reliable pedicle. The anatomic configuration is excellent; the gracilis has a useful tendinous origin for attachment proximally and a long tendon of insertion that provides flexibility in its insertion. The donor site is easily hidden, since it lies in the upper half of the medial aspect of the thigh, and there is no functional deficit from removal of the muscle. The anatomy and operative technique have been described in detail elsewhere.

Technique of Muscle Transplantation

A two-team approach allows simultaneous preparation of the recipient arm and the donor muscle for transfer, thereby minimizing the operative time. There are many details of technique that are important to the eventual functional outcome.

Preparation of the Arm

The recipient area dissection is frequently tedious as a result of extensive scarring. The dissection is done to elevate flaps that will accept and cover the muscle, to identify vessels and prepare them for microanastomoses, to find a suitable motor nerve and clarify its capability of regeneration, and to prepare the site of muscle origin and tendons of insertion.

Technical points of importance are as follows:

1. Preparation of vessels is carried out from proximal to distal, beginning in an undamaged area.
2. Since arterial repairs in a zone of injury are prone to spasm, this problem is minimized by placing the anastomoses proximal to the injury when possible or by using end-to-side repairs.
3. Suitable recipient vessels in the flexor forearm for end-to-end repairs include the ulnar recurrent and anterior interosseous arteries. For end-to-side repairs, the radial and ulnar arteries are preferred. Extensor forearm muscles are usually revascularized by end-to-side repairs to the proximal radial artery.

   Venous repairs are usually end-to-end using superficial veins or venae comitantes.

   For revascularization of the upper arm, direct end-to-side repairs to the brachial artery and vena comitans or transfer of the thoracodorsal or other small arteries to the site of anastomosis provide useful vascular recipient pedicles.
4. The distal part of the muscle tendon unit must be housed under intact skin and subcutaneous tissue to allow tendon gliding.
5. Selection of a suitable motor nerve requires a detailed knowledge of the local neural anatomy and its variations.

The anterior interosseous nerve is the most suitable for reinnervation of a finger flexor muscle transfer. Suitable branches of the posterior interosseous nerve are

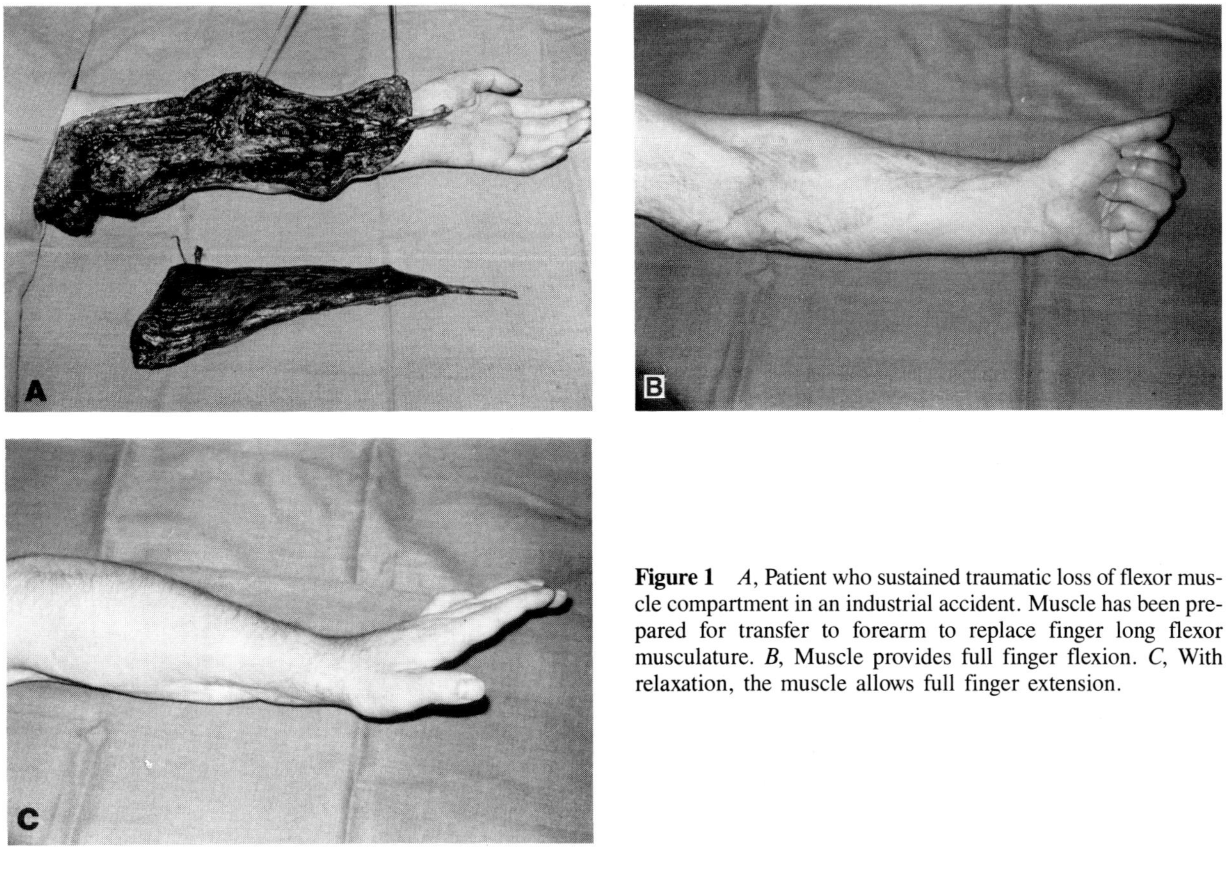

Figure 1 *A*, Patient who sustained traumatic loss of flexor muscle compartment in an industrial accident. Muscle has been prepared for transfer to forearm to replace finger long flexor musculature. *B*, Muscle provides full finger flexion. *C*, With relaxation, the muscle allows full finger extension.

preferred for finger extensor muscle transfer. The motor branches of the musculocutaneous nerve are used for elbow flexion transfer and the motor branches of the circumflex nerve are used for deltoid muscle reconstruction.

If there is significant intraneural fibrosis when the selected nerve is divided, the nerve should be trimmed proximally until an undamaged area of nerve is identified. Neurohistologic quick section analysis may be helpful in determining the usefulness of the nerve for reinnervation.

Muscle Transfer

The forearm should be completely prepared prior to muscle transfer in order that the muscle can be placed in the forearm and promptly revascularized. Vessel anastomoses should be precise because thrombosis and revision of the anastomosis are likely to produce detrimental ischemic damage to the muscle.

The important technical considerations are as follows:

Revascularization. Prior to revascularization, the muscle's origin is held fixed, the insertion is stretched distally, and the movements of the pedicle are observed relative to the intended site of anastomosis on the arm. This procedure ensures that the anastomoses will be undamaged with excursion of the muscle during contraction and relaxation.

After revascularization, the muscle is observed. Any distal musculature that is not viable must be removed and the cut surfaces of the muscle reinserted into the intramuscular portion of its own tendon.

Nerve Repair. The nerve repair is placed as close as possible to the neuromuscular hilum to minimize the duration of paralysis. A fascicular repair is required as the motor nerve of muscles such as the gracilis may contain up to 60 percent fatty connective tissue.

Balanced Tendon Fixation. When the muscle is being used to power more than one tendon, such as the five flexor tendons to the fingers and thumb, each of these tendons must be inserted into the muscle in such a position that a balanced grip will be produced with all fingers flexing in unison when the muscle contracts. By sewing the four profundus tendons side by side in a balanced position prior to attaching the transferred muscle, a balanced mass flexion can easily be produced.

When the flexor pollicis longus is to be motored with the same transfer as the fingers, its tendon should be sewn to the finger flexor tendons with some slackness; this is so that, upon muscle contraction, the fingers start to form a fist before the thumb moves. This placement will bring the thumb against the radial surface of the index in a key pinch position rather than flex it into the palm under the fingers, as would happen if the thumb flexor was placed too tightly.

Muscle Positioning for Optimum Tension. The technique of muscle positioning has been worked out in detail. Marking sutures are used on the muscle prior to its removal from its normal site. These marking sutures are placed with the muscle at its maximum physiologic stretched length.

With transfer of the muscle to the recipient area, it is then possible to plan the muscle's excursion and make use of the marking sutures to identify the normal maximum extended length of the muscle. In view of the normal length-tension curve of muscle function, the muscle should be transferred in a tension that allows an excursion in the more extended range of the muscle's excursion capability.

Flap Coverage. Closure of the recipient skin over the muscle must be done with care in order to provide good coverage of the distal half of the muscle tendon unit to allow muscle tendon gliding. The proximal skin flap should not be closed tightly over the muscle or compression and obstruction of the pedicle may occur. The muscle will function well with a split-thickness skin graft on its proximal half; this will not impede excursion of the muscle.

Postoperative Care

Successful revascularization without anastomosis thrombosis requires maintenance of normal peripheral perfusion in the immediate postoperative period. Adequate intravenous intake and maintenance of body temperature are the most important factors.

The extremity should be positioned so that the muscle is relaxed. It should remain splinted in this position for 3 weeks. Following this period, the joints that will be activated by the muscle are actively and passively moved in order to stretch the muscle to its fully stretched length and to develop tendon and muscle gliding. This mechanism of gliding will be used by the muscle during active motion when reinnervation occurs.

When clinical signs of reinnervation occur, the patient should be encouraged to actively use the muscle as much as possible. When a good range of excursion is developed, the patient should be placed on an active resisted exercise program that will significantly improve the strength of the muscle.

TIMING OF TRANSFER

I have used this procedure in patients whose injuries were sustained many years previously and good results were obtained. It is interesting that a motor nerve that has not functioned for up to 25 years has the capability of reinnervating a functioning muscle and providing good muscle contraction.

THERAPEUTIC OUTCOME

A review of our first 36 functioning muscle transfers reveals the following applications and results.

When used to replace the long finger flexors to provide useful grip, the gracilis muscle is outstanding in its capability. A review of our first dozen muscle transfers to the forearm revealed that the muscle was capable of producing a full range of finger excursion in both wrist

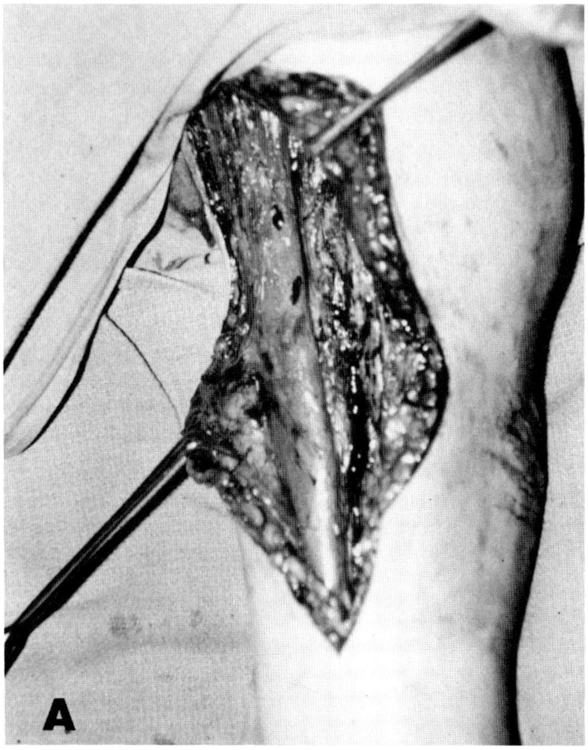

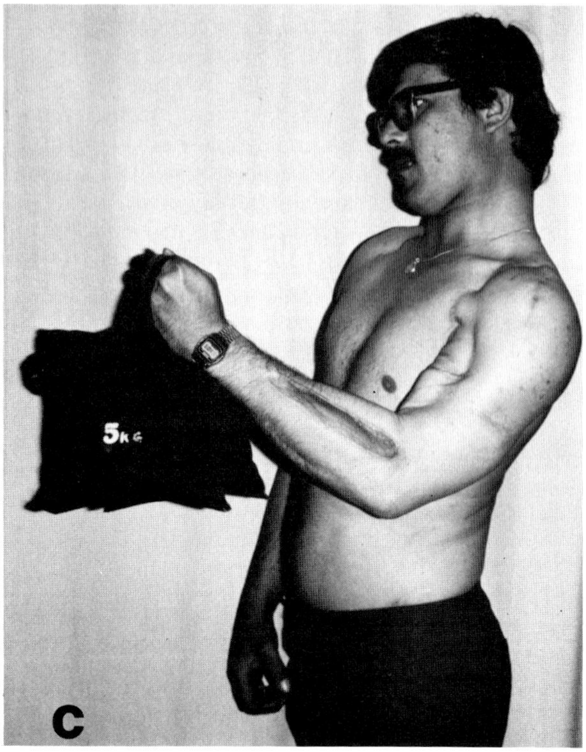

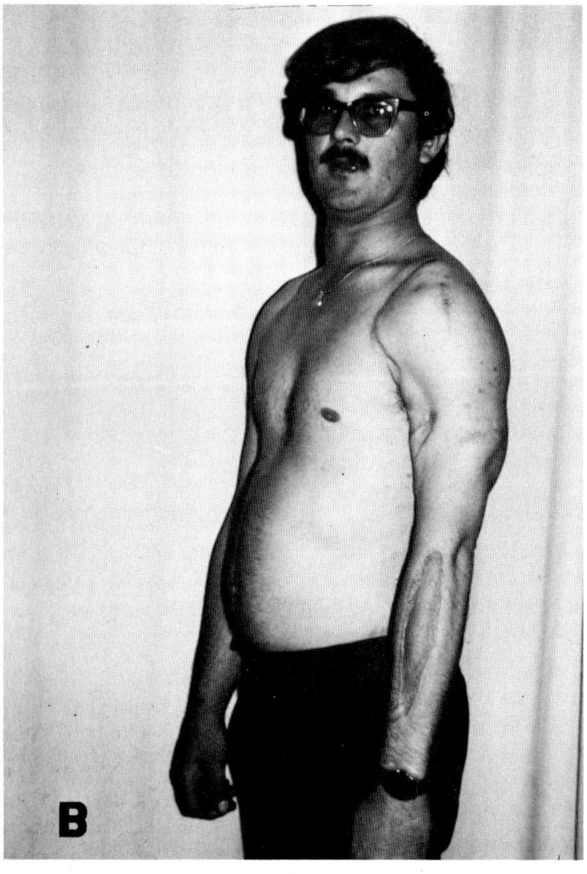

Figure 2 *A*, Patient received a crush injury to upper arm with loss of biceps and brachialis musculature. Gracilis muscle was transferred to anterior compartment and innervated with motor portion of the musculocutaneous nerve. Muscle origin was attached to the coracoid and insertion was attached to biceps tendon. Muscle is seen 4 months postoperatively at incidental exposure when the muscle was separated from surrounding structures during bone grafting of nonunion of humerus. *B*, Patient is seen 1½ years postoperatively with full elbow extension. *C*, Muscle provides full elbow flexion and patient can lift 7 kg held in his hand from a fully extended position.

flexion and extension. The extent of grip strength varied from patient to patient, but in adults the transferred gracilis developed a maximum potential of 50 percent of that of the opposite normal arm. Patients were able to use the extremity for persistent heavy manual activities, such as heavy construction and farm labor, and did not notice undue muscle fatigue (Fig. 2).

PROCEDURE'S STRENGTHS AND WEAKNESSES

The advantages of this procedure are its flexibility in reconstructive design and the functional results achieved. The procedure provides a range of excursion and strength that is frequently greater than that available from standard tendon transfers.

The weaknesses of this procedure are related to its complexity and the duration of time before maximum benefit is obtained. The potential for error in this operative procedure is greater than that in most surgical and microsurgical procedures. Improper patient selection, errors in surgical technique, and incorrect postoperative care will result in a failed procedure and a disappointed surgeon and patient. Many patients are not suitable for this procedure because the addition of a single muscle to an already severely compromised extremity will not make a significant difference in the functional value of the extremity. Caution must be applied to the surgeon's enthusiasm for carrying out this exciting operative procedure.

SUGGESTED READING

Carlson FD, Wilkie DR. Muscle physiology. Englewood, NJ: Prentice-Hall, 1974.

Gordon AM, Huxley AF, Julian FJ. The variation in isometric tension with sarcomere length in vertebrate muscle fibers. J Physiol 1966; 184:170–192.

Manktelow RT. Microvascular reconstruction: anatomy, applications and surgical technique. Heidelberg: Springer Verlag, 1986.

Manktelow RT. Muscle transplantation. In: Green DP, ed. Operative hand surgery. New York: Churchill Livingstone, 1987.

Manktelow RT, McKee NH. Free muscle transplantation to provide active finger flexion. J Hand Surg 1978; 3(5):416–426.

Manktelow RT, Zuker RM, McKee NH. Functioning free muscle transplantation. J Hand Surg 1984; 9A:32–39.

IMPLANTS IN THE HAND AND WRIST

VERNON L. YOUNG, M.D.
BARRY FERNANDO, M.D.
R. EVAN CRANDALL, M.D.

Autogenous and alloplastic materials have been used in the hand and wrist to replace bones and joints and to resurface articular surfaces. Bone replacement has been performed for avascular necrosis, fractures, nonunion, and arthritis. Joint replacement has been performed for traumatic destruction of all or portions of the articular surface, degenerative or osteoarthritis, rheumatoid arthritis, postinfectious arthritis, and several less common arthritides. Proper choice of arthroplastic technique can result in dramatic relief of pain, functional improvement measured by increased movement and strength, and improved appearance. Autogenous materials have included tendons, ligaments, joints, and cartilage. Tendons are used primarily as space occupiers following resection of bones. The only common use of ligaments is proximal interphalangeal (PIP) joint hemiarthroplasty. Joint transfers have included the use of metatarsophalangeal and interphalangeal joints of toes and portions of joints harvested from fingers undergoing amputation. Both free and vascularized joint transfers have been performed. Free joint transfers have produced poor results because of failure of union and avascular necrosis. Hemijoint transfers have suffered from similar problems. Even when these transfers have survived, joint mobility has been poor as a result of capsular scarring and tendon adhesions. The transfer of vascularized joints has eliminated the problem of survival and nonunion; however, joint mobility remains a major problem. Vascularized joint transfers are largely restricted to the pediatric age group, where joint mobility is better. Open epiphyseal plates are included here as part of vascularized joint transfer; these plates continue to grow after transfer. We have not used cartilage grafts to resurface joints in the hand or wrist.

A number of alloplastic materials have been used for joint or bone replacement in the hand and wrist, but only silicone has achieved widespread use. Silicone has been used to replace the metacarpophalangeal and proximal interphalangeal joints in the fingers, the trapezium, the lunate for Kienböck's disease, the scaphoid for fracture nonunion and avascular necrosis, and for resectional wrist arthroplasty. Functional results following these arthroplasties and bone replacements have been variable. Proximal interphalangeal joint replacement has been moderately successful; results are often influenced by scarring of the joint capsule, tendon adhesions, and the individual's response to silicone. Metacarpophalangeal (MP) joint replacement for rheumatoid arthritis combined with soft tissue release, realignment of the extensor tendons, and balance of the intrinsic muscles has resulted in cosmetic and functional improvement. Resection of the trapezium and replacement with a silicone joint spacer—either a great toe prosthesis or trapezium implant—for degenerative arthritis at the carpometacarpal (CMC) joint has produced excellent results with relief of pain and good motion. The main functional drawback has been decreased strength, particularly in opening jars or in rotary movement. Complications have included dislocation, fracture and wear of the prosthesis, and silicone rubber synovitis. Resectional wrist arthroplasty for rheumatoid arthritis has produced good functional and cosmetic results. The main drawbacks to this procedure include fracture, dislocation, and migration of the prosthesis. Currently, the prostheses are fitted with titanium metal grommets to avoid these complications. However, there is no proof that this innovation has solved these problems. Replacement of the lunate and scaphoid has been less successful and has been plagued with problems of dislocation, alteration of the carpal architecture, and silicone rubber synovitis.

Silicone rubber synovitis has resulted in recent important changes in the use of silicone implants. The mechanism of development of silicone rubber synovitis is wear and fragmentation at the surface of the implant, which results in shedding of microparticles of silicone ranging from 0.5 to 1 μm in diameter. As the microparticles are shed, they are phagocytized by giant cells, which subsequently produce a synovial reaction. This synovial proliferation and hypertrophy subsequently invades adjacent bones and produces cystic lesions (Fig. 1). Silicone synovitis can also spread to noncontiguous carpal bones and to the radius. The mechanism of spread of the silicone synovitis to nonadjacent bones is unclear. Patients with silicone synovitis may remain asymptomatic for months to years. Once wrist pain develops, removal of the implant and curetting of the cystic lesions is required to arrest the process. Reinsertion of a new silicone implant is contraindicated because it results in recurrence of the syndrome. The incidence of silicone rubber synovitis for various joints and bones is 75 percent for scaphoid implants, 55 percent for lunate implants, and 3 percent for trapezium implants. The syndrome is much less common with proximal interphalangeal, metacarpophalangeal joint, and wrist arthroplasties. The lower incidence in these joints is probably because the joints are exposed in different load and shear forces than carpal bones. In 25 patients evaluated with roentgenograms 1 to 7 years following trapezium replacement, we found 92 percent of the patients had radiographic changes that were attributable to silicone arthroplasty. Three of those patients developed symptomatic silicone synovitis that required removal of the implant and curetting of multiple cystic lesions. To date we have not had any patients who have developed silicone synovitis following PIP joint, MP joint, or wrist arthroplasty. As a result of our experience and that of others, we no longer recommend replacement of the trapezium, scaphoid, or lunate with silicone prostheses. We still perform silicone replacement arthroplasty for the PIP joint, MP joint, and wrist. The remainder of this chapter is devoted to the management of joint replacement at each joint.

DISTAL INTERPHALANGEAL JOINTS AND THUMB INTERPHALANGEAL JOINTS

We do not use silicone replacement arthroplasty in the distal interphalangeal (DIP) joints in the fingers or in-

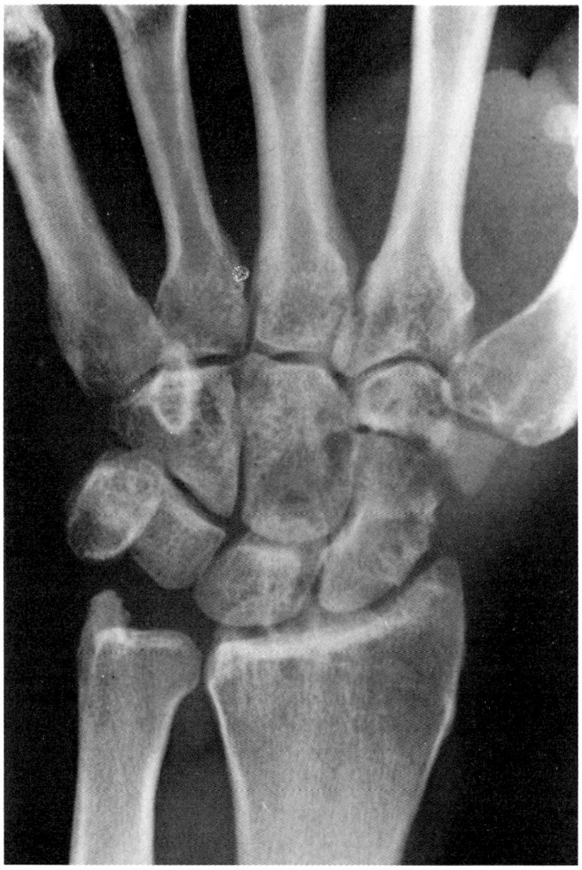

Figure 1 Multiple cystic lesions in the carpal bones associated with silicone synovitis.

terphalangeal (IP) joint in the thumb because stability of pinch is critical at these joints. Silicone replacement arthroplasty can result in unstable pinch at this joint level. Our management of painful arthritis in these joints is initial treatment with nonsteroidal, anti-inflammatory drugs. When that management fails, we perform joint fusion. Because joint fusion at this level is unpredictable and can require prolonged immobilization, we combine bone grafting with fusion. This results in a shorter period of immobilization and an increased incidence of primary fusion.

PROXIMAL INTERPHALANGEAL JOINTS

Joint Replacement with Silicone Joint Spacers

The indications for PIP joint arthroplasty with silicone joint spacers include degenerative or osteoarthritis, traumatic joint destruction, and rheumatoid arthritis. All PIP joints can be replaced in individuals who do not perform physical labor. Replacement of the PIP joint of the index finger in some individuals results in unstable pinch. If the patient is a manual laborer and has multiple joints involved, it is usually best to fuse the PIP joint of the index finger at 30 degrees to 40 degrees. Stability of pinch in the long and ring fingers is less important; PIP joint replacement here produces satisfactory results. Movement is critical for strength in the little finger, and PIP joint replacement is ideal for that finger. Contraindications to PIP joint replacement include inadequate skin coverage and bone stock and irreparable destruction of the flexor or extensor tendon mechanisms. Joint replacement can be performed through either a palmar or a dorsal approach. The joint should be approached through a dorsal incision if the flexor tendon mechanism does not require surgery. A curved dorsal incision is made over the PIP joint, extending from the proximal midphalanx to the midproximal phalanx. The extensor tendon mechanism is split longitudinally, thus allowing exposure of the PIP joint. The attachment of the central slip to the base of the middle phalanx is preserved. The head of the proximal phalanx is resected with a saw, preserving the collateral ligaments if possible. The medullary cavity of the proximal phalanx is reamed out in a rectangular shape to accept the prosthesis. The cartilage is removed from the base of the middle phalanx and a guided burr is used to create a rectangular cavity in the middle phalanx. Sizing implants are used to achieve a proper-fitting prosthesis. A proper-fitting prosthesis should allow the hinge of the prosthesis to fit flush with the end of the proximal phalanx and the base of the middle phalanx. The joint should be moved through a complete range of motion to be sure that the bone edges do not impinge on the prosthesis or block flexion or extension. Metal grommets can occasionally be used in PIP joint replacement, but their use is not routinely possible because of the size of implants used in these joints. The average range of motion following PIP joint replacement for degenerative arthritis and rheumatoid arthritis is 65 degrees to 75 degrees. The range of motion is less when these implants are used for joint replacement at the time of replantation or following traumatic injuries. Injuries to the flexor and extensor tendon mechanisms and soft tissues limit the range of motion in these patients.

Advancement of the Volar Plate

The other arthroplasty that we use in the PIP joint is advancement of the volar plate onto the articular surface of the middle phalanx. This is used following fractures that involve the articular surface of the middle phalanx with loss of a significant portion of the articular cartilage or destruction of the volar aspect of the middle phalanx. The joint is approached through a volar zigzag incision that identifies the digital nerves and tendon sheath. The tendon sheath is opened and the volar plate is detached distally and freed proximally. The surface of the middle phalanx is smoothed with a rongeur or burr. The surface of the proximal phalanx must be smooth and even to allow the PIP joint to move in a normal arc. Any irregularities will impair movement, thus resulting in angulation and subsequent pain. When the surface of the middle phalanx is smooth, the joint is flexed, and the volar plate is advanced to the surface of the middle phalanx and attached there with sutures. Secure, smooth attachment usually requires drilling small holes through the base of the middle phalanx and passing sutures through this bone to anchor the volar plate. At the completion of the procedure, the joint should be flexed approximately 40 degrees. It is left in that position for approximately 3 weeks, during which time active flexion is carried out. An extension block splint is used to prevent full extension. Thereafter, extension of the finger is progressively increased at approximately 10 degrees per week. The functional results of this type of arthroplasty are excellent.

METACARPOPHALANGEAL JOINTS

The main indications for replacement arthroplasty in the metacarpophalangeal joints of the fingers are rheumatoid arthritis and, less commonly, degenerative arthritis and posttraumatic deformities. We use silicone joint spacers for MP joint replacement. Patients chosen for this procedure should be well motivated and have adequate bone stock to allow resection of the metacarpal head and insertion of the prosthesis. Replacement of a single joint is uncommon, but when necessary, is performed through a curved dorsal incision. Typically, multiple joints are replaced at the same time and the incision used is a transverse one over the dorsum of the distal hand. In the index and little fingers, the joints are exposed through an incision between the independent and common extensor tendons. In the ring and long fingers, a longitudinal incision is made through the ulnar aspect of the dorsal hood. Each of these incisions allows relocation of the extensor tendons at the completion of the procedure. The metacarpal head is resected and the medullary cavity is reamed in a rectangular fashion to allow insertion of the implant. The attachments of the collateral ligaments should be preserved if possible. The cartilage is resected from the base of the proximal phalanx and the medullary cavity is reamed in a similar rectangular fashion. If the base of the proximal phalanx is deformed from chronic subluxation, it should be converted to a smooth transverse surface. The volar plate and fibro-osseus tunnel should be mobilized from the base of the proximal phalanx prior to the contouring. The soft tissues are released to allow proper relocation of the proximal phalanx on the metacarpal. The ulnar intrinsic tendons are identified and divided. Sufficient tendon length should be maintained to allow transfer of the ulnar intrinsic to the radial intrinsic of the adjacent finger to help correct ulnar drift. When soft tissue release is completed, a proper-sized implant is chosen. The dorsal surface of the metacarpal is recontoured for insertion of a titanium metal grommet; the volar surface of the proximal phalanx is similarly contoured.These grommets are press fitted into the defect in the respective bones. Once the grommets are in place, a proper-sized implant is inserted and the soft tissue is reconstructed. This should include reinsertion of the radial collateral ligaments, ulnar intrinsic transfer, and extensor tendon realignment. The radial collateral ligaments should be adjusted to correct ulnar drift of the fingers. Transfer of the ulnar intrinsic of one finger to the radial intrinsic of the adjacent finger also helps prevent ulnar drift. The extensor tendon mechanism should be reefed in an overlapping fashion so that the extensor tendon is brought slightly to the radial side of the center of the joint. Postoperative care consists of a bulky dressing applied at the time of surgery. In 3 to 5 days, the dressing is removed, and movement and splinting are initiated.

Metacarpophalangeal Joint of the Thumb

We do not routinely perform silicone replacement arthroplasty in the MP joint of the thumb. However, thumb MP joint replacement is necessary if both the CMC and IP joints require fusion. Fusion of all three joints results in severe disability, and it is critical to preserve motion at either the CMC or the MP joint. If CMC joint function is adequate, MP joint fusion is a better procedure because it relieves pain and provides stable pinch. Silicone joint arthroplasty can result in unstable pinch. The technique of joint replacement is similar to that of MP joint arthroplasty. The joint is approached through a curved-dorsal incision. The adductor aponeurosis is divided, and the extensor pollicis longus is retracted radially. The head of the metacarpal is resected and the medullary cavity is reamed to accept a prosthesis. The collateral ligaments should be preserved if possible. If these ligaments are divided, the ulnar ligament should be reattached or reconstructed with a tendon graft to provide stable pinch. The medullary cavity of the proximal phalanx is reamed with a guided burr. Sizing implants are used to determine the proper size. Titanium grommets are used if possible. Therapy is initiated 5 to 7 days postoperatively.

Fusion of the thumb MP joint is performed through a curved dorsal incision. The adductor aponeurosis is divided and the extensor pollicis longus is retracted to expose the joint. The articular surface is removed from the head of the metacarpal, taking more off the volar aspect. The articular surface of the proximal phalanx is removed, and this leaves a smooth transverse surface. Power tools should not be used to contour bones for fusion, as the heat generated both kills cells and can interfere with fusion. The bony surfaces are fitted together to access the angle of fusion. The desired angle is between 15 degrees to 30 degrees. After final contouring with a rongeur, a radial to ulnar hole is drilled through both bones with a 1-mm Kirschner wire. A 26-gauge wire is passed through these holes and tightened. This provides both compression and control of rotation. A 1-mm Kirschner wire across the fusion site completes stabilization. Bone grafting is usually not necessary, but can salvage nonunions. Fusion is usually complete in 2 to 3 months and provides stable, pain-free pinch.

CARPOMETACARPAL JOINT OF THE THUMB

Degenerative arthritis is the most common indication for arthroplasty of the CMC joint of the thumb. This is primarily a disease of middle-aged women. The initial management consists of analgesics and nonsteroidal anti-inflammatory drugs; surgery is reserved for failure of conservative therapy. In the recent past, our preferred surgical treatment of CMC arthritis of the thumb was resection of the trapezium and replacement with a silicone great toe prosthesis. Recent experience with silicone synovitis associated with this joint arthroplasty has convinced us that this procedure should not be performed until the natural history of silicone synovitis is better understood. We recommend follow-up at yearly intervals with roentgenograms in patients who have undergone trapezium resection and silicone joint arthroplasty. In a recent review of these patients, we found ulnar wear of the prosthesis in 44 percent, radial scaphoid depression in 44 percent, scaphoid lucencies in 32 percent, loosening of the stem in 28 percent, implant resorption in 8 percent, and lucencies in other carpal bones in 12 percent. Three patients out of our series of 100 have developed symptomatic silicone synovitis requiring removal of the implant and curetting of cysts from multiple carpal bones. The majority of patients have remained asymptomatic. In general, they have a good range of motion and good strength. The main functional disability that patients have expressed is difficulty in opening jars.

Our current method of management is resection of the trapezium and replacement with a tendon "rolled anchovy"—usually the palmaris longus. There is no proof that a tendon rolled anchovy is essential following resection of the trapezium. Some authors comparing this procedure to resection alone have shown no difference in range of motion or strength. We use it because we think it occupies the space resulting from resection of the trapezium and prevents proximal migration of the thumb metacarpal. The trapezium is approached through a curved incision over the base of the thumb at the first dorsal compartment. The radial artery and the sensory branches of the radial nerve are identified and protected. The first dorsal compartment is opened and the extensor pollicis brevis and abductor pollicis longus retracted. The joint capsule of the CMC joint is opened longitudinally and reflected from the trapezium. Preservation of the capsule is critical to postoperative joint stability. The entire trapezium is resected piecemeal with a rongeur. Failure to resect the entire trapezium can result in recurrent pain because of subsequent development of arthritis between the residual trapezium and other carpal bones. The palmaris longus is harvested with a tendon stripper, the muscle is removed, and the tendon is sutured into a roll "anchovy" with 4–0 Supramed. The anchovy is packed into the cavity resulting from trapezium resection and the joint capsule is closed. The thumb and wrist are kept immobilized for 6 weeks, after which time hand therapy is initiated. This procedure provides excellent pain relief, and mobility and strength are equal to that achieved with replacement with a great toe prosthesis.

WRIST

The indications for implant replacement arthroplasty in the wrist include advanced rheumatoid arthritis and, less commonly, posttraumatic and osteoarthritis. The results of this arthroplasty have been excellent in patients with rheumatoid arthritis. There is good correction of the cosmetic deformity and pain relief. However, improvement in strength and motion are less dramatic. Complications associated with silicone replacement arthroplasty include fracture, dislocation, and migration of the prosthesis. The use of titanium grommets to correct this problem is unproven. Silicone synovitis is rare with this arthroplasty. Young, active patients with posttraumatic arthritis are more likely to have problems with fracture and migration of prosthesis and should be warned that they may eventually need wrist fusion.

Implant arthroplasty in the wrist is approached through a curved dorsal incision, in order to identify and protect the sensory branch of the radial nerve and the dorsal sensory branch of the ulnar nerve. Superficial veins are preserved where possible. The extensor retinaculum is elevated as a radially-based flap to expose the extensor tendons. A synovectomy is performed if necessary. Retraction of the tendons exposes the radiocarpal joint capsule, which is elevated from the radius, ulna, and proximal carpal bones as a distally-based flap. The distal radius is resected; this produces a smooth transverse surface. The head of the ulna is resected in a similar manner, thus preserving the periosteum. The ulna should be resected, thus preserving a portion of the attachment of the pronator quadratus to minimize subsequent subluxation. The remains of the scaphoid and lunate are removed along with the proximal portions of the capitate and triquetrum. The medullary cavity of the radius is reamed to accept the implant and a dorsal titanium grommet. A 2-mm Kirschner wire is driven through the capitate into the base of the long finger metacarpal. This forms a channel that is subsequently used to ream the capitate and metacarpal for the implant and a volar grommet. The sizing implants are used to determine the appropriate implant, and small holes are drilled in the dorsal radius to reattach the wrist capsule. The grommets are press fitted, the implant is inserted, and the wrist capsule is reattached with preplaced 3–0 nonabsorbable sutures. The periosteum is closed over the distal ulna. No ulnar cap is added. The dorsal retinaculum is sutured beneath the extensor tendons and the skin is closed over a drain. The wrist is immobilized for 4 weeks, after which time hand therapy is begun.

Lunate

Replacement of the lunate with a Silastic joint spacer has been a standard treatment for Kienböck's disease. Problems associated with this arthroplasty include dislocation and fracture of the prosthesis, proximal migration of the capitate, compression of the prosthesis, and silicone synovitis (50 percent). We currently do not recommend the use of a silicone joint spacer for lunate replacement for Kienböck's disease. Some authors are currently recommending continued use of this joint spacer, protecting it from shear and loading forces by performing a triscaphoid fusion. There is no evidence that the addition of a joint spacer to a triscaphoid fusion improves functional results or diminishes pain. Our current management of Kienböck's disease is dependent on the stage of the disease. In Stages O through II, where the lunate architecture is maintained and there is no arthritis or loss of scapholunate ligament integrity or instability pattern, treatment involves unloading the lunate by performing a triscaphoid fusion. In more advanced stages where there is cystic degeneration or fragmentation of the lunate with loss of architecture or development of radiocarpal arthritis, we remove the lunate and perform a triscaphoid fusion. Failure to remove a damaged lunate in which there are cystic changes can result in persistence of pain. We have had patients in which the lunate was not removed, and the patient continued to complain of pain; subsequent removal of the lunate resulted in relief of the pain.

Scaphoid

Silicone replacement arthroplasty has been recommended for nonunion of scaphoid fractures, degenerative arthritis at the radiocarpal joint, and avascular necrosis of portions of the scaphoid. The problems associated with this arthroplasty include dislocation of the prosthesis and silicone synovitis (75 percent). Because of the frequency of silicone synovitis and other associated problems, we do not recommend the use of silicone prostheses at this time. For nonunion of the scaphoid, we perform bone grafting. For degenerative arthritis that fails management with analgesics, we perform a wrist fusion. We do not recommend proximal row carpectomy because the long-term results are unsatisfactory.

SUGGESTED READING

Beckenbaugh RD. Total wrist arthroplasty: review of current concepts. In: Lightman DM, ed. The wrist and its disorders. Philadelphia: WB Saunders, 1988.

Bieber EJ, Weiland AJ, Volenec-Dowling S. Silicone-rubber implant arthroplasty of the metacarpophalangeal joints for rheumatoid arthritis. J Bone Joint Surg 1986; 68-A:206–209.

Brase DW, Millender LH. Failure of silicone rubber wrist arthroplasty in rheumatoid arthritis. J Hand Surg 1986; 11-A:175–183.

Burton RI, Margles SW, Lunseth PA. Small-joint arthrodesis in the hand. J Hand Surg 1986; 11-A:678–682.

Eaton RG, Glickel SZ. Trapezoimetacarpal osteoarthritis: staging as a rationale for treatment. Hand Clin 1987; 3(4).

Fatti JF, Palmer AK, Mosher JF. The long-term results of Swanson silicone rubber interpositional wrist arthroplasty. J Hand Surg 1986; 11-A:166–175.

Pellegrini VD, Burton RI. Surgical management of basal joint arthritis of the thumb: 1. Long-term results of silicone implant arthroplasty. J Hand Surg 1986; 11-A:309–324.

Swanson AB, Swanson G. Implant arthroplasty in the carpal and radiocarpal joints. In: Lightman DM, ed. The wrist and its disorders. Philadelphia: WB Saunders, 1988.

Watson HK, Brenner LH. Degenerative disorders of the carpus. In: Lightman DM, ed. The wrist and its disorders. Philadelphia: WB Saunders, 1988.

NAILBED INJURIES

ELVIN G. ZOOK, M.D.

Injury to the fingertip is the most common hand injury and roughly half involve the nailbed. Injuries to the nailbed occur when force is applied to the nail and the bed is compressed between the nail and the underlying bone and thus crushed apart. The vast majority of nailbed injuries are crushing injuries rather than lacerations, since a blow from a sharp object with enough force to penetrate the nail usually amputates the tip. The anatomy and physiology of the perionychium should be reviewed for maximum understanding.

SUBUNGUAL HEMATOMA

Subungual hematomas are the result of disruption of the nailbed with bleeding beneath the nail. The hematoma, under pressure, causes dissection of the nailbed from the nail and, usually, severe throbbing pain. As a rule, the larger the nailbed disruption, the larger the subungual hematoma. If more than 25 percent of the visible nail is undermined by hematoma, serious consideration should be given to removal of the entire nail, repair of the nailbed wound, and replacement of the nail. If throbbing pain occurs and it is elected not to remove the nail, it can be perforated to relieve the pressure. Perforation is accomplished by heating the tip of a straightened paper clip with an alcohol lamp until red-hot. The heated tip is pressed against the nail over the hematoma. The paper clip rapidly penetrates the nail and the tip is cooled when it strikes the hematoma, thus preventing further injury to the nailbed. Another excellent technique for nail perforation is the ophthalmologic cautery available in most emergency rooms. Both methods leave a round, smooth, permanent hole in the nail, which will stay open and continue to drain for several days. The use of a nail drill is painful. A needle or scalpel blade makes only a small slit that evacuates the hematoma initially, but allows clot to obstruct effective drainage from beneath the nail. Prior to nail perforation, the finger should be prepped with a standard surgical preparation to decrease chances of infection.

SIMPLE AND STELLATE LACERATIONS

When a localized force is applied to the nail, the compression usually causes a single, straight, crushing laceration. When the force is over a larger area, stellate or bursting lacerations occur. Both are treated in a similar fashion.

If the proximal nail is avulsed from the nail fold, it should be removed because injury to the nailbed is almost always present. The nail is removed from the nailbed by dissection either with a small, smooth-edge periosteal (Kutz or Freer) elevator (Fig. 1) or by gentle spreading of fine iris scissors. Dissection is from the hyponychium proximally and beneath the eponychium. Nailbed injuries may be treated in the emergency room with finger block and careful surgical preparation and drape. The nail is removed and the nailbed explored. If the edges of the nailbed wound are irregular, they may be trimmed carefully. However, since the nailbed is so adherent to the underlying bone, it is difficult to remove nailbed without causing tension on the closure. If there is any question, it is better to reapproximate the jagged edges of the nailbed carefully than to trim them smooth and then approximate with tension. It is difficult to approximate the nailbed without tension if more than 1 mm of nailbed has been removed. Even with the removal of 1 mm, the nailbed should be elevated from the surrounding periosteum to allow tension-free approximation. The nail is washed with soap and water; the undersurface is scraped to remove fragments of nailbed, and soaked in Betadine solution while the nailbed is repaired.

Loupe magnification facilitates and improves the repair of the nailbed. My suture preference is 7–0 chromic suture on a double arm microspatula ophthalmic 3/8 cutting needle. Division of the suture in the center provides two needles in case one is bent during suture. The knot tails of the 7–0 chromic suture are cut short to avoid interference with the molding of the nailbed by the replaced nail. A perforation for drainage is made in the nail in an area away from the repair. The cleaned nail is replaced over the repaired nailbed and into the nail fold. A 5–0 nylon suture is placed through the nail and the tip of the finger to maintain the nail in the nail fold.

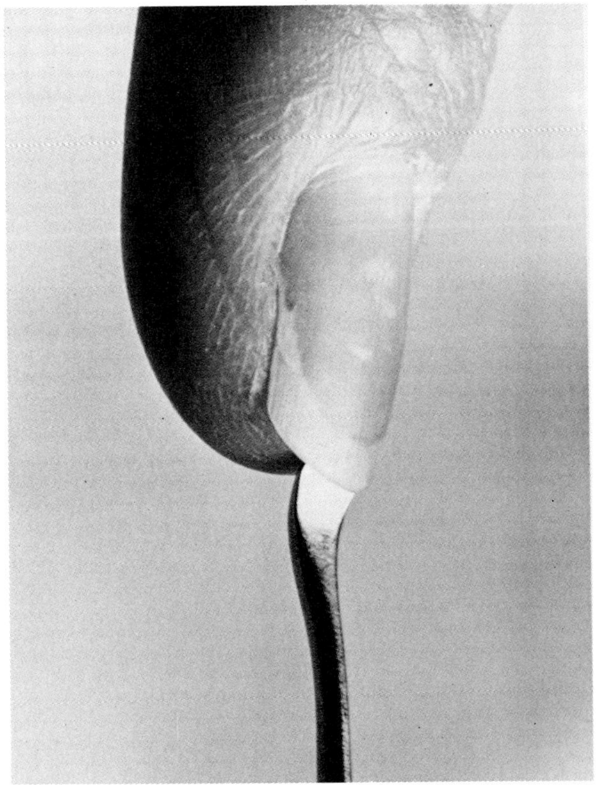

Figure 1 A Kutz elevator is used to separate nail from nailbed.

Lacerations through the dorsal roof of the nail fold and dorsal skin should be carefully repaired to prevent synechia in the fold, with resultant split nail. The dorsal roof is approximated with 7–0 chromic suture, with the knots in the fold not buried in the tissue, and the skin is sutured with 6–0 monofilament nylon. Nail, silicone sheet, or gauze must be placed and maintained in the fold to keep the raw surfaces of the roof and floor apart until healing occurs.

SEVERE CRUSH

In severe crush injuries, the area of compression between the nail and the distal phalanx is wide, thus causing multiple lacerations and partially or completely free fragments of nailbed. It is important that no nailbed be discarded, for it cannot be replaced with anything else. Small fragments of nailbed attached to the nail should be removed and replaced on the avulsion site. Lacerations and fragments should be approximated as accurately as possible with fine chromic sutures.

If the nail is intact, or enough remains to cover the repair site, it should be used. The nail molds the approximated edges, reduces pain, improves sensation, keeps the nail fold open, and maintains reduction of fractures of the distal phalanx and tuft. Otherwise, a nail-shaped piece of .020 silicone sheet, or nonadherent gauze, is placed in the nail fold and over the nailbed repair. Silicone sheet has a tendency to slide out of the fold so it should be maintained in place by a fine nonabsorbable suture. It is placed from the dorsal surface of the finger into the proximal nail fold, through the sheet and back out in horizontal mattress fashion, as shown in Figure 2, other than the sheet is sutured rather than the nailbed. The suture is removed in 2 to 3 weeks.

AVULSION

Approximately 15 percent of nailbed injuries involve its avulsion. It varies from avulsion of the proximal nailbed from the nail fold to complete avulsion and loss of the fragment.

Avulsion of a flap occurs because the nailbed is a continuum with the nail. When the nail is avulsed from the nail fold, the nailbed may be torn from the periosteum rather than from the nail. When this occurs, it is essential that the nailbed be replaced in the nail fold as accurately as possible. This is best achieved by removal of the nailbed from the nail if it is still attached. If the nail fold is deep and the laceration is at its proximal extent, incisions to open the nail fold to allow access may be necessary. These are best done at the proximal lateral aspects of the eponychium and at a 90 degree angle from the eponychium (Fig. 3). If the laceration in the nail fold is straight and

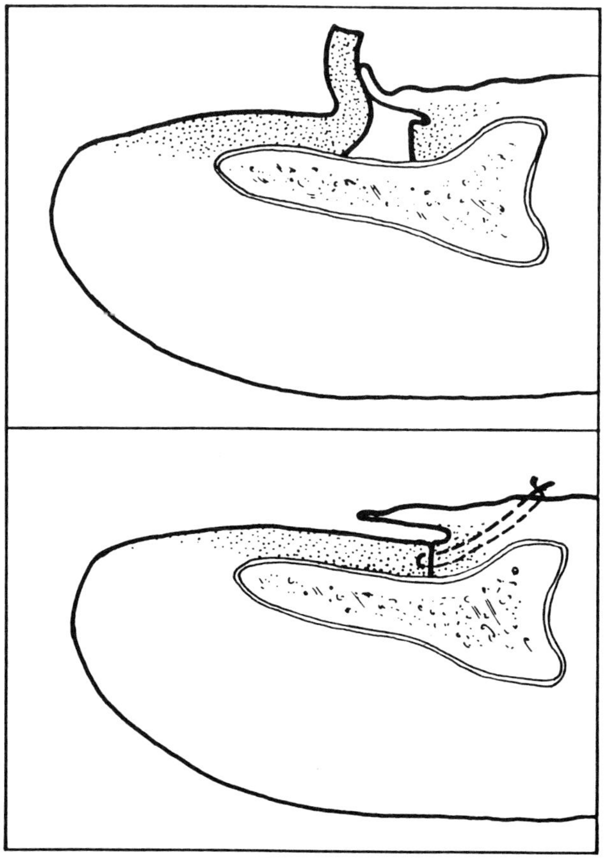

Figure 2 Mattress sutures to replace and maintain nailbed in fold or silicone sheet in the nail fold.

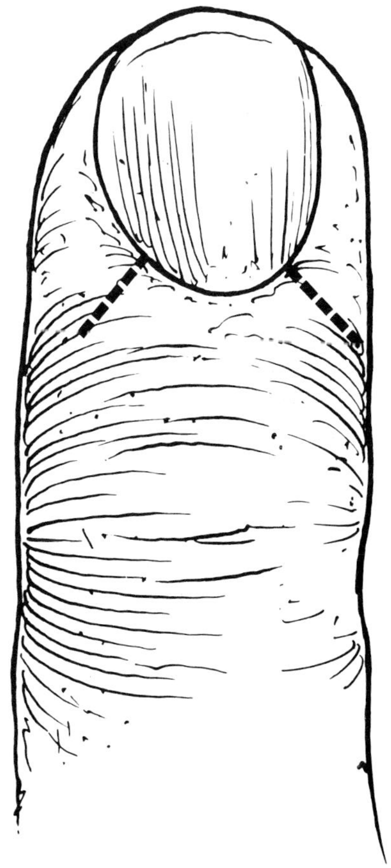

Figure 3 Incisions for exploration of the nail fold.

at the most proximal border of the nailfold, horizontal mattress sutures of 6–0 nylon may be placed through the nail wall in a horizontal mattress fashion, in the middle and at both corners, to pull the nailbed back into position in the nail fold and maintain it there (see Fig. 2). The nail is then cleaned and replaced in the nail fold to approximate further the edges of the laceration.

An attempt should be made to find avulsed fragments of nail, for they may have attached pieces of nailbed that can be used as grafts. If a small area of nail with the underlying nailbed has been avulsed, it may be replaced accurately and held there for several days with a dressing. More injury will be done to the nailbed by trying to remove these small fragments from the nail than by leaving them in place (Fig. 4).

In larger avulsions, the nail may be removed from the outer 2 mm of nailbed to allow accurate suturing of the nailbed into place. If approximation can be carried out accurately, the result is usually excellent since these injuries are frequently sharp.

If the avulsed fragment is missing (Fig. 5A), Shepard has shown us that the use of a split-thickness nail graft from the adjacent nailbed or from a toenail can give excellent results. After the wound has been cleaned and

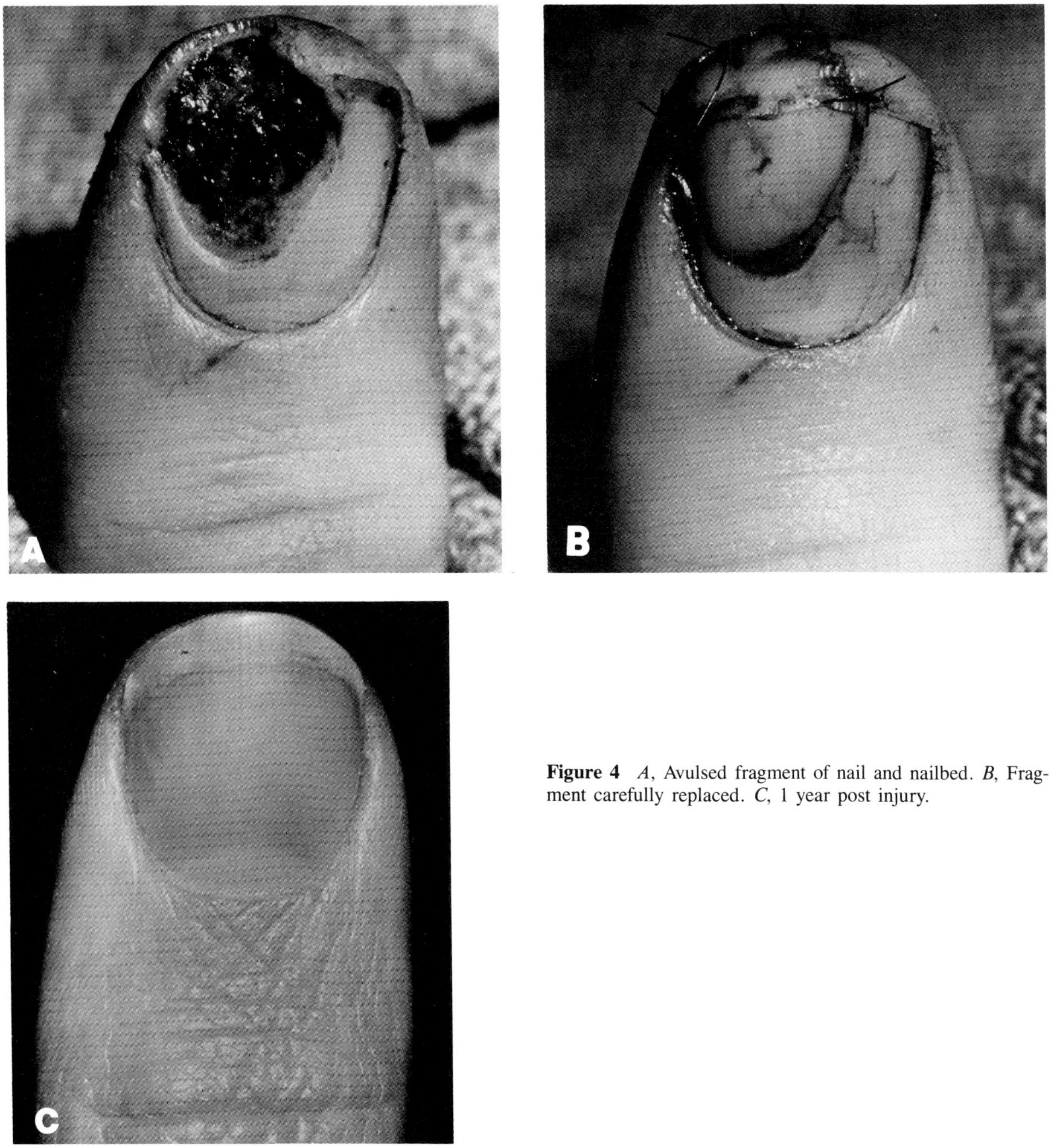

Figure 4 *A*, Avulsed fragment of nail and nailbed. *B*, Fragment carefully replaced. *C*, 1 year post injury.

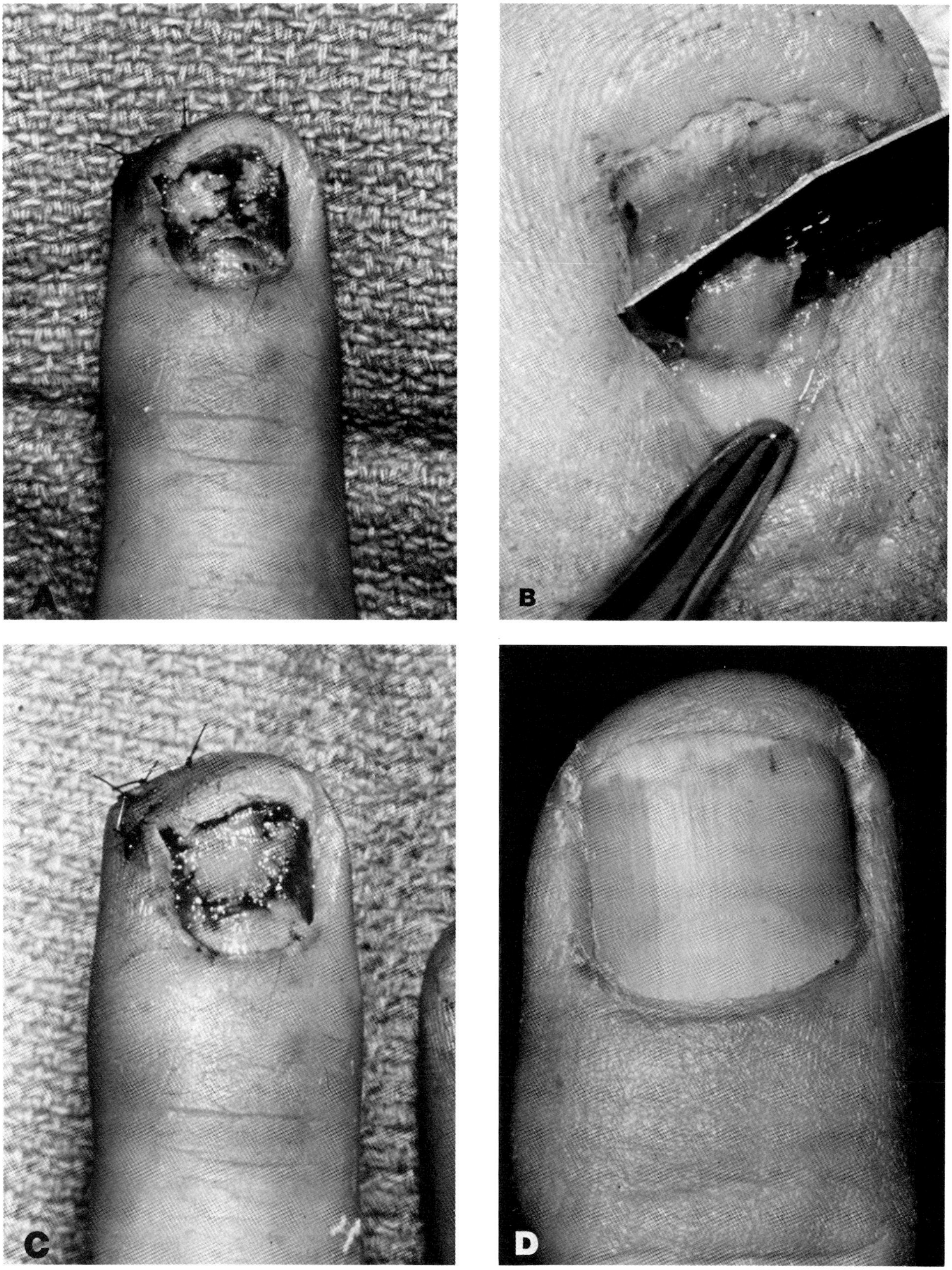

Figure 5 *A*, After suture of lacerations approximately 25 percent of the sterile matrix is missing. *B*, A split-thickness sterile matrix graft is removed from the large toe. *C*, Graft sutured into the defect. *D*, 1 year post injury.

examined under tourniquet, and it has been determined that nailbed is missing, the remainder of the nailbed is examined. If the nailbed of an adjacent area of the same nail is large enough for the harvesting of the split-thickness nailbed graft, this is used to cover the defect. The split-thickness nailbed graft is removed with a 15 scalpel blade and loupe or microscope magnification (Fig. 5B). The side or tip of the blade is used and an attempt made to remove the nailbed approximately .012 to .014 of an inch thick. Shepard's experience, as well as mine, has shown that if done carefully, no further deformity of the nailbed occurs. The nailbed graft is then placed over the defect and sutured with 7–0 chromic suture (Fig. 5C). The nail, Silastic sheet, or gauze is placed over the graft. The dressing is left in place for 7 to 10 days before removal of the dressing to allow adherence of the graft, since movement may disrupt it (Fig. 5D).

In my experience, if there is not enough surface available on the adjacent nailbed to cover the defect, there will not be enough nailbed graft available on any but the large toe. The large toenail is removed with an elevator or scissors; a split-thickness nailbed graft is removed from the toenail bed, as previously described and the large toenail is replaced and sutured distally. Harvest of a split-thickness nail bed graft from the large toe gives surprisingly little discomfort, and the patient is usually able to ambulate with little difficulty in a few days. A new nail will grow and force the old toenail distally. It takes 6 months to a year for the toenail to grow out completely.

It takes approximately 3 to 4 months for full growth of a fingernail, and about three full growths before maximum smoothness occurs. Therefore, the patient should be warned that it will take at least a year for maximum recovery and any revision should not be contemplated before then.

A split-thickness graft of germinal matrix will not grow nail. Only a full-thickness germinal matrix graft will do so, and its harvest deforms a toe.

It must be remembered that nowhere is the timely care of an acute injury more important than in nailbed injuries. Reconstruction and revisions of nail deformities are never as successful as appropriate early care.

SUGGESTED READING

Ashbell TS, Kleinert HK, Putcha S, Kutz JE. The deformed fingernail, a frequent result of failure to repair nailbed injuries. J Trauma 1967; 7:177–190.

Schiller C. Nail replacement in fingertip injuries. Plast Reconstr Surg 1957; 19:521–530.

Shepard GH. Treatment of nailbed avulsions with split-thickness nailbed grafts. J Hand Surg 1983; 8:49–54.

Zook EG. Complications of the perionychium. Hand Clin 1986; 2:407–427.

Zook EG. Injuries of the fingernail. In: Green DP, ed. Operative hand surgery. New York: Churchill Livingston. 1st ed., 1982:895 and 2nd ed. 1988:1331.

Zook EG. Nail bed injuries. Hand Clinics 1985; 1:701–716.

Zook EG, Guy RJ, Russell RC. A study of nailbed injuries: causes, treatment and prognosis. J Hand Surg 1984; 9A:247–252.

FINGERTIP INJURIES

ROBERT R. SCHENCK, M.D.

Though fingertip injuries occur extremely commonly, treatment is often less than ideal. The aim of fingertip reconstruction should be to provide stable, painless skin coverage that has both adequate sensory function and acceptable appearance. My preferred method to accomplish these objectives is the hypothenar full-thickness skin graft.

THERAPEUTIC ALTERNATIVES

Numerous methods can be used to treat fingertip injuries. These include composite replacement, open method, split-thickness and full-thickness skin grafts, revision with direct closure, local advancement flaps, cross finger flaps, thenar flaps, distant pedicle flaps, and free microneurovascularized flaps. All of these have particular advantages and disadvantages; however, the simpler methods usually suffice for the more common injuries.

PREFERRED APPROACH

The hypothenar full-thickness skin graft technique is easy to use, predictable in its results, and satisfying to both patient and surgeon. An elliptical skin graft is excised from the ulnar aspect of the palm, designed so that its longitudinal axis is parallel and only slightly volar to the lateral axis of the hand (Fig. 1B). Sharp dissection is used to remove as much subcutaneous fat as possible from the graft as it is taken (Fig. 1C). The donor area is closed with 3–0 Nylon sutures, alternating between vertical mattress and simple types (Fig. 1D). Any remaining fat is removed by using two hemostats to secure the corners of the free graft, draping the inverted skin over the surgeon's index finger, and then applying the convexity of a curved scissors against the dermal side of the graft (Fig. 2A).

Minimal debridement of the injured fingertip is performed as indicated, and any protruding bone is removed with a rongeur to a level slightly lower than the surrounding soft tissue. The defatted skin graft is then tailored to match the area of skin loss and sutured in place with 4–0 silk sutures that are left long, to be tied later over a bolus

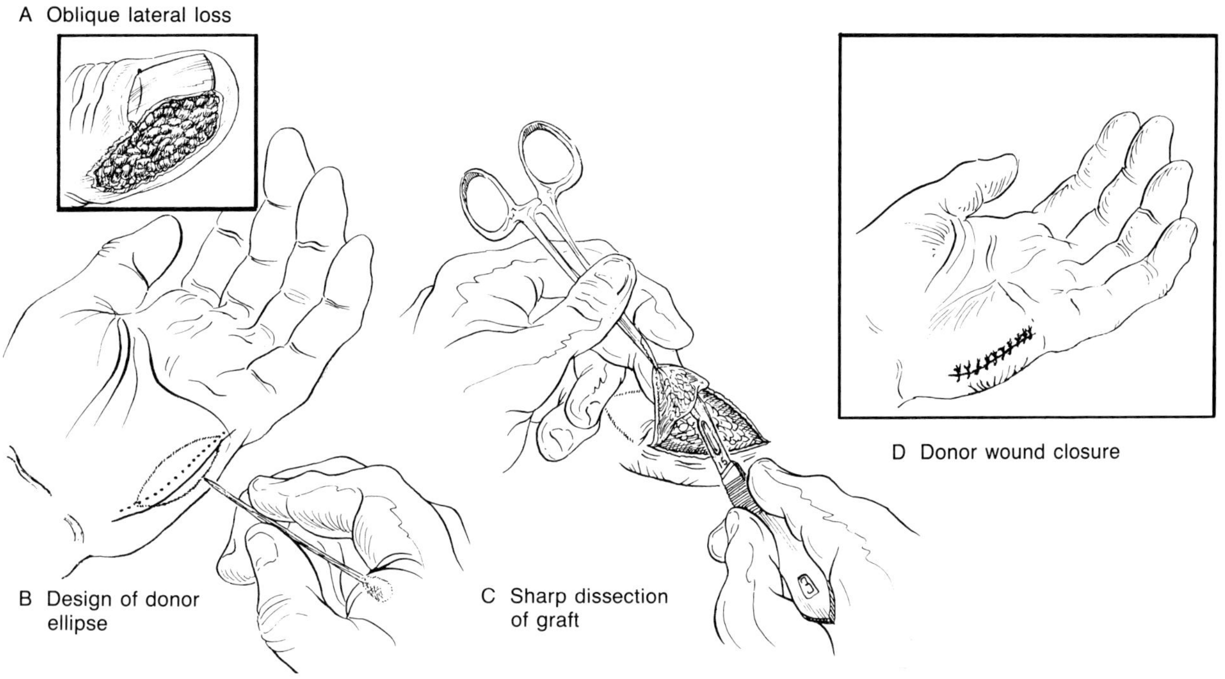

Figure 1 *A*, Oblique lateral loss of tissue is one particularly appropriate use for the hypothenar full-thickness skin graft. *B*, The longitudinal axis of the donor ellipse closely parallels the midlateral axis of the hand. The design is drawn by methylene blue using the bevelled end of a cotton swab. *C*, The full-thickness skin ellipse is placed on traction and sharply dissected, leaving the graft dermis as free as possible of subcutaneous fat. *D*, The donor wound is closed using 3–0 Nylon sutures.

dressing (Fig. 2B and C). A layer of Xeroform is applied on the skin graft. Templates of plain gauze dressing are then designed with Mayo scissors, the first layer being the same size as the graft and moistened with saline for better conformity. The dry, slightly larger second layer and smaller third layer are then applied. The silk sutures are tied, using an assistant with a needle holder to keep the proper tension in the first throw, a surgeon's knot, until the final second knot has been placed.

The finger tip dressing is complete using a 4″ by 4″ gauze cut to fit around the bolus dressing and is followed by application of a padded aluminum splint applied over the tip for a shorter length volarly than dorsally (Fig. 3). One inch-wide Elastoplast tape is used to cover the entire splint and dressing. This provides secure protection until the time of the first dressing change and bolus dressing removal, which are usually done 10 days after grafting. Donor site sutures must remain for 3 weeks in order to ensure full healing of the donor wound. No crosshatch marks result because of the thickness of the palmar skin. Antibiotics are not routinely used.

PATIENT SELECTION OR REJECTION

Many varieties of fingertip injuries may be successfully treated with the hypothenar full-thickness skin graft. Exposed bone is not a contraindication, for it can simply be removed with a rongeur as needed, provided there is sufficient soft tissue surrounding the bone. The skin graft will heal over a small area of bone due to the "bridging" effect. However, if the level of amputation is through the proximal one-third of the distal phalanx, it may be simpler to excise the remaining bone and to perform primary closure at the distal interphalangeal joint level. Digits with greater tissue loss dorsally than volarly can also be treated by direct primary closure.

Some patients have a favorable level and angulation of the amputation site so that a local advancement flap (i.e., a "V-Y" advancement flap) may be satisfactory. However, digits with a proximal, volar angulation of tissue loss are not suitable for an advancement flap because of inadequate tissue volarly distal to the distal interphalangeal joint crease. In those digits, the hypothenar full-thickness skin graft becomes extremely useful, as it also avoids the necessity for the cross finger flap. The latter requires immobilization which can cause joint stiffness, not only in the initially injured digit, but also in the adjacent donor digit.

Hypothenar full-thickness skin grafts are quite useful for palmar and lateral tissue loss in the digits—circumstances in which "V-Y" flaps are often impractical.

In digits with less than 1.0 cm loss of skin, and in young children, no procedure is needed. The open (dressing) method can be used, and the wound heals by a combination of re-epithelialization and scar contracture.

TIMING OF THERAPY

Reconstruction of fingertip injuries should be performed as soon after injury as is possible. With proper

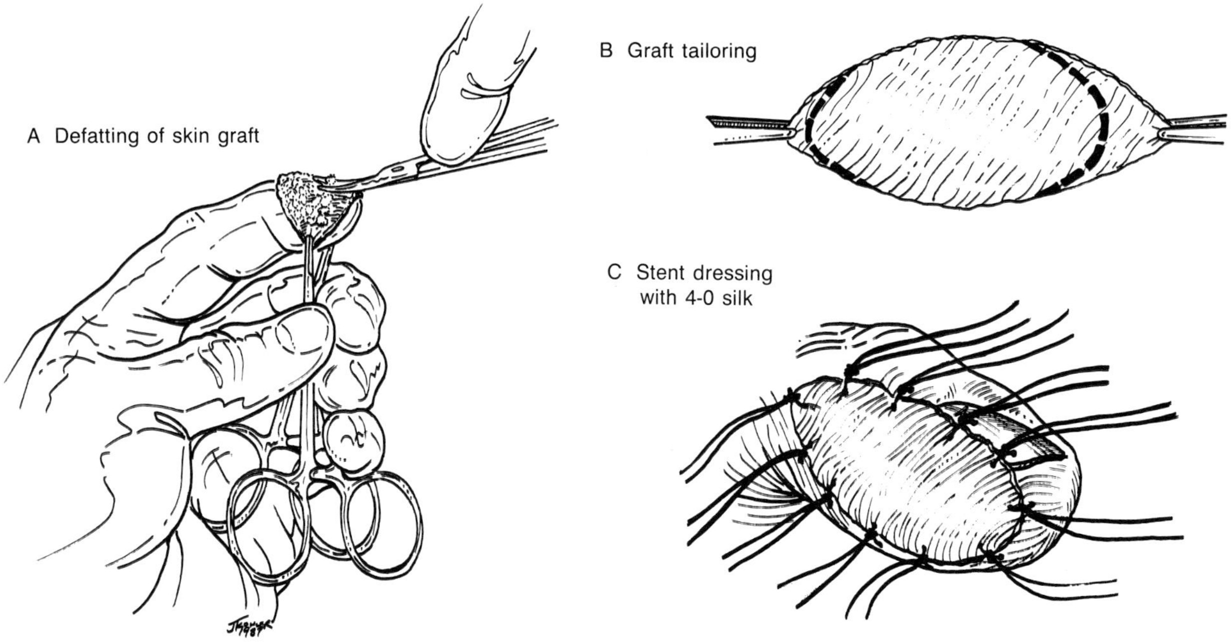

Figure 2 *A*, The inverted skin graft is held by two hemostats draped over a finger and is defatted with the application of the convexity of a pair of fine scissors. *B*, The graft is tailored to exactly match the size of skin loss. *C*, The skin graft is secured with 4–0 silk sutures which will be tied over the dressing bolus.

cleansing and debridement, primary skin grafting may be the definitive procedure. Once the skin graft has been applied, however, there is usually little urgency to change the dressing. Leaving the dressing undisturbed for 10 days gives the graft time to become securely attached, and after a further week, hand therapy may be begun.

PRINCIPLES OF TREATMENT APPROACH

Full-thickness skin grafts have an inherent advantage over split-thickness skin grafts by providing a thicker protective layer, as well as contracting less later. In addition, palmar full-thickness skin differs from the hair-bearing skin of the rest of the body in that it has a thicker epidermis and keratin layer. Pigment cells containing melanin are few in number, and the sebaceous glands are absent. Palmar full-thickness skin has a more compact, and thus less elastic, connective tissue. These characteristics allow greater resistance to pressure, friction, and trauma. The quality of return of sensibility in a grafted area depends in part on the nature of the grafted skin. The pattern of nerve plexus just below the basal layer of the epidermis is largely responsible for the quality and extent of the grafted area's reinnervation.

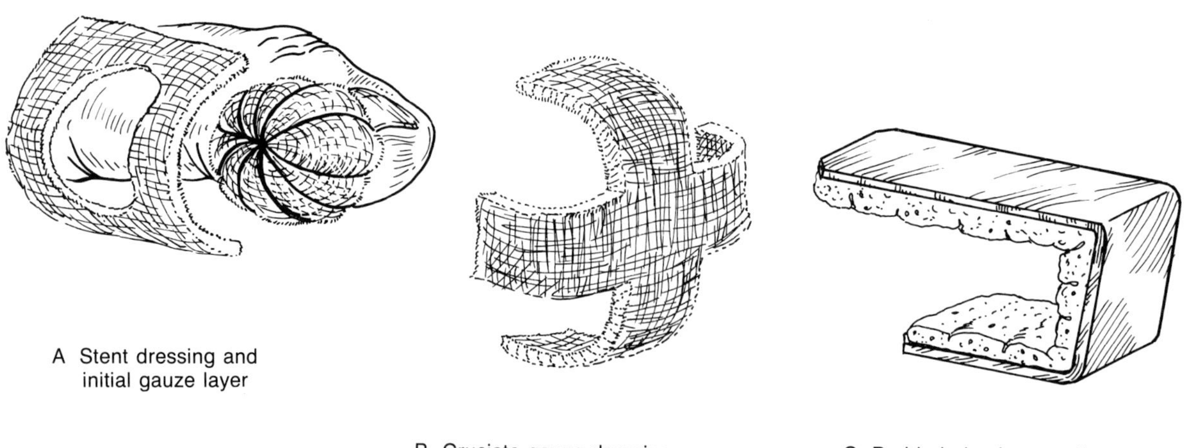

Figure 3 *A*, The initial gauze layers are cut out to fit around the stent dressing. *B*, A cruciate gauze dressing covers all sides of the digit. *C*, A foam padded aluminum splint is secured by 1″ elastic tape application.

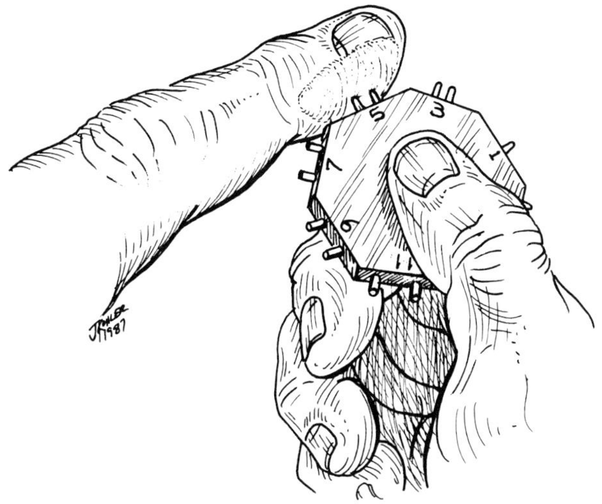

Figure 4 Later sensory testing confirms the basis for an excellent functional result.

Skin from the ulnar border of the hand provides a donor site conveniently placed within the same operative field. Because the donor area is well away from the grasping surface of the hand, the hypothenar skin graft thus avoids both the midpalmar donor site tenderness noted when the patient grips tools, and the cosmetic problem of scarring on the wrist or arm from donor sites at those areas. The donor area on the ulnar border of the hand usually leaves a faint scar, which in its position is usually hidden from view by either the patient or others. The scar is rarely symptomatic.

The hypothenar skin graft is ideal in patients with racial skin pigmentation, for it avoids the contrast of darkly pigmented skin grafts from other donor sites with the lighter skin of the fingertips.

Lastly, in those patients with extensive skin loss or in those with multiple fingertip involvement, the hypothenar donor skin can be obtained with an ellipse length of as much as 8 or 9 cm and a width of 2 cm (Fig. 4A and B).

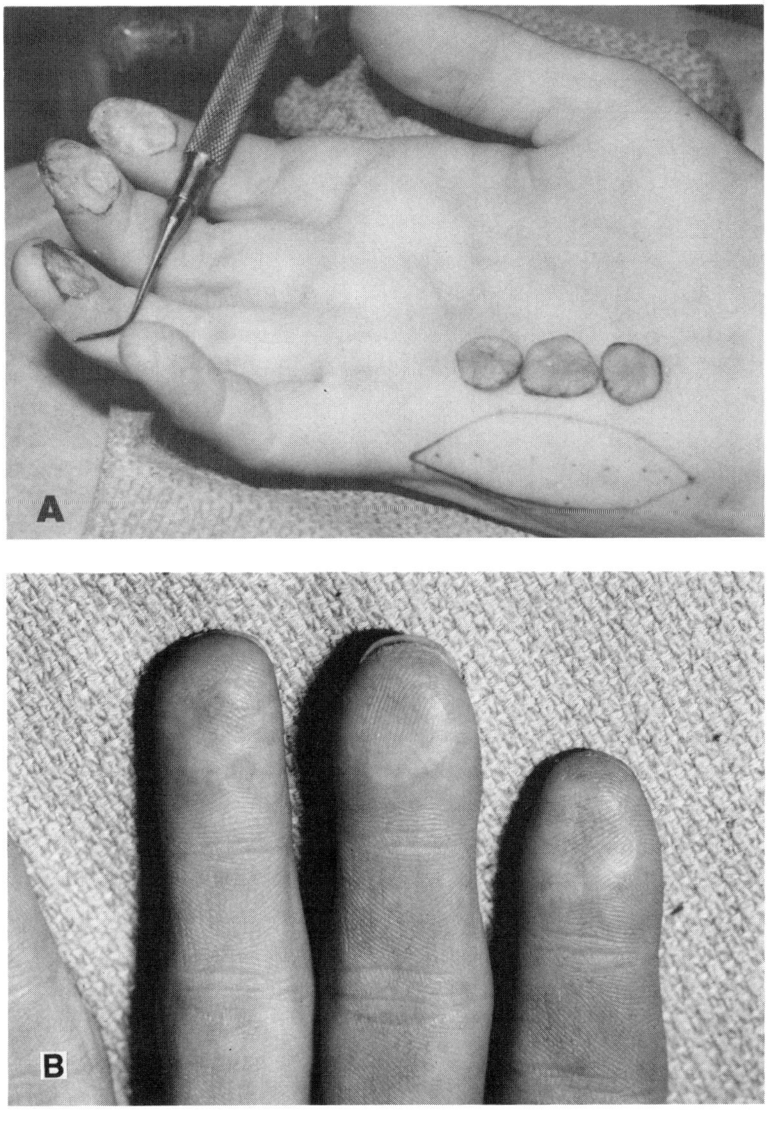

Figure 5 *A*, A 10-year-old male had groin full thickness skin grafts applied that ended 2 years later with dry, cracked skin. These areas were excised and are shown next to the outline for the donor site, which is adequate to resurface multiple fingers. *B*, The excellent cosmetic result is seen. The patient had 4 mm two point discrimination, providing excellent function.

TRICKS AND TRAPS OF THERAPEUTIC APPROACH

A common error of those inexperienced in the technique is to place the donor site too volarly onto the grasping surface of the palm. If this occurs, not only is the donor wound harder to close, but the ultimate scar will be more visible and tenderness bothersome. Therefore, it is important that the longitudinal central axis of the graft ellipse be placed parallel to, and very near, the axial line of the ulnar border of the hand. This skin has the same desirable characteristics described, but it is more mobile than skin from other areas of the palm.

Undermining the margins of the donor wound is neither advised nor necessary. However, the width of the graft should normally not exceed 2 cm to allow easy primary closure of the donor wound. Closure is most easily accomplished by suturing first from each end of the elliptical area and gradually advancing toward the center.

THERAPEUTIC OUTCOME

The expected result of use of the hypothenar full-thickness skin graft for fingertip injuries is cosmetically pleasing skin coverage with good sensibility, thickness, and durability. The donor area can barely be distinguished and is otherwise asymptomatic.

In my series, 86 percent achieved two-point discrimination of 10 mm or less with one-half of those achieving 6 mm or less two-point discrimination (Fig. 3D). Patient satisfaction with the procedure was of a similarly high degree.

BENEFIT-RISK ANALYSIS

The stated benefits for the hypothenar full-thickness skin graft method of fingertip reconstruction are endangered by the usual risks to any skin graft. These are the hazards of improper immobilization, infection, or bleeding. If the reader meticulously follows the technique I have described, these risks should be minimal.

A particular caution should be given against removing the sutures too early from the donor site (21 days is preferred), for this could cause a dehiscence that necessitates healing by secondary intention.

The procedures of greater complexity, such as those using cross-finger flaps or distant flaps, have a much greater risk of complications than the hypothenar full-thickness skin graft. The latter has high benefit potential with minimal risk.

In my experience, the hypothenar full-thickness skin graft has provided the best functional and esthetic results of all skin grafting techniques. As the method is more widely used, it should become a favorite treatment approach for fingertip injuries.

SUGGESTED READING

Allen MJ. Conservation management of fingertip injuries in adults. Hand 1980; 12:257–265.

Atasoy E, Ioakimidis E, Kasdan ML, Kutz JE, Kleinert HE. Reconstruction of the amputated fingertip with a triangular volar flap. A new surgical procedures. J Bone Joint Surg 1970; 52A:921–926.

Beasley RW. Local flaps for surgery of the hand. Orthop Clin North Am 1970; 1(2):219–225.

Elsahy N. When to replant a fingertip after its complete amputation. Plast Reconstr Surg 1960; 26:80–90.

Johnson RK, Iverson RE. Cross-finger pedicle flaps in the hand. J Bone Joint Surg 1971; 53A:913–919.

Patton HS. Split skin graft from hypothenar area for fingertip avulsions. Plast Reconstr Surg 1969; 43:426–429.

Schenck RR, Cheema TA. Hypothenar skin grafts for fingertip reconstruction. J Hand Surg 1984; 9A-5:750–753.

Smith RJ, Albin R. Thenar "h-flap" for fingertip injuries. J Trauma 1976; 16(10):778–781.

EXTENSOR AND FLEXOR TENDON INJURIES

PAUL G. PIN, M.D.
PAUL M. WEEKS, M.D.

Normal hand function is dependent upon the integrity of extensor and flexor tendons. Following injury, appropriate management may lead to complete recovery, whereas deficient care is usually associated with poor results. This chapter describes our therapy for specific extensor and flexor tendon injuries.

EXTENSOR TENDON INJURIES

Injuries to extensor tendons differ from injuries to the flexor tendons in many ways. The extensor tendons are more superficially located and thus are more easily damaged. Distal to the metacarpophalangeal (MP) joint, the extensor mechanism is thin and difficult to suture. Fortunately, at this level retraction of the ends of the divided tendon is seldom significant. Satisfactory healing can be frequently attained without surgery by splinting the digit in extension. Treatment of injuries to the extensor mechanism requires rebalancing of the system. This can be complicated as the extensor mechanism is constructed of two integrated sub-systems, an extrinsic one which consists of the extensor tendon proper, and an intrinsic one which consists of the lumbrical and the interosseus muscles. Chronic injury to the extensor mechanism may lead to a collapse deformity in the digit due to an imbalance between flexor and extensor forces. Consequently, old extensor tendon injuries are less amenable to treatment than are old flexor tendon injuries. Given the complexity of the extensor mechanism and the difficulty in treating old lesions, all extensor injuries should be treated acutely and with the same care afforded flexor tendon injuries.

The management of extensor tendon injuries is dictated by the level of injury. An outline for their care is presented based on the various levels of injury.

Distal Forearm to Wrist

All of the extrinsic extensors leave their respective muscle bellies in the forearm and pass through one of six fibro-osseous tunnels covered by the extensor retinaculum. This arrangement prevents "bowstringing" of the tendons with wrist extension. Repair of injured extensors at this level must maintain or restore a functional retinaculum or "bowstringing" will occur postoperatively.

Retrieval of the tendon ends is facilitated by wrist extension and elbow flexion. Tendon repair is preferably accomplished by a modified Kessler suture using 3–0 or 4–0 nonabsorbable suture, such as Prolene. Following repair, the wrist is flexed and extended to ascertain whether the suture line will pass beneath the retinaculum. If not, the repair is modified or that portion of the retinaculum is excised.

In general, repaired extensor tendons require and tolerate more immobilization than do flexor tendons. For specific recommendations on postoperative care, please refer to the chapter entitled *Role of Physical Therapy.*

Wrist to Metacarpophalangeal Joint

Injuries at this level can occasionally be difficult to diagnose. Junctura tendinum connect the individual slips of the extensor digitorum communis at the metacarpal level. Lacerations of this tendon proximal to these juntura may result only in partial loss of extension as the connecting bands can transmit the extension force around the site of injury. Repair of lacerations is performed using a modified Kessler suture when possible. Since the extensor becomes thin at this level, this suture is sometimes not practical and a horizontal mattress suture is a reasonable substitute.

Metacarpophalangeal Joint

Extensor mechanism injuries at the MP joint level can damage the tendon itself and/or associated structures, such as the sagittal bands. Tendon repair is performed using several horizontal mattress sutures of 4–0 Prolene. The sagittal bands are also meticulously repaired to prevent subluxation of the central tendon resulting in extensor lag and digital deviation.

Proximal Phalanx Joint

Division of the extensor apparatus at the proximal phalanx level is usually incomplete and managed by simple suture using 4–0 or 5–0 Prolene. Difficulty arises only when the injury involves skin loss, tendon loss, or fracture.

Proximal Phalangeal Joint

Normally, the extensor force is distributed over the MP joint and the proximal (PIP) and distal (DIP) interphalangeal joints. Loss of extension at one joint results in a redistribution of the force to the remaining two joints, which can result in hyperextension at these joints. Injury to the central slip of the extensor tendon at the PIP joint is a classic example. Loss of extension causes a flexion deformity at the PIP level. Over time, the lateral bands sublux volar to the axis of joint rotation. Additional extensor force transmitted to the DIP joint results in hyperextension and the boutonniere deformity. This lesion is seldom present acutely and its development depends on the PIP joint being flexed while tension is placed on the extensor tendon. Diagnosis is made by inspection and the patient's inability to actively extend the PIP joint.

Open injuries at the PIP joint are treated by simple suture repair of the extensor apparatus. The skin is closed separately. Excellent results can be expected, except when there is significant loss of tendon substance. We know of no single technique that yields consistently good results in this setting. Closed disruption of the central slip most commonly occurs when there is forced flexion of the extended PIP joint. Treatment is based on the fact that significant retraction does not occur and that splinting results in healing with slight elongation of the mechanism. The preferred treatment of the acute injury is splinting the PIP joint in extension. A Kirschner wire across the joint may be used to add further support. Throughout the 6 weeks required for healing, the DIP joint is to be actively flexed and extended.

Distal Interphalangeal Joint

Loss of extensor tendon continuity at the DIP joint level results in a flexion deformity (mallet finger). The extensor force is referred proximally and can lead to hyperextension of the PIP joint and a swan-neck deformity. Most commonly, tendon disruption occurs as a result of forced flexion of the extended digit. Rupture may arise within the tendon substance or at the insertion resulting in small bony avulsions. Alternatively, hyperextension of the DIP joint can cause fracture of the dorsal base of the distal phalanx.

When the associated fracture constitutes less than one-third of the joint surface, and when there is no subluxation of the DIP joint, closed injuries are best managed by splinting the DIP joint in full extension for 6 weeks. Due to the absence of tendon retraction, joint extension allows apposition of the severed ends. Immobilization must be continuous and may be accomplished by plaster, by Kirschner wire, or by Stack finger splint; we prefer the latter. To avoid IP joint stiffness, only the DIP joint should be immobilized and hyperextension of the DIP joint should be avoided. Open repair of closed injuries is strongly condemned as results are inferior. Even when a lag develops after 6 weeks of immobilization, we prefer to reinstitute splinting rather than perform surgery.

With displaced fractures greater than one-third the joint surface and with joint subluxation, surgery is the preferred treatment. The joint is reduced and fixed with a longitudinal Kirschner wire. Through a dorsal incision, the fracture fragment is reduced and fixed to the distal phalanx with a pull-out wire. Open lacerations which disrupt the tendon invariably enter the joint. After thorough irrigation, the tendon is repaired with 5–0 Prolene sutures; the skin is repaired separately. Immobilization may be achieved with a longitudinal Kirschner wire or with a Stack finger splint. Immobilization is continued for 6 weeks.

FLEXOR TENDON INJURIES

Despite great technical advances in hand surgery, flexor tendon lacerations continue to represent a therapeutic challenge. Early, accurate diagnosis, meticulous repair, and aggressive hand therapy are requisites for a good result. Substandard care invariably leads to permanent disability.

Patients with volar lacerations to the hand and wrist should all be suspected of having flexor tendon lacerations. Integrity of the superficialis tendons is assessed by observing active flexion of the PIP joint, while the other digits are held in full extension to block the action of the profundus tendons. Failure to flex the PIP joint fully indicates at least a partial laceration to the superficialis tendon, except in the little finger. Profundus tendons are individually tested by blocking PIP motion and observing active DIP flexion. Incomplete flexion reflects a profundus injury. All suspected tendon injuries are explored.

Exploration of possible tendon injuries takes place in the operating suite under axillary block or general anesthesia. A cephalosporin is administered preoperatively and a pneumatic tourniquet is employed after exsanguinating the extremity. Exposure is gained by incorporating any laceration into a zigzag incision that crosses flexion creases obliquely. Nerves in the vicinity of the laceration are explored and, when lacerated, are repaired using standard microsurgical techniques after tendon repairs have been completed. Partially injured tendons are evaluated for their potential to produce triggering; small flaps of tendon are excised. The wound is irrigated and when possible, the tendon sheath is repaired using a 5–0 absorbable suture, such as Vicryl. Postoperative care of partial flexor tendon lacerations consists of guarded, early active motion, and protective splinting for 6 weeks. Unrestricted motion predisposes to "spontaneous" tendon rupture.

Completely severed flexor tendons are handled as atraumatically as possible. Care is taken to avoid injury to the vincular blood supply. Tendon ends are squared off using a No. 11 blade, and repair of the tendons is accomplished using either the modified Kessler or the modified Bunnell suture technique. The suture material should be nonabsorbable and we prefer Prolene, usually 4–0. Edges of the tendons may be further approximated using a 6–0 Nylon continuous suture (Fig. 1). The tendon sheath is closed when possible. The tourniquet is released, hemostasis is obtained, and the wound is closed with interrupted 5–0 Nylon simple sutures. A bulky dressing is placed, and hand therapy begins 3 to 5 days postoperatively.

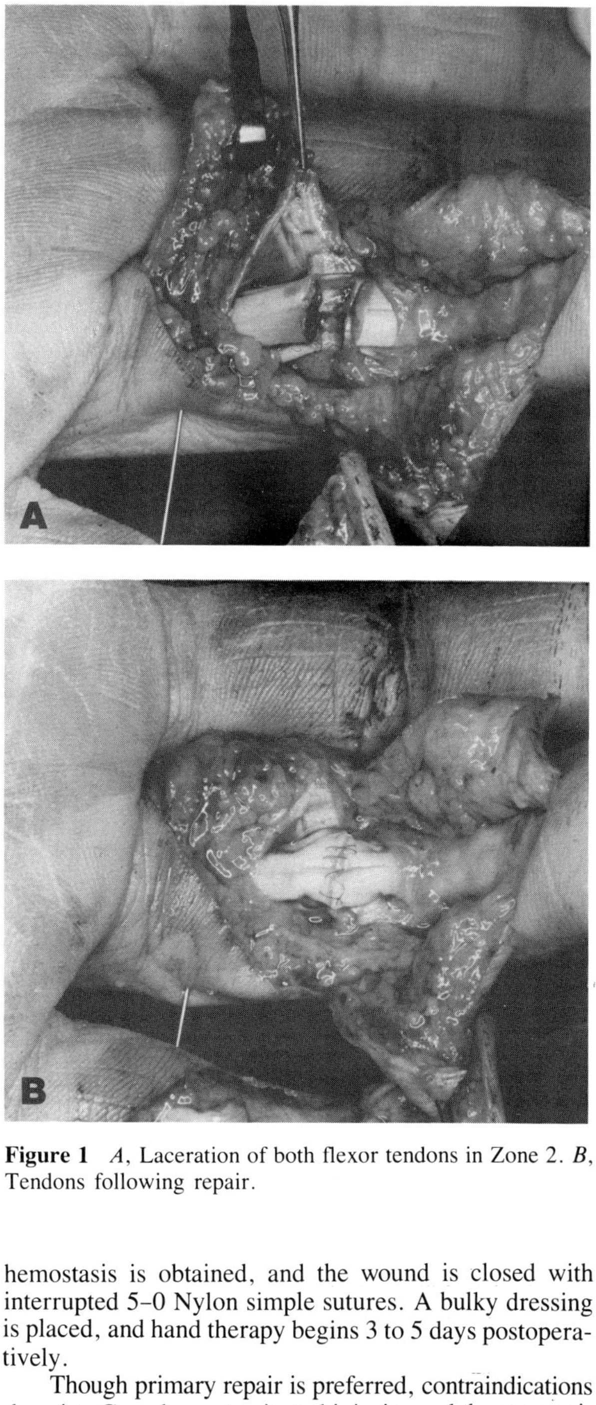

Figure 1 *A*, Laceration of both flexor tendons in Zone 2. *B*, Tendons following repair.

Though primary repair is preferred, contraindications do exist. Grossly contaminated injuries and those associated with loss of soft tissue cover are not repaired immediately; once the wound is clean and coverage is obtained, delayed primary repair may be considered. Since tendon function is dependent on an adequate pulley system, primary tendon repair should not be performed in the presence of complete loss to the A2 or A4 pulleys. In this instance, we reconstruct the pulley using a portion of the lacerated tendon and place a Hunter rod for staged flexor tendon reconstruction.

A final contraindication to primary tendon repair occurs when there has been loss of over 1 cm of tendon substance. This most commonly is seen in delayed primary repair when the tendon has contracted. Repair in this setting will obstruct full flexion of the other digits and impair full extension of the injured finger.

Postoperative positioning places the wrist in 40 degrees of flexion, the MP joints in 70 degrees of flexion, and the interphalangeal joints in 10 degrees of flexion. Reliable patients are placed on protocols that emphasize early mobilization of the repair site, as described by Kleinert and Duran. Small children and unreliable adults are immobilized continuously for at least 3 weeks.

SPECIFIC INJURIES

Flexor tendon lacerations are frequently classified according to zone. Zone 1 begins distal to the insertion of the superficialis tendon, and by definition, Zone 1 injuries involve only the profundus tendon. Retrieval of the proximal stump is facilitated by the fact that it is usually tethered by the intact vinculum. When the laceration is more than 1 cm proximal to the tendon insertion, direct repair is performed as previously described. It is mandatory that the repair site be able to pass beneath the A4 pulley otherwise tendon excursion will be limited. When the injury is in the distal 1 cm of the tendon, the profundus is advanced and sutured to the distal tendon stump. The fundamental concept governing management of Zone 1 injuries is that the normal function of the PIP joint and superficialis tendon should not be disturbed. For this reason, early active flexion of the PIP joint is employed while blocking flexion of the DIP joint by holding adjacent fingers in full extension.

Zone 2 begins at the proximal border of the tendon sheath and extends to the superficialis insertion. Injuries in this area have traditionally been associated with the worst prognosis due to the development of adhesions between the two tendons and the fibro-osseous tunnel. Yet the results of primary repair of both tendons in Zone 2 generally surpasses those seen with tendon grafting. Position of the tendon ends is in part determined by the position of the digit at time of injury. The distal stump can frequently be brought into the wound by flexing the IP joints. Retrieval of the proximal end can be more difficult. Several attempts are made to find it by milking the sheath while flexing the wrist and the MP joints. Blindly passing a clamp into the sheath is tempting, but should be discouraged as it can inadvertantly injure the tendon stump and the sheath. Instead, we make a small counterincision at the level of the distal palmar crease to retrieve the tendon. The proximal end is sutured to a tendon rod and passed distally into the wound. Care is taken to keep the tendons moist during repair. In cases where repair of the superficialis tendon is not technically feasible, a portion of the tendon should be sutured to the distal end of the A2 pulley to prevent the late development of a swan-neck deformity.

Zone 3 corresponds to the origin of the lumbricals; Zone 4 coincides with the carpal tunnel; and Zone 5 represents the wrist level. Results of flexor tendon repair in these zones are fairly comparable in our experience. Tendon retrieval requires only extension of incisions proximally and distally. Repair is performed as previously described.

COMPLICATIONS

Acute complications of tendon repair are mainly caused by infection. Postoperative infections are rare in our experience, but must be treated like any other hand infection. Rupture of the tendon repair is the most common subacute problem and occurs anywhere from several days to several weeks postoperatively. Though rupture can be caused by poor technique, it frequently occurs in patients who perform their therapy enthusiastically and who seem to form very few adhesions. Patients who seem on the verge of obtaining an excellent result are at greatest risk for rupture. When disruption is detected early, it should be treated as soon as possible by direct repair. Occasionally, tendon rupture is hard to distinguish from severe adhesions. However, the intact tendon should produce at least some DIP joint motion even with extensive adhesions.

Late complications consist of poor tendon gliding manifested by little active motion and joint stiffness, which results in poor passive motion. Causes of each include poor technique, inadequate hand therapy, and a tendency of the patient to excessive scarring. Treatment consists of tenolysis and capsulotomy followed by aggressive hand therapy. To limit the chance of recurrent adhesions by operating on an active wound and to allow the tendon to establish a vigorous blood supply, we usually defer such surgery for 6 months. Hopelessly scarred tendons can be salvaged by staged flexor tendon grafting.

FLEXOR TENDON GRAFTING

In general, primary tendon repair is the preferred method for restoring tendon function. When primary or delayed primary tendon repair is not feasible, tendon grafting should be considered, as should alternatives such as DIP joint tenodesis and fusion. Tendon grafting can be performed as a single stage procedure provided skin coverage is adequate, joints are supple, the tendon bed is unscarred, and at least the A2 and A4 pulleys are intact. When these conditions are not met, placement of a graft is preceded by tendon rod insertion with pulley reconstruction and/or capsulotomy as indicated. A mallet finger and a previous failed tendon graft are relative contraindications to tendon grafting.

Tendon Graft

The ideal donor tendon for grafting has the following characteristics: (1) its presence can be detected by examination; (2) its use results in no functional loss; (3) it is thin, thus allowing the total revascularization; (4) it is present within the operative field; (5) it has adequate length; and (6) it is easy to suture. For these reasons, the palmaris longus is our preferred source for tendon grafts. Harvesting is performed through an incision over the tendon insertion at the distal wrist crease. The tendon is divided and removed with a tendon stripper. When the palmaris is absent or of insufficient length, the plantaris tendon is favored, though this requires general anesthesia and a separate operative field; additionally, its presence cannot be determined preoperatively. Use of the extensor digitorum longus to the middle three toes is our third choice but is avoided whenever possible.

Single-Stage Grafting

When primary repair is not possible and when there are no contraindications, tendon grafting can be performed as a single stage. Exposure is gained through a volar zigzag incision exposing the digital sheath. The proximal end of the profundus tendon is drawn into the palm. The sheath is opened over the DIP joint and the distal stump is withdrawn. A Silastic rod is passed into the digital sheath from the palm to the distal phalanx. When the superficialis tendon is intact, it does not matter if the rod passes around one of the slips, or through the chiasm. When the superficialis is irreparably disrupted, the sheath is opened between the A2 and A4 pulleys, and the distal end of the superficialis tendon is sutured to the A2 pulley with the PIP joint in 10 degrees of flexion. This prevents future hyperextension of the joint.

The tendon graft is sutured to the proximal end of the tendon rod and advanced into the sheath by pulling the rod distally. The proximal suture is performed using a standard end-to-end repair, when no size discrepancy exists, or with a weave technique, when a discrepancy is present. Graft tension is set by extending the digit and pulling on the graft to fully relax the muscle. The intersection of the graft and the tendon stump is marked. A modified Bunnell suture is passed in the end of the graft and is then threaded through a drill hole in the distal phalanx and tied over a button. At completion of the procedure, the digit should be slightly more flexed than normal to allow for inevitable elongation at the repair site.

In children and uncooperative adults, postoperative care consists of complete immobilization for 4 weeks. In reliable patients, therapy is dictated by the status of the superficialis tendon. When the tendon is intact, motion is begun 3 to 5 days postoperatively. The grafted finger is positioned with the MP joint in 70 degrees of flexion, the PIP in 20 degrees of flexion, and the DIP at zero degrees. The adjacent fingers are held in extension. Active motion of the PIP is encouraged, but not at the DIP. If the superficialis tendon is missing, complete immobilization in a position of repose is used for 4 weeks, before beginning progressive exercises.

Two-Stage Grafting

When the conditions for single-stage grafting are not met, two-stage grafting is performed. In stage I, the entire digital sheath is exposed to define the status of the A2 and A4 pulleys. The profundus tendon is resected at least as far proximally as the lumbricals, and a 1- to 2-cm stump is preserved distally. Capsulotomy is performed when indicated. When the superficialis is intact, tenolysis is accomplished as necessary. When the superficialis is irreparably severed, PIP joint tenodesis is performed as previously described. A tendon passer is then inserted from the distal tendon sheath into the wrist. Through a counter incision, a tendon rod is attached to the passer and advanced distally. The rod is carefully sutured beneath the tendon stump to prevent erosion through the pulp. Missing pulleys are reconstructed. Postoperative therapy begins 3 days later and is continued for 3 months. By this time, a pseudosheath is usually adequately formed and stage II can be performed.

At the second stage, a small incision is made over the distal phalanx to expose the rod and the profundus stump. A second incision is made over the wrist to expose the rod and the proximal profundus stump. The proximal repair is performed and the graft is inserted. Tension is adjusted and distal repair is accomplished. Postoperative care is identical to that following single-stage repair.

SUGGESTED READING

Blue AI. Spira M, Hardy SB. Repair of extensor tendon injuries of the hand. Am J Surg 1976; 132:128–132.

Elliott RA. Splints for mallet and boutonniere deformities. Plast Reconstr Surg 52:282–285.

Kleinert HE, Lubahn JD. Current state of flexor tendon surgery. Ann Chir Man 1984; 3:1–17.

Schneider LH. Staged flexor tendon reconstruction using the method of Hunter. Clin Orthop 1982; 171:164–171.

Strickland JW, Glogovac SV. Digital function following flexor tendon repair in zone II: a comparison of immobilization and controlled passive motion techniques. J Hand 1980; 5:537–543.

INTERNAL FIXATION OF METACARPAL AND PHALANGEAL FRACTURES

MICHAEL E. JABALEY, M.D.
ALAN E. FREELAND, M.D.

A quiet revolution in the treatment of hand fractures is being driven by the confluence of (1) a better understanding of bone healing and its relation to ultimate function, (2) the availability of precision instruments and implants, and (3) an increased awareness of the importance of aggressive therapy in the postoperative result. The effect of this convergence of ideas and implants is that fracture treatment is no longer a passive activity and is now very much an active process.

The fracture dictum of immobilization of the fracture, as well as the joint above and the joint below, usually results in healed fractures, but functionally poor results may occur because of joint stiffness and adjacent tendon adhesion. An appreciation of the importance of outcome led Richard Smith to observe, "Perhaps nowhere is it as important as in the hand and wrist to achieve maximum motion and strength in concert with accurate alignment and stable union."

Heretofore, plaster or Kirschner wire fixation have been the benchmarks against which fracture treatment has been measured. As experience has grown, we feel that we can now identify fractures in which treatment by stable internal fixation and early mobilization yields results that equal or exceed those obtained by the older, traditional methods. Return of function is faster and ultimately better.

The goal of stable internal fixation is primary bone healing. It requires rigid immobilization and compression of fracture fragments. When these goals are successfully accomplished, no external callus forms and there is no phase of enchondral ossification; the implant replaces the external callus. More importantly, moving parts can be mobilized immediately, and the unstable fracture can be neutralized as a factor in the management of the overall wound. A new dictum has emerged in which the fracture is stabilized while adjacent tendons and joints are moved.

INDICATIONS

Many hand fractures can be managed by closed reduction and plaster fixation, or by simple techniques of percutaneous pinning. In some patients, however, such techniques often result in stiff, painful hands and poor functional recovery, known as "fracture disease." This may be partly due to the injury, but these effects are sometimes compounded by the treatment. It was the victims of "fracture disease" who inspired the search for better fixation techniques.

Operative fracture treatment is not for all fractures, nor for all surgeons. They are precision techniques that must be precisely applied. As one becomes more familiar with the methods and gains experience in their application, the indications for their use can be expanded into areas where one might not otherwise employ them.

The setting in which the fracture occurs is always an important consideration in planning treatment. For example, one may choose not to open an isolated fracture, but one might internally fix the same fracture when it is associated with tendon or nerve damage. Contrary to what some may think, open wounds are an indication, not a contraindication, to the use of implants and they are frequently employed in this setting.

Some indications for internal fixation of hand fractures are:

1. Open fractures with associated tendon, nerve, or vessel injury.
2. Intra-articular fractures.
3. Periarticular fractures.
4. Unstable subcapital fractures.
5. Displaced fractures with unstable configuration.
6. Unstable configuration with comminution.
7. Fractures with bone loss.
8. Multiple fractures in the same hand.
9. Hand fractures in the polytrauma patient.

Smith further noted, "Ultimately, the purpose of the treatment is always to reduce and immobilize any fracture about the hand that is displaced and unstable in order to permit early and complete motion. The purpose of stable fixation, simply put, is to lay the groundwork for successful wound management and early rehabilitation. Toward this end, fracture fixation is the beginning of a treatment continuum that must then proceed to intensive and concentrated therapy on a daily basis. This means that moving parts must be moved and kept moving during the period of scar formation when capsular tightness, joint stiffness, and tendon adhesions occur. When these secondary shortcomings can be successfully avoided, the functional result seems better and is reached earlier.

PREFERRED APPROACH

When fractures that require fixation occur in the presence of an open wound, one should always do as much as possible through the existing wound(s). When necessary, we do not hesitate to enlarge such wounds along functional lines. If such extension is not feasible, separate incisions can be made to allow adequate exposure. Fracture fixation is best accomplished through elective incisions placed on the dorsum or dorsolateral aspects of the fingers or hand. It is better, where possible, to have an intact flap of skin over gliding structures, such as the extensor mechanism. For this reason, we favor zigzag or curvilinear incisions, placed so that the scar does not lie directly over tendons. Longitudinal incisions over long bones give the best exposure, but the worst scar. In some fractures we even use a transverse skin incision in combination with longitudinal incision of the deeper structures. Such an incision protects nerves and permits adequate access for the insertion of lag screws or a tension band; it causes minimum restriction of motion by adhesion, and it produces the most esthetically acceptable scar.

Distal phalanx fractures rarely require fixation. The middle phalanx can be approached dorsally between the lateral bands, or from either side. The proximal phalanx can be exposed by splitting the central band of the extensor mechanism through the interval between central and lateral bands, or by lifting the lateral band on either side. This latter technique can be facilitated by the removal of a triangular wedge (the Littler release) from the lateral band. The metacarpals can be exposed by reflecting the extensor tendons and incising the underlying periosteum longitudinally. The metacarpophalangeal (MP) and proximal interphalangeal (PIP) joints are entered much the same as for a capsulectomy, by taking down various collateral ligaments, sagittal bands, and other structures.

A variety of anesthetics are satisfactory for fracture fixation. Many of our patients are treated with regional blocks as outpatients. Postoperative pain is minimized by local infiltrations of long-acting anesthetics such as bupivacaine (Marcaine). We prefer to treat fractures early, before edema and stiffness develop, but surgical fixation can be performed at any time within the first several weeks after injury when necessary to correct an unacceptable fracture position.

PRINCIPLES OF TREATMENT

Successful treatment is directed toward two goals: stable fixation, and compression of bone fragments. To accomplish these ends, we rely on a modification of Lambotte's sequential principles of fracture management, the four Rs—reduction, retention, rigid fixation, and rehabilitation. From a practical standpoint, these goals can be accomplished by three techniques, or combinations thereof: tension band wiring, lag screws, or plate and screw fixation.

Tension Band Wiring

Although a tension band can be constructed with a plate and screws, stainless steel wires are frequently suited to hand fractures (Fig. 1). Several technical variations have been described. These usually consist of combina-

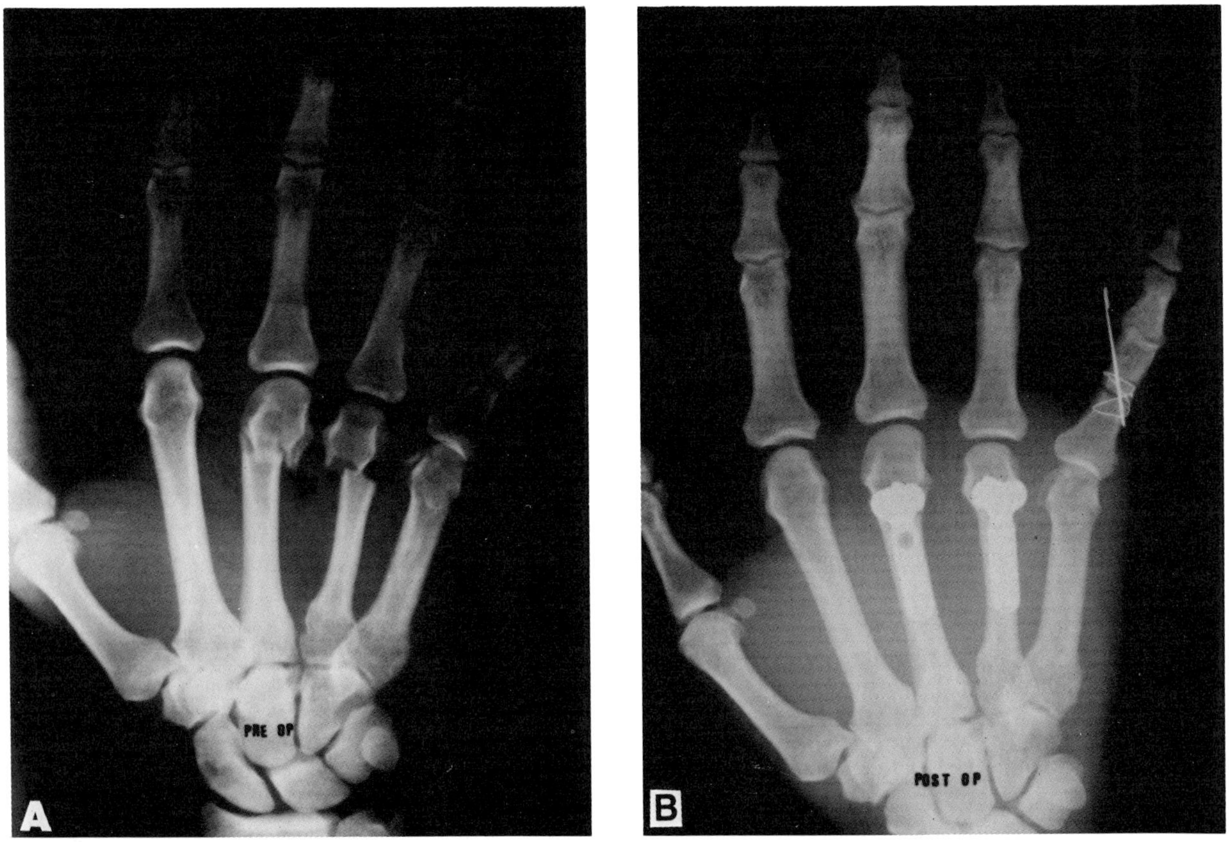

Figure 1 *A*, A 41-year-old man suffered a crush injury when his right hand was caught between a heavy pipe and a forklift. There were transverse, unstable, subcapital fractures of the 3rd and 4th metacarpals, a stable fracture of the head of the 5th metacarpal, and a transverse unstable fracture of the diaphysis of the proximal phalanx of the small finger. There was a transverse bursting wound of the palm, and the dorsal skin was raised as a large flap. *B*, The fractures of the 3rd and 4th metacarpals were provisionally fixed with K-wires, and T-plates applied. The screw holes were offset so that the bone fragments were compressed. The 5th metacarpal fracture was stable and required no fixation. A tension band was constructed on the dorsum of the proximal phalanx with No. 28 gauge wire and a 0.035 K-wire was inserted to prevent rotation.

tions of Kirschner wires and stainless steel wires. We use No. 28 gauge wire in the phalanges and No. 26 gauge in the metacarpals. The technique to be described uses a dorsal figure-of-eight wire, with or without one or two Kirschner wires to control rotation. It *must* be applied on the tension (dorsal) side of the bone. The essentials are: no bone loss; an intact or minimally-comminuted volar cortex; transverse drill holes passed dorsal to the midaxis of each fragment; and a malleable wire crossed in figure-of-eight fashion over the dorsum of the fracture. Other texts provide details of techniques.

Tension bands are best suited for transverse or slightly diagonal fractures through the diaphysis of a long bone such as a phalanx or a metacarpal. Among their advantages are the minimal bulk, little interference with motion, no necessity to remove the implant, and the minimal exposure required for insertion. In practice, tension bands work very well in all three phalanges or the metacarpals, and they meet the criteria for stable fixation.

A tension band is a dynamic fixation technique and depends on active flexion of the fingers for compression. Such motion complements the overall goal of rehabilitation. As fingers bend and flexor tendons glide, they apply a force through their pulleys that is transferred to bone fragments and results in their axial compression. Stability is sufficient to allow active motion, but the fracture should not initially be stressed beyond the preload of the implant lest fatigue failure occur. As noted, 26-gauge wire is preferred for the metacarpals; 28 gauge is sufficient in phalanges.

A tension band controls flexion and extension, but *not* rotation, and many transverse fractures of the phalanges or metacarpals tend to rotate. If the fracture edges are jagged and interdigitate, an anatomic fit may be sufficient to prevent rotation. If there is still a tendency to rotate, as in an osteotomy or when fracture edges are smooth, a single diagonal or two longitudinal Kirschner wires will prevent it. K-wires are best inserted *before* the tension band is tightened by drilling retrograde from the fracture line through one fragment and out of the skin, then the K-wire is passed back through the other fragment *after* the tension band has been tightened. The purpose of the K-wire is not fixation, and the tension band need not be disturbed while the K-wire is being passed. The Kirschner wire can be removed relatively early, once motion has been started and x-ray studies have confirmed that the fixation is stable.

Lag Screw Fixation

Lag screw fixation is a cornerstone of internal fixation techniques (Figs. 2 and 3). When correctly applied,

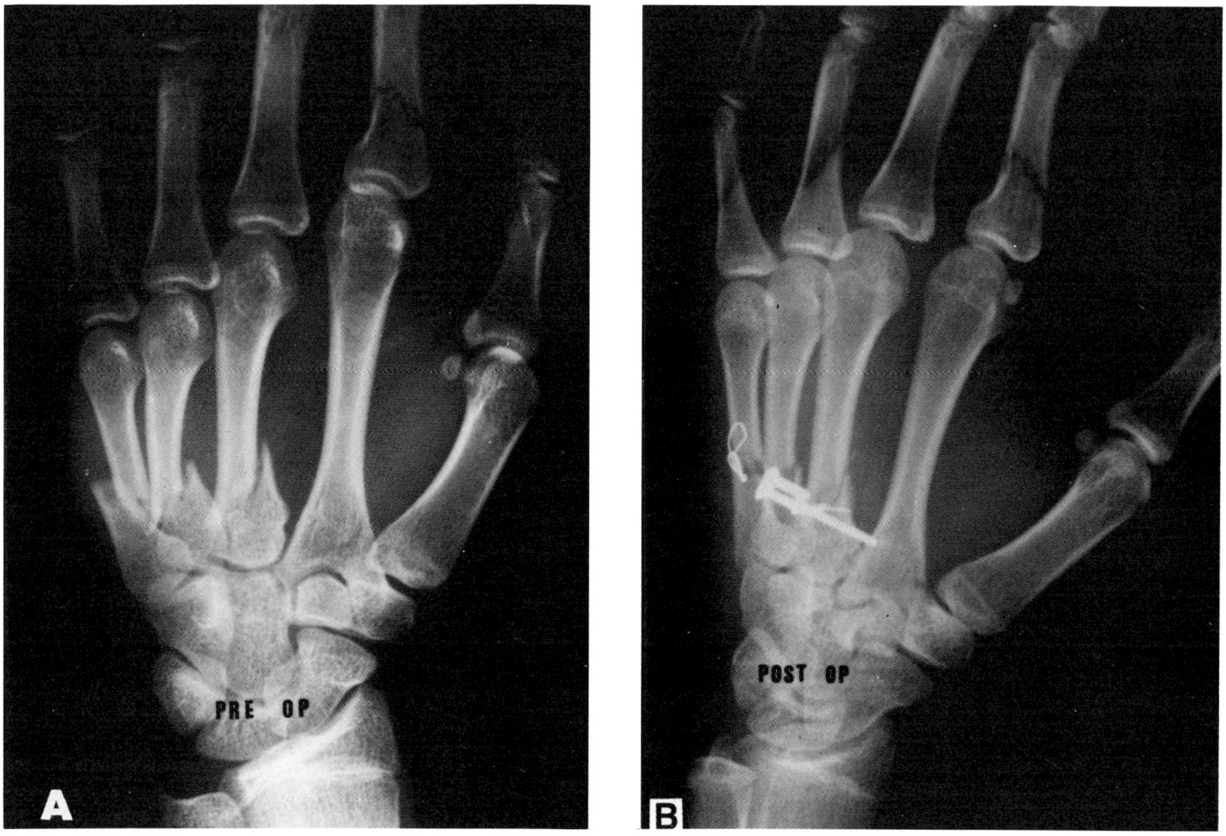

Figure 2 *A*, A 16-year-old girl suffered closed spiral oblique fractures at the bases of the 3rd, 4th, and 5th metacarpals, with instability and overriding, when she was thrown from a horse. There is also an undisplaced stable fracture of the proximal phalanx of the index finger. *B*, All three metacarpal fractures were fixed by a variety of techniques. A tension band was constructed for the 5th metacarpal, two lag screws were used for the 4th, and a lag screw and tension band was inserted in the 3rd metacarpal. Healing was uneventful, and there was full recovery of function.

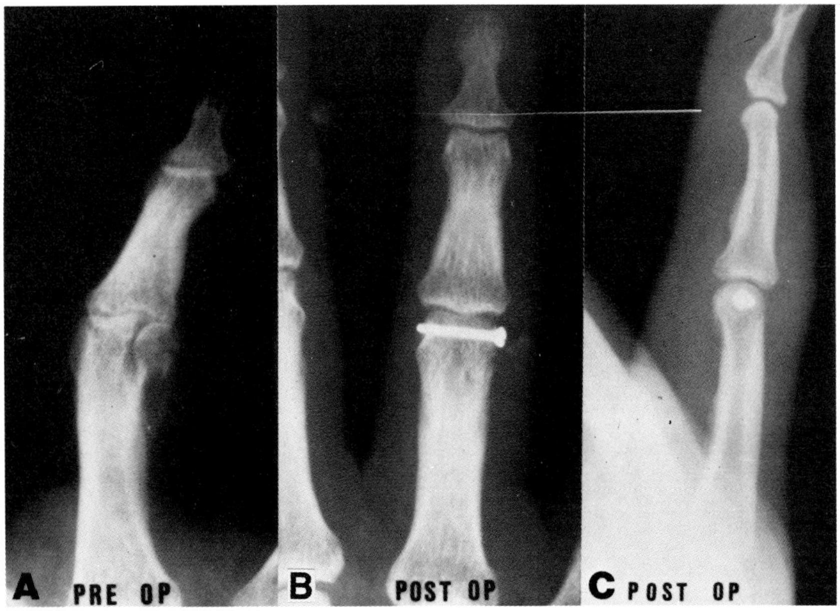

Figure 3 *A*, A 34-year-old man was injured water-skiing. He suffered an unicondylar intra-articular fracture of the proximal phalanx in which the fragment was rotated 180 degrees. *B*, The fracture has been opened through a midaxial incision and the fragment reduced. A single 2.0 mm screw was passed transversely to hold the reduction. *C*, Lateral view with screw in place shows anatomic restoration of articular surface.

a lag screw, which is based on the principle of the inclined plane, can both compress and rigidly fix two fragments of bone. To achieve these goals, one first drills a hole through both cortices. The hole in the near cortex must be large enough for the outer diameter of the screw (core + threads) to pass (or glide) without grasping. A concentric hole, with diameter the same as the core of the screw, is drilled in the far cortex. This hole is then threaded (or tapped) so that the screw will turn precisely and firmly grasp the far cortex. As the screw glides through the near cortex and grasps the far cortex, the two cortices are drawn toward each other, compressed, and rigidly fixed.

Lag screws are ideal for diagonal or oblique fractures of the diaphysis or for intra-articular fractures of the metaphysis (see Fig. 3). They are also useful in reattaching "butterfly" fragments in complex fractures. To use lag screws effectively in an oblique fracture, the fracture line should be twice as long as the diameter of the bone. Two small screws are preferable to one large one. We recommend 1.5 or 2.0 mm screws in the phalanges and 2.0 or 2.7 mm screws in the metacarpals. To accept a screw successfully, the diameter of the fragment should be three to four times the diameter of the proposed screw hole. When correctly inserted, one thread of the screw should be visible on x-ray film beyond the distal hole in the cortex. 1.5 and 2.0 mm screws have flat heads and can be left in place without risk. If one uses the 2.7 mm screw, it is necessary to gouge (countersink) a concavity in the cortex to accommodate the spherical screw head. Otherwise, it will stand too high and be palpable through the thin skin. Even when countersunk, 2.7 mm screws are usually better removed because of their bulk.

Concern is sometimes voiced about the presence of metal implants beneath moving structures such as tendons, ligaments, and joint capsules. Soft tissue does not adhere to metal, but reacts by encapsulating it and gliding easily over it. Because of its smooth surface, it is unlikely that metal will result in fraying and rupture of tendons. That this is true is borne out by our experience with over two hundred patients, in whom we have not seen tendon rupture or tendon attrition from the presence of one or more screw heads. In contrast, wires may result in tendon fraying and care should be taken that the twisted portions are placed away from gliding tendons. They are best bent so that the ends are buried in bone and not allowed to impinge on tendons.

Plate Fixation

Metal plates and screws have a long history of use in larger bones, but acceptance in the hand has been slow and their use has been limited. Their main drawbacks have been the extensive dissection required for implantation, their bulk, the eventual need to remove them, and the idea that they somehow impinge on moving structures and limit ultimate mobility. These criticisms are not entirely unwarranted, but they have been addressed, in part, by the production of smaller screws and plates. Although plates are not used as commonly as tension band wires and lag screws, they play an important role and meet certain needs that cannot otherwise be addresed. Their role in the treatment of hand fractures is becoming increasingly well-defined.

From a practical standpoint, plates find their greatest application in the metacarpals and in the proximal phalanges (see Fig. 1). Although they may occasionally be used in the middle phalanx of fingers and distal phalanx of the thumb, such applications are rare and probably constitute less than 1 percent of the total applications in our series.

In the simplest sense, a plate offers a method for spanning an unstable or missing segment of bone and obtaining fixation to stable segments at one or both ends. Plates of different shapes and thickness are available, depending on whether the fracture is in the diaphysis or the metaphysis. They may be straight, L-shaped, T-shaped, or cloverleafed. They also have different hole configurations, and they take different size screws.

A plate can perform one or more of three basic functions, depending on the character of the fracture and the mode in which it is applied. It can compress, neutralize, and buttress. Sometimes there is functional overlap, and a single plate may play more than one role. When a plate is described, one should always state both its name and its function because neither may otherwise be apparent, either clinically or on x-ray film.

General Principles About Plates

Flat or quarter-tubular plates are usually satisfactory in the fingers. Quarter-tubular or dynamic compression plates (DCP) can be used on the metacarpals. Screw sizes are those previously described for the lag screw. In the metacarpal, one should strive to insert two screws and grasp four cortices on either side of a fracture line. This rule also applies in the phalanges, although the screws can be smaller. One sometimes obtains satisfactory fixation in either case with a single screw on one side of a fracture. If a screw is inserted through a plate and across a fracture line, it should be in the lag mode. Plates can be bent to the contour of a bone and we offer plate removal to patients after 6 months or later for cause.

Situations for the clinical use of plates cannot be strictly defined but depend in part on the ingenuity of the surgeon who applies them. A compression plate can be a *tension band* when it is applied on the tension side of a bone and meets the other criteria previously described for tension bands. When one takes advantage of the elliptical shape of the holes and the spherical shape of the screw head to produce interfragmentary compression, the plate is a *compression plate*. A plate can be passed over an area of bone loss or great comminution in such a way as to bridge the section of instability. In this fashion, it serves as a *bridge plate*. Bridge plates are often used in conjunction with bone grafts. If the area of instability occurs in the cancellous portion of the metaphysis, a T-shaped or cloverleaf plate can be used to envelop or buttress the unstable portion and become *a buttress plate*. Finally, a *neutralization plate* can be applied in conjunction with interfragmentary lag screw(s) so as to neutralize rotation and bending forces on the screw, thereby protecting it. As noted, a plate sometimes suits dual purposes.

TRICKS AND TRAPS

The surgeon who would apply the principles of internal fixation that we have described is forewarned that this is not an approach to be learned in the operating room on living patients. The precision steps are better perfected in the skills laboratory with artificial bones. To this end, the reader is referred to books on the subject and courses where techniques can be mastered and skills honed. Once gained, however, the techniques are limited only by the surgeon's experience and ingenuity.

Intraoperative control using x-ray studies is essential, particularly in the early stages of one's mastery of the techniques of internal fixation. It assists in assessment of the reduction and visualization of the length and location of screws, as well as their purchase (or lack thereof) on bone.

Only the surgeon knows how firmly the fracture is fixed. If the fixation is adequate, rehabilitation can safely begin immediately. The dictum "Know thy fixation" is critical. If fixation is less than perfect (and this is sometimes the case, particularly in small bones), the rehabilitation program must be modified to avoid excessive stress.

The surgeon should always have a lifeboat. Small bone fixation is fraught with pitfalls, some irreparable. If a segment of bone is not much larger than the screw hole, it must be correctly drilled the first time. Otherwise, there is no second chance. In many such instances, a 0.028 Kirschner wire, or an interosseous wire, may salvage the situation. Although such fixation is not rigid, it may nevertheless provide enough stability and alignment to allow healing and cautious rehabilitation. In the hand, fixation need only be good enough to maintain alignment and permit motion. Although less than perfect, many fractures do surprisingly well with less than rigid fixation.

Postoperative Care

In stable fixation, the purpose of the treatment is always to reduce and immobilize any fracture that is displaced and unstable, in order to permit early and complete motion. In other words, the objective is to neutralize the fracture(s) as a factor in the rehabilitation of moving parts. If this can be done successfully, joints show less tendency to stiffen and tendons are more likely to glide than might otherwise be the case.

From the standpoint of rehabilitation, several techniques enhance the ultimate function and are integral parts of our postoperative program. Among these are: minimization and early resolution of edema; scar massage and manipulation; early, load-free motion of joints; active range of motion exercises as soon as tendon integrity permits; and application of load to the bone as healing allows it to relieve the implant of its stress.

No technique is a panacea and internal fixation is no exception. Open fracture fixation and poor postoperative management combine the worst of both techniques. The patient has more scar and stiffness and would have been better left alone.

Tendolysis and Capsulectomy

In many patients, despite our best efforts, motion does not return as completely as either we or the patient would like. In such instances, we take the opportunity when we are removing implants to perform tendolysis, capsulectomy, or both. Continuous passive motion machines show promise for maintaining motion gained by these procedures, and appear to minimize pain and swelling. These have all been extremely useful adjuncts and can reliably increase motion with a minimum of additional effort, surgical trauma, and expense, since they are usually performed in the outpatient setting. We recommend an arbitrary wait of 6 months before these procedures are performed.

SUGGESTED READING

Dabezies EJ, Schutte JP. Fixation of metacarpal and phalangeal fractures with miniature plates and screws. J Hand Surg 1986; 11A:283–288.

Freeland AE, Jabaley ME, Hughes JL. Stable fixation of the hand and wrist. New York: Springer-Verlag, 1986:3.

Heim V, Pfeiffer KM (in collaboration with Meuli HC). Small fragment set manual. Technique recommended by the ASIF group (Swiss Association for Study of Internal Fixation). New York: Springer-Verlag, 1974:1.

Jabaley ME, Freeland AE. Rigid internal fixation in the hand: 104 cases. Plast Reconstr Surg 1986; 77:288–297.

Segmuller G. Surgical stabilization of the skeleton of the hand. Baltimore: Williams & Wilkins, 1977.

Smith R. Foreward. In: Freeland AE, Jabaley ME, Hughes JL. Stable fixation of the hand and wrist. New York: Springer-Verlag, 1986: vii, viii.

REPLANTATION SURGERY

WILLIAM W. SHAW, M.D., F.A.C.S.
WILLIAM E. POWERS Jr., M.D.

For centuries, when surgeons were called upon to treat severely injured limbs, the main concern was whether the limb was sufficiently viable or salvageable to avoid the need for amputation. The experimental replantation of limbs in dogs by Hoefpner and Carrel finally became reality in the 1960s with the successful replantations of arm, hand, thumb, and digits in humans. The feasibility of replantation introduced a new dimension to our surgical options. More important, the ability to regain sensation or motion by nerve repairs, to restore critical tissue losses by direct microvascular tranplantation of tissue from elsewhere (free flaps), and to improve function by custom-designed high performance prostheses has created a more dynamic concept of limb reconstruction. No longer is the level of amputation determined solely by the level of viability, nor do replantation or reconstruction eliminate the need for rehabilitation or prostheses. Today, with optimal surgical reconstruction and postoperative rehabilitation, many limbs can be saved and made useful that once were routinely discarded or allowed to survive as useless appendages. On other occasions, unreplantable distal parts may be replanted as a free flap to achieve a more functional lower amputation. The goal today is maximal esthetic and function restoration compatible with the extent of the injury (Fig. 1).

GENERAL CONSIDERATIONS

Proximal Versus Distal Replantations

Because of differences in the nature of injuries, the reconstructive goals, and the surgical techniques, replantation surgery can be discussed under two categories: (1) the proximal (major) limbs, which include injuries above the wrist or ankle and (2) the distal parts, which include the digits, hand, toes, and penis.

Distal amputated parts contain little or no muscle mass and have a high surface area to mass ratio. Surface cooling with ice results in rapid effective tissue cooling and extends the tolerable ischemic time before irreversible changes occur. This permits the surgeon to work in a more orderly fashion to complete the tedious microscopic repairs of many small vessels and nerves. Frequently, 6 to 8 hours of ischemia go by before the circulation is restored, and the total operating time may be two or three times longer. In rare cases, successful replantations of fingers have been accomplished after more than 30 hours of ischemia.

Proximal amputations, on the other hand, must be handled differently in that the substantial muscle mass tolerates, at best, only 4 to 6 hours of warm ischemia. Due to the thick subcutaneous fat insulation of limbs, surface cooling reduces the core temperature rather slowly. Reperfusion after prolonged ischemia may result in sudden acidosis and myoglobinemia, with serious systemic and renal consequences. Perfusion of the limb with cold heparinized lactated Ringer's solution can rapidly bring down the core temperature, but it may have minor undesirable effects on the microcirculation, and the methodology is presently not totally worked out. Finally, the nature of these injuries is such that the patient may be hypovolemic or have associated multiple injuries. The surgeon, therefore, must work rapidly to stabilize the patient, to assess and debride the wounds, and to restore circulation. This is facilitated by the fact that the vessels involved are much larger and, therefore, easier to repair. When needed, temporary shunt catheters may be utilized to restore circulation for a short period to gain the additional ischemic time needed for proper bone fixation and harvesting of vein grafts. It may help to allow the initial dark venous blood to bleed out before releasing the venous clamps, in order to minimize systemic acidosis. Finally, the functional goals of proximal replantations are, by necessity, less precise, and the surgery tends to involve fewer structures.

Upper Limb Versus Lower Limb

The hand and the entire upper limb need precision, dexterity, and power if they are to be useful. The demand for adequate restoration of sensation and motion is there-

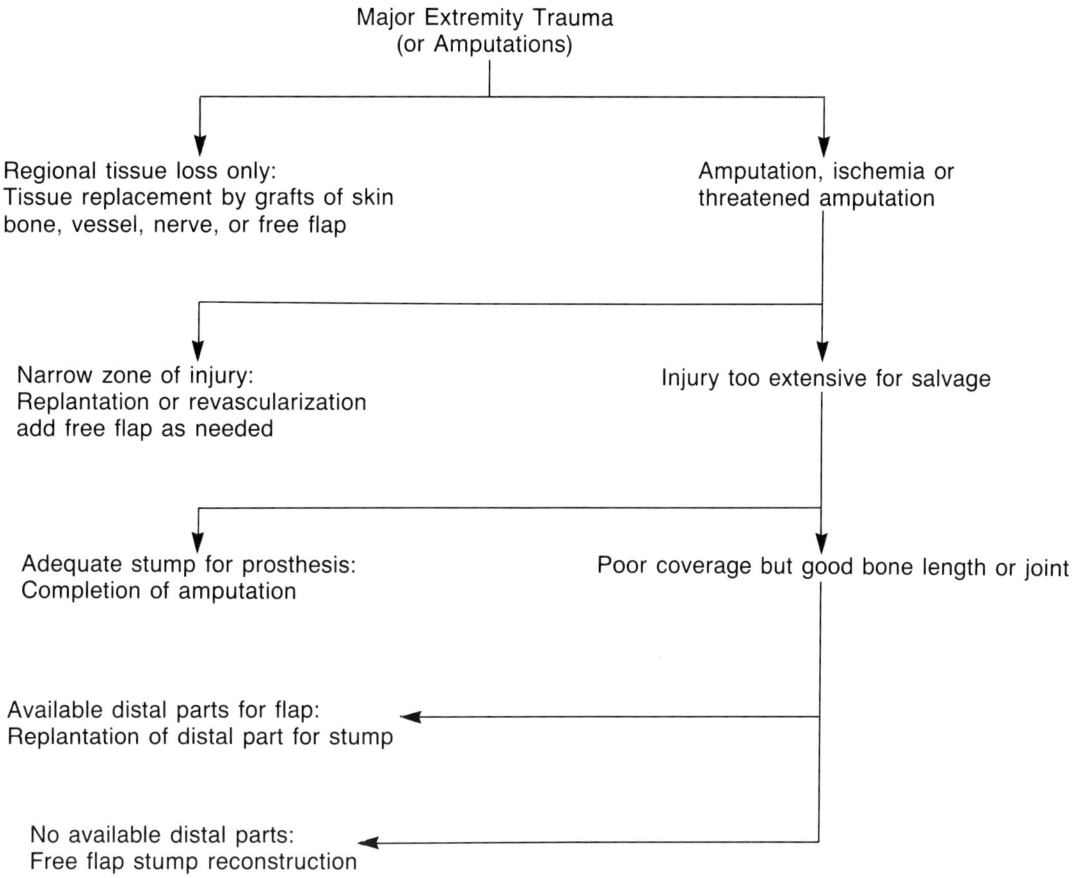

Figure 1 Decision tree showing the reconstructive options available in major limb trauma or amputations.

fore, high (Fig. 2). Detailed attention is needed to ensure proper bone position, tendon length, joint immobilization, and nerve repair. The lower limb, on the other hand, neither performs dexterous manipulations nor requires delicate sensory discrimination. Stability, durable weight-bearing surface, and protective sensation of the foot are important. Since prostheses do not need ankle or toe motions to be effective, many times a replanted leg with compromised motion or sensation can still function well as a "living prosthesis." The loss of length in replantation of an upper limb is generally well tolerated, both functionally and esthetically. On the other hand, it becomes increasingly more difficult to compensate for discrepancy of greater than 2 inches in the lower limb. For bilateral lower limb amputations, however, shortening of greater than 2 inches may be tolerated. If the amputations are at dissimilar levels, one may consider replanting a foot to the opposite leg—the so-called "foot switch" procedure.

Associated Injuries

Either proximal or distal amputations may be associated with other injuries at multiple sites or levels, due to the nature of injury or to the reflex reaction from the injury. All of these need to be fully assessed to determine the overall surgical strategy. Major limb amputations are invariably due to high energy trauma and the patient often arrives at the hospital hypotensive from external or internal bleeding. Blood volume resuscitation and management of any life-threatening emergency obviously take precedence over considerations for replantation. At times, technically feasible replantations may have to be abandoned to avoid compromising the patient's chance for survival.

Ideally, there should be full cooperation and experienced coordination between the replant surgeon, the trauma surgeon, and other surgical specialists. The decision to proceed with replantation must be made with optimal input from everyone, so that no life is endangered by the replantation effort and no salvageable limb is unnecessarily wasted due to poor management of systemic problems. For example, the trauma surgeon could be doing a laparotomy while the replant surgeon debrides the amputated limb with the intention to replant. The decision to complete the replantation, however, depends upon the total consideration of the magnitude of the abdominal injury, the condition of the patient, and the likelihood of a good anatomic and functional result from replantation. Even with distal replantations, there may be additional blood loss incurred in an already unstable patient; therefore, the aggressiveness and extent of surgery must always be tempered with awareness of the patient's overall condition.

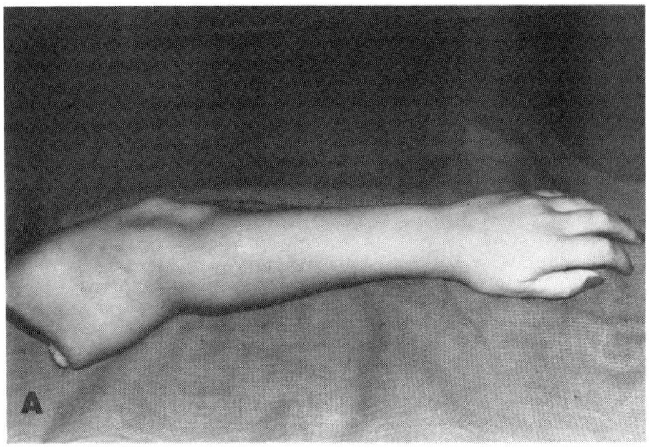

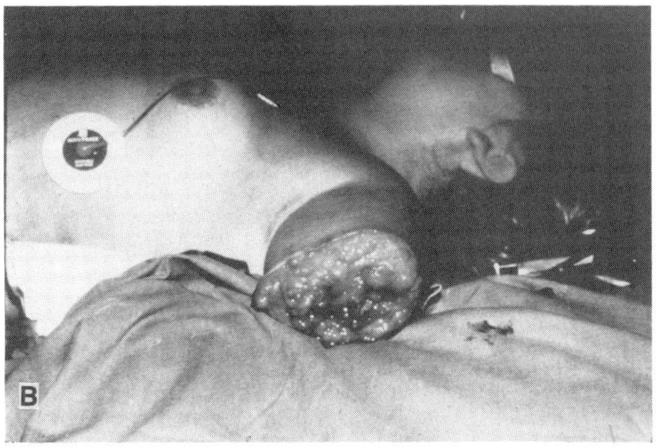

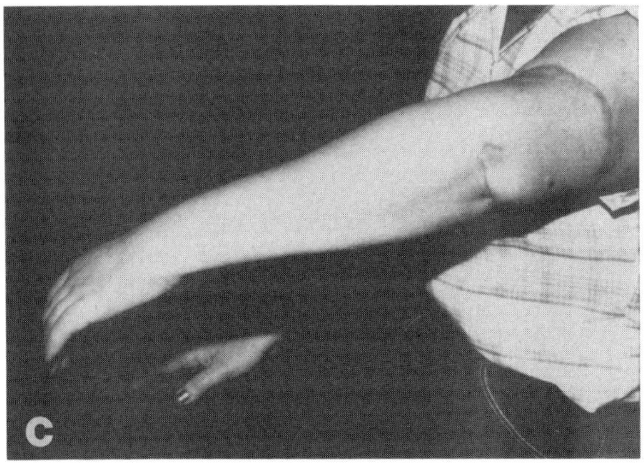

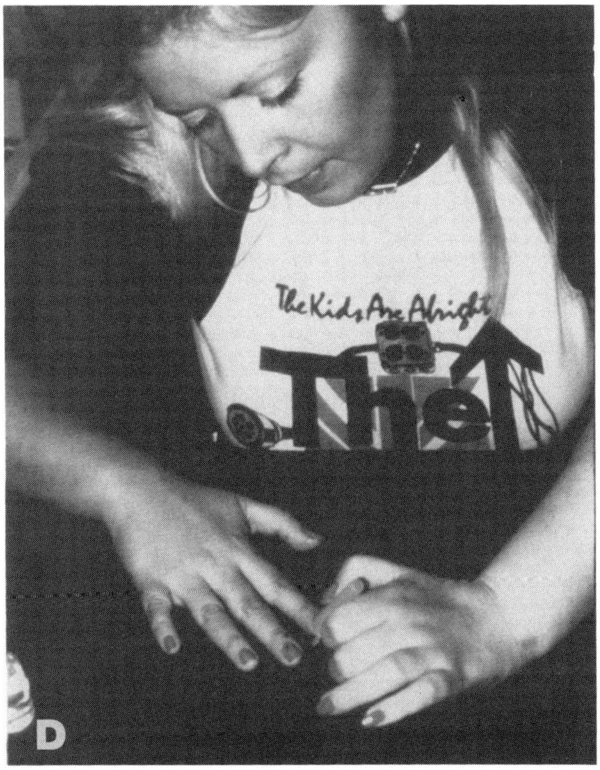

Figure 2 A midarm amputation with primary neurovascular replantation and no additional surgery. *A*, The amputated arm with limited crush and *B*, the proximate stump. *C*, One year after replantation, with independent wrist extension, and *D*, there is useful finger motion and sensation 1½ years after replantation.

Care of the Amputated Part and Stump

The majority of replantation patients are brought in from a distance or referred from another hospital. The emergency care of the amputated part and the patient is critically important (Table 1). For the amputated part, prompt cooling to about 4° C is ideal to lower metabolic rate and prolong tolerable ischemic time. For most smaller amputated parts, such as hands and fingers, this cooling is done by rinsing the part with water or saline to remove gross contamination and then wrapping it with a thin dry gauze to protect it from freezing. The wrapped part is then sealed in a plastic bag and placed in a bucket of ice and water. Saline is not used with ice because it may result in subzero temperature. Liquid nitrogen or dry ice (liquid CO_2) are also to be avoided because of the freezing injury to the tissue. For a large portion of an extremity, not suitable for the plastic bag and bucket, one can simply wrap it with a layer of towel and place ice packs around the limb. It is important that the amputated part be properly labelled and transported with the patient to avoid inadvertent loss or mix-up.

The amputation stump should be covered with gauze and wrapped with ace bandages to control surface bleeding. A tourniquet is used only if there is uncontrolled bleeding and must be removed at the earliest possibility to avoid iatrogenic ischemic injury at a higher level. Unstable fractures need to be splinted to avoid pain and additional injuries from the bone edges. All available medical information or x-ray films should accompany the patient to expedite his entry to the operating room. Unstable patients may require helicopter or attendant physician for the

TABLE 1 Initial Management of Extremity Amputations

Patient	*Amputated Part*
Vital signs Control bleeding by pressure Transfer to nearest trauma center if patient unstable Contact and transfer to replant center	Rinse to rid of gross contamination Wrap in clean gauge or cloth Pack with ice bags for large limb, seal in plastic bag and cover with ice for digits

transfer. Such transfers should be carefully screened and coordinated so as to avoid unwarranted travel that may endanger the patient's life in a poor attempt to save a limb.

INDICATIONS FOR REPLANTATION

As experience is gained with replantations, we have learned that there are no simple rules for surgical indications for all patients. Economics, psychology, and other nonsurgical factors are also important and must be kept in mind when deciding what is best. Also, experience and an appreciation of the long-term results are essential before the subject can be approached realistically. The surgeon must be able to look beyond survival and assess whether the replanted part will contribute to or delete from hand function. Every case is unique and should be decided on an individual basis. Nonetheless, there are general guidelines that should be well-known to all surgeons who see such patients (Tables 2 and 3).

There is continued skepticism regarding the value of a single digit replantation (excluding the thumb) in an otherwise normal hand. Single digit replantations at, or proximal to, the insertion of the superficialis tendon onto the middle phalanx are particularly questionable because of the frequently associated proximal interphalangeal (PIP) joint stiffness. Replantations distal to the sublimis insertion, though not as critical to hand function, usually do not detract from it, and therefore, may be considered more favorably. Any thumb amputation should be considered for replantation because of its obvious importance along with a lessened need for interphalangeal (IP) joint motions. Ring avulsion amputations present a particularly difficult challenge. Not only are they technically more difficult to reattach than a clean amputation, but, if they survive, they are also more apt to have severe disturbances of sensation and stiffness. Replantation should be attempted for multiple amputated fingers, or those in previously damaged hands, so as to have the best chance for some useful function.

Major upper limb replantations are associated with wide zone of injury, higher complications, and poorer functional results. In general, replantations are still highly preferable to the prosthetic alternatives. The problems with extensive high energy trauma are even more severe with lower limb amputations, and few cases are suitable for replantation. Frequently, soft tissue free flaps are needed to permit salvage replantation. Also, lower limb prostheses work fairly well and should always be considered as an alternative.

A dogmatic approach to indications for replantation is not warranted, and one should retain a flexible attitude. The definitive chapter on decisions for replantation surgery will never be written, except, perhaps, by naive bureaucrats from the government or insurance companies. The accumulation of experience and the reassessment of results are always helpful.

SURGICAL TECHNIQUE

The need to maintain a flexible surgical plan and be prepared to deal with the unexpected problem, or seize on a creative reconstructive opportunity of the moment, is particularly important in replantation surgery. Nonetheless, it helps to follow a pattern that has proved efficient after many years of replantation surgery (Table 4). The basic principles of microsurgical techniques are well described in standard texts.

Preoperative Preparation

In the initial comprehensive history and examination, particular attention is paid to the patient's occupational needs and his expectations regarding surgery. Such information becomes important when the surgeon must make critical decisions for the patient in the operating room as regards the ultimate goals of reconstruction, based on the findings after debridement. Appropriate laboratory tests and consultations are quickly obtained. X-ray films of both the amputated part and the stump are obtained to begin the decision making and surgical planning. Arteriography is obtained only when there is a special need and when a good quality study is readily available without delay. It is not necessary with most sharp, open injuries. The patient should be expedited into the operating room to give the surgeon more time for an orderly replantation. In many cases, the amputated part can be taken to the operating

TABLE 2 Indications for Upper Extremity Replantation

Strong	*Borderline*	*Weak*
Arm	Single digit	Avulsion injuries
Hand	Digit of special significance	Extensive crush
Thumb		
Multiple digits		
Clean and sharp injuries		

TABLE 3 Indications for Lower Extremity Replantation

Medically stable
<3 inch bone shortening
Bilateral amputations
Adequate soft tissue and nerve restoration
Well-motivated patient
Children

TABLE 4 Steps in Hand Replantation Surgery

Debridement and identification of structures
Bone fixation
Extensor tendon repairs
Dorsal vein repairs*
Flexor tendon repairs
Digital nerve repairs
Digital artery repairs
Skin closure
Cast or splint application

* If ischemic time is long the flexor side repairs are done first to provide reperfusion of the finger prior to venous repair.

room first for debridement while the patient is still in the examining room.

Debridement and Identification

All damaged or contaminated tissues must be excised meticulously, both grossly and microscopically. High pressure jet lavage irrigation is used in contaminated cases to decrease the bacteria count. Inadequate debridement is the most common reason for infection after successful vascular repair and frequently results in delayed failure of replantation. Four patterns of injuries are often recognized. The easiest to deal with is the sharp clean *guillotine* amputation such as from a paper cutter or from a machete (surprisingly, not uncommon in New York City; Fig. 3). *Localized crush* amputations result from table saws or industrial press machines with blunt edges. The zone of injury may be very narrow or wide and occasionally, multileveled depending upon the wounding instrument. *Extensive crush* amputation occurs when the limb is caught between two large flat surfaces, such as two automobile bumpers or a falling concrete block. With an increasing zone of injury, it becomes progressively less feasible to replant or reconstruct with good results. Unfortunately, many crush injuries also have a significant avulsion component that occurs when the patient tries to withdraw the limb by reflex. Such *crush-avulsion* amputations often have rupture of the tendons from the muscles at a higher level and extensive stretch injuries of the vessels and nerves. Frequent examples are seen from punch press accidents at work or trash compactors around the home. Fasciotomies and extensive resections of the injured nerves and vessels are mandatory, and nerve and vein grafts are usually needed. The overall functional results are also severely compromised in such cases.

During debridement, the corresponding structures on the two sides are tagged with sutures or clips to facilitate later identification for repairs. Tendon sutures or K-wires may be replaced on one side of the tendons or bone to expedite the final repair, as well as to minimize later manipulation of the parts.

Skeletal Fixation

Skeletal stabilization is usually done first to allow a fixed frame for subsequent repair of smaller structures. This may require shortening of the bone to allow for tension-free closure of skin as well as repair of vessels and nerves. In some circumstances, vessels and nerves can be lengthened with interpositional grafts to overcome gaps and eliminate tension. When an entire joint is too severely damaged, it may be better to accept a permanent fusion. Most commonly, the fixation of small bones is done with K-wires and interosseous wires, while larger bones are fixed with internal plates or external fixators through pins above and below the fractures.

Tendon Repairs

The extensor and flexor tendons are usually repaired next, after osseous fixation, so as to avoid the later need for gross movements after the microsurgical repairs. It is often difficult to place the tendon repair junctures at a site remote from the bone repair. Scar tissue tends to fill the wound completely and cement the tendons and bone into a common dense cicatrix. Replantations proximal to the wrist do better with motion, but adhesions between the muscles and scars may still prevent full motion.

Microsurgical Repairs

The veins, nerves, and arteries are then repaired with the aid of the operating microscope. The sequence can be varied to suit the conditions. If the ischemia time has been long, it may be preferable to repair an artery and allow the part to perfuse promptly. It is preferable to repair one or more veins, then the nerves, and, lastly, the artery. The excessive bleeding after the arterial repair makes subsequent venous or nerve repairs more difficult. Interpositional grafts should be used if there is any hint of tension on the repairs.

Skin Coverage

Last but not least, skin coverage is obtained. The most important principle with limb trauma is to obtain primary wound healing. It may be necessary to use small skin grafts, or even a distant flap from an adjacent finger, to accomplish the desired tension-free closure. Efforts should be made to cover the vessel anastomoses with local tissue. Tight closure, use of compromised skin, and residual dead space are common causes of later breakdowns, infections, and failure.

Repair Priorities

When more than one digit is to be replanted, a priority of reattachment must be determined. Long operations are fatiguing to the surgeons as well as potentially harmful to the patient. It is preferable to put effort early in the operation where it will do most good. Some unlucky individuals have multiple digital amputations that include their thumbs. The thumb is the most important digital and should generally be restored first (Fig. 4). It needs adequate length, stability, and basilar joint mobility. When debridement of the thumb leaves it too short or

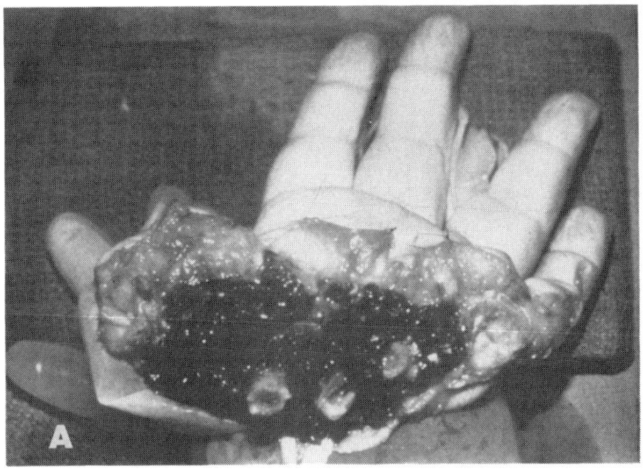

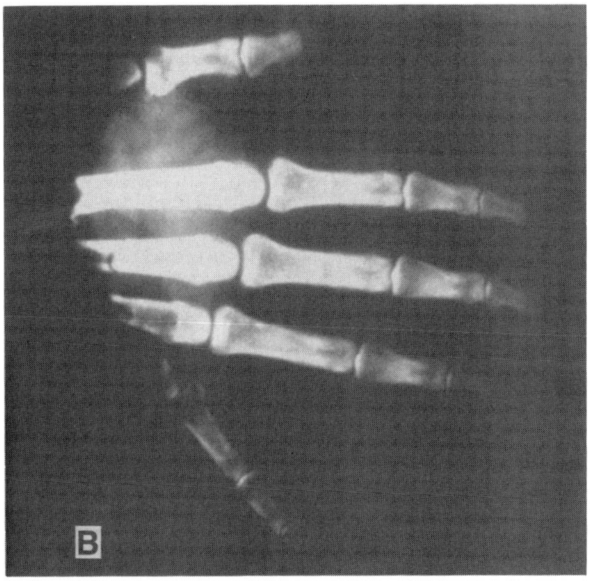

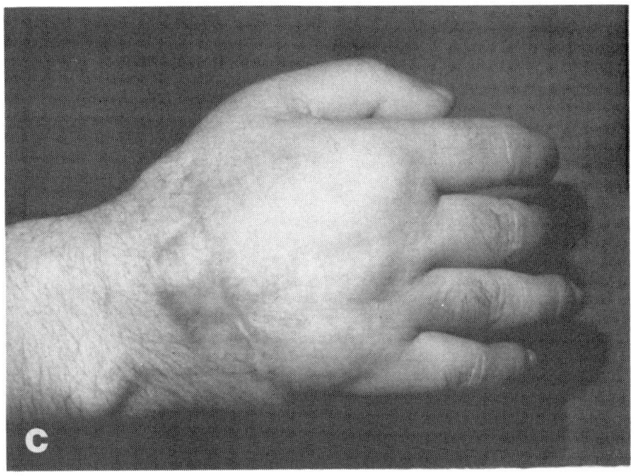

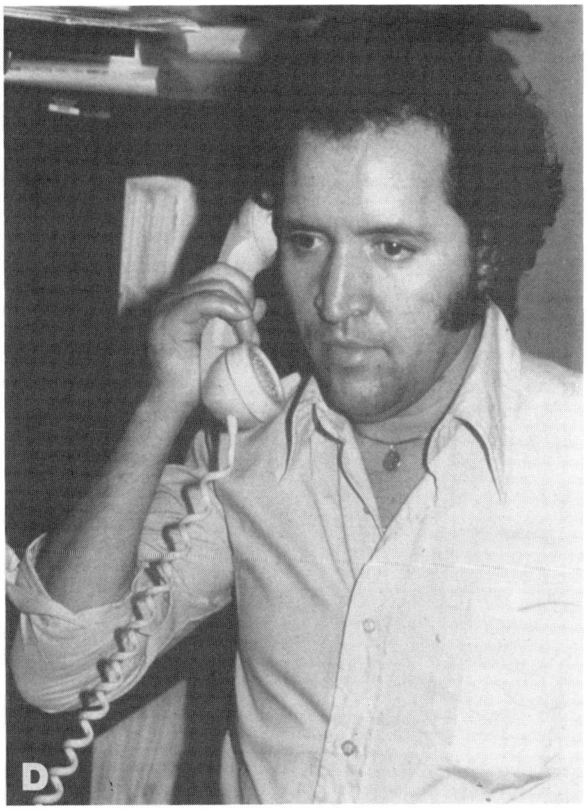

Figure 3 Paper cutter caused a palmar amputation. *A* and *B*, the distal part and an x-ray film of it. *C*, the hand is shown 6 months after replantation and, *D*, another six months later there is good use of the replanted dominant hand.

too restricted, one may consider attaching one of the other amputated fingers to the thumb position. The alternative is to preserve the stump and cover it with a soft tissue flap, as needed, to facilitate a later toe transfer or pollicization. It helps to complete one digital reattachment before starting the next. In general, a good finger in the long or ring position is more useful than one in the index position therefore, the index finger is usually replanted last.

Dressing and Splints

Sometimes, it is difficult to splint the extremity in the protective position because of concern for the vessel repairs. This is a violation of basic hand care principles, but can be excused in the interest of preserving circulation. The tendency towards a flexion contracture of the wrist and extension contractures of the metacarpophalan-

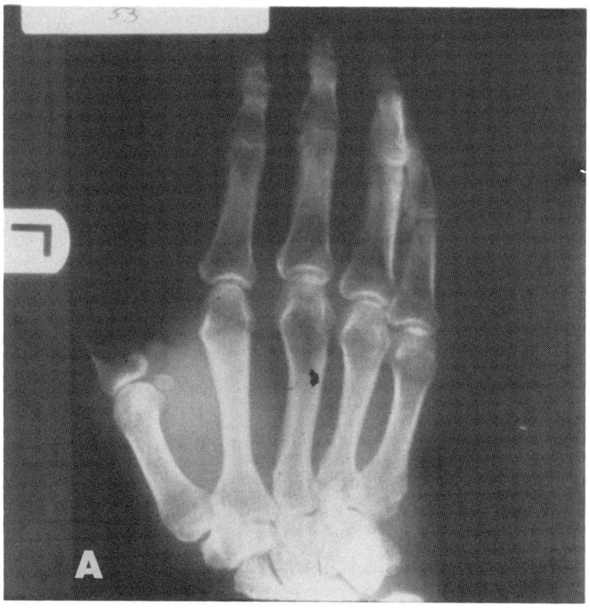

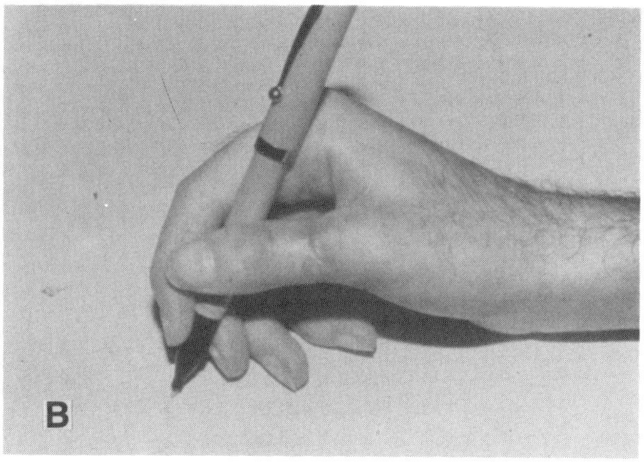

Figure 4 *A* and *B*, Thumb was successfully replanted after amputation.

geal joints, however, must be watched carefully and timely remedied with aggressive hand therapy. These problems have to be dealt with by the hand therapist.

Free Tissue Transfers

There are several roles for free tissue transfers in the care of the patient with a replantation. Acutely, a free flap may be required for wound closure. This may be where a major replantation is otherwise successful but lacks skin closure. It is worth investment of a latissimus dorsi or rectus free flap to achieve this. Somewhat more frequent is the situation where a free flap is needed to keep an amputation at a below knee level. Late ulceration and breakdown is not uncommon after major lower extremity replantations. A free flap may be the only means of correction.

POSTOPERATIVE REHABILITATION AND ADJUSTMENTS

Human replantations, unlike machines, cannot be expected to function immediately after reattachment. The survival of the replanted part promises only the potential for function. Time is needed for wounds to heal. The patient must be motivated to relearn the use of the part. A comprehensive rehabilitation program is essential to regain function. The specific rehabilitation needed should be customized according to the patient's injury, his surgical reconstruction, and his personal needs. Psychological and social adjustments are also forced upon the patient. A general pattern is described below.

Postoperative Management

Anticoagulation is generally not needed with major limb replantations, as the vessels are large and the risk of bleeding considerable. With crush injuries of the finger and hand, however, the vessel sizes are much smaller and the zone of injury difficult to assess. Aspirin or dextran often are given routinely. In marginal cases, or after prior thrombosis, heparin usually is used. Occasionally, in patients with suggestions of vasospasm, a calcium-channel blocker or other vasodilators may be used.

In all patients, it is important to keep the systemic blood volume and hydration adequate to avoid hypotension and vasoconstriction. The ambient and body temperatures should be kept warm to ensure optimal peripheral vasodilations and avoid vasoconstriction. Antibiotics are routinely given during the perioperative period, but not continued unless specifically indicated.

Occupational and Physical Therapy

During the first week or two, the primary concern is for survival and wound healing. Because both the flexor and extensor components are involved, forceful active or passive movements would risk rupture of the repairs. Generally, the replanted part is immobilized and elevated to minimize pain, hemorrhage, vasospasm, and edema. A routine, postoperative, respiratory therapy and general conditioning program, however, may help to hasten the patient's overall recovery from the anesthesia.

After the first 2 weeks, the vascular survival of the part is usually no longer a problem and the main concern becomes the regaining of motion. The race is between getting the tendon and joints to move and the tendency toward restricted movement as the wound heals by scar formation. Customized splinting may be helpful to separate the tendon repair sites from the bone fractures in order to avoid the "one wound" scar contracture. Gentle active and passive motions, along with judicious splinting, must be carefully supervised to prevent excessive tension on the tendon repairs. Also, physical therapy with whirlpool, hot packs, or ultrasound is often beneficial, both for wound healing and motion. Early motion during this period sets the stage for a favorable recovery of movement.

By 4 to 6 weeks postreplantation, tendon rupture is unlikely and more vigorous active and passive motion can gradually begin, as well as muscle strengthening exercises. Within 2 to 4 months, most of the ultimate motion and strength has usually been established.

Useful nerve regeneration usually becomes evident by 3 to 5 months, depending upon the level of the replantation. Sensory re-education should start as soon as the patient begins to have any kind of sensation, so as to develop optimal sensibility as well as minimal pain symptoms. When electrical activities of muscle contractions can be picked up by cutaneous electrodes, a biofeedback exercise program may get the patient started on relearning how to use the formerly denervated muscle.

Once basic functions are somewhat restored, the patient needs to regain confidence in using the limb to perform daily living and occupational activities. In cases where the patient cannot be expected to return to previous work that requires heavy labor or great dexterity, vocational rehabilitation should be recommended.

FUNCTIONAL IMPLICATIONS

The surgeon who performs a replantation of an amputated part should consider not only the technical side of the operation but also the total rehabilitation of the individual. It is important to recognize the various functional patterns and anticipate how the final surgical result may contribute to hand function. Beasley has identified four patterns of upper extremity functions. First, a patient may use his upper limb as a *pusher and stabilizer.* A disarticulation at the elbow may achieve this. Second, a patient with an amputation through the midforearm may use the elbow as a *hook* to carry a suitcase. This justifies replantation of an amputation through the upper arm even if the hand is not useful. The third pattern, *grasp*, is still more important. A hand with poor sensation may act as a vice and be extremely helpful. Of the more than 200 varieties of upper limb prostheses, none does more than act as a vice. Fourth, the most refined function of the upper limb is *precision manipulation.* This requires normal sensation, along with adequate mobility and stability. For instance, because of age and the nature of the injury, the replanted digit in an adult often achieves only basic protective sensation and meager discriminative sensibility. It is incapable of precision manipulation and may become a liability to the adjacent fingers that have better sensibility. It may be better to concentrate on replanting a digit to the ulnar aspect of the hand where it can better contribute to power grasp.

Aside from basic structural restorations, the most important determinant to the ultimate function of a replanted hand or finger is the return of nerve function. Surgeons are gradually learning that the nerves should be repaired with the same careful attention to detail that is used for the vessels. Secondary nerve reconstructions, nerve grafts, and neurovascular island flaps may be important secondary operations to improve sensation.

The key to motility of the finger is the proximal interphalangeal joint. In the absence of relatively normal motion in the PIP joint, a finger cannot contribute to precision manipulation and has limited power grasp. This is why replantation of a single digit at, or proximal to, the insertion of the sublimis tendon into the middle phalanx is rarely indicated because of the certainty of PIP joint stiffness. A patient may be grateful for a hypesthetic finger that moves only at the metacarpophalangeal joint, but it probably does not contribute to hand function. A different situation exists when multiple fingers have been amputated.

Finally, there are instances when a replanted digit or limb interferes and limits total performance. Peter Keblish calls this "dysfunctional salvage." Thoughtful amputation at a level consistent with good prosthetic function can spare the patient many years of emotional and physical suffering.

PSYCHOLOGICAL IMPLICATIONS

A highly complex psychology is involved with replantation surgery, which is different from the routine care of extremity injuries. Surgeons should be well-acquainted with the psychodynamics involved with each patient in order to achieve better results and avoid unnecessary problems.

For most patients, the amputation injury and the loss of parts or functions represent the most traumatic event in their lives. The patient is ill-prepared for the ensuing emotional avalanches related to the circumstances of the injury; the threatened career plans, strained relationships with loved ones, and the doubts as to self-worth or image. The adaptation process is similar to that which follows the death or loss of loved ones: a sequence of denial, anger and grief, acceptance, and optimal adaptation. Courage, intelligence, guidance, and material support are essential to avoid poor adjustment and lifelong problems.

Invariably, the patient is angry that the accident should happen to him or her. Someone must be blamed for this! "If only...did not make me do..., this would not have happened, ...etc." The hostility is also frequently directed toward those who are taking care of his or her injuries; particularly those who made the critical decisions. If the replantation was not attempted or failed, the referring emergency physician may become suspected of unnecessary delays or poor management. Also, a number of nuisance lawsuits have been brought by patients against surgeons, claiming that the decision not to replant was because of "my inadequate insurance," "he didn't care," "he was too busy," and so on. Even after the best surgical efforts, minor inconsistencies in nursing care, wound management, operative procedures, or communications become monumental inadequacies that the patient may insist are the reasons for his poor outcome. It is vitally important that the patient perceives his surgeon as understanding, competent and interested in achieving the best result for him. Also, the feeling of having received the best possible care helps the patient accept the outcome, thereby avoiding unwarranted litigations.

The majority of patients are referred to a replantation center by a physician from another hospital who, in many instances, could have competently assessed and performed the needed repairs or amputations. Yet the idea of restoration of the severed part is like magic: the promise of total negation of the clumsy act that produced the injury. The replant surgeon has the impossible task of living up to the fantasy of the patient who says, "Doc, I know you can put me back together like before. I have faith in you!" It is often difficult to talk a patient out of replantation in cases where shortening of the bone and skin closure may be more practical and functional. If the part survives, both the surgeon and the patient are tempted too frequently to consider the operation a success and forget that it is just the first step toward rehabilitation. Uninjured parts may stiffen and unhealed wounds become indolent. The patient's unrealistic expectations can be difficult to change and the replanted finger often becomes the central focus of the patient's life. Instead of reassessment of his or her many remaining capabilities and an attempt to return to normalcy, convalescence is prolonged and rehabilitation is undermined. Unpublished data of James May of Boston show that patients who have undergone "successful" replantations are much less likely to have returned to work several years after their injury than similar patients who have undergone amputation. The surgeon, therefore, has the obligation to guide the outcome of surgery toward the best overall result rather than mere tissue survival.

It should be said, however, that most patients are delighted with their replanted fingers or limbs, and rarely is secondary elective amputation of the replanted part requested. Most patients can be guided to realize eventually that, despite the unfortunate accident, they have much left for which to be grateful. In fact, most patients can function remarkably well with considerable disability. On occasion, such injuries have prompted individuals to redirect their life goals and perform beyond their prior expectations.

THE ROLE OF PROSTHETICS

There are two basic types of prostheses: functional and esthetic. The functional type acts as a hook or a vice while the esthetic prosthesis emphasizes the passive substitution of the lost appearance. The available functional prostheses, particularly those for the lower extremity, are well-described in standard text and are not elaborated here.

In the past, many hand surgeons felt that there was only a limited place for esthetic prostheses. First, the quality was frequently poor, and the appearance unsatisfactory and unnatural. In particular, fingernails were poorly reproduced. In addition, the materials were hard to keep clean. Second, our understanding of function was incomplete. It was assumed that a stiff, unnatural, hypesthetic, and functionless finger was preferred to an artificial one. Now we have learned that the appearance of our hands is secondary in importance only to that of our faces. The handicap from a deformed hand is frequently the result of the individual not wanting it seen by others; not because of stiffness or poor sensation. In addition, there have been great advances in the fabrication of hand and digital prostheses. The new silicone rubber prostheses, which are easy to keep clean, are constructed as mirror images from the contralateral hand. The coloring is accurate even to duplication of the dorsal venous pattern. The detail of fingernail construction is uncanny. In addition, pressure and position sense are transmitted to the stump, thus allowing individuals to use a typewriter without difficulty. Some even return to playing musical instruments such as the flute and guitar. The prostheses can be passively positioned to aid in grasp. Patient acceptance of these fabricated parts is excellent. Although prostheses do not replace the lost hand or finger, they may be vastly preferable to a visible deformity.

CONCLUSION

At present, we can anticipate an 85 percent survival in most centers for replantation or revascularization. In time, the survival rate will be improved still further and the surgery will become more routine with improved results. First, advances in organ preservation will greatly extend the tolerable ischemia time, thereby permitting the replantations to be done semielectively under optimal conditions. Second, we will have a much greater understanding as to which patients will benefit from the surgery, and this will allow us to focus our indications more clearly. Finally, because of increasing government regulations and concerns for cost-effectiveness, we will be forced to be more selective in our replantation efforts.

What was considered a surgical miracle only a few years ago, is now a routine and well-established procedure. Our thinking has matured beyond considerations of technique or survival to that of well-defined indications. In fact, replantation is not a unique discipline, but is simply one aspect of total reconstruction and rehabilitation of a severely traumatized limb.

SUGGESTED READING

Aldea P, Shaw W. The evolution of the surgical management of severe lower extremity trauma. Clin Plast Surg 1986; 13:549–569.

Beasley R. Alternatives to replantation. Presented at Microsurgery for Extremity Trauma: Decisions and Techniques. New York: Bellevue Hospital Center, 1986.

Beasley R. Hand and finger prostheses. J Hand Surg 1987; 12A:144.

Buncke HT, Castleton KB, Daniel RK, et al. Replantation surgery in China. Plast Reconstr Surg 1973; 52:476–489.

Colen S, Romita M, Godfrey N, Shaw W. Salvage replantation. Clin Plast Surg 1983; 10:125–131.

Keblish P. Amputation alternatives in the lower limb, stressing combined management of the traumatized extremity. Clin Plast Surg 1986; 13:595–618.

Shaw W. Forward. Lower extremity trauma and reconstruction. Clin Plast Surg 1986; 13:xix–xxii.

Shaw W. Microvascular surgery. In: Haimovici H, ed. Vascular surgery. East Norwalk: Appleton & Lange, 1985:289.

Shaw W. Microsurgery—looking ahead. Clin Plast Surg 1986; 13:319–326.

USE OF LEECHES IN PLASTIC SURGERY

BRUCE A. KRAEMER, M.D.
KENNETH E. KORBER, M.H.S.

Leeches have been used clinically for over 2,500 years to treat a variety of medical conditions. In England, during the tenth century, because of the widespread use of leeches, Anglo-Saxon physicians were actually called "Leeches." Today, leeches are used at many microsurgical centers to provide critical venous outflow for compromised tissue replantations and transfers which would otherwise be unsalvageable. Leeches have also been suggested as an indicator of tissue viability since they will not attach themselves to a dead flap or to a flap with very poor arterial inflow. Furthermore, failure of a leech to rapidly attach to a replanted part and poor feeding behavior (poor sucking or consuming less than a full meal) prognosticates poor tissue survival despite a favorable skin color.

LEECH BITES

The leech uses its three jaws to pierce the skin to a depth of up to 1.5 mm (Fig. 1). The leech administers salivary gland secretions, which promote bleeding in the host, primarily through terminal salivary ductules at the leading edge of the jaw. In addition, active pharyngeal peristalsis and sucking during feeding further promote the egress of venous blood. After detachment, the leech leaves a characteristic "Y-shaped" or trefoil wound. Leeches usually feed until there is a six to 11-fold increase in their weight before detaching. A blood meal averages eight to nine times the leech's initial weight. Feeding lasts for 20 to 60 minutes. The feedback for cessation of feeding is related to distension of the gut wall.

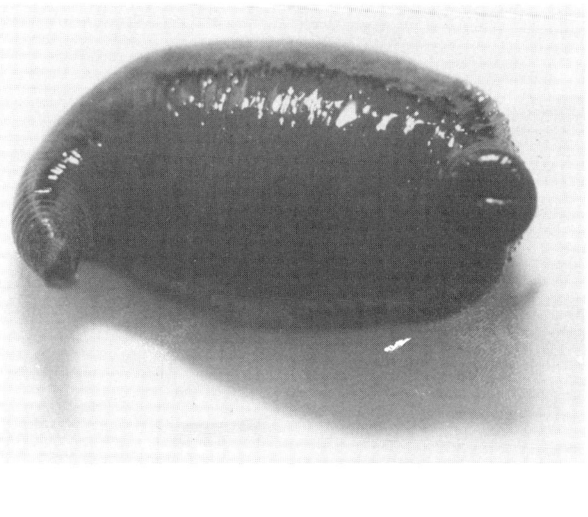

Figure 1 The leech has two suckers: the larger sucker (right) is at the caudal end and supports the leech while it "looks" for a suitable host with its smaller anterior sucker (left). The tripartite jaw is withdrawn into the anterior sucker during the resting state.

Leeches possess properties that make them uniquely able to assist with venous compromised tissue. The saliva of *Hirudo medicinalis* contains an anticoagulant, hirudin, which is a low molecular weight polypeptide composed of 65 amino acids. It is an extremely specific nonenzymatic inhibitor of thrombin, which it inactivates by blocking its substrate binding groups and preventing its binding to saturable sites. In vitro studies have also suggested that it inhibits active Factor X. Hirudin has advantages over heparin in that hirudin does not require the presence of antithrombin III for its effect, is not bound by the heparin-neutralizing platelet factor 4, and works locally in the wound inhibiting clotting at the wound. The prolonged bleeding that occurs from a leech bite cannot be solely explained by the presence of hirudin. A histamine-like vasodilator has also been identified in the saliva which also promotes bleeding. The hyaluronidase present in salivary glands not only increases tissue permeability to the other salivary secretions but has antibiotic properties, presumably due to its bacterial capsule dissolving properties.

CARE OF THE LEECHES

We obtain leeches from Leeches, U.S.A. (300 Shames Drive, Westbury, New York), who distribute *Hirudo medicinalis* in the United States for Biopharm. Biopharm leeches are raised on a leech farm in Swansea, South Wales. They are fed bovine blood until they are shipped to the United States for subsequent distribution. Our pharmacy department stocks the leeches and is responsible for periodic reordering so that a supply of at least 5 to 8 leeches is available at all times. Leeches are obtained as clinically needed from the pharmacy department. When the leeches are used, the pharmacy orders a fresh supply, which is usually obtained within 24 hours.

Leeches are best kept in a glass or plastic container, which has a tightly fitting nylon stocking covering it to prevent their escape. A portion of the water in the container should be replaced on a weekly basis with dechlorinated water. Leeches U.S.A. recommends that leeches be kept in distilled water to which a salt mixture they offer (Hirudosalt) is added. The water temperature should be approximately 10° C, at which temperature leeches may live for many months without feeding. The leeches respond and perform well after warming to room temperature. Hungry leeches position themselves with their anterior sucker slightly out of the water whereas well-fed leeches position themselves deeper in the container—a fact to keep in mind as one selects a suitable leech for a treatment.

CONSENT FOR USE

We obtain a separate written consent for leech treatment. Other institutions find a verbal consent to be sufficient for treatment. Alternative therapies, such as systemic heparinization or removal of the fingernail and heparin-soaked sponge administration to the nail bed, are presented to the family as part of the informed consent as less optimal alternatives to leech therapy for venous congestion.

The patient and family should be informed of the following possible complications.

Infection. *Aeromonas hydrophilia* lives endosymbiotically in the gut of *Hirudo medicinalis* and produces digestive enzymes for the leech, as well as an antibiotic that restricts the growth of other bacteria. In addition, there are reports that leeches can carry some viruses in their gastrointestinal (GI) tract for as long as 4 months. A poorly described infection in one of 14 digital replants in which leeches were used and an *Aeromonas hydrophilia* constitute the only possible leech related infections reported in the literature. We have not experienced any infections in our patients. To minimize patient risk, leeches are used only once and the patient is placed on intravenous antibiotics during the course of treatment.

Allergic reaction. While there are no reports in the literature of allergic reactions to *Hirudo medicinalis*, the possibility exists that a patient could manifest local allergic symptoms. Local, self-limited allergic reactions have been reported with the use of other leech species. The use of *Hirudo medicinalis* in the United States may be more safe than in Europe (where the leech is endemic) because a patient is unlikely to have had prior exposure to this species of leech.

Bleeding. Although the leech consumes only 5 to 10 cc of blood during its 30 to 60 minute feeding, the wound is stimulated to bleed by the nursing staff for many hours after the leech treatment. Leech treatments may be needed for as long as 7 to 14 days (usually 4 to 7 days). The use of leeches may increase the possible need for postoperative blood transfusions. Therefore, the patient and the family should be made aware that blood transfusions may be required if leech therapy is to be used.

PROTOCOL

The following protocol is a combination of published protocols and personal experience. Success and acceptance of therapy depends upon continued physician support of both patient and nursing staff. It is important for a physician to be present at the initiation of treatment and to evaluate the patient every 12 to 18 hours to determine the need for continued treatment.

Intravenous antibiotics are used during the course of leech therapy. Treatment is based on use of a broad spectrum antibiotic which protects against *Aeromonas hydrophilia, Pseudomonas, Proteus, Enterobacteraciae* as well as gram-positive organisms, which the leech may harbor. Adults are given ceftriaxone (Rocephin), 1 g twice daily, and children are given 50 mg per kilogram per day in divided doses during the course of leech therapy. Pretreatment of the leech with chloromycetin has been shown to inhibit the *Aeromonas hydrophilia*, but since infection has not been a problem for us, we have not adopted this into our treatment program.

1. Cleanse the site for the proposed leech attachment with saline. The skin must have all traces of antiseptics, dried blood, ointments, and petrolatum removed as their presence may discourage or distract the leech. It is important to not have the leech positioned directly over a blood vessel. Marked bleeding has been reported after a leech pierced a communicating artery in the forearm.
2. Place a saline-moistened gauze sponge around the proposed site of leech attachment to cover any areas that may have blood and thus distract the leech from his purpose. Use towels or other covering to prevent the leech from crawling into the recesses of the wound or dressing.
3. The leech should be handled with protective gloves. Before the leech is applied to the patient, it should be gently wiped off with a lightly saline moistened gauze sponge to remove excess mucus and secretions.
4. The site for leech attachment is pricked with a 20 gauge needle and then compressed until a drop of blood forms. The anterior leech sucker (smaller end) (Fig. 2) is then coaxed to attach to this site with a gloved finger or a cotton swab.
5. The leech may need encouragement to begin feeding. Several drops of a 5 percent glucose-saline solution may help encourage the leech to attach to the desired site. In addition, warming of the site of attachment may promote leech attachment because leeches bite best when the contact surface is 37 to 40 ° C. Caution should be exercised in warming the tissues to avoid thermal damage to the already compromised tissues. One might also isolate the leech to the desired "bite site" with a glass tube until it is attached.
6. After attachment, the leech should be observed until it demonstrates active muscular pharynx peristalsis, an indication that attachment has been successful and

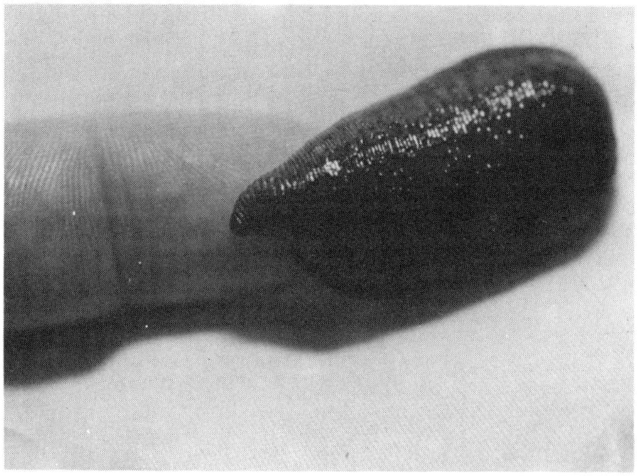

Figure 2 The leech's anterior head is initially small when it contacts a suitable host. The head then enlarges as the leech brings its jaws into contact with the host and begins to bite.

that the leech is interested in feeding (Fig. 3). In addition to pharyngeal peristalsis, the leech body occasionally peristalses as feeding progresses.

7. Once attached, the leech should be allowed to feed uninterrupted until it drops off. The leech should be monitored at least every 5 to 10 minutes while it is feeding, which usually lasts for 20 to 40 minutes. On rare occasions, a leech may not release after it is engorged. One should not grab or squeeze the leech as it may cause the leech to regurgitate its crop contents (containing *Aeromonas hydrophilia*) into the wound or to leave one or more of its jaws in the wound leading to wound complications. Stroking the leech with an alcohol wipe or applying salt to the leech causes it to release.
8. Although a replanted digit may be well served by a single leech at each treatment, a flap may need several leeches. The exact number and location of the leeches depends upon the degree and location of venous obstruction. As not all leeches feed equally well, one may need to apply several leeches for a single treatment.
9. Depending upon the amount of tissue being treated and the vascular status, a leech may be reapplied to the same site or to a new site. Distal digital replants, especially in children, often necessitate use of the same site which is usually on the side opposite the vessel repair. The site of reattachment is stimulated to bleed by pressing a small amount of blood out of the wound or by repricking the skin.
10. Used leeches are euthanized by placing them in small containers of 70 percent alcohol before they are disposed of.
11. The leech bite sites are periodically examined for signs of either allergic complications or infection. The physician is contacted when there is any concern about unusual swelling, ecchymoses, or petechial hemorrhages. Bacterial cultures are performed, should there be concern about an impending infection.
12. Serial hematocrit tubes are spun from the free-flowing blood from the leech bite site every 6 hours, and these values are recorded on a flow sheet. As these values may vary depending upon the blood flow, a complete blood count is performed daily., The physician is notified if either the serial hematocrits or the daily complete blood count is less than 27 percent. Crossmatched blood should be readily available if needed.
13. The nursing staff should record and chart the frequency of leech application, how often bleeding needs to be stimulated from the wound, the frequency that congestion redevelops, and serial hematocrits.

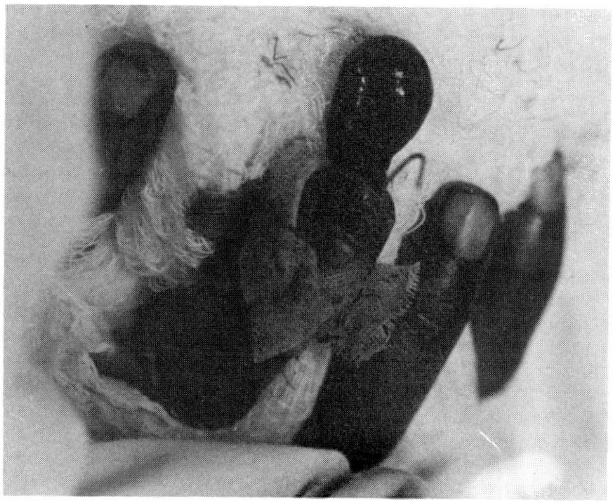

Figure 3 After the leech attaches to a host site, the leech everts its jaws, and the anterior sucker enlarges as the leech begins active pharyngeal suction. The leech often bends its posterior sucker around and attaches it adjacent to the anterior sucker.

SUGGESTED READING

Adams SL. The medicinal leech: a page from the annelids of internal medicine. Ann Int Med 1988; 109:399–405.

Batchelor ACG, Davidson P, Lully L. The salvage of congested skin flaps by the application of leeches. Br J Plast Surg 1960; 37: 358–360.

Foucher G, Henderson HR, Maneau M, Merle M, Braun FM. Distal digital replantation: one of the best indications for microsurgery. Int J Microsurg 1981; 3(4):263–270.

Green C, Gilby JA. The medicinal leech. J Royal Soc Health 1983; 103(1):42–44.

Leeches U.S.A., Ltd. Medicinal leeches restoring venous circulation in cosmetic and reconstructive surgery. Product Information, Westbury, New York, 1987.

Rao P, Ballie FB, Bailey BN. Leechmania in microsurgery. Practitioner 1985; 229:901–905.

Raubenheimer O. Leeches: how to dispense them. J Am Pharm Assoc 1923; 12:338–340.

Sawyer RT. Leech biology and behavior. Vol. 1, 2, and 3. New York: Oxford University Press, 1986.

POLLICIZATION FOR THE APLASTIC THUMB

JOSEPH UPTON, M.D.

During the past decade, no area within hand surgery has changed as dramatically as thumb reconstruction. Microvascular reattachment of the cleanly-amputated part is routine, and results following avulsion injuries are promising. If the carpometacarpal joint and a portion of the first metacarpal are present, excellent results can be achieved with transfer of an entire great toe, a debulked great toe, or a portion of the great toe as a wrap-around flap.

Despite these tremendous advances, pollicization is still the treatment of choice for congenital absence or severe hypoplasia of the first ray. The early contributions of Gosset and Hilgenfeldt have been artistically refined by Littler and Buck-Gramcko to the point where this is a predictable, functional, and esthetic procedure.

INDICATIONS

Any child with severe bilateral absence or hypoplasia of the thumb is an excellent candidate for pollicization, barring any accompanying major cardiovascular, hematologic, or central nervous system deficiency that would prevent the child from using the upper limbs effectively. Most experienced surgeons recommend pollicization for unilateral, as well as bilateral, deficiencies. Patients with severe retardation, or proximal limb deficiencies such as hand-to-shoulder phocomelia, may not be good candidates. An important consideration is the motion status of the ipsilateral shoulder and elbow, as well as arm and forearm length, because the child must be able to position the hand in space in order to use the thumb effectively.

Esthetic considerations are also important and are usually expressed by teenage children who have not had reconstructions. Creation of a deep, broad web space, and the bulk of the intrinsic muscle cone are key variables that impact upon the final appearance of the pollicized index finger, which, distally, will always be thinner than a normal thumb.

The decision to ablate a hypoplastic thumb to provide space for a more functional pollicization may be difficult. However, most of these patients have bilateral, yet asymmetrical, deformities, and it is best to pollicize the most efficient side first so the parents' subsequent decision becomes easier with a good functional result. Attempts to provide excellent function by reconstructing a hypoplastic thumb with no carpometacarpal joint can be frustrating. Microvascular transfer of joints, tendons, and skin have been performed, but long-term comparisons of their results with pollicizations are not available.

TIMING

Some controversy still exists regarding the optimal time for pollicization. Although Buck-Gramcko and Riordan have performed the procedure expertly at 6 months of age, most other experienced surgeons perfer to wait until 18 to 36 months of age. The advantages of waiting include improved cooperation of the child and an increased likelihood of performing precision surgery on a much larger hand. This age range is also consistent with our limited knowledge of neuromuscular maturation and conditioning of the cerebral cortex.

PRINCIPLES

In pollicization, the index digit is transferred as a neurovascular island into a new position that strategically simulates the thumb. To provide normal length, position, stability, and appearance, various maneuvers are necessary. New thumb length requires a significant recession and shortening of the transferred digit, accomplished by resection of almost the entire metacarpal with destruction of the epiphysis. Simultaneously, the ray is rotated 100 to 120 degrees and placed in a position of palmar abduction with the metacarpal head anterior to its base and acting as the new trapezium. This placement simulates the normal metacarpal arch, which is absent in these patients (see Fig. 4). Other important principles include proper incisions, meticulous soft tissue dissection with preservation of all intrinsic muscles, rebalancing of muscle-tendon units, and, of course, the application of a conforming dressing with proper immobilization.

OPERATIVE TECHNIQUE

Incisions

In contrast to post-traumatic thumb reconstructions, adequate skin cover is present in congenital cases, and the need for skin grafts usually indicates poor incision planning. A racquet-shaped incision is made at the base of the index finger just proximal to the digitopalmar flexion crease, with a radial extension that continues into the palm toward the new thenar flexion crease (Fig. 1). The rotation-recession movement of the index finger then invites a Y-to-V advancement of tissue from the radial border of the hand into either the radial or dorsal portion of the transferred index finger (see section on skin closure). The exact placement of this incision within the index finger often cannot be determined preoperatively and depends upon the tissue available. The esthetic appearance is more pleasing if a gradual web exists between the new thumb and long finger. This requires advancement of dorsal and ulnar tissue from the index finger up toward the long finger (Fig. 2). .

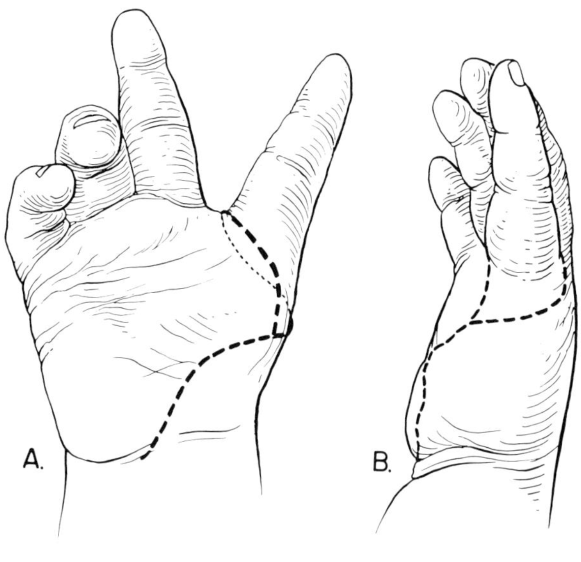

Figure 1 Outline of preferred incision at the level of the digitopalmar flexion crease on the palmar side and at the level of the metacarpophalangeal joint dorsally.

Pouce Flotant (Floating Thumb)

Although small nonfunctional thumbs, attached by soft tissue pedicles, should be ablated in the newborn nursery, it is occasionally useful to preserve the hypoplastic thumb and use its filleted soft tissue to augment radial bulk. This tissue can effectively be advanced into the dorsal aspect of the index finger to allow advancement of tissue for web construction (Fig. 3). It is best to plan incisions first as though there were no thumb remnant, and then see how one can incorporate this extra tissue into the original design. The level of hypoplastic thumb placement along the index ray, as well as the amount of tissue available, varies tremendously.

Often in the Holt-Oram syndrome (congenital heart disease and radial dysplasia), a hypoplastic thumb is joined through a simple, complete syndactyly to the index finger. This remnant can be excised as a separate procedure prior to pollicization, or at the same time. The advantages of the latter include increased exposure, which facilitates intrinsic muscle reattachment, and the avoidance of dissection of scar tissue during formal pollicization.

Soft Tissue Dissection

After incision marking, limb elevation and exsanguination, and inflation of a pneumatic tourniquet to 200 mm Hg, the first incisions are made around the base of the index finger and extended into the palm. Careful elevation of dorsal skin to expose the areolar plane between the dermis and subcutaneous fat facilitates dissection and the preservation of dorsal veins and sensory nerves. Palmar flaps are raised above the level of the palmar aponeurosis, which is then incised longitudinally over the flexor sheath. Any intrinsic muscles to the hypoplastic thumb, when present, are detached distally and raised on their proximal origin. The hypoplastic thumb, when present, is filleted from its skeletal remnants.

Isolation of the superficial palmar arch delineates the common digital artery and its two venae comitantes to the index-long web space, and, usually, the radial digital artery to the index finger as well. Approximately half of the patients have a well-formed radial neurovascular bundle. Digital sensory branches from the median nerve are identified, but are *not* dissected from their vascular partners. The arterial bifurcation to the radial side of the long (middle) finger is isolated, tied, and incised, followed by transsection of the intravolar plate ligament (transverse metacarpal ligament), which affords increased mobility to the index ray. The digital nerve to the long finger is then teased proximally to separate it from the index bundle. Vascular and neural loops may commonly be found within this bundle and must be manipulated carefully under magnification.

The hand is pronated 180 degrees, and the dorsal soft tissue dissected. The large veins and dorsal sensory branches of the radial nerve are identified and left within the soft tissue bed as the overlying skin is elevated. Occasionally, the largest and dominant dorsal vein runs in an ulnar direction over the long metacarpal and requires isolation.

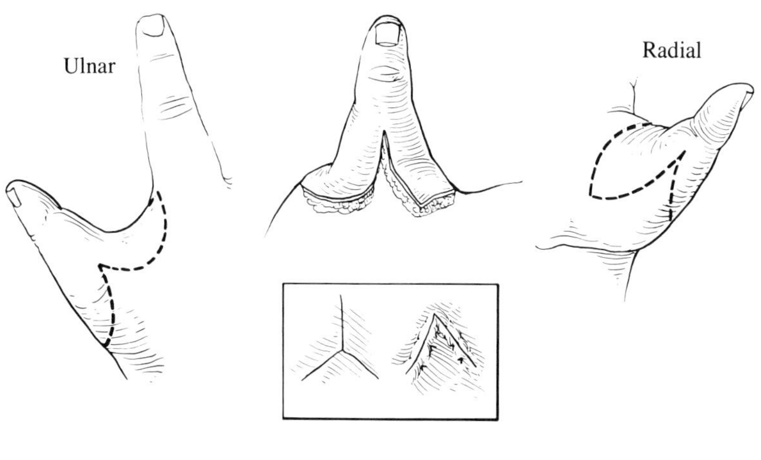

Figure 2 A Y-to-V closure principle improves contour, brings tissue in abundance into deficient areas, and improves first web space construction. The soft tissue flap from the radial border of the hand can be advanced into the index finger in one of three ways.

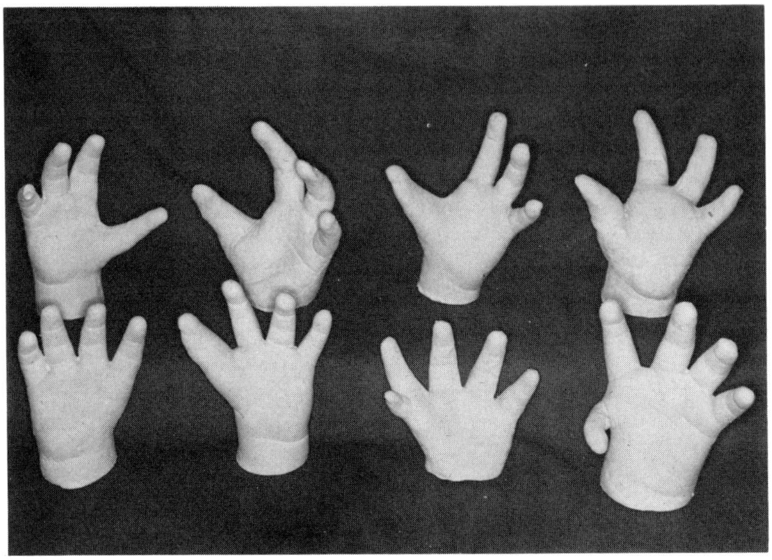

Figure 3 Pre- (bottom), and postoperative (top) hand molds demonstrate first web space reconstructions. The middle two hands are from patients with the Holt-Oram syndrome. A hand with a floating thumb is on the right.

The insertions of intrinsic muscles to the index finger are then detached and the muscles raised and mobilized. The first palmar interosseus (1st PI, or ulnar interosseus) is consistently present and will become the new adductor pollicis (AddP). Distal bone and tendinous insertions are carefully incised so that at least 1.0 to 2.0 cm of tendon is present for future reattachment by use of interweave junctures. The first dorsal interosseus (1st DI), also called the abductor indicis or radial interosseus, is detached in a similar fashion. More than one muscle belly occasionally is seen, especially in patients with hypoplastic thumbs. The lumbrical to the index finger is not dissected.

The extrinsic tendons are then prepared. The first annular and cruciate pulleys (A–1, C–1), as well as a small portion of the second annular pulley (A–2), are incised along the palmar midline of the flexor sheath, so that the flexor tendons to the new thumb approach at a more favorable angle. The index extensor digitorum communis and extensor indicis proprius are isolated dorsally, incised proximal to the extensor hood, and *freed* proximally well beyond the dorsal aspect of the index metacarpal. They are reattached following skeletal repositioning.

Skeletal Shortening and Repositioning

Once soft tissue dissection has been completed, the index metacarpal is exposed dorsally, and subperiosteal dissection is completed from metacarpal base to epiphysis. Intrinsic muscle attachments to periosteum are left intact. The collateral ligaments and palmar plate at the metacarpophalangeal joint also remain intact. A transverse osteotomy is made at the epiphysis. With deep retraction, the metacarpal base is cut obliquely to serve as a pillar to support the metacarpal head, which will be positioned anterior to it (Fig. 4). The metacarpal head, as part of an ovoid joint, becomes the trapezium as a substitute for the toroidal or universal saddle joint.

The index finger is then rotated and recessed in what becomes the most difficult maneuver of this operation. Adequate retraction is mandatory so that the metacarpal head (now a trapezium) can be fixed with either K wires passed from dorsal to palmar, or nonabsorbable sutures with the joint held in a position of hyperextension. The joint positioning advocated by Buck-Gramcko avoids excessive hyperextension of the new thumb. Superior function results are achieved when there is a stable skeletal union at this level instead of a mobile pseudoarthrosis. The positioning of the metacarpal head must be precise so that the new thumb now lies: (1) with the metacarpal head pronated 100 degrees, (2) flexed 35 to 40 degrees relative to the long (middle) metacarpal, and (3) abducted 20 degrees in a radial position.

The wound is covered with a moist sponge and the tourniquet deflated for a 25-minute respite at this point in the operation.

Intrinsic Muscle Rebalancing

Not only does skin closure reinforce this new position, but also muscle reattachments provide dynamic balance. Through intrinsic muscles, the child must be able to stabilize the repositioned new thumb.

At this point, after limb re-exsanguination and tourniquet reinflation, a decision is made regarding the first web construction. The cut-back incision is made within either the dorsal or radial surface of the new thumb to accept soft tissue from the radial border of the hand as a Y-to-V advancement flap (see Fig. 3). This maneuver also facilitates exposure of the extensor mechanism for reattachment of the intrinsic muscles.

The extensor index digitorum communis is advanced to become the abductor pollicis longus and is sutured with nonabsorbable stitches into the periosteum of the index proximal phalanx (now thumb metacarpal) under moderate tension. If eccentrically placed on the ulnar side of the phalanx, this transfer also serves both to extend and pronate the base of the new thumb. The extensor indicis proprius is then shortened and reattached to the central

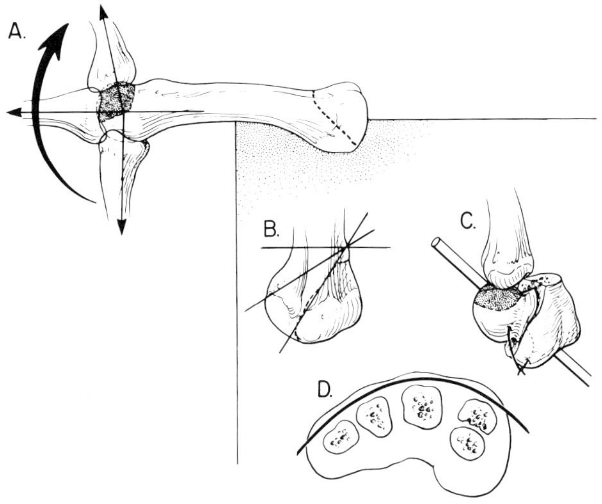

Figure 4 *A,* The eventual working surface of the hyperextended metacarpal head is darkly shaded. *B,* An oblique osteotomy is made at the metacarpal base to aid with extension of the metacarpal head (*C*), which can be stabilized with either nonabsorbable sutures or K wires. *D,* The new transverse metacarpal arch now exists.

portion of the extensor mechanism to become the extensor pollicis longus. End-to-end, simple overlap, or interweave tendon junctures work equally well.

The intrinsic muscles are then reattached. The 1st PI becomes the adductor pollicis and is attached to periosteum of the middle phalanx (now the thumb proximal phalanx). Some authors prefer to interweave this into the radial side of the extensor mechanism. This muscle is often small with poor mechanical advantage and can be reinforced with transfer of the flexor digitorum superficialis at a later date. The 1st DI (radial interosseus, abductor indicis) is then advanced and interwoven into the lateral band portion of the extensor mechanism at the level of the middle phalanx (now thumb proximal phalanx). If two muscle components are present, one is attached to the extensor mechanism and the other to the base of the phalanx to simulate the abductor pollicis brevis, thereby providing both palmar abduction and flexion-pronation for the new thumb. This muscle also provides some stability against excessive hyperextension.

The extrinsic flexor tendons are not altered as they will shorten and adjust to proper tension with time and growth. Within 18 months, strong flexion is present. This is not true for the extensor muscle-tendon units, which must be shortened (Fig. 5).

Despite careful rebalancing with what is available, some prime movements may be deficient and can be reinforced with future transfers; namely, the abductor digiti quinti transfer for palmar abduction (Huber transfer) or the flexor digitorum superficialis for adduction and pronation.

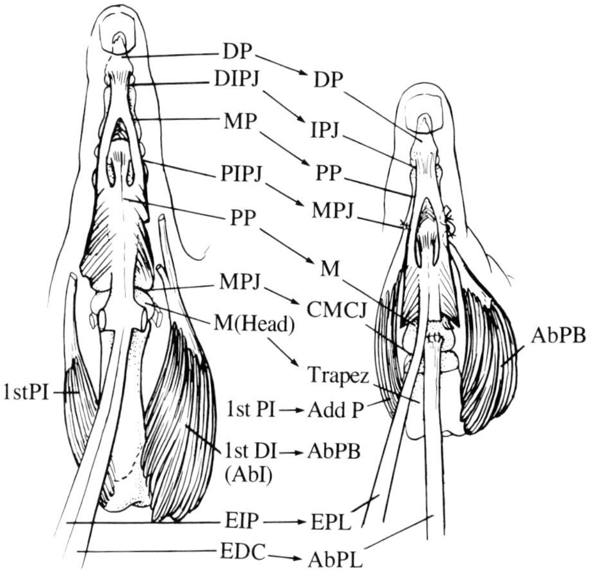

Figure 5 Rebalancing of the intrinsic and extrinsic muscles from index finger *(left)* to new thumb *(right)*. DP = distal phalanx, MP = middle phalanx, PP = proximal phalanx, M = metacarpal, DIPJ = distal interphalangeal joint, IPJ = interphalangeal joint, MPJ = metacarpophalangeal joint, M(head) = metacarpal head, CMC - carpometacarpal joint, EDC = extensor digitorum communis, EPL = extensor pollicis longus, EIP = extensor indicis proprius, 1st PI = first palmar interosseus (ulnar interosseus), 1st DI = first dorsal interosseus (radial interosseus, abductor indicis), ABPB = abductor pollicis brevis, ADDP = adductor pollicis, FPB = flexor pollicis brevis, ABPL = abductor pollicis longus.

Skin Closure

Although all incisions have been made, minor adjustments may be necessary to position scars so that healing and contracture do not impair function (Fig. 6). The upper portion of the skin within the first web space is closed first, followed by the palmar incision, and then by the dorsal or radial inset flap. Creation of a gentle web curvature to the base of the long (middle) finger is the ideal, and depends upon the amount of soft tissue available after the Y-to-V advancement (see Fig. 2, Fig. 7). If an excess of soft tissue bulk in the form of fat is present dorsally, it should be left and trimmed as a secondary procedure in order to avoid injury to, or kinking of, the dorsal venous outflow. Closure of the palmar incision dramatically stabilizes the new position of pronation and palmar abduction. Absorbable 5–0 and 6–0 chromic sutures are used. No drains are placed.

Dressing

One layer of impregnated gauze dressing is placed over the incision and covered by a one-inch layer of moist

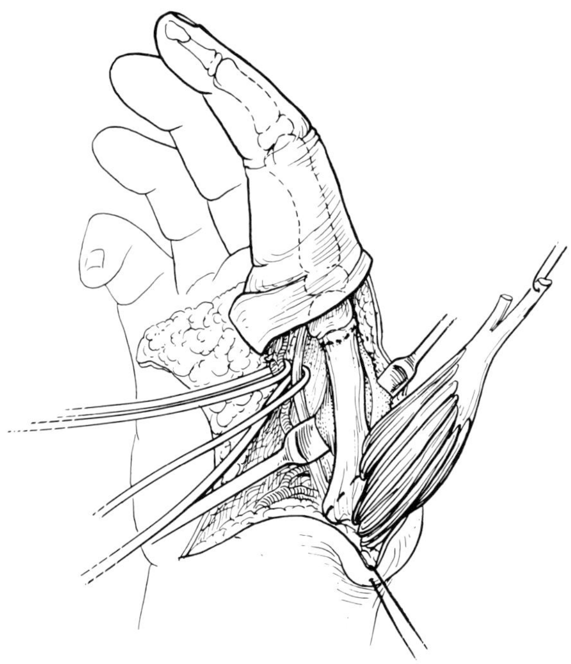

Figure 6 Placement of osteotomies within the metacarpal, designed to ablate the epiphysis and to provide a pillar for interior placement of the metacarpal head.

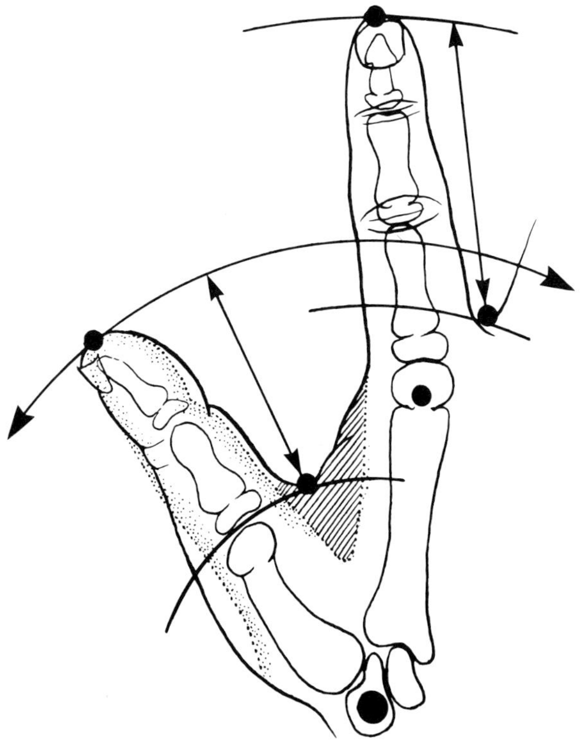

Figure 7 Comparison of metacarpal and phalangeal lengths of the normal thumb and index fingers demonstrates the slender configuration and very deep web space that exists if the index is superimposed (stippled within thumb). The darkly striped region represents the more distal and normal first web, which must be created with local tissue advancement. The distance from the tip of the thumb to the first web space is much less than that of the index finger to the second web space.

cotton, kneaded to match the thumb conformity. A firm hand dressing is then applied, and the entire limb is immobilized in a long arm fiberglass cast that extends well proximal to the elbow, which is flexed at 90 degrees. This position of flexion must be maintained while the dressing is applied, in order to avoid antecubital pressure, which can occur when the elbow is first wrapped with webril in extension before it is placed in a position of flexion.

The top of the thumb is left exposed, and parents are instructed to call if the thumb tip disappears; a signal of a loose dressing and/or cast. Four to 5 weeks postoperatively, the cast, pins, and sutures are removed. A thumb spica night-resting splint, molded with aquaplast, is then fabricated, and the child is started on an exercise regimen. No restraints are required at school or during play.

FOLLOW-UP

Following the immediate postoperative period, it is important to see these children yearly to assess function. Additional procedures, as indicated, may be necessary and, often, adaptive early intervention programs may be needed in school, particularly for children with multiple anomalies and severe handicaps. These children should not be denied placement with their peer groups on the basis of musculoskeletal anomalies alone.

The new thumb will never be normal; although it is perceived by the child as a thumb. Pinch strength and adduction will be deficient. Nail width, pulp volume, phalangeal lengths, joint relationships, and curvatures will never

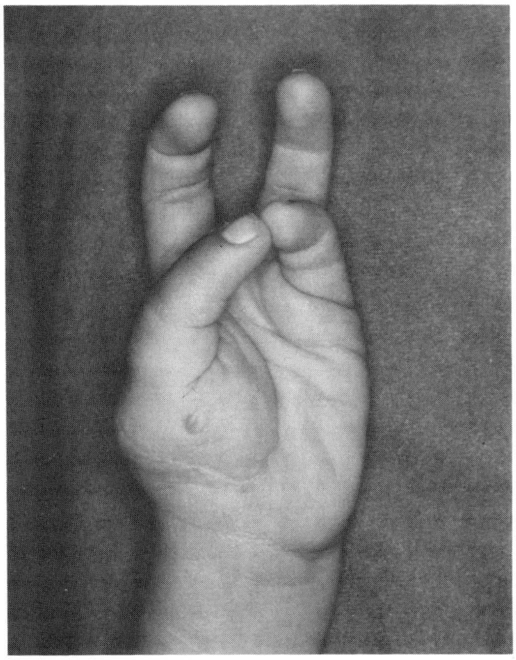

Figure 8 Postoperative appearance 3 years after pollicization demonstrates excellent pinch and palmar abduction due to a very functional intrinsic (first dorsal interosseus to abductor pollicis brevis) transfer.

precisely mimic the normal thumb (Fig. 8). Despite these minor drawbacks, the pollicized index digit is still the best and most predictable substitute for the congenitally absent thumb.

SUGGESTED READING

Buck-Gramcko D. Pollicization of the index finger. J Bone Joint Surg 1971: 53A:1605–1617.

Foucher G, Denuit P, Braun FM, et al. Le transfert total ou partiel du deuxieme orteil dans la reconstruction digitale. Acta orthop Belg 1981; 47:854–866.

Gosset J. La pollicization de l'index. J Chir 1949; 65:403.

Hentz VR, Littler JW. The surgical management of congenital hand anomalies. In: Coverse JE, ed. Reconstructive plastic surgery. 2nd ed. Philadelphia: WB Saunders, 1977:3306–3349.

Hilgenfeldt O. Operativer Daumenersatz, Stuttgari: Ferdinand Enke Verlag, 1950.

Littler JW. Neurovascular pedicle method of transposition for reconstruction of the hand. Reconstr Surg 1953; 12:303–319.

Morrison WA, O'Brien BM, MacLeod AM. Thumb reconstruction with a free neurovascular wrap-around flap from the big toe. J Hand Surg 1980; 5:575–583.

PAINFUL HAND SYNDROME

VERNON L. YOUNG, M.D.
BARRY FERNANDO, M.D.

The hand serves the individual as a primary point of contact with the environment. This important function, however, makes it highly susceptible to injury. The painful hand or wrist, regardless of the cause, is often an incapacitating problem that results in prolonged absence from work and permanent disability. Discomfort and disability are minimized by early diagnosis and proper treatment.

Establishment of the correct diagnosis is dependent upon a thorough, systematic history and physical examination and an understanding of hand anatomy. Subsequent radiologic and laboratory evaluations are directed by this initial examination.

This chapter outlines our approach to the painful hand and wrist. In addition, some of the common causes of wrist and hand pain will be discussed.

HISTORY AND PHYSICAL EXAMINATION

As in any medical evaluation, a complete, pertinent history must be obtained. Important historical points include: the onset of symptoms, the mechanism of injury (when applicable), prior hand or wrist problems, and associated medical illnesses. The patient's age, occupation, hobbies, and dominant hand should also be noted. Adequate examination of the hand and wrist requires attention to four principles: (1) observation, (2) palpation, (3) evaluation of the joints through a complete range of motion, and (4) a thorough neurologic examination.

The examination begins by exposing both upper extremities from the elbow distally. The presence of edema, inflammation, asymmetry, masses, and scars from prior operations is noted, as well as overall muscular development. Palpation always begins in areas removed from the points of maximal tenderness. The wrist is placed through a complete range of motion including flexion, extension, radial and ulnar deviation, pronation, and supination. Active and passive flexion and extension of the digits, and determination of collateral ligament stability, complete this portion of the examination. Limitations in motion with associated pain, popping, clicking, or instability are noted. Sensation in the median, ulnar, and radial nerve distributions is then evaluated. At this point in the examination, one can frequently localize the patient's discomfort to a specific anatomic structure. A tentative diagnosis can then be established to categorize the complaint into a bone, joint, ligamentous, tendon, soft tissue, neurologic, or vascular problem. Further studies are directed by this preliminary diagnosis and can include roentgenograms, bone scan, nerve conduction velocities, plethysmography, angiography, and pertinent laboratory tests. Sympathetic blockade can also be a useful diagnostic tool in certain patients.

X-ray films should be obtained for possible bone, joint, or ligamentous injuries. Appropriate views of the affected structure, in addition to radiographs of adequate quality, are essential. The minimum number of views for a finger includes posteroanterior (PA) and lateral; for the hand a PA, lateral and oblique; and for the wrist a four-view series that includes a PA, a lateral, and views with the wrist in radial and ulnar deviation. Failure to obtain appropriate roentgenograms can result in misdiagnosis caused by inadequate profile of a fracture line or joint. If these routine x-ray films do not establish a diagnosis, a bone scan is obtained. The bone scan is an extremely sensitive test that identifies almost all bony injuries, most ligamentous injuries, and many joint, vascular, or inflammatory problems. Positive findings on the bone scan can be further pursued by more sophisticated radiologic techniques such as wrist arthrograms, computerized tomography, and magnetic resonance imaging.

Nerve conduction studies are obtained for evidence of neurologic dysfunction. If the patient's primary complaint is pain, and the nerve conduction tests are nondiagnostic, a bone scan should also be obtained. A normal bone scan under these circumstances necessitates either close follow-up or referral to a neurologist.

Vascular diagnostic tests such as plethysmography or angiography are helpful in patients who demonstrate a vasospastic or ischemic etiology as a source for their hand pain.

Laboratory tests are rarely needed to establish the diagnosis of pain in the hand or wrist. They are primarily used to determine if systemic disease processes such as rheumatoid arthritis, collagen, vascular disease, or calcium pyrophosphate disease are the source of the patient's symptoms.

BONY INJURIES

Fractures are a common cause of wrist and hand pain. Almost all phalangeal and metacarpal fractures, and most fractures of the carpal bones, are demonstrated on routine x-ray films. However, some fractures are frequently overlooked because findings on routine films are subtle or absent. Failure to diagnose these injuries can result in persistent pain, decreased strength and motion, degenerative arthritis, and persistent nonunion. Establishment of the diagnosis requires suspicion and a systematic approach—as outlined in this chapter. The following are examples of fractures in the hand and wrist that are often overlooked or misdiagnosed.

The most commonly-missed phalangeal fracture is an avulsion fracture of the volar lip of the middle phalanx. These avulsion fractures are associated with rupture of the volar plate. The bone fragment may only be 2 to 3 mm at its greatest diameter and can be mistaken for a sesamoid. The diagnosis and treatment of this problem is discussed under ligament injuries.

Fractures of the scaphoid, dorsal avulsion fractures of the triquetrum and hook of the hamate, fractures of the dorsal ulnar aspect of the trapezium, ulnar or radial styloid, and pisiform are frequently not demonstrated by routine x-ray films. These fractures will be briefly discussed in the following paragraphs.

The scaphoid is the most commonly fractured carpal bone. This fracture usually results from a fall on an outstretched hand. Scaphoid fractures should be suspected in a patient with a history of wrist trauma, and pain or tenderness in the anatomic snuff box. This fracture, however, may not be obvious on initial radiologic examination. Management of a patient with a history of wrist trauma, tenderness over the scaphoid, and nondiagnostic x-ray films should consist of immobilization in a short-arm thumb spica cast for approximately 2 weeks. X-ray films repeated at the end of this 2-week interval usually demonstrate a fracture if present. If pain and tenderness persist and the film is negative, a bone scan should be performed. This also provides information regarding the vascularity of the proximal pole of the scaphoid. If the bone scan shows increased uptake in the region of the scaphoid, tomography should be obtained to confirm or refute the presence of a fracture. Although a negative bone scan essentially rules out the presence of a fracture, it does not exclude a ligamentous injury. Under these circumstances, wrist arthrography is necessary. Failure to diagnose and treat scaphoid fractures properly can result in a painful nonunion and is a major source of litigation.

Triquetral fractures comprise approximately 20 percent of carpal fractures. They are usually associated with other carpal injuries. An avulsion fracture of the dorsal triquetrum is the most common type of triquetral fracture. These fractures are caused by traction, and the resulting bone fragment is often small. This diagnosis should be suspected in a patient with a history of wrist trauma and tenderness over the triquetrum. If routine x-ray films fail to demonstrate the fracture, a bone scan should be obtained. This will show increased uptake in the area of the triquetrum when a fracture is present. The diagnosis can be confirmed by tomography or fluoroscopic spot films. Treatment consists of cast immobilization for 2 to 3 months. Tomography may be necessary to demonstrate healing. Nonunions are rare.

Fractures of the dorsal ulnar tubercle of the trapezium are rare. We have treated only four cases at our institution. The mechanism of injury is unclear. There is usually a history of injury followed by pain at the base of the thumb. Routine roentgenograms usually do not demonstrate this fracture, but a bone scan will show increased uptake in the area of the trapezium. Once again, fluoroscopic spot films or tomography are usually necessary to confirm the diagnosis.

Fractures of the hook of the hamate result from direct blows to the hypothenar area—usually caused by a golf club, baseball bat, or a tennis racquet. This diagnosis should be suspected following an injury to the hypothenar area that produces persistent pain. Patients present with pain in the hypothenar area and a deep, poorly defined tenderness to palpation over the region of the hook of the hamate. Symptoms of ulnar nerve compression may also be present. Routine four-view radiologic examination often fails to demonstrate this fracture. A carpal tunnel view often demonstrates it and should be obtained as part of the evaluation of pain in the hypothenar area. A bone scan will demonstrate increased uptake at the fracture site, and tomography can be used to confirm the diagnosis.

Nondisplaced fractures of the ulnar or radial styloid may not be apparent on routine wrist x-ray films. If there is localized tenderness in these regions despite normal film findings, a bone scan should be obtained.

Pisiform fractures are uncommon. The mechanism of injury is usually a fall on the outstretched hand, resulting in localized tenderness over the pisiform. If no fracture is seen on routine roentgenograms, fluoroscopic spot films or tomography should be obtained to confirm or refute the presence of a fracture.

KIENBÖCK'S DISEASE

Kienböck's disease, or avascular necrosis of the lunate, is a rare cause of wrist pain. Various etiologies have been proposed, but to date a definite cause has not been established. The current, most widely-accepted theory proposes that repetitive compressive forces alter the internal bony architecture and result in avascularity of the lunate, with subsequent necrosis. The presence of an ulnar mi-

nus variant (short ulna with respect to the distal radius) appears to make individuals more susceptible to compressive forces. Approximately 50 percent of the normal population have an ulnar zero variant and 20 percent have an ulnar minus variant. However, 80 percent of people who develop Kienböck's disease have an ulnar minus variant; 5 percent have an ulnar zero variant; and Kienböck's disease rarely occurs in the presence of an ulnar plus variant. Susceptibility is also increased in individuals in whom the blood supply to the lunate is derived solely from volar sources.

Symptoms typically consist of vague wrist pain that is exacerbated by use of the wrist. There is usually a history of trauma or of work that requires repetitive wrist motion. Often, there is tenderness over the lunate on physical examination. Establishment of the diagnosis depends on the stage of the disease. Stage 0: wrist pain, tenderness over the lunate, normal x-ray film and positive bone scan. Stage I: wrist pain, tenderness over the lunate, increased density of the lunate on film, and a positive bone scan. Stage II: pain, tenderness, cystic changes with retention of shape of the lunate on film, and a positive bone scan. Stage III: pain, tenderness, collapse or fragmentation of the lunate without radiocarpal arthritis shown on film; under these circumstances a bone scan is not necessary. Stage IV: pain, tenderness, collapse and fragmentation of the lunate, and perilunate arthritis. The role of magnetic resonance imaging (MRI) in the diagnosis and staging of Kienböck's disease is unproven. Early results indicate that MRI may identify Stage 0 and Stage I Kienböck's disease in some patients before the bone scan and x-ray films become positive. However, long-term follow-up of patients with positive MRI and negative bone scans and x-ray films is needed to clarify the role of MRI in Kienböck's disease.

The treatment of this disease is controversial. Stages 0 and I are currently treated by triscaphoid fusion, with the lunate left in place. In Stages II and III, a triscaphoid fusion is performed and the lunate is excised. Failure to excise the lunate in these stages has resulted in persistent pain. Stage IV usually requires wrist fusion because of radiocarpal arthritis. We do not currently use silicone prostheses for Kienböck's disease because of the high (50 percent) incidence of silicone synovitis associated with this arthroplasty.

CARPAL BOSS

A carpal boss is an osteoarthritic spur that usually develops at the base of the index or long finger metacarpal at its articulation with the trapezoid and capitate respectively. Most carpal bosses are congenital and asymptomatic. They occur approximately twice as commonly in women and are usually not symptomatic prior to the third or fourth decade. Carpal bosses present in two ways: (1) a painless mass on the dorsum of the hand, or (2) pain in the wrist. Patients who present with a painless mass are simply concerned about the mass, which is usually firm and immobile. The diagnosis can be confirmed by a lateral x-ray film taken with the wrist flexed. The asymptomatic carpal boss does not require treatment. Carpal bosses that are painful have developed degenerative arthritis between the opposing bony spurs. Trauma and repetitive motion often precede the onset of pain. The diagnosis can be established by a history of pain localized to the boss and a positive bone scan. Routine films usually demonstrate the bony overgrowth, but fail to answer whether the boss is responsible for the symptoms of wrist pain. Treatment is removal of the bony overgrowth down to normal articular cartilage. A ganglion is also present in approximately 30 percent of the cases.

BONE CYSTS

Radiolucent areas within the bone are not true cysts but areas of fibrosis. Although there are many reports in the literature of interosseous ganglia, we have never been able to establish histologically this diagnosis in any of our patients. Often, patients present complaining of wrist or hand pain with radiologic evidence of a lucent area in one or more carpal bones. Symptoms in these patients may be related to ligament injury, or a microfracture within the wall of the cyst. Evaluation should include a bone scan and arthrogram to rule out an occult fracture or ligament injury. When these other causes are eliminated, surgical removal of these radiolucent areas frequently eliminates the pain.

LIGAMENTOUS INJURIES

Ligament injuries in the hand and wrist are often missed because x-ray films do not show fracture or dislocation. Failure to recognize and treat ligament injuries properly can result in chronic pain and permanent disability. Ligament injuries should be suspected whenever patients have joint centered pain and tenderness following trauma. Routine films may show soft-tissue swelling or avulsion fractures, but are often normal. Arthrography and bone scans are the keys to establishing the diagnosis and should be obtained whenever persistent pain is unexplained by the history, physical examination, and roentgenograms.

The following is a discussion of the common ligament injuries encountered in the hand and wrist.

Injuries to the collateral ligaments and the volar plate of the proximal interphalangeal (PIP) joints, and avulsion of the ulnar collateral ligament of the thumb metacarpophalangeal (MP) joint (gamekeeper's thumb) are the most common ligamentous injuries to affect the digits. The collateral ligaments of the PIP joints are frequently injured during athletic endeavors. The typical complaint is of a jammed joint that is swollen and tender. There is often a history of a dislocation that was reduced on the playground by the patient or a friend. The joint is fusiformly swollen and tender over the injured collateral ligament. The ligaments usually rupture at the attachment to the base of the middle phalanx. The diagnosis can be established by radial and ulnar stressing of the joint under digital block anesthesia. If the ligament is completely torn, the joint will open on the side of the injury. The joint should also be stressed by attempting to hyperextend it to rule out an associated volar plate injury. X-ray films should be obtained to rule out an articular fracture. Proper treatment consists of reinsertion of the ligament.

Volar plate injuries result from forced hyperextension of the PIP joint. The joint is usually fusiformly swollen and tender over the volar surface. The diagnosis can be established by hyperextension of the joint under digital block anesthesia. If the ligament is completely torn, the joint will hyperextend. X-ray films should be obtained to rule out an avulsion fracture of the base of the middle phalanx and subluxation. Treatment depends on the presence or absence of subluxation and fractures of the articular surface. In the absence of the subluxation of the middle phalanx, the best treatment is extension block splinting. If subluxation is present, the middle phalanx should be reduced and fixed with a Kirschner wire and the volar plate reinserted. Nondisplaced fractures of the base of the middle phalanx are treated with extension block splinting. Displaced fractures that involve one-fourth to one-third of the articular surface should be reduced as anatomically as possible and internally fixated.

Rupture of the ulnar collateral ligaments of the thumb (gamekeeper's thumb) results in unstable pinch and chronic pain. The joint is fusiformly swollen and tender over the injured ligament. X-ray films should always be obtained prior to stressing the joint in order to avoid displacement of an associated fracture. Casting is the preferred treatment when an avulsed bone fragment is demonstrated at or near the base of the proximal phalanx. A displaced bone fragment indicates entrapment of the ligament beneath the adductor aponeurosis and this requires surgical reinsertion of the ligament. If no bone fragment is seen, the thumb should be stressed under digital block anesthesia. If the joint opens 40 or more degrees, the ligament has been completely avulsed. The ligament is almost always trapped beneath the adductor aponeurosis and requires reinsertion. Joints that open less than 40 degrees have partial tears or contusions and are best treated with casting. Injuries to the radial collateral ligament of the thumb occur less frequently and are evaluated and treated similarly.

Tears of the intercarpal ligaments are often incapacitating injuries that can be misdiagnosed for extended periods of time. Improper management leads to degenerative arthritis of the carpal bones and chronically painful wrist. In our practice, the scapholunate ligament is the most commonly injured carpal ligament, followed by the lunotriquetral ligament. Occasionally, both of these ligaments are torn. Tears of the triangular fibrocartilage are another cause of wrist pain. It is not uncommon for ligament injuries to occur after minor trauma. The patient often provides a history of preceding injury and may describe a popping sensation. On examination, there is usually localized tenderness over the injured ligament, or dynamic instability between the associated carpal bones. The entire wrist can be diffusely tender, with limitation of motion secondary to pain and swelling. Routine x-ray films are usually normal, but occasionally demonstrate abnormal widening of the scapholunate space or an instability pattern characterized by dorsal or volar angulation of the lunate and rotation of the scaphoid. If routine films are normal, a bone scan should be obtained to rule out the presence of a fracture. Most ligamentous injuries also produce a positive bone scan; however, a negative bone scan does not exclude a ligament problem. The next test in the diagnostic algorithm is a wrist arthrogram. This will demonstrate a tear in the area of the affected ligament.

A complete discussion of the surgical management of these injuries is beyond the scope of this chapter. Many controversies exist in the literature for management of ligamentous injuries. The goal of surgery is to provide the patient with a functional, pain-free wrist. Scapholunate ligament tears are commonly treated with a triscaphoid fusion and lunotriquetral injuries with a lunotriquetral fusion. Combined tears of the scapholunate and lunotriquetral ligament often require wrist fusion for pain relief. Unfortunately, in the active individual this option is less than ideal. Management of triangular fibrocartilage tears is controversial and, currently, we are enlarging the defect.

ARTHRITIS

Degenerative joint disease and rheumatoid arthritis are the two most common forms of arthritis that cause pain in the hand and wrist. Degenerative arthritis usually manifests itself in the distal interphalangeal (DIP) joints of the fingers and the carpometacarpal joint of the thumb. Pain at the base of the thumb in a middle-aged woman is the most common presentation of degenerative arthritis involving the carpometacarpal joint. Joint space narrowing and the presence of Heberden's nodes, are characteristic radiologic findings in degenerative arthritis. The changes that show up on film at the carpometacarpal joint of the thumb are also diagnostic; however, these findings often do not correlate well with the clinical symptoms. Typically, these patients have pain at the base of the thumb, are tender over the joint, and have a positive grind test. A grind test is performed by grasping the thumb and rotating the metacarpal while it is compressed against the trapezium. In patients with carpometacarpal (CMC) arthritis, this maneuver produces intense discomfort. If changes shown on x-ray film are minimal, a positive bone scan will confirm the diagnosis.

Initial management of osteoarthritis consists of treatment with aspirin or nonsteroidal antiinflammatory agents. This approach is usually adequate for treatment of DIP joint disease and for initial management of patients with CMC arthritis. Surgery is reserved for patients who fail conservative therapy. The trapezium is resected and replaced with a tendon anchovy. Silicone arthroplasty replacement of the trapezium is no longer recommended because of silicone synovitis.

Rheumatoid arthritis affects the MP joints and the wrist more commonly than the distal joints. The diagnosis can be confirmed by a positive rheumatoid factor and characteristic radiologic findings. The treatment of rheumatoid arthritis is primarily medical. When extensive destruction of the joints or severe synovitis occurs, management consists of arthroplasty or synovectomy.

INFECTION

Chronic osteomyelitis is a rare cause of pain in the hand and wrist. The diagnosis can be confirmed by bone scan or x-ray film, with appropriate cultures.

TENDONS

Suppurative tenosynovitis and nonspecific tenosynovitis of the flexor tendon sheath are the two most common pathologic processes that involve tendons.

Suppurative tenosynovitis is relatively simple to diagnose. Typically, there is a history of penetrating injury with fairly rapid onset of pain, erythema, and swelling of the involved digit. There are, characteristically, five clinical signs of tenosynovitis: (1) fusiform swelling of the digit, (2) maintenance of the involved finger in a flexed position, (3) pain on passive extension, (4) tenderness to palpation over the tendon sheath, and (5) erythema and increased warmth. There may also be purulent drainage from the associated puncture wound.

Roentgenograms are an essential part of the evaluation and occasionally demonstrate a foreign body. Surgical treatment consists of drainage, insertion of an irrigation catheter into the tendon sheath, and parenteral antibiotics.

Nonspecific tenosynovitis is much more common. Patients present with a history of pain involving either the flexor or extensor tendon compartments, or with a history of trigger digit. The diagnosis of trigger digit is relatively easy to make based on the history and physical examination. Patients complain of intermittent locking of the digit, which is occasionally painful. The examiner can frequently elicit a popping sensation in the area of the A1 pulley with active flexion and extension of the finger. Trigger digit is commonly associated with carpal tunnel syndrome, and symptoms of median nerve compression should be sought. It is also important to remember that trigger digit may be congenital.

Initial therapy of acquired trigger digit is injection of the tendon sheath in the area of the A1 pulley with a water-soluble steroid such as Celestone. Approximately 80 percent of patients obtain relief of symptoms with one to three steroid injections. Surgical release is reserved for failure of conservative therapy, locked digits, and congenital trigger digit.

Nonspecific tenosynovitis can also involve the tendon compartments of the wrist or hand. The first dorsal extensor compartment (de Quervain's disease), the area where the abductor pollicis longus and extensor pollicis brevis cross the radial wrist extensors (intersection syndrome), or involvement of the wrist flexor or extensor tendons are common sites for this form of tenosynovitis. Patients present with complaints of pain over the involved tendons, exacerbated with use. There is tenderness to palpation over the tendon sheath and pain with active and passive motion of the tendons. Therapy can consist of immobilization, steroid injection, or surgical release. Most patients respond to 2 to 3 weeks of immobilization or one to three steroid injections. Surgical treatment is reserved for those patients who fail conservative therapy.

SOFT TISSUES

Soft-tissue problems are usually limited to bruises, bites, contusions, or superficial infections. A thorough history and physical examination establish the diagnosis. X-ray films and a bone scan are useful to eliminate the presence of bone, joint, or ligament pathology.

NERVES

Compression neuropathies of the upper extremity occasionally present with wrist and hand pain as the primary complaint. The most common of these is compression of the median nerve at the carpal tunnel. Other less common forms of neuropathy include compression of the ulnar nerve at the elbow (cubital tunnel syndrome) and neuromas of the sensory branch of the radial nerve or the digital nerves.

The diagnosis of carpal tunnel syndrome can be established in patients who demonstrate characteristic history and physical examination findings. Nerve conduction studies aid in confirmation of this diagnosis. Symptoms of median nerve compression include nocturnal paresthesia, intermittent numbness, and pain in the hand that often radiates to the elbow or forearm. Carpal tunnel syndrome can be associated with rheumatoid arthritis, pregnancy, and trigger digit. On physical examination, patients usually exhibit a positive Tinel's sign over the median nerve at the wrist. Phalen's, or reverse Phalen's, test can be positive within 1 minute, and in extreme situations patients may demonstrate thenar atrophy. In 90 percent of the cases, nerve conduction studies show abnormal conduction across the carpal tunnel.

Standard therapy consists of surgical decompression of the median nerve at the wrist. Medical management, which includes splinting, steroid injections, and vitamin B_6, does not provide lasting relief. Nighttime splinting may be useful for symptomatic relief during pregnancy, or prior to surgery. Some patients have classic historical and physical examination findings of median nerve compression with normal nerve conduction velocities. Steroid injection of the carpal tunnel may aid in confirmation of the diagnosis, but if the latter remains questionable, neurologic consultation is indicated.

Compression of the ulnar nerve at the elbow is much less common than carpal tunnel syndrome. Typically, there is a history of numbness in the ring and little fingers. Pain in the hand is uncommon. In extreme cases, atrophy of the interosseous muscles can occur. The diagnosis can almost always be confirmed by nerve conduction studies.

The wearing of a tight bracelet or wristwatch can cause compression of the radial nerve at the wrist. There is usually pain at the site of compression and numbness in the distribution of the sensory branch of the radial nerve. Physical examination reveals a positive Tinel's sign at the point of compression and altered sensation in the thumb-index web space. Resolution of the symptoms occurs with removal of the wristwatch or bracelet.

Neuropathies that involve the digital nerves are usually related to sports activities such as bowling (bowler's thumb). The history is characteristically that of pain at the site of chronic irritation or compression of the nerve. A positive Tinel's sign over the site of nerve irritation can usually be elicited. A neuroma may be palpable. Discontinuation of the offending activity usually results in resolution of the symptoms.

VASCULAR PROBLEMS

Vascular problems such as ulnar artery thrombosis,

Raynaud's phenomenon, and collagen vascular disease can all be sources of hand and wrist pain. Ulnar artery thrombosis usually results from repetitive trauma due to vibration exposure or the use of the hand as a hammer (hypothenar hammer syndrome). It can also occur in a more insidious fashion with gradual occlusion of the artery in association with atherosclerosis or collagen vascular disease. Patients complain of pain in the hand, more pronounced in the ring and little fingers. There may also be a history of cyanosis and cold intolerance. Concomitant ulnar nerve involvement at the wrist can also occur and may present as altered sensation in the ring and little fingers. The ulnar pulse is absent, and the Allen's test is positive. A Doppler can confirm absent ulnar arterial flow. Arteriography is usually not necessary but can differentiate diffuse occlusive disease.

Treatment consists of either thrombectomy or resection of the thrombosed segment. Acute cases that present within 1 to 2 days can usually be treated with thrombectomy. Chronic cases require resection of the thrombosed section of artery. Vein grafting is usually unnecessary. Fifty percent of these interposition grafts thrombose within 1 year. Vein grafting should be performed if there is inadequate circulation to the ring and little fingers after resection of the thrombosed segment.

Raynaud's phenomenon is a vasospastic disorder associated with overactivity of the sympathetic nervous system. It can be idiopathic (Raynaud's disease) or related to other systemic disease processes such as collagen vascular disease. The patients complain of episodic hand pain with digital pallor and cyanosis, exacerbated by cold exposure. Immersion of the hand in cold water usually triggers the vasospasm and reproduces the symptoms. Digital plethysmography can be used to differentiate diffuse from isolated vascular occlusion. Pulse volume plethysmography, used in conjunction with a cold immersion test, is used to predict the therapeutic efficacy of surgical sympathectomy in these patients. Conservative therapy consists of abstinence from smoking, protection from cold exposure, and the use of calcium channel blocking agents. Biofeedback has also been shown to be helpful in early therapy. In refractory cases, digital sympathectomy often alleviates the symptoms. Thoracic outlet syndrome is also a cause of Raynaud's phenomenon, and treatment of this problem improves the vasospastic symptoms. Laboratory tests for collagen vascular diseases such as in lupus erythematosus preparation, and for erythrocyte sedimentation rate and rheumatoid factor should also be obtained.

REFLEX SYMPATHETIC DYSTROPHY

Reflex sympathetic dystrophy (RSD) is a poorly understood but relatively common cause of hand and wrist pain. The pathogenesis is unclear and the clinical picture variable. The combination of a susceptible personality, a persistent painful condition, and abnormal sympathetic reflex are required for development of RSD. The initiating painful condition can range from a minor injury such as a smashed fingertip to a gunshot wound that involves the median nerve. Common examples include carpal tunnel syndrome, blunt hand trauma, penetrating injuries to major peripheral nerves, and Colles' fracture. Susceptible individuals are usually emotionally labile, chronic complainers, passive-aggressive, insecure, fearful, and suspicious. They also demonstrate sympathetic overactivity, manifested by decreased pain tolerance, cold, clammy, sweaty hands, and fainting. The abnormal sympathetic reflex arc produces local vasoconstriction and is out of proportion to the apparent painful stimulus. Symptoms include pain, swelling, stiffness, and discoloration. The patient's description of the pain is the most typical feature of the syndrome. The pain is severe, out of proportion to the cause, burning, and constant. RSD should always be suspected in patients who complain of constant burning pain. Movement and exposure to cold tend to exacerbate the pain. The hand and wrist are usually swollen, shiny, and sweaty. Pallor, erythema, or cyanosis may be present. Roentgenograms are usually normal except for the soft-tissue swelling.

The diagnosis is established by the presence of the cardinal findings of typical pain, swelling, stiffness, and discoloration. It is confirmed by relief of pain when the abnormal sympathetic reflex is interrupted. The most reliable way to interrupt the sympathetic reflex is to use a stellate ganglion block. When a good response is obtained, repeated blocks, physical therapy, and elimination of the painful stimulus usually result in resolution of the problem. Psychotherapy may also be needed.

Early diagnosis and prompt treatment are the keys to avoiding permanent pain and disability.

PAINFUL TUMORS

Glomus tumors, angiolipomas, hemangiopericytomas, and angioleiomyomas are tumors that can present as pain in the hand and wrist. Of these, the glomus tumor is by far the most common. Glomus tumors are about twice as common in women and usually occur in the fourth through the sixth decades. At least 50 percent are subungual and symptoms consist of severe pain, tenderness, and cold intolerance. Large lesions can produce ridges in the nail, and a blue or red spot may be present in the nailbed. The key to diagnosis and treatment is point tenderness over the tumor. Surgical excision, using magnification, is usually curative.

SUGGESTED READING

Almquist EE, Kienbock's disease. Clin Orthop 1986; 202:68–78.

Palmar AK, Levinsohn EM, Kuzma GR. Arthrography of the wrist. J Hand Surg (Am) 1983; 8(1):15–23.

Peimer CA., Medige J, Eckert B.S. Wright JR, Howard CS. Reactive synovitis after silicone arthroplasty. J Hand Surg (Am) 11(5):624–638.

Pellegrini VD Jr, Burton RK. Surgical management of basal joint arthritis of the thumb. Part I. Long-term results of silicone implant arthroplasty. J Hand Surg (Am) 1986; 11A(3):309–324.

Pin PG, Semenkovich JW, Young VL, Bartell T, Crandall RE, Gilula LA, Reed K, Weeks PM, Seigel BA. The role of radionuclide imaging in the evaluation of wrist. J Hand Surg 1988;

Rockwell WB, Destouet JM, Gilula LA, Young VL, Weeks PM. Radiographic approach to the painful wrist. Orthopaedic Rev 1985; 14(5):270–279.

Smith RJ, Atkinson RE, Jupiter JB. Silicone synovitis of the wrist. J Hand Surg (Am) 1985; 10(1): 47–60.

Watson HK, Hempton RF. Limited wrist arthrodesis. I. The triscaphoid joint. J Hand Surg (Am) 1980; 5(4):320–327.

Young VL, Bartell T, Logan SE. Ganglions in the hand and wrist. Southern Medical Journal 1988; 81(6):751–760.

LOWER EXTREMITY

DIABETIC FOOT

LAWRENCE B. COLEN, M.D.
WILLIAM D. MORAIN, M.D.

Many plastic surgeons are playing a new role in managing the diabetic foot. Reasons for this include a new understanding of the microvasculature in diabetes, an increased ability of vascular surgeons to revascularize ulcerated extremities, and new reconstructive methods for transferring arterialized tissue. Since one in five diabetic patients entering the hospital does so for foot problems and 50 to 75 percent of nontraumatic amputations occur in diabetics, the numerical magnitude of this problem is large.

Until recently a certain negative fatalism existed in dealing with the diabetic foot, in large measure because of the prevailing myth of small vessel disease. The puzzling juxtaposition of indolent ulcers in a foot with palpable pulses was for many years explained by postulating that diabetic patients suffered distal ischemia because of widespread occlusive disease of small arterioles. However, this entire small vessel disease theory of etiology has at last been set aside by a body of new surgical experience and by several lines of investigation. This is well summarized by LoGerfo and Coffman.

Clinically, this new understanding has erased the hopeless attitude toward diabetic foot ulcers and has resulted in a more aggressive approach to management. With the recognition that these indolent wounds are neurotrophic in origin and carry adequate arterial inflow, the application of the surgical principles of debridement, bacterial control, and wound closure has paid healthy dividends.

PREOPERATIVE EVALUATION

Work-up of the ulcerated diabetic foot begins with vascular evaluation of the affected extremity. Although there is no diabetic-specific small vessel occlusive disease, there is a characteristic lesion in the infrapopliteal arteries. Diabetics frequently develop atherosclerotic occlusive disease in the tibial vessels with sparing of the iliofemoral system. Noninvasive work-up should therefore include directional Doppler wave form assessment and measurement of ankle/brachial pressure indices. The latter may be falsely elevated because of noncompressible calcification within the media of the diabetic arteries. Angiography should be undertaken when indicated by the noninvasive examination. If the infrapopliteal disease is so severe that runoff would be too feeble to permit successful surgical repair, distal bypass should be undertaken by the vascular surgeon prior to any attempt at wound closure. This may be best accomplished with the use of an in situ saphenous vein.

Radiologic assessment is also mandatory to rule out concurrent osteomyelitis. Plane films may demonstrate erosive changes, but it may be difficult to distinguish active bony infection from postsurgical or pressure-induced alterations. Bone scans and gallium scans, although useful, do not appear to offer a consistent advantage over plane films because of a high rate of false positive findings in the presence of soft tissue inflammation. An accurate diagnosis of osteomyelitis is established only by bone culture and histologic examination.

PREOPERATIVE WOUND CARE

The principles of wound management are no different for the diabetic than for the nondiabetic patient. Strict bedrest with foot elevation must be prescribed for as many preoperative days as are required to gain control of the edema. Wide drainage of purulence, sharp debridement of devitalized tissue, and culture of involved bone must be carried out, often repeatedly, until the wound is surgically clean. Aggressive paring of any hyperkeratotic plantar callus around the ulcer is essential to permit apposition of vascularized surfaces during subsequent wound closure. Topical antibacterial agents should be used in appropriate fashion. During the period of incomplete debridement, a cream with excellent tissue penetrability, such as silver sulfadiazine, is the most efficacious. When the wound is fully debrided, a program of frequent moist dressing changes with quarter-strength Dakin's solution maintains excellent bacterial suppression.

WOUND CLOSURE

Forefoot Wound

Ulcers of the distal third of the foot (the forefoot) are best managed by local flaps or by distal amputation. Conservation of tissue is paramount in the management of this region since amputation as far proximally as the distal tarsal row still permits normal ambulation without the need for a prosthesis. Therefore, every effort must be made to achieve closure at or beyond this critical level, even if this means consideration of free tissue transfer. Although it seems inappropriate that local tissue transfer should be the procedure of choice in such a distal location, the approach is sound because of the axiality of arterial flow in this region and because small vessel disease is not a feature of diabetes.

Infections of single or multiple toes are best managed by amputation. Usually plantar and/or dorsal flaps of the proximal toe skin may be fashioned for simple linear closure. However, if insufficient skin remains for direct closure, an adjacent toe may be filleted and transposed into the resulting defect. In general, plantar skin is preferred to dorsal skin for this purpose because it is better vascularized through the proper digital vessels and because it has greater length. If the dorsal skin is to be used, it is important to resect well proximally around the base of the nail so as not to incorporate any portion of the nail matrix into the reconstruction. Ray amputation is usually required if the ulcer or infection extends as far proximally as the metatarsal head.

A common lesion in diabetic patients is the indolent neurotrophic ulcer on the plantar surface underlying one of the metatarsal heads. Although split-thickness skin grafts often achieve wound closure in this location, they are usually unable to withstand the shearing stresses associated with weight-bearing and ambulation. Local tissue transfer with plantar skin is therefore the procedure of choice in this situation. Among the many methods described for locally transferring plantar skin, three are clearly superior because of their relatively minimal disruption of the important restraining structures of the plantar pad. These methods are: (1) the neurovascular island toe flap; (2) the total plantar island toe flap with toe sacrifice; and (3) the plantar V–Y advancement flap.

The plantar V–Y advancement flap is particularly easy and reliable for closure of wounds up to 2 cm in diameter (Fig. 1). Larger wounds may be closed with two such flaps advanced toward each other from opposing sides. This flap is unusually well perfused because of the rich array of fine perforating arteries linking the plantar fascia to the overlying skin. Once it is divided circumferentially with the flap in a local area, the fascia will slide a considerable distance without vascular compromise and will carry its overlying skin satisfactorily.

As is the case with other pressure-related ulcers, it is necessary to relieve the pressure from the underlying bony prominence to prevent recurrence. Should the ulcer involve the first metatarsal head, a conservative debridement of the bony prominence should be carried out prior to flap inset. The fifth metatarsal head should be resected through a dorsal approach if the ulcer involves this digit. If the ulcer underlies the second, third, or fourth metatarsal heads, a free-floating osteotomy should be carried out with an osteotome through the neck of the involved metatarsal via a linear dorsal incision. In each case, the offending metatarsal head will support less of the total weight-bearing load as a result of the procedure, thus permitting redistribution in a manner less likely to promote recurrence of the ulcer.

Midfoot Wound

The majority of wounds of the middle third of the foot, the midfoot, are the result of Charcot's joints in diabetics. This form of neuroarthropathy is present in 0.1 to 0.5 percent of the diabetic population and involves the tarsometatarsal joints in 30 percent and the intertarsal joints in 24 percent of cases. The early stages are characterized by mild effusions, joint instability, crepitus, and soft tissue swelling. However, by the time of plastic surgical consultation, the acute episode has usually resolved, leaving a fixed deformity of the foot. The arch of the instep has been ablated, and a plantar ulcer has resulted either beneath the navicular/first cuneiform/first metatarsal base or laterally at the cuboid/fifth metatarsal junction.

Midfoot wounds may be closed either by local flaps or by free tissue transfer. As in the case of the forefoot, split-thickness skin grafts do not reliably take; when these grafts do take, they do not long withstand the stresses of weight-bearing. For defects of less than 3 to 4 cm in diameter, the plantar V–Y advancement flap (single or double) is the most reliable option in most instances. Other options include plantar rotation flaps with split-thickness skin grafts, neurovascular island flaps, toe fillet flaps, or abductor hallucis muscle flaps, provided that the patient's vascular status will permit these.

Defects of 4 cm and larger must be closed by free tissue transfer. Selection of the donor flap must be undertaken with care, as the presence of atherosclerosis in the donor vascular pedicle can be problematic at the time of wound closure. Experience has shown that harvesting flaps from the upper trunk and torso is less likely to result in atheromatous donor vessels than flaps from the lower extremity. The serratus anterior muscle flap, in particular, has been found to be a suitable option because of its long vascular pedicle and its thin, broad expanse.

Hindfoot Wound

Microvascular tissue transfer is usually required for hindfoot wounds in the diabetic. These wounds are characteristically large in size and may be associated with osteomyelitis of the calcaneus or desiccation of the Achilles tendon. Again, the serratus anterior muscle has been a favorite option with its thin, pliable texture and its long vascular pedicle that will reach to the dorsalis pedis artery when indicated (Fig. 2). Although it has been proposed that sensate tissue be introduced by microneurovascular transfer, it is the very neuropathy that precludes this solu-

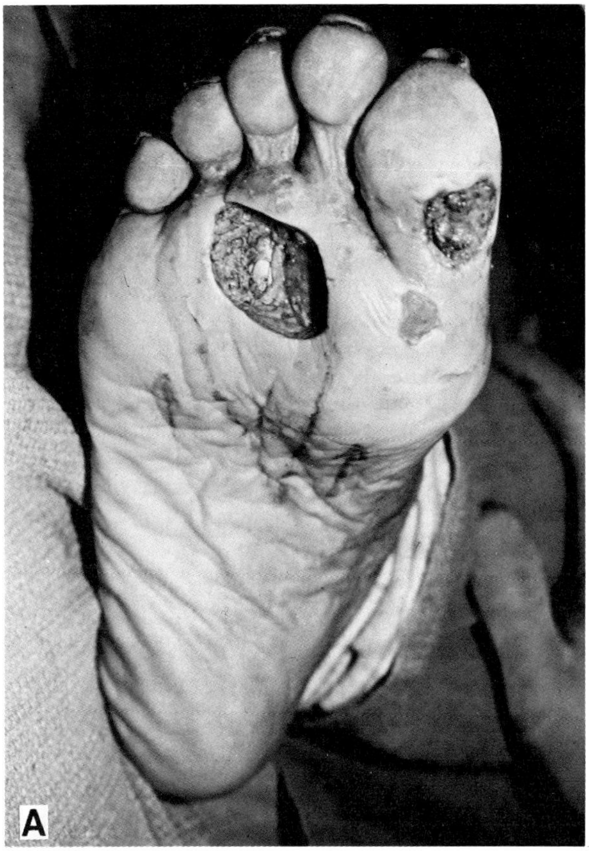

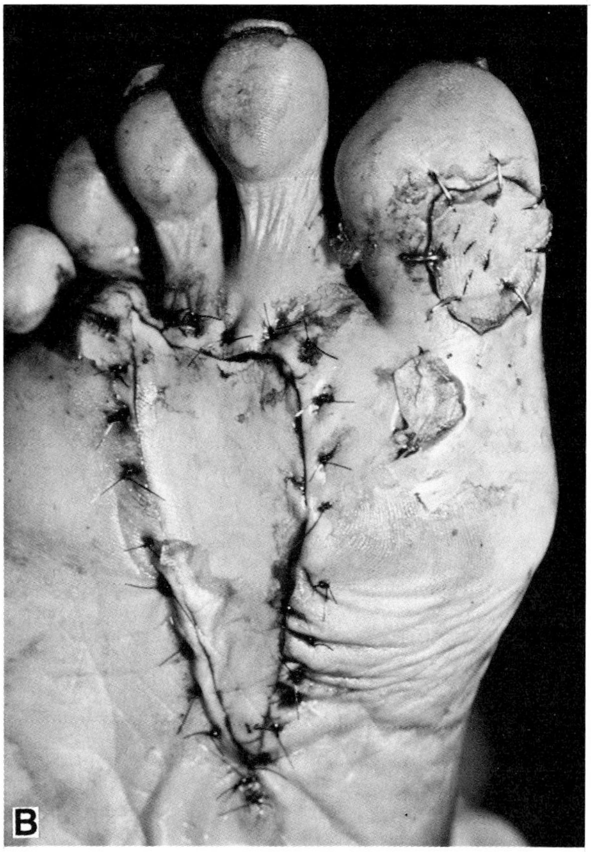

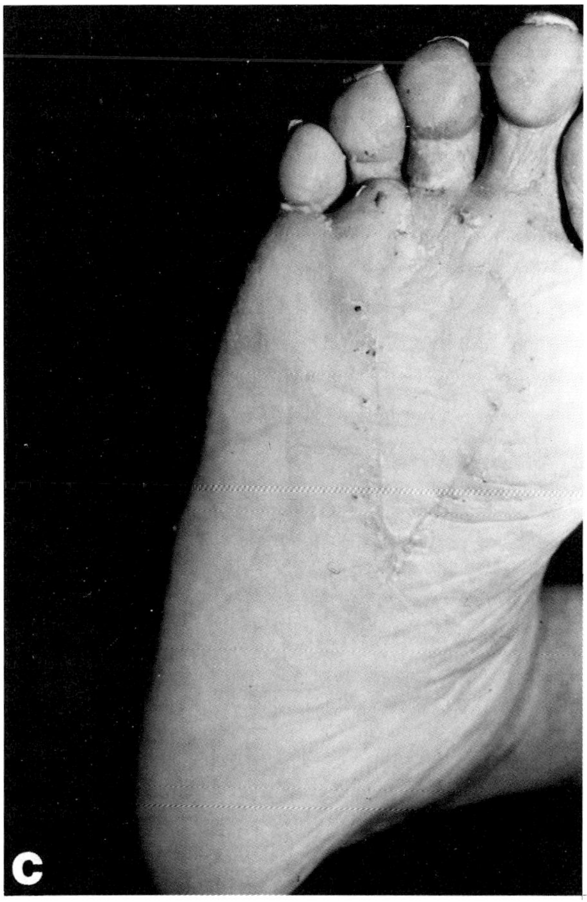

Figure 1 *A*, Large third metatarsal head ulcer following debridement. A great toe ulcer is also present. *B*, V–Y plantar advancement flap sutured into place. Third metatarsal neck osteotomy has also been performed. *C*, The healed wound.

tion. It is usually fruitless to attempt an anastomosis to a poorly functioning nerve. However, should examination disclose significant sparing of a major nerve of the foot or ankle, such a nerve transfer might be considered.

Rarely, a small ulcer of less than 3 cm may be amenable to closure by local flap techniques. Because of the local arterial anatomy of the hindfoot, small V–Y advancement flaps are not usually available. The heel pad may frequently be rotated posteriorly, based either on its medial or lateral circulation (Fig. 3). Alternatively, selected wounds may be closed by the use of the instep island flap on the medial plantar vessels, the lateral calcaneal artery flap, the abductor hallucis muscle flap, the flexor digitorum brevis muscle flap, or a neurovascular island toe flap.

ROLE OF NERVE COMPRESSION

Dellon and MacKinnon have demonstrated strong evidence for a prominent role of nerve compression in diabetic extremities, especially in the tarsal tunnel. It is therefore advisable, and usually extremely simple, to divide the lacinate ligament (flexor retinaculum) overlying the tibial nerve just distal to the medial malleolus. This often can be done in conjunction with flap surgery in the

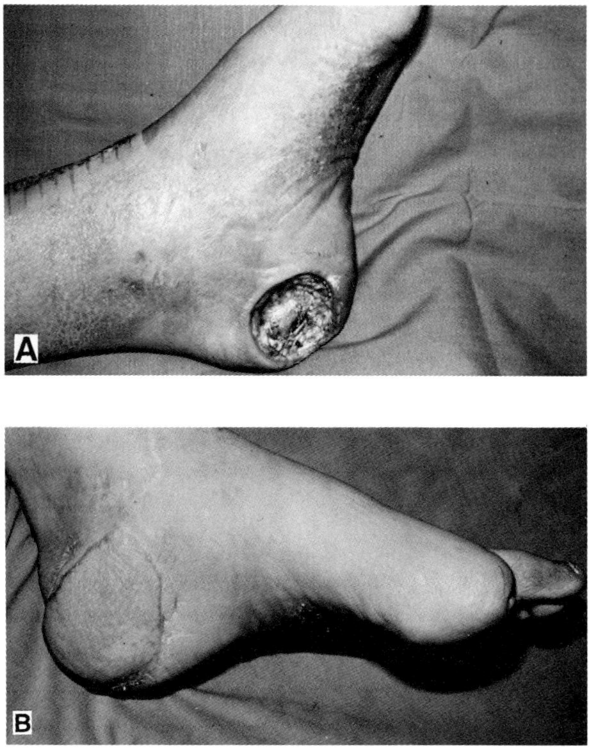

Figure 2 *A*, Large neurotrophic heel ulcer with calcaneal osteomyelitis. *B*, Thin, durable coverage achieved by a free serratus anterior muscle transfer and split-thickness skin graft.

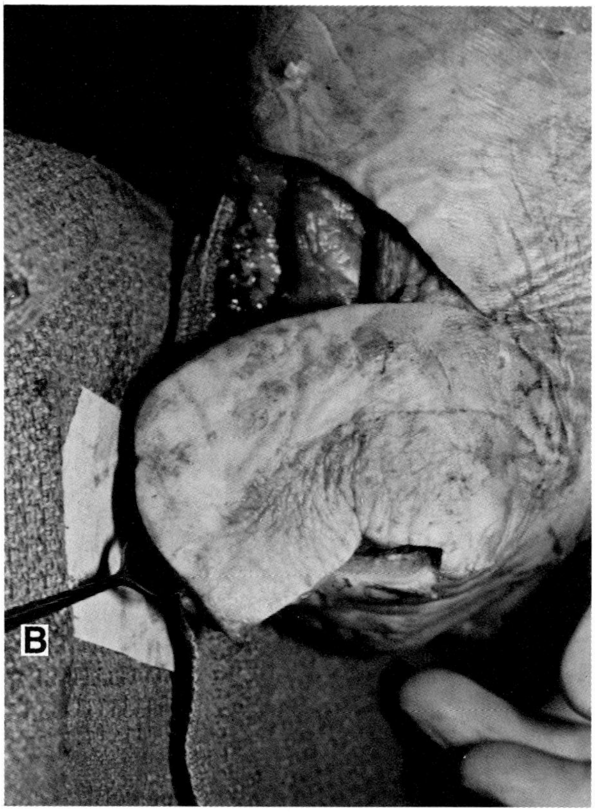

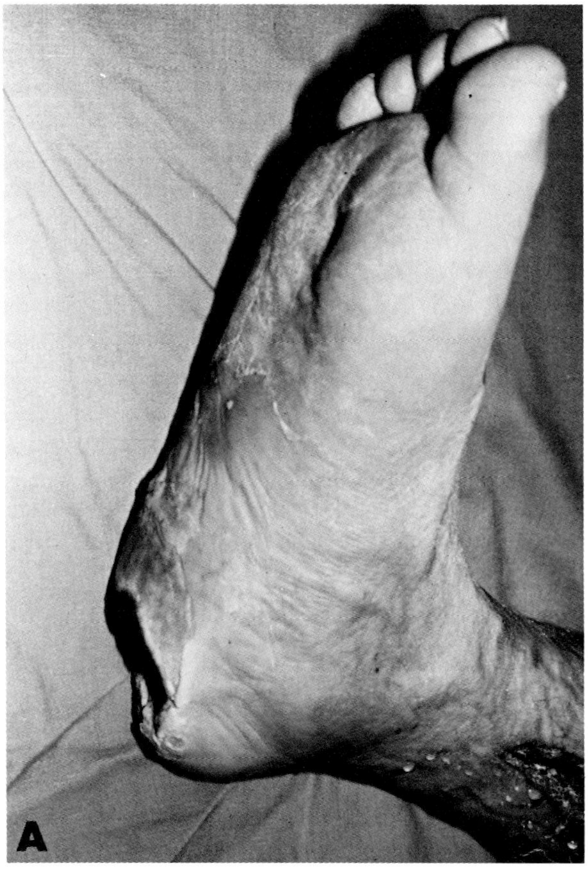

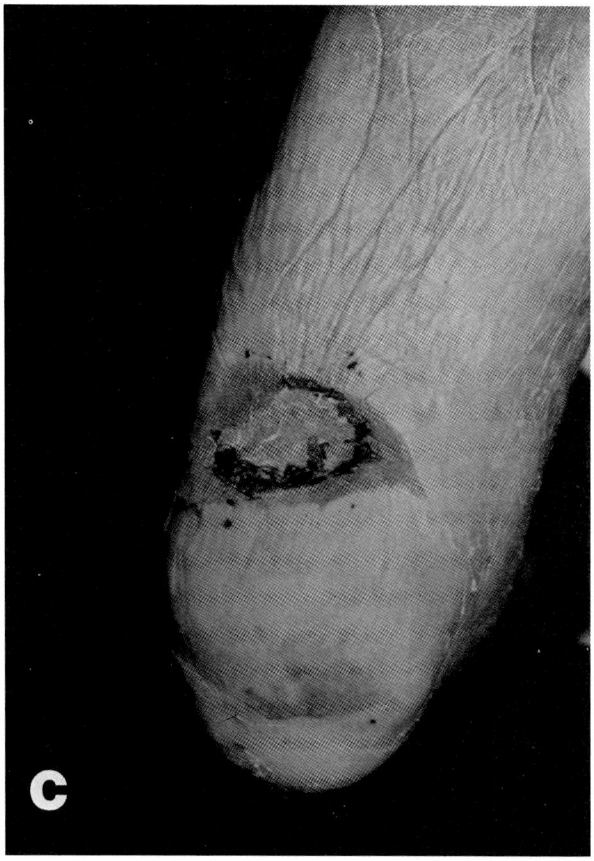

Figure 3 *A*, Plantar heel ulcer. *B*, Medially-based flap of the remaining heel pad to provide a weight-bearing surface. *C*, The closed wound with adjacent split-thickness skin graft.

area and is analogous to release of the transverse carpal ligament over the median nerve at the wrist. If necessary, release at the ankle can include the origin of the abductor hallucis muscle.

IMPROVING BLOOD RHEOLOGY

There is growing evidence that "stiff" red blood cells in the diabetic play a major role in impeding flow in the microcirculation. Elevated serum glucose levels induce specific membrane changes that render the red cell less deformable and therefore more resistant to passage through capillaries. Based on this evidence, pentoxifylline (1.2 g per day) should be used adjunctively in diabetic patients throughout the perioperative period. By a direct effect on intracellular ATP concentrations, pentoxifylline renders the red cell less rigid and probably improves flow characteristics. The theoretic case for use of this drug in diabetic surgery is sufficiently strong that we have adopted its use clinically while awaiting laboratory confirmation of its specific efficacy.

WEIGHT REDISTRIBUTION

Despite the best efforts of the plastic surgeon, the vascular surgeon, and the orthopaedist, success in the closure of the diabetic foot wound is short-lived without prompt attention to the fitting of custom footwear. The podiatrist should be promptly called upon to provide weight dispersion devices within the patient's footwear to redistribute the external pressures and to help prevent recurrence. Regular follow-up visits with both the plastic surgeon and the podiatrist are essential on a long-term basis if recurrence is to be avoided. Although amputation below or above the knee is always available, the conscientious patient may today face a more optimistic future as success in limb-sparing surgery is extended to diabetic patients in more aggressive ways.

SUGGESTED READING

Buncke HJ, Colen LB. An island flap from the first web space of the foot to cover plantar ulcers. Br J Plast Surg 1984; 33:242–244.

Colen LB, Replogle SL, Mathes SJ. The plantar V–Y fasciocutaneous flap for reconstruction of the forefoot. Plast Reconstr Surg 1988; 81:220–227.

LoGerfo FW, Coffman JD. Vascular and microvascular disease of the foot in diabetes: implications for foot care. N Engl J Med 1984; 311:1615–1619.

Morain WD. Island toe flaps in neurotrophic ulcers of the foot and ankle. Ann Plast Surg 1984; 13:1–8.

Morain WD, Dellon AL, MacKinnon SE, Colen LB. Reconstructive surgery in the diabetic extremity. Adv Plast Surg 1987; 4:1–35.

RESTORATION OF STABLE SOFT TISSUE COVERAGE IN WOUNDS OF THE FOOT

THOMAS R. STEVENSON, M.D., F.A.C.S.

Plantar skin and soft tissues of the foot are specialized to withstand the pressure and shear forces exerted during walking. Loss of these tissues through avulsion injury, burn, or tumor excision results in significant functional impairment. The goals of reconstruction include closure of the open wound, replacement of missing tissues, restoration of sensibility, and establishment of a durable wound site. Achievement of satisfactory appearance and shoe fit is also important.

THERAPEUTIC ALTERNATIVES

Many patients with extensive foot wounds either seek or are referred for reconstruction. Selection of the appropriate patient for operation is not based solely on the simple presence of a wound. The patient, or his caregiver, must be able to manage and protect the wound postoperatively.

Numerous options are available for the treatment of the soft tissue wound of the foot. Selection of a particular reconstructive technique is based on the location and size of the defect (Table 1). When alternative operations are available for a given wound, the simplest is the first choice. Failure of one treatment modality requires progression to a more sophisticated reconstructive procedure.

Preoperative preparation of the patient with an extensive foot wound includes management of all preexisting medical problems. Diabetes mellitus is a predisposing factor in lower extremity ulceration and must be adequately controlled before proceeding with reconstruction. If arterial or venous insufficiency is present, and amenable to surgical therapy, it is treated before the foot wound is addressed. Wound cultures are obtained, and the patient is placed preoperatively on appropriate antibiotics. Antibiotic coverage is continued for 1 week postoperatively.

Split-thickness skin grafting is useful in treatment of wounds on the non-weight-bearing surface of the foot, as well as smaller (<5 cm) wounds of the weight-bearing plantar heel. The area to be grafted should be free of necrotic tissue and infection. This is accomplished by serial debridement and the use of culture-specific antibiotics. The wound bed must be well vascularized to permit take of the skin graft; a graft will fail if placed over bone denuded of periosteum, or tendon stripped of its peritenon.

Once the recipient bed is properly prepared, graft-

TABLE 1 Selection of Reconstructive Technique Based on Location and Size of Defect

Location of Wound	*Size (diameter)*	*Treatment*
HEEL		
Posterior, non-weight-bearing	< 5 cm	Lateral calcaneal artery island flap
	> 5 cm	Free muscle graft with split-thickness skin graft
Plantar surface	up to 1/3 of surface	Split-thickness skin graft
	1/3 to 2/3 of surface	Local rotation flap, plantar muscle, or musculocutaneous flap
	2/3 of surface	Free muscle graft with split-thickness skin graft
INSTEP	Entire non-weight-bearing surface	Split-thickness skin graft
FOREFOOT		
Plantar surface	< 5 cm	Local rotation flap, toe fillet, or ray amputation
	> 5 cm	Free muscle graft with split-thickness skin graft Forefoot amputation

ing is undertaken. The procedure is performed under local, regional, or general anesthesia. Final wound preparation is done with tourniquet hemostasis. Either an intact or meshed (1½:1) split-thickness skin graft, 15/1000 inch in depth, is raised and transferred to the wound. A bolster dressing is placed to provide compression. The dressing is removed after 5 days and the wound inspected. An elastic wrap is applied, and crutch-walking without weight-bearing is resumed 1 week postoperatively. The patient is allowed to bear weight on the involved foot graft 6 weeks after reconstruction. Subsequent care includes daily observation of the graft for evidence of trauma or infection. It is common for callous formation to occur at the junction between grafted and uninjured skin. A skin graft applied to the appropriate foot wound is durable.

A small (< 3 cm) wound of the forefoot, typically over one metatarsal head, is treated by transposition of a local skin flap, with skin grafting of the donor site. If one or more toes are involved in a traumatic wound, the phalangeal bones can be removed (toe fillet) and the soft tissues approximated to cover the defect. When chronic osteomyelitis is present in the metatarsal bone(s) underlying a forefoot ulcer, removal of the involved metatarsal(s) can be performed with closure as a ray amputation. The defect left after metatarsal excision may be large enough to require additional coverage by a toe fillet or local flap.

The larger heel ulcer that comprises one-third to two-thirds of the plantar heel surface is best treated by a medially-based local rotation flap. Such a flap is vascularized through the proximal plantar subcutaneous plexus, as described by Shaw. With this design, an innervated flap of skin and subcutaneous tissue is elevated superficial to the plantar fascia. This technique allows preservation of branches of the medial and lateral plantar nerves. The flap is transposed posteriorly, and the donor site skin grafted. Weight-bearing is resumed in 6 weeks. If a previous traumatic or surgically-created wound precludes elevation of this medially-based flap, a musculocutaneous flap consisting of the flexor digitorum superficialis and its overlying instep skin can be employed. The flexor digitorum superficialis is supplied by branches from the lateral plantar vessels, and its associated skin island is innervated by plantar cutaneous nerves. After transposition, the donor site is likewise skin grafted.

A defect of the posterior, non-weight-bearing heel less than 5 cm in diameter can be successfully closed by transposition of a lateral calcaneal artery island flap. This flap is elevated from the dorsolateral aspect of the foot, based on the lateral calcaneal artery and branches of the lesser saphenous vein. The sural nerve is included in the flap and innervates the transposed skin. After elevation of the flap as an island, the bridge of skin that separates donor site from wound is undermined and the flap is passed into the posterior heel defect. A skin graft is applied to the donor site. Ambulation, with weight-bearing, is begun 4 weeks postoperatively.

Wounds of the posterior heel greater than 5 cm in diameter, plantar heel wounds that involve more than two-thirds of the weight-bearing surface, and plantar forefoot defects greater than 5 cm in diameter are managed by microvascular muscle transfer (Fig. 1). The muscle adds padding to absorb local stresses and bulk to improve contour. The two muscles most frequently employed are the gracilis and latissimus dorsi. The gracilis is selected when a smaller muscle is required, while the latissimus dorsi is chosen if a larger muscle or longer vascular pedicle is needed. A split-thickness skin graft is applied simultaneously to the transferred muscle.

Gracilis muscle transfer is performed with the patient in the supine position. It is usually most convenient to harvest the muscle from the thigh opposite the foot wound. The donor site wound is closed primarily. Frequently, the gracilis vascular pedicle has two draining veins in addition to its single nutrient artery. The artery and both veins (if possible) are anastomosed at the recipient site. The most common recipient vessels are the posterior tibial artery and concomitant veins at the ankle.

The latissimus dorsi is removed with the patient in the lateral position. The muscle on the side contralateral to the foot defect is commonly selected. The chest wall donor site is closed primarily after insertion of a suction drain.

The microvascular portion of the free tissue transfer operation, although time-consuming, is not the only important phase. Once the muscle (gracilis or latissimus dorsi) has been revascularized, it is carefully tailored to minimize redundancy. A bulky reconstruction is prone to instability, shear forces, and ulceration. An intact or meshed split-thickness skin graft is applied to the muscle. A large absorbent dressing is placed for warmth and protection.

Four weeks after muscle transfer, the patient is allowed to crutch-walk without weight-bearing and with the extremity wrapped in an elastic bandage. Weight-bearing is permitted 6 weeks postoperatively. The wound is observed for evidence of breakdown. Most patients are fitted with a shoe liner when ambulation is initiated, to minimize shear forces and permit more even distribution of weight. Harris mat studies have shown that the majority of patients alter their gait to shift weight away from the reconstructed site. The free muscle graft with split-thickness skin graft is durable and can withstand the pressure of ambulation (Fig. 2).

Chronic osteomyelitis of the tarsal or metatarsal bones often complicates foot wounds. The deficit created after debridement of the infected bone may be filled by a transferred muscle that provides the elements necessary for wound healing.

In some patients, amputation either of the forefoot, foot, or entire limb below the knee is preferable to attempted reconstruction. The completely insensate foot, accompanied by a stiff ankle, is often plagued by ulceration, regardless of the reconstructive technique employed. Unreconstructible, ischemic, vascular disease often precludes limb salvage. Every reasonable effort toward wound closure is made. However, when faced with the prospect of multiple operative procedures with little hope of success, the patient usually selects amputation and an early return to ambulation with use of a prosthesis.

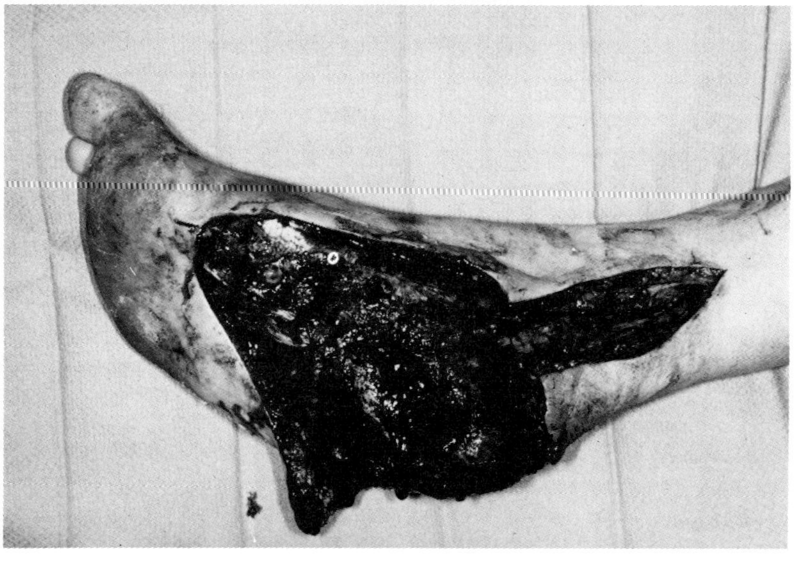

Figure 1 Heel avulsion.

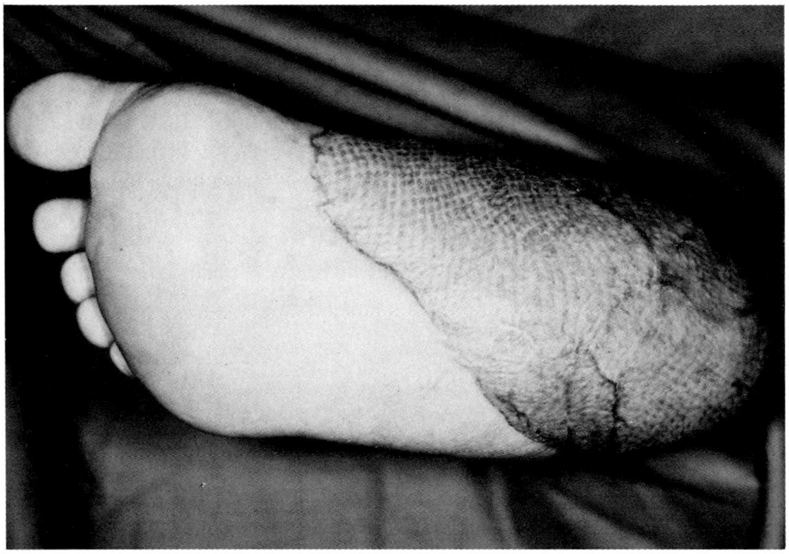

Figure 2 Wound seen 6 months after coverage with the latissimus dorsi muscle and split-thickness skin graft.

SUGGESTED READING

Hartrampf CR, Scheflan M, Bostwick J. The flexor digitorum brevis muscle island pedicle flap: a new dimension in heel reconstruction. Plast Reconstr Surg 1980; 66:264–270.

Hidalgo DA, Shaw WW. Anatomic basis of plantar flap design. Plast Reconstr Surg 1986; 78:627–636.

May JW, Halls MJ, Simon SR. Free microvascular muscle flaps with skin graft reconstruction of extensive defects of the foot: a clinical and gait analysis study. Plast Reconstr Surg 1985; 75:627–639.

Morrison WA, Crabb DM, O'Brien BM, Jenkins A. The instep of the foot as a fasciocutaneous island and as a free flap for heel defects. Plast Reconstr Surg 1983; 72:56–63.

Reiffel RS, McCarthy JG. Coverage of heel and sole defects: a new subfascial arterialized flap. Plast Reconstr Surg 1980; 66:250–260.

Shaw WW, Hidalgo DA. Anatomic basis of plantar flap design: clinical applications. Plast Reconstr Surg 1986; 78:637–649.

Stevenson TR, Mathes SJ. Management of foot injuries with free-muscle flaps. Plast Reconstr Surg 1986; 78:665–669.

Woltering EA, Thorpe WP, Reed JK, Rosenberg SA. Split thickness skin grafting of the plantar surface of the foot after wide excision of neoplasms of the skin. Surg Gynecol Obstet 1979; 149:229–232.

ACUTE FLAP COVERAGE OF OPEN FRACTURES OF THE LOWER EXTREMITY

MICHAEL J. YAREMCHUK, M.D.

Historically, open fractures of the lower extremity, in conjunction with extensive soft tissue damage, have been associated with a high incidence of infection, nonunion, and amputation. At the Shock Trauma Center of the Maryland Institute for Emergency Medical Services Systems (MIEMSS), over 100 open fractures of the tibia are managed annually. Approximately 65 of these fractures are associated with soft tissue damage severe enough to be categorized as Type III injuries by the Gustilo classification (Table 1). To treat this large number of injuries effectively, often in patients with multisystems trauma, a management protocol was developed. The key components in the MIEMSS approach are: close collaboration between orthopaedic and plastic surgeons; external fracture stabilization; the radical and serial debridement of all devitalized soft tissue and bone; acute, local, and free muscle flap soft tissue closure; and staged bone reconstruction. This chapter outlines the MIEMSS regimen for management of the open, lower extremity fracture with emphasis on soft tissue management.

MANAGEMENT PROTOCOL

The treatment of open fractures of the lower extremity can be divided into four separate stages:

1. Emergency evaluation, debridement, and stabilization.
2. Wound management.
3. Soft tissue coverage.
4. Bone reconstruction.

TABLE 1 Gustilo Classification of Open Fractures Based on Extent of Soft Tissue Damage

Type I	—laceration less than 1 cm long and clean
Type II	—laceration greater than 1 cm
Type III	—extensive soft tissue damage

It is emphasized that the functional rehabilitations of the open fracture with severe soft tissue damage must be a collaborative effort between plastic and orthopaedic surgeons.

Emergency Evaluation, Debridement, and Stabilization

The American College of Surgeons' Advanced Trauma Life Support (ATLS) evaluation and resuscitation for trauma patients, which systematically evaluates all organ systems, is strictly adhered to in our unit.

Upon admission to the hospital, information is obtained concerning the injury mechanism, contamination at the scene, and tetanus immunization status. It is important for the surgeon to understand the implications of the mechanism of injury. The mechanism of injury determines the energy absorbed by the extremity, the severity of the injury, and, hence, the prognosis of that extremity. Calculations made by Chapman based on the following equation:

$$E = \frac{1}{2} mv^2$$

help illustrate the implications of the mechanism of injury in terms of energy imparted to the extremity. He determined the forces involved in four common mechanisms of fracture (Table 2). These calculations make it clear as to how the mechanism of injury influences the prognosis of the extremity, and how devastating injuries related to the mechanization of our society can be.

Thorough examination of the extremity is performed with special attention to the neurovascular status. A sterile dressing is applied and appropriate x-ray studies obtained. All patients are administered intravenous antibiotics. It has been shown that between 45 and 75 percent of patients with extensive soft tissue damage injuries (Gustilo Type III) have contaminated fractures at the time of admission. These injuries are treated as surgical emergencies. Consistent with the ATLS multisystems trauma evaluation and resuscitation, these patients are taken to the operating room as soon as possible after the accident.

Attempts are made to salvage all extremities unless there is obvious irreparable nerve damage in the plantar distribution and/or irreparable devascularization. Emergent amputation may be necessary as part of the multiply-injured patient's resuscitation. If warranted by the high-energy fracture location, nerve deficit, or diminished pulses, angiography is performed to evaluate the limb vasculature. Compartment pressures are measured in all injured extremities since traumatic lacerations do not effectively decompress the swollen muscle compartments. It has been documented that compartment syndrome accompanies 9 percent of open tibial fractures. If compartment pressures exceed 30 mm of mercury, all four compartments are decompressed by fasciotomies performed by double-incision exposure. A jet lavage irrigation system is then used to remove gross environmental and bacterial contamination. Low-pressure volume irrigation is inadequate to remove fine particulate matter. After irrigation, all devitalized tissue, including all devascularized bone fragments, is debrided.

Both the bone and soft tissues are reduced and rigidly immobilized by use of the external fixation device. The external fixator provides rigid stabilization while avoiding further devascularization of structures in its application. The anterior half-frame construct is most frequently used. This unilateral frame requires pin insertion into the subcutaneous crest of the tibia, and thereby avoids damage to muscle compartments and neurovascular structures. Such frames are much less bulky than bilateral frames, and allow easy access for bedside wound care and for gastrocnemius and soleus muscle flap harvest, as well as access to the posterior tibial and popliteal vasculature if free tissue transfer reconstruction is required (Fig. 1).

With rare exception, no attempts are made at wound closure at the time of initial evaluations and debridement.

TABLE 2 Forces Involved in Four Common Mechanisms of Injury*

Fall off curb	100 ft. lb.
Skiing (20 mph)	300–500 ft. lb.
Gunshot Wound	2,000 ft. lb.
Bumper Injury (20 mph)	100,000 ft. lb.

* As determined by Chapman.

Wound Management

As has been the experience of others, I have found it difficult to define the zone injury in high-energy induced trauma upon presentation. Marginal tissues often do not declare themselves until the second or third re-exploration. Patients are, therefore, returned to the operating room every 48 to 72 hours for reevaluation and further debridement until the wound is stable. In the interim, the wounds are dressed with wet-to-wet saline dressings at the bedside, if possible. In situations where the wound is defined, and the effects of multisystem trauma demand

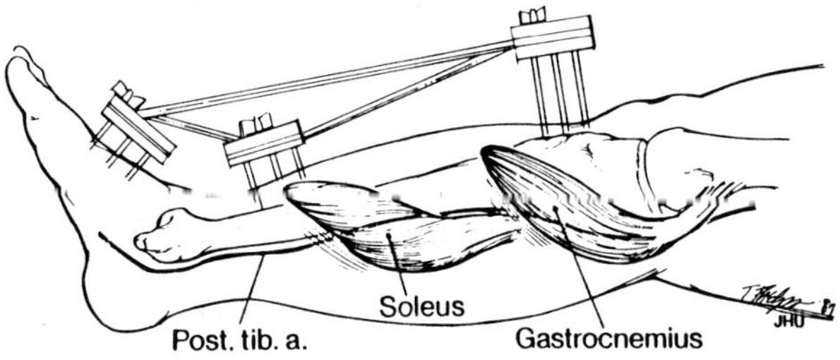

Figure 1 Schematic diagram of lower extremity stabilized with external fixator in anterior half-frame configuration. This construct allows access for bedside wound care. It also allows easy exposure of the gastrocnemius and soleus muscles if they are required for wound closure. If a free muscle flap reconstruction is necessary for soft tissue closure, the posterior tibial vessels are easily accessible. Note that foot is included in construct to prevent tendon excursion and, hence, soft tissue movement.

a delay in definitive extremity reconstruction, cadaver allograft skin has been a useful adjunct in management of large, open wounds. These biologic dressings provide a closed and, therefore, pain-free, mechanically-clean wound.

Timing of Coverage

Because the zone of soft tissue injury that results from high-energy mechanisms is difficult to define upon presentation, I rarely attempt definitive soft tissue coverage at the time of presentation. An average of three debridements is performed at 48- to 72-hour intervals before the definitive debridement and muscle flap closure is performed. In general, most wounds can be closed within 7 to 10 days after injury. Recovery from multisystems trauma frequently results in a delay in flap coverage. If appropriate local care is performed, wound closure can be delayed another 1 to 2 weeks without ill effect. Adequate debridement, particularly of all free bone fragments, lessens the likelihood of infection and, hence, the constraints on the timing of closure.

Soft tissue wounds that are not closed within the first week, if healthy, inevitably develop some granulation tissue, and exposed bone may undergo some desiccation. At the time of definitive debridement, which is done under tourniquet control, a new wound is created. All granulation tissue is removed, and the bone is debrided until it bleeds. This allows primary healing between the recipient bed and the undamaged well-vascularized muscle flap. The cost of this primary healing situation, when cell tissue closure is delayed, is the loss of small amounts of soft tissue and, often, some bone. I believe that a low incidence of infection outweighs this small cost of tissue loss. Similarly, the benefit of primary soft tissue healing and early bone union, made possible by my orthopaedic colleague's confidence and expertise in bone grafting, far outweighs the relatively small cost of bone loss to desiccation.

The posthumous report of the excellent results achieved with emergent free flap coverage of extensive soft tissue defects of the extremities, is a tribute to the judgment and expertise of the late master microsurgeon, Marco Godina. Emergent coverage can be appropriate in well-selected patients. It requires the around-the-clock availability of a microsurgery team.

Soft Tissue Coverage

When possible, the soft tissue wounds that accompany open fractures of the lower extremity are managed with delayed primary closure or split-thickness skin grafting. When there is insufficient local tissue available for this type of management, the wounds are closed with skin-grafted muscle flaps. As has been described classically, defects of the upper third of the tibia are managed with the medial gastrocnemius flap, and middle third defects are managed with the soleus flap. Free muscle transfers are used for defects of the lower third of the tibia and significant defects of the foot.

Very large defects are best managed with skin-grafted, free muscle transfers. Free muscle transfers provide a virtually unlimited supply of undamaged conformable tissue for reconstruction. Although the rich vascularity of muscle flaps makes them effective in controlling subclinical infections, their conformability and, hence, their ability to fill dead space, is, in large part, responsible for their success in the management of these wounds (Fig. 2). In very high-energy wounds, the gastrocnemius and soleus muscles are often involved in the injury zone, thereby making them unsuitable for local transfer. If uninjured, they are, too often, inadequate to fill the large defect.

Cutaneous and fasciocutaneous free flaps are avoid-

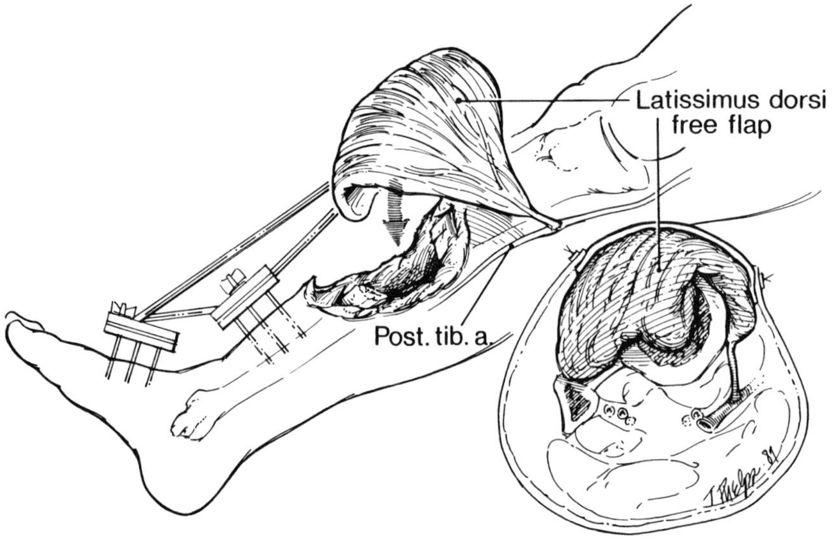

Figure 2 Schematic diagram showing free muscle transfer being used to close large defect. Note preferred end-to-side anastomosis to posterior tibial vessels. Inset with cross-sectional view shows how muscle flaps have the ability to conform to the three-dimensional configuration of a wound, thereby obliterating all dead space.

ed, because these flaps are less able to conform to the three-dimensional configuration of a wound. Furthermore, as opposed to muscle flaps, cutaneous and fasciocutaneous flaps are theoretically less tolerant of a given bacterial inoculum.

When the appropriate debridement of devitalized soft tissue and bone results in a true segmental osseous defect, a gastrocnemius or soleus muscle flap usually does not provide sufficient bulk to fill these large wounds. Segmental osteocutaneous defects, therefore, usually require closure with a free muscle transfer. One-stage bone and soft tissue reconstructions with free osteocutaneous flaps are avoided in these situations. The geometry of an osteocutaneous flap, with its relatively fixed bone and soft tissue relationship, too often prohibits the flap from absolute conformation to the configuration of the wound in the way muscle flaps conform.

The Latissimus Dorsi

The latissimus dorsi muscle was one of the first muscle and musculocutaneous free flap donor sites described. This muscle's large size, long vascular pedicle of wide diameter, intramuscular vascular anatomy, and minimal donor site morbidity make it the donor muscle preferred for free transfer. The latissimus' large dimensions (30 × 40 cm) allow it to cover very large defects. Furthermore, in defects of unusual configuration or size, it can be combined with the serratus anterior muscle, the pedicle of which also arises from the thoracodorsal artery and vein. Furthermore, the thoracodorsal artery and vein reliably split into two branches within the latissimus muscle. This consistent anatomy allows a portion of the muscle to be harvested and used for small defects. This branching also allows the muscle to be split, thus allowing further flexibility in orientation of the muscle at the time of flap inset. The thoracodorsal pedicle is a long one that ranges from 7 to 9 cm, and thereby allows the microvascular anastomosis to be done well out of the zone of injury. The latissimus donor site is remote from the lower extremity and so permits two surgical teams to work simultaneously in extremity preparation and flap harvest. Finally, sacrifice of the latissimus has little morbidity associated with it. The latissimus is harvested without an overlying skin component. It is my experience that the skin-grafted muscle ultimately provides a superior contour and allows greater flexibility at the time of flap inset. The flap is positioned to obliterate all dead space rather than to conform a predetermined skin paddle.

The gracilis and the rectus abdominis muscles are alternative donors for free muscle transfer. The gracilis has virtually no donor site morbidity and is very useful for small defects. The rectus abdominis is the most accessible free muscle donor site. It can be used both for very small and long defects. Like the gracilis, it is more difficult to fold on itself, an attribute that is often necessary in the obliteration of large spaces. The latissimus can be harvested and tailored in a manner to mimic these muscles' attributes.

There are several features that I believe optimize the chances for successful free tissue transfer. Preoperative angiography is routinely performed prior to soft tissue reconstruction. Angiographic definition of the limb vasculature helps define the zone of injury and the applicability of recipient site vasculature, as well as the possible use of local muscle flaps. Microvascular anastomoses are always done, using end-to-side technique in vessels proximal to the injury. Care is taken never to use vessels in the zone of injury. A new skin incision is virtually always made to isolate recipient site vasculature, thus assuring undamaged vessels. Use of the latissimus dorsi, with its long vascular pedicle and considerable muscle length, usually allows these anastomoses to be done without the use of interposition vein grafts. Use of anterior half-frame external fixator apparatus allows easy access to the posterior tibial and popliteal vasculature and, therefore, makes these the preferred recipient vessels. The saphenous vein is avoided as a recipient vein, because spasm of this relatively thick-walled vessel may result in inadequate venous drainage from the well-arterialized flap and in the need for revisional surgery.

Bone Reconstruction

Bone reconstruction is usually performed when the soft tissue envelope is healed and stable—at about 4 to 6 weeks after flap closure. Defect size determines the type of graft used. In general, defects that are less than 8 cm in length are bridged with cancellous grafts placed through a posterolateral approach, and defects greater than 8 cm are bridged by vascularized fibula transfers. Increasing experience has made it apparent that a previously placed free muscle transfer provides such a rich vascular milieu that cancellous grafting is a reasonable alternative for certain bone defects longer than 8 cm.

Based on an earlier experience in which there was a high incidence of nonunion in the type III tibial fractures, any bone defect greater than one-third the cortical circumference is grafted 4 to 6 weeks after soft tissue coverage. Because virtually all cancellous grafts are placed from a posterolateral approach, it is not necessary to elevate the flaps at the time of bone grafting nor is it necessary to prepare a space for subsequent bone grafts with bone substitutes.

Due to its bone configuration, vascular pedicle, and ease of dissection, the vascularized fibula is my preference to bridge massive bone defects. The fibula is a straight cortical bone, 22 cm in potential length, with a vascular pedicle 4 to 5 cm long and vessel diameter of 2 to 3 mm. The iliac crest osteocutaneous flap, supplied by the deep circumflex iliac system, is an alternative one-stage reconstruction for skin and bone defects of the lower extremity. However, the curvature of the iliac crest usually limits its use for bone defects 10 cm in length or less. Furthermore, the relatively fixed relationship between the bone and soft tissues of the flap creates geometric constraints that may preclude its exact fit to the osteocutaneous defect. Rather than compromise debridement or the obliteration of dead space, a staged soft tissue and bone reconstruction is preferred. Simultaneous cancellous grafting and muscle flap closure is avoided because of dissatisfaction with limited earlier clinical experience. Although not clinically infected, these wounds are invariably contaminated with bacteria at the time of wound closure. The addition of cancellous graft to the wound makes the flap fit less precise and hematoma formation more likely, thereby complicating an already difficult wound and making infection more likely.

CLINICAL EXPERIENCE

At the Shock Trauma Unit of MIEMSS, approximately 2,000 acute trauma victims are managed annually. Ninety percent of these patients are victims of blunt trauma. This patient population presents for acute care a high incidence of high-energy-induced open lower extremity fractures and many of these patients have multisystems injury. When the approximately 100 open tibia fractures, managed annually, are categorized by the classification system of Gustilo (see Table 1), 19 percent are type I, 17 percent are type II, and 64 percent are type III. The predominant mechanisms of injury are three: 30 percent of the patients are pedestrians struck by automobiles; another 30 percent are motorcyclists; and 26 percent are occupants in automobile accidents. The remaining 14 percent are victims of miscellaneous injury mechanisms.

In a three-year period beginning in July of 1983, 100 type III open tibia fractures required flap coverage (Table 3). All were closed with muscle flaps: 44 percent of these wounds were closed with gastrocnemius or soleus flaps, and the remaining wounds were closed with free muscle flaps.The latissimus dorsi provided coverage in 80 percent of those cases in which free flaps were used. Four soleus and five free flaps failed. This includes a patient who developed malignant hyperthermia intraoperatively with resultant loss of his free flap. The overall acute infection rate has been 9 percent. One patient presented with a late infection after a bone grafting procedure. Four legs have been amputated. One of these extremities belonged to the patient who developed intraoperative hyperthermia, described above. Another patient required amputation for socioeconomic reasons, after successful soft tissue closure and prior to bone reconstruction. No patient who has undergone successful soft tissue and bone reconstruction has subsequently requested amputation.

The average time to full weight-bearing is ultimately dictated by the severity of injury and resultant bone defect. Patients who do not receive bone grafts heal in approximately 35 weeks, while those who require a graft for any size defect ambulate overall without assistance devices in 40 weeks. Patients with segmental defects of less than 8 cm ambulate on the average in 42 weeks, while those with defects greater than 8 cm heal in an average of 70 weeks after injury.

TABLE 3 Results of Flaps Used to Cover Soft Tissue Defects Associated with Type III Open Tibia Fractures in 100 Patients

	Flaps	*Failed*	*Acute Infection*	*Late Infection*	*Amputation*
TOTAL	100	8 (8%)	9 (9%)	1 (1%)	4 (4%)
LOCAL	44	4 (9%)	6 (14%)	0	0
FREE	56	5 (9%)	3 (5%)	1 (2%)	4 (7%)

ILLUSTRATIVE CASE

A high-energy-induced open tibial fracture with extensive soft tissue damage, managed by the protocol outlined in this chapter, is presented in Figure 3.

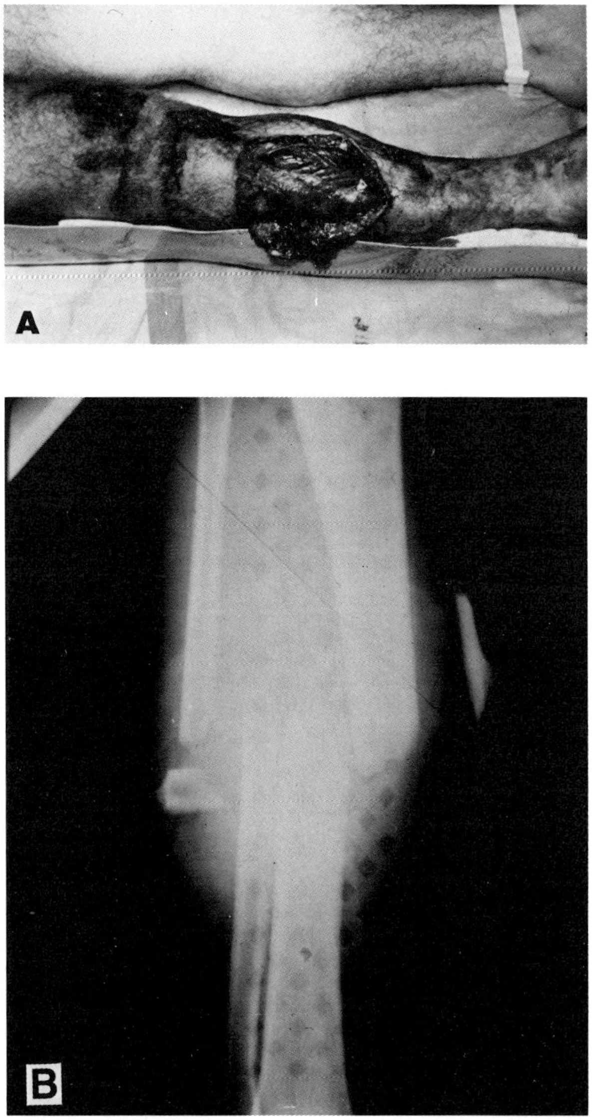

Figure 3 A high-energy induced open tibial fracture with extensive soft tissue damage. *A*, Appearance of 18-year-old motorcyclist's lower extremity at presentation. *B*, Appearance of extremity on x-ray film. Note high-energy fracture pattern with comminution and marked displacement.

Figure continues on opposite page

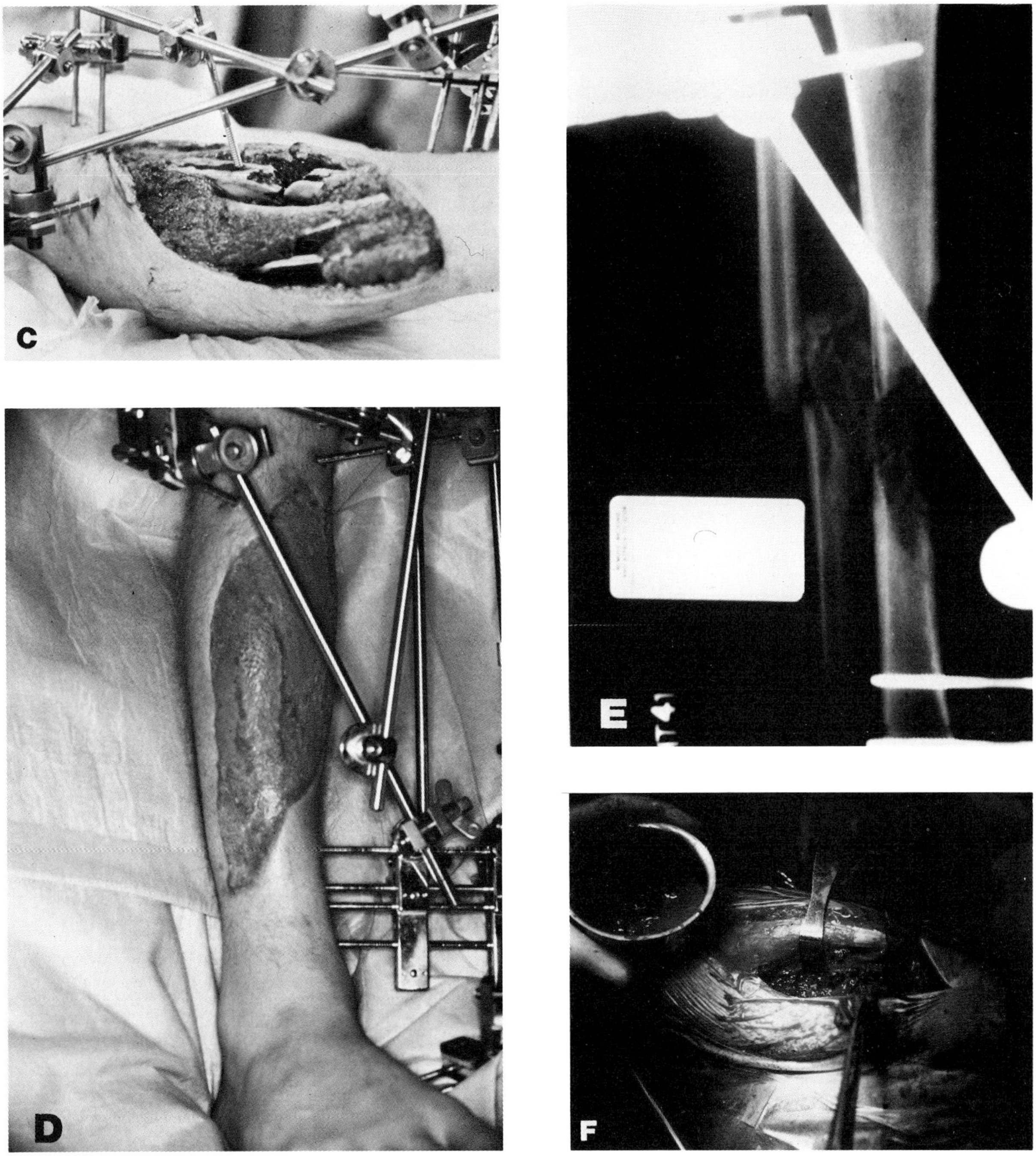

Figure 3 (continued) *C*, Appearance of extremity on day 6, prior to definitive debridement and flap closure. *D*, Appearance 3 weeks after skin-grafted free latissimus dorsi muscle flap closure. *E*, X-ray film showing resultant bone defect after definitive debridement. *F*, Cancellous grafting performed 8 weeks after muscle flap closure through posterolateral approach. A total of three cancellous grafts were required.

Figure continues on following page

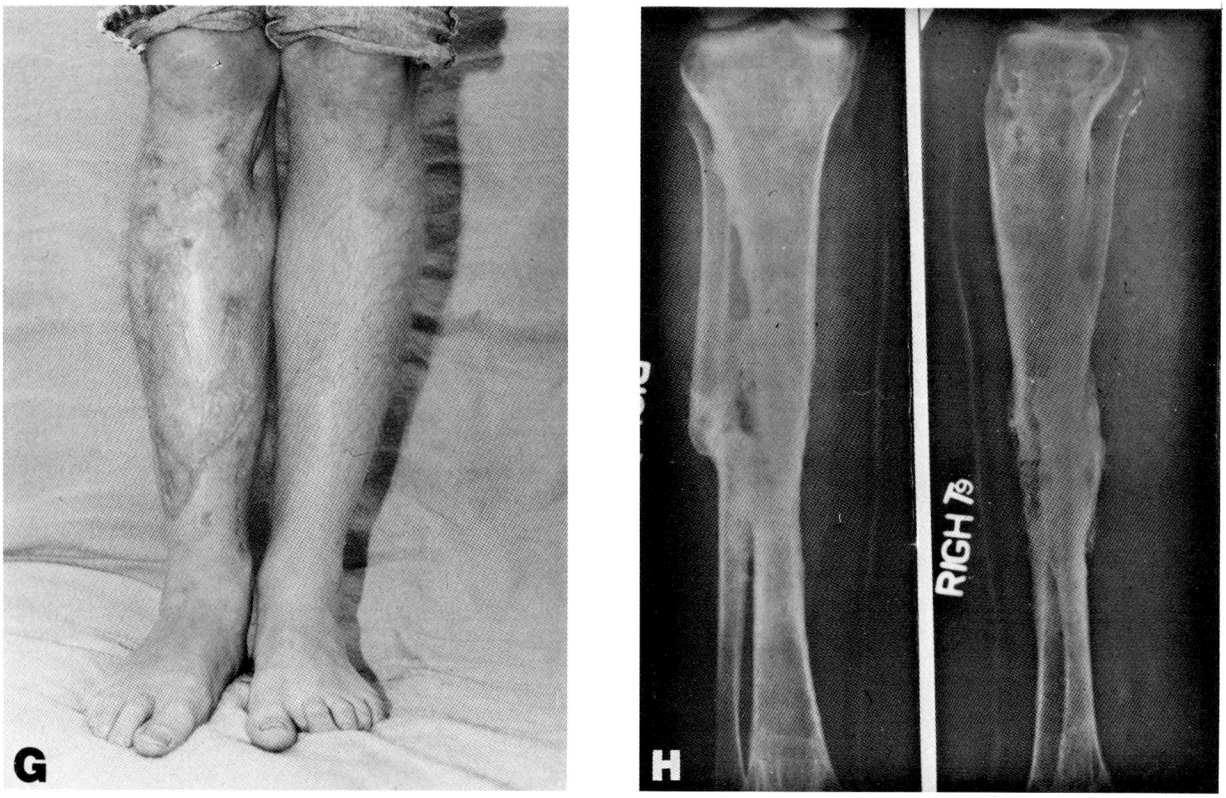

Figure 3 (continued) *G*, Healed extremity is shown 2 years after injury. *H*, Posteroanterior and lateral appearance on x-ray film 2 years after injury.

SUGGESTED READING

Bartlett SP, May JW Jr, Yaremchuk MJ. The latissimus dorsi muscle: a fresh cadaver study of the primary neurovascular pedicle. Plast Reconstr Surg 1981; 67:631–636.

Godina M. Early microsurgical reconstruction of complex trauma of the extremities. Plast Reconstr Surg 1986; 78:285–292.

Gustilo RB, Mendoza RM, Williams DN. Problems in the management of type III (severe) open fractures: a new classification of type III open fractures. J Trauma 1984; 24:742–746.

Maxwell GP, Hoopes JE. Management of compound injuries of the lower extremity. Plast Reconstr Surg 1979; 63:176–185.

Neale HW, Stern PJ, Kreilein JG, Gregory RO, Webster KL. Complications of muscle-flap transposition for traumatic defects of the leg. Plast Reconstr Surg 1983; 72:512–515.

Weiland AJ, Daniel RK. Microvascular anastomoses for bone grafts in the treatment of massive defects in bone. J Bone Joint Surg 1979; 61A:98–104.

Yaremchuk MJ, Brumback RJ, Manson PN, et al. Acute and definitive management of traumatic osteocutaneous defects of the lower extremity. Plast Reconstr Surg 1987; 80:1–12.

CHRONIC TRAUMATIC LOWER EXTREMITY WOUNDS: FREE MUSCLE TRANSFER AND SKIN GRAFT

JAMES W. MAY Jr., M.D.
BURT M. GREENBERG, M.D.

A chronic wound in the lower extremity is defined as one that has existed for longer than 6 weeks. In many of these circumstances following trauma, the wound remains unhealed for prolonged periods of time related to a variety of wound-healing inhibitory factors that are present in the local area. In the lower extremity, these factors may include devitalized soft tissues or exposed and devitalized bone. Both may occur in relation to traumatic devascularization of the extremity. In addition, an exposed bony fracture may exist.

DIAGNOSIS

When faced with a nonhealing wound in the lower extremity, the surgeon must ascertain the factors that are inhibiting wound healing. Although factors such as venous and/or arterial insufficiency and diabetes can play a role, the most common cause of chronic traumatic wounds in the lower extremity is exposed, devitalized bone. Under these circumstances, the periosteal or periosteal and endosteal blood supply to a segment of bone may be disrupted during the initial traumatic event. As the wound begins to heal, avascular segments of cortical bone, complicated by bacterial contamination, fail to pick up blood supply from the surrounding soft tissues. The contaminated devitalized bone becomes an etiologic factor in the persistence of the chronic lower extremity wound.

These factors must be evaluated in order that appropriate steps toward the goals of reconstruction can be taken. In some circumstances, there may be other complicating factors in addition to the wound, such as lack of bony continuity and dennervation of important weight-bearing skin, joints, and bony structures of the foot. These factors may make the process of reconstruction long and arduous and may shift the balance toward an expeditious amputation and prosthesis fitting. It is important for the lower extremity reconstructive surgeon to be experienced and conversant with the prosthetic alternatives. The patient and surgeon must be convinced that all possible alternatives have been discussed and that the process of rehabilitation is most practical and efficacious in treating the patient's problem. Although the decision between amputation and reconstruction must be individualized, it is important to explain to each patient the realistic steps and timetable required in order to achieve their lower extremity reconstruction. It is also important to discuss the caliber of the lower extremity that the patient is apt to have after the reconstructive process is complete. Armed with this information, the patient can then play an active role in the decision as to whether or not to proceed with reconstruction. In borderline circumstances, it may be helpful to meet with patients who have lower extremity prostheses or who have undergone reconstruction. Whether the right decision is made or not is impossible to answer for an individual patient, but it is clear that the patient must feel they were active in selecting the ultimate course. The patient's feeling of involvement can make the most arduous and difficult reconstructive steps much more palatable to the most demanding of patients.

SURGICAL MANAGEMENT

Wound Evaluation

After a careful history has been obtained, the leg and wound should be thoroughly examined. The location and size of the wound should be noted and the nature of the exposed tissue determined. Roentgenograms are essential in checking for healing fractures and for evidence of osteomyelitis. However, roentgenograms and even tomograms cannot usually determine the exact extent of nonliving infected bone. In our institution, chronic wounds usually are debrided formally in the operating room before a full definite reconstructive plan is outlined. This allows the full extent of the wound to be determined and the edges of the wound to be evaluated for carcinoma, especially when the wound has been open for years. This is an important issue in treating chronic wounds. In the operating room, all nonliving tissues should be debrided. This frequently includes nonliving bone, which is best managed by sequential debridement with a power drill under loupe magnification accompanied by copious saline irrigation. The irrigation system prevents bone destruction from the heat of the power drill, while bleeding is recognized under loupe magnification. Bleeding is the most reliable method of evaluating bone viability. Cultures are taken from the depths of the wound and post-debridement roentgenograms are taken in several views to assess the extent of the remaining bone or the size of the defect created. The debridement process itself may require several procedures as, on occasion, tissue that appear questionable will benefit from a second look and further debridement.

When soft tissues alone are needed in reconstruction, a skin graft or local flap may be adequate. When bone is exposed then flap coverage is usually needed. Often a local muscle flap is the best option as skin muscle or fasciocutaneous flaps may have a significant donor deformity. When significant weight-bearing bone is debrided and a large gap is created, then amputation versus reconstruction should be fully discussed. The reason for this is that the most time-consuming and difficult part of lower extremity rehabilitation in a chronic wound setting is that of bony reconstruction; this is particularly true where a significant gap is created in the femur or tibia. Therefore, plastic surgeons and orthopaedic surgeons should work closely together to give the patient the best option involving soft tissue and bony reconstruction.

With an intact long bone in the lower extremity, it is

emotionally difficult for the surgeon to continue the debridement process to a point where a gap exists. In our own patients, it is this circumstance that leads the surgeon toward an inadequate bony debridement in the greatest number of patients. Nonetheless, the surgeon must recognize that inadequate debridement at this stage can spell disaster if wound sepsis emerges following debridement and wound closure, particularly if the wound sepsis returns after bone graft reconstruction has been undertaken.

In general, if a local muscle flap or free flap is needed, angiography is performed to assess not only specific recipient vessel sites in the lower extremity, but also the degree of vascular injury remaining in that same extremity. Angiography may not be needed if a local muscle flap is adequate and the primary pedicle is outside the zone of trauma. The angiography is normally done at least several days prior to the planned soft tissue reconstruction. Although we do not hesitate to reconstruct a lower extremity that has only a single artery, it is not uncommon to reconstruct damaged longitudinal vessels with a vein graft at the time of free flap transfer.

The choice of soft tissue for reconstruction varies greatly depending on the size, location, and damage to the remaining tissues of the lower extremity. It is common to see a patient in whom a local muscle flap, such as a gastrocnemius or soleus, is adequate to move into a well-debrided soft tissue and bony defect, especially if the defect is in the upper half of the leg and can be completely closed by the volume of tissue available. On the other hand, it is increasingly common that severely damaged lower extremities have no ideal local muscle flap available below the knee. Rather than further inhibit lower extremity function in these patients, our preference increasingly has been to utilize free tissue transfer for these complex reconstructions. In addition, we tend to favor a two-stage reconstruction supplying a sepsis-free soft tissue envelope at the first stage followed by an elective bony anatomic reconstruction at the second procedure.

The reasons we perform these procedures in two stages rather than in a single combined soft and bony tissue reconstruction are related to a number of patient care factors. In general, osteocutaneous flap donor sites leave the patient with a more morbid donor site than do standard muscle and nonvascularized bone donor sites. We also prefer not to put the relatively poorly vascularized bone of an osteocutaneous flap into a bed that has recently had a high bacterial count. In addition, the dead space surrounding an osteocutaneous reconstruction can be problematic, especially in a contaminated field. Finally, we find that most bony requirements in the lower extremity can be solved by standard cancellous bone graft reconstructive techniques, particularly when an intact or healed fibula is seen in the lower extremity. Although an in-depth discussion of this topic is beyond the scope of this chapter, on the uncommon occasion where free fibula transfer is needed, we still prefer to do this type of vascularized tubular cortical bone reconstruction at a second stage after complete soft tissue healing has been achieved. It should be noted that no bony reconstruction is carried out until 6 weeks following soft tissue closure; under these circumstances, careful inspection is made deep to the soft tissue closure before the bone graft is harvested to rule out any obvious persistent sepsis.

If local muscle flaps cannot be used to close the wound, we usually prefer to proceed immediately with a free muscle transfer. Our willingness to do this is related to our growing experience with the safety and reliability of these transfers and with the fact that we have lost only a single free muscle flap in over 90 such cases involving chronic bony wounds.

In the leg, depending on the size of the wound, our muscle flaps of choice include the gracilis muscle for small dead space filling requirements and the latissimus dorsi muscle for larger requirements. The rectus abdominus muscle is an ideal muscle in terms of length, width, and dominance of its inferior vascular pedicle. However, this muscle is not usually our first choice since the long-term effects of the loss of the rectus muscle in the donor site are still unknown. However, we do have extensive experience with the transfer of this muscle in breast reconstruction; when attention is paid to the maintenance of the arcuate line fascia and total abdominal wall fascial reconstruction, with mesh augmentation, the morbidity from the donor site of this flap has, to date, been very low.

Since 1980, it has been our preference, when possible, to use free muscle flaps with skin grafts because the scar in the donor site is less conspicuous than if a skin-muscle flap is taken. More importantly, the ultimate contour in the lower extremity is far superior in most cases with this procedure than with a skin muscle flap.

Preoperatively, the patient must be counseled as to the possible need for vein graft reconstruction and alternative muscle dissection if an intraoperative mishap occurs. As much as possible, all potential problems should be anticipated and discussed with the patient such that appropriate alternatives can be executed if complications are encountered.

Surgical Procedure

Once the flap has been chosen, the surgical team should be assigned in such a way that each member knows which portion of the operation he or she is to perform. This allows anatomic familiarity and preplanning by the individual surgeon. If the surgeon has a lack of experience at procuring any of these donor tissues, then the cadaver lab is the place where that experience and confidence should be established.

The night before surgery, the patient's lower GI tract should be cleared because bed rest will be required postoperatively. In addition, the night before surgery, the patient is begun on rectal aspirin suppositories and the flap donor site is prepared with Phisohex washes.

The morning of surgery in the operating room, after induction of anesthesia, a Foley catheter is instituted and culture-specific intravenous antibiotics are begun. An alternating air mattress is placed on the operating table to avoid pressure difficulties with a prolonged procedure. The position of the patient is important as both donor and recipient muscle sites must be created to allow full exposure of both operative areas. In the right lower leg, for example, if the posterior tibial vessels are to be used, one might consider using the right gracilis muscle for small defects or the left latissimus dorsi muscle for larger defects. Under these circumstances, with the left abdomen up, the left rectus abdominus muscle can also be used; this muscle can be harvested through a transverse abdominal lipectomy-type incision, although a vertical incision makes the exposure of the muscle more expeditious.

As the flap donor team begins the dissection of the flap donor site, the recipient site team begins to explore and expose the recipient vessels. The vessels to be used for the recipient site are dependent upon information gleaned from the angiogram and any venous studies thought to be necessary. Usually we prefer an end-to-side arterial anastomosis into a single dominant arterial vessel in the leg rather than using a damaged end vessel stump. When all vessels are patent, our first choice for distal lower extremity reconstruction is usually the distal posterior tibial artery. Venous anatomy can be more difficult to sort out than arterial anatomy since venous thrombosis may have occurred in relation to the original trauma. As much as possible, the surgeon should avoid the zone of trauma as scar tissues and vascular injury within this area can lead to ultimate vessel thrombosis. We generally prefer end-to-side venous repairs. If a large defect resides in the upper portion of the lower leg, rather than approach the popliteal artery or the upper posterior tibial artery, we often bring the vascular repairs of the flap above the knee and use the superficial femoral artery and vein at the adductor canal as the vascular repair site. If this is done, the latissimus dorsi length is used in part to prolong the vascular pedicle, and thus the upper part of the muscle is simply laid in the deep tissue dissection plane, which has the effect of prolonging the length of the vascular pedicle. The more distal part of the muscle then closes the defect. It is important not to use so much of the muscle length that the portion of the muscle that closes the wound fails to survive. This same concept can also be used for the rectus abdominis muscle flap.

Once the recipient arteries and veins are dissected out, they are bathed in 2 percent Xylocaine to avoid vessel spasm. As soon as the muscle flap is harvested from the donor site, the muscle is taken to a separate table and the nerve of the neurovascular bundle is used as a handle to help control manipulations of the vascular pedicle. The artery and vein are irrigated with heparin to avoid blood stasis and thrombosis during the flap positioning stage. In some cases, the muscle is then fitted into the recipient site, and with a marking pen one can decide which portions of the muscle need to be thinned or trimmed and which portions can remain full. The vascular characteristics of the muscle flap itself will have been determined in the donor site prior to muscle removal. It is important to be certain that the dominant vascular pedicle of the muscle (those vessels which will be repaired) are adequate to perfuse the desired extent of the muscle to be used in the reconstruction. If not, the muscle should be debrided and tailored such that only the muscle tissues that are alive and are reliably perfused by the vascular pedicle are left for the ultimate reconstruction.

Before the muscle is set into the wound, a redebridement of the wound is carried out, and the scarred margins of the wound are reexcised. It is important to uplift the margins of the wound to allow inset of the muscle as though the defect were being created to fit the muscle rather than the reverse. The reasons for this are related to ultimate wound healing and the esthetic result that ensues if the muscle is carefully set into the recipient defect. This is usually done with pledget sutures, which are brought out at a distance from the remaining surface of the wound (Fig. 1). Once the muscle has been secured into the recipient site and large, adequate drains are placed in the depths of the bed, the vascular pedicle is led over to the region of the recipient vessel dissection and the artery and vein repairs are completed. It is important to use well-placed suture bites with thickened arteries and veins in the lower extremity. The most important part of the repair itself is cutting appropriately sized side holes in the artery and vein such that the holes are slightly larger than the dilated vessels of the free flap. Once the vessels are repaired, the artery is released initially after a 1,000 bolus of IV heparin is given. As soon as the vein is filled, the venous clamps are removed as well. Thermocouple

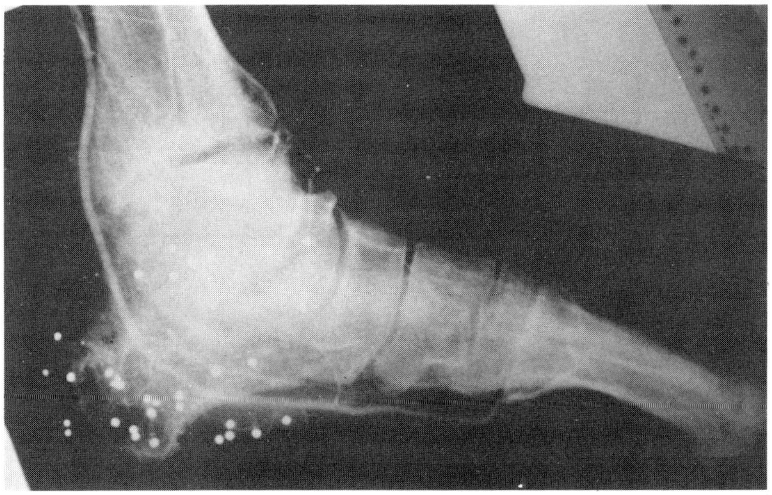

Figure 1 Lateral angiogram of right foot. Note osteomyelitis of os calcis and open posterior tibial artery.

probes are secured adjacent to the donor and recipient arteries and are brought out parallel to these vessels percutaneously. At this point, the fascia of the free muscle flap is sutured to the dermis of the inset side such that there is smooth continuity between the flap and the adjacent skin when the skin graft is placed over the flap. We no longer make any effort to overcorrect the volume of the flap, as we have learned from 7 years of experience that, although the flap does atrophy, it never assumes a concave healed appearance in the lower leg. In addition, at the time of skin graft placement, a sterile doppler is used to locate the primary vascular pedicle, and therefore a spot on the muscle flap near the junction of the primary vascular pedicle is designated as a listening window. As a result, postoperative monitoring of the flap can include not only direct clinical inspection and thermocouple monitoring, but also direct doppler evaluation. It is important to locate the point of doppler listening properly in the operating room so that other vascular noise will not be confused for patent vessels.

The skin graft is harvested at this point after an appropriate interval of flap perfusion and hemostasis. The skin graft is taken of moderate thickness and sutured carefully around the circumference of the free flap. Mesh skin is usually not used. However, if significant oozing occurs and mesh is indicated, it is not spread. In the free muscle flap donor site, great care is given to drain placement and to secure hemostasis. In cases where the latissimus dorsi muscle has been split to allow a portion of the muscle to remain in the donor site, the cut edge of the muscle is run with 3-0 locking chromic sutures prior to large suction catheter wound closure to secure hemostasis.

Postoperative Care

Postoperatively most patients are maintained on low molecular Dextran at 30 cc per hour; heparin is not routinely continued. Patients usually are not transfused as they will be at bed rest and will usually tolerate a hematocrit of 20 percent without difficulty. When the patient is elderly or has some evidence of myocardial ischemia, a higher hematocrit is favored. As a final maneuver, a plaster splint is prepared not only to support the lower leg, but also to support the foot and ankle and thus to prevent foot drop. It is of greatest importance to be certain that the calf and ankle regions bear most of the weight of the lower extremity and that the examining finger can be placed behind the heel such that no heel tissue pressure necrosis will ensue.

When the patient returns to the floor, the postoperative monitoring flow sheet is initiated for hourly documentation of clinical inspection and temperature monitoring and doppler probe data. Any change in any of these parameters requires a visit by the covering physician, who routinely examines the flap on an alternating hour basis the first evening after transfer. Although vascular problems in free tissue transfers are usually confirmations of intraoperative suspicions, there is no doubt that careful clinical monitoring is the most reliable current method for monitoring free tissue transfers.

A free muscle flap covered with a skin graft turns blue and weeps dark venous blood when an early venous congestion problem is encountered. On the other hand, the muscle does not bleed and does not look pink when an arterial inflow problem exists. Although these observations may be subtle, it is incumbent upon the monitoring physician to make sure that the muscle flap bleeds red blood if there is any question about its viability. This is accomplished on the floor by simply lifting the window of the skin graft and snipping the muscle to be sure it is alive. It is uncommon for a free muscle transfer that has been totally successful and problem-free for 24 hours to have any vascular difficulties in the ensuing postoperative period.

On the floor postoperatively, the operated extremity is elevated with several pillows and constant attention is paid to Foley catheter output and patient fluid resuscitation in addition to respiratory toilet.

Usually within the first week postoperatively, the patient is taken back to the operating room for a dressing change and for careful assessment of skin graft viability. Under most circumstances, thermocouple probes are removed between 5 and 7 days transcutaneously and the Jackson-Pratt drains are similarly removed.

CASE REPORT

Mr. JB is a 50-year-old machine operator who sustained a shotgun injury to his right heel and lower leg with subsequent skin breakdown over the os calcis of his right foot. Over a period of 6 months in 1983, the patient sustained continuous breakdown with an enlarging wound despite close attention to dressing changes and wound management. This eventuated in a 3 by 5 cm wound centered over the os calcis with a partially devitalized and exposed area of Achilles tendon (Fig. 2). Preoperative evaluation revealed his pulses to be 0 to 1+ in the pos-

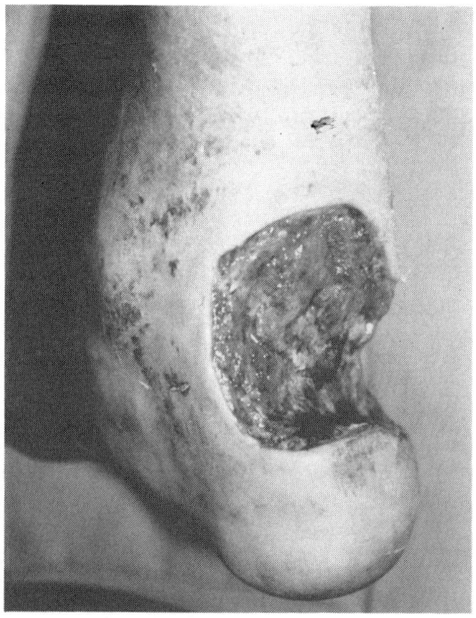

Figure 2 Open chronic wound involving calcaneous and Achilles tendon. Heel to left, posterior medial view.

terior tibial, dorsalis pedis, and popliteal distribution. An arteriogram revealed patent posterior tibial artery in the right lower extremity with minimal arthrosclerotic changes (see Fig. 1). Additional radiographic evaluation revealed chronic osteomyelitis of the calcaneus (see Fig. 1).

Debridement was performed with removal of all necrotic and nonviable tissue including the entire margins of the ulcer to the base of the ankle and nonbleeding regions of the calcaneus. The entire Achilles tendon involved in the necrosis was removed, as well as its insertion, to the calcaneus. Bone debridement was continued until brisk bleeding surfaces were noted. Debridement resulted in a wound measuring 8 by 14 cm. One week after debridement a microvascular transfer of the right gracilis muscle was performed (Fig. 3), with end-to-side vessel anastomosis between the gracilis artery and posterior tibial artery and with end-to-side venous repair between the gracilis venae comitans and posterior tibial venae comitans. A split-thickness skin graft measuring 0.018 of an inch with a surface area of 10 by 16 cm was harvested from the left lateral buttock and placed over the viable gracilis muscle (Fig. 4). Technical points of the transfer include adequate inset of the gracilis muscle beneath a 2 cm skin-elevated edge surrounding the wound and adequate approximation of the gracilis fascia to the surrounding dermis to recreate a smooth skin muscle interface (see Fig. 4). In this case, no attempt to reconstruct the Achilles musculotendinous unit was performed. Postoperatively, the patient was placed in a posterior plaster splint to maintain some plantar foot flexion, and previously placed Jackson-Pratt suction drains were positioned to wall suction.

Postoperative monitoring via temperature probes was performed for 1 week with differential temperatures between the proximal and distal probes of less than 0.05 °C. Probes and Jackson-Pratt drains were removed 1 week postoperatively and ambulation was gradually initiated 4 weeks postoperatively. Continual ace wrap conforming support was used to expedite lymphatic egress and to minimize edema. The foot was gradually brought up into neutral position with return of "Achilles" tendon function. The con-

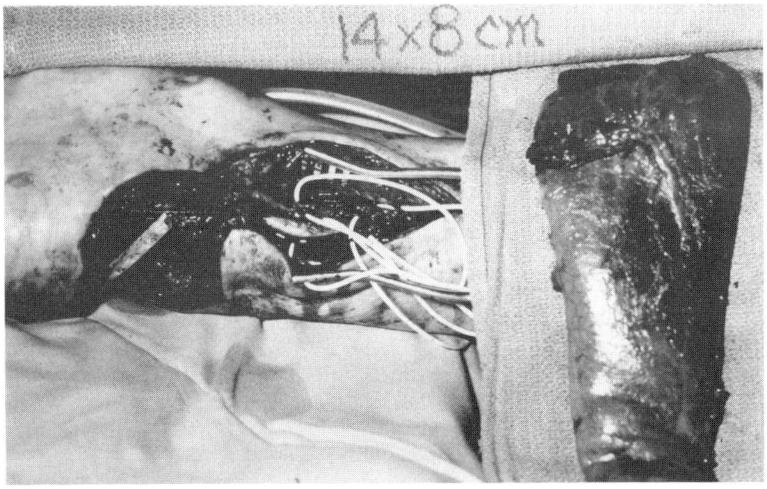

Figure 3 Open debrided wound with gracilis muscle ready for inset. Posterior tibial vessels have been dissected.

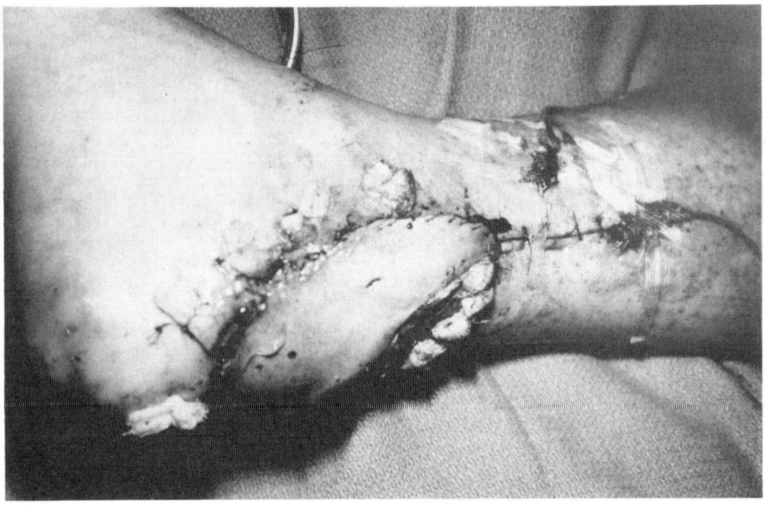

Figure 4 Skin-graft covered muscle. Right leg, heel to left view.

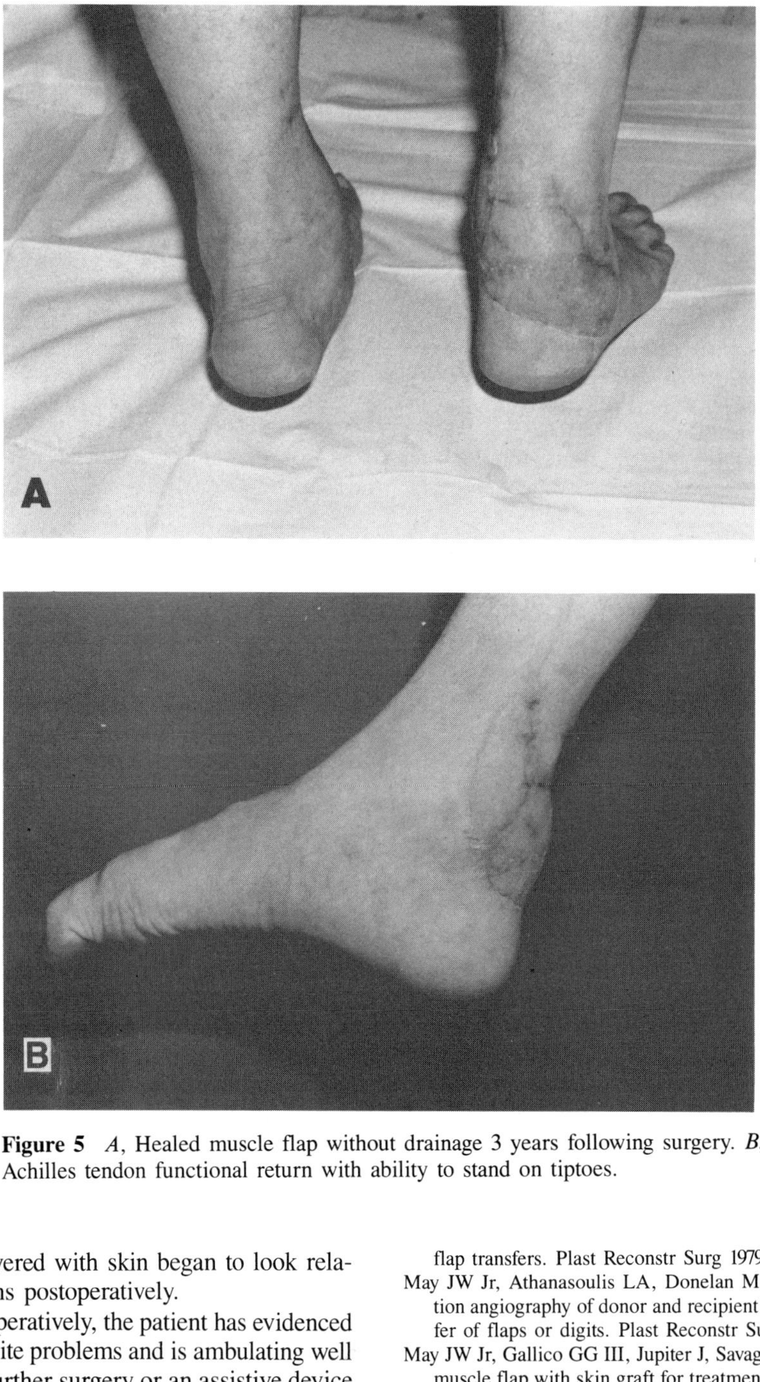

Figure 5 *A*, Healed muscle flap without drainage 3 years following surgery. *B*, Achilles tendon functional return with ability to stand on tiptoes.

tour of the muscle covered with skin began to look relatively normal 3 months postoperatively.

Three years postoperatively, the patient has evidenced no donor or recipient site problems and is ambulating well without the need for further surgery or an assistive device for walking (Fig. 5).

The authors would like to thank the residents and fellows in Plastic Surgery at the Massachusetts General Hospital for their help in the care of this patient. We also appreciate the assistance of Ms. Jeanne M. Spindler in manuscript preparation.

SUGGESTED READING

Bas L, May JW Jr, Handren J, Fallon J. End-to-end versus end-to-side microvascular anastomosis patency in experimental venous repairs. Plast Reconstr Surg 1986; 77(3):442–448.

Godina M. Preferential use of end-to-side arterial anastomoses in free flap transfers. Plast Reconstr Surg 1979;64:673–682.

May JW Jr, Athanasoulis LA, Donelan MB. Preoperative magnification angiography of donor and recipient sites for clinical free transfer of flaps or digits. Plast Reconstr Surg 1979; 64:483–490.

May JW Jr, Gallico GG III, Jupiter J, Savage RC. Free latissimus dorsi muscle flap with skin graft for treatment of traumatic chronic bony wounds. Plast Reconstr Surg 1983; 73:691–699.

May JW Jr, Gallico GG III, Lukash FN. Microvascular transfer of free tissue for closure of bone wounds of the distal lower extremity. N Engl J Med 1982; 306:253–257.

May JW Jr, Lukash FN, Gallico GG III. Latissimus dorsi free muscle flap in lower extremity reconstruction. Plast Reconstr Surg 1981; 68:603–607.

May JW Jr, Lukash FN, Gallico GG III, Stirrat CR. Removable thermocouple probe microvascular patency monitor: an experimental and clinical, study. Plast Reconstr Surg 1983; 72:366–379.

Moore JR, Weiland AJ. Vascularized tissue transfers in the treatment of osteomyelitis. Clin Plast Surg 1980; 13(4):657–662.

Rosenthal RE, MacPhail JA, Ortiz JE. Nonunion in open tibial fractures: analysis of reason for failure of treatment. J Bone Joint Surg 1977; 59A:244.

LYMPHEDEMA

TIMOTHY A. MILLER, M.D., F.A.C.S.

Lymphedema of the extremity remains one of the more resistant clinical problems in surgery. The etiology of the edema process remains obscure and the pathophysiology is poorly understood. As a result, operative procedures designed to reconstruct lymphatic flow are completely unsuccessful. It is a discouraging reality that we are unable to cure lymphedema by either medical or surgical means.

Because of our inability to cure lymphedema, varying amounts of postoperative swelling inevitably occur. As a result of the lack of an objective end point, the evaluation of surgical results is frequently subjective and inexact. In addition, because most of the operative procedures designed for lymphedema are anatomically unexciting and recurrence inevitable, most surgeons' interest in this problem wanes rather quickly. Few long-term studies of patients followed for periods greater than a few years exist in the literature. The lymphedema patient is frequently relegated to the uncomfortable position of being sent from physician to physician and advised of a number of conflicting methods of care. They are frequently offered unrealistic expectations of success from operative procedures that offer only modest improvement.

We have a very imperfect understanding of the lymphedema process. While it is likely that congenital lymphedema represents a group of patients with a fewer number ("hypoplastic") of lymphatics, the occurrence of lymphedema following regional node dissection or irradiation is puzzling (Fig. 1). Two questions immediately come to mind with regard to the appearance of secondary or "acquired" lymphedema:

1. Why does not *every* patient develop lymphedema following a standard anatomic dissection?
2. Why is there always a delay of 6 months to 1 year before the edema process begins? What is the status of lymphatic flow in that interval of time?

When these questions can be answered, a more realistic and physiologically sound approach to lymphedema of the extremity can be undertaken.

SURGICAL THERAPY

At this time, there are many operative choices. In general, these operative procedures can be divided into two categories: physiologic and excisional procedures. Physiologic procedures are those that attempt to reconstruct lymphatic flow by introducing a pedicle of omentum, skin flap, prosthetic material (e.g., nylon threads), or buried dermis. This approach attempts to create a bridge to drain the involved edematous extremity into the trunk area. Although success has been reported sporadi-

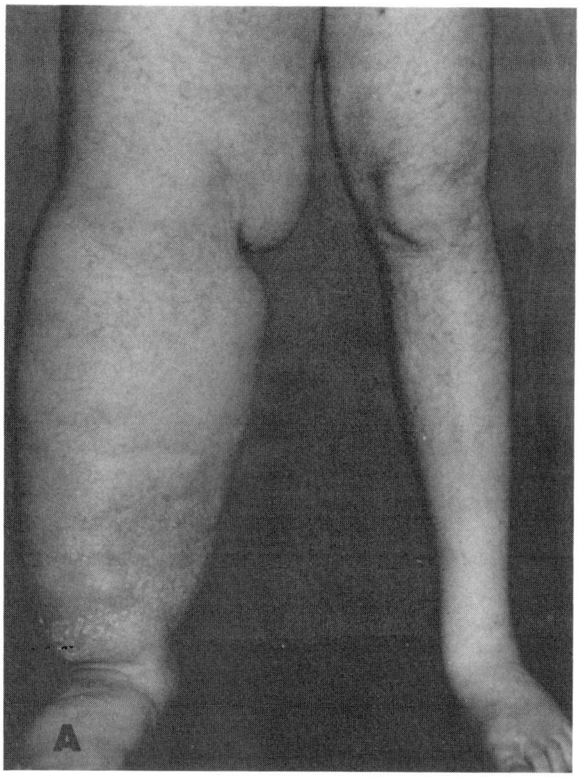

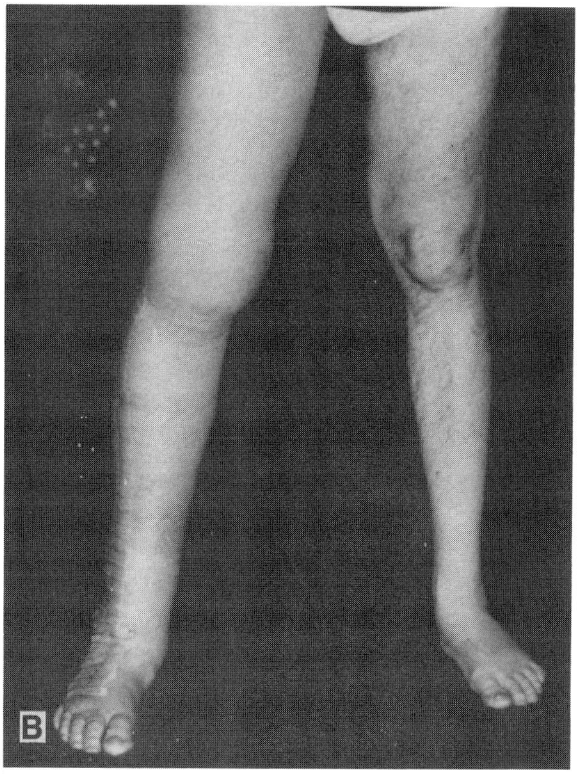

Figure 1 The patient is a 42-year-old white male who developed lymphedema of the right leg (*A*) post inguinal node dissection and radiation for testicular carcinoma. The same patient is shown (*B*) 8 months following medial and immediately postlateral reduction surgery.

cally, these operations have, in general, been found to be less than optimal in their success. In addition, it should be pointed out that there has been no documentation that the newly reconstructed lymphatic channels actually improve lymph drainage of the extremity.

Promising results have now been reported with lymphatic–lymphatic and lymphatic–venous microsurgical techniques. While these reports are encouraging, complete resolution of the edema process has not been seen and these microsurgical methods are frequently supplemented by excisional operative procedures.

The latter procedures remove varying amounts of skin, subcutaneous tissue, and deep fascia. The most radical procedure is the operation named after Charles, originally described in 1917. This procedure excises all of the involved skin, subcutaneous tissue, and fascia, and split-thickness skin grafts are placed on the extremity. This operation is mentioned only in order to strongly condemn its use. The presence of split-thickness skin grafts on the lower extremity of a patient with lymphedema is, in itself, such a deforming and hazardous procedure that, in my experience, the operative procedure is far worse than the original disease process.

Favorable reports of full-thickness skin grafts utilized to cover these defects have appeared in the literature. It is a substantial technical challenge to obtain complete graft take of full-thickness grafts over the entire lower extremity.

For these reasons, it is my opinion that the best available operative procedure is to remove as much skin and subcutaneous tissue as possible and close the defect beneath skin flaps. This operative procedure (erroneously referred to as the Kondolean procedure) was first described by Sistrunck in 1917. By this method, early wound closure is accomplished and substantial amounts of tissue can be removed. The operative procedure is usually performed in two stages; first operating on the medial side of the extremity and, 3 months later, on the lateral aspect (see Fig. 1).

The results of this operation are consistently good—although patients are never cured. It is not uncommon for the swelling of the extremity to be relieved by 50 percent after this operation. Other than the creation of a scar, and areas of reduced sensation over the skin of the flaps developed from the midmedial and midlateral areas, the complications of this operative procedure are extremely low.

All patients wear an elastic stocking during the postoperative period and are urged to avoid periods of prolonged standing to periodically elevate the involved extremity. It has been found that approximately 80 percent of patients have substantial improvement by this method and a significant reduction in the incidence of cellulitis (30 percent preoperatively to 9 percent postoperatively).

It should be emphasized that this method of therapy is the best available at this time. It should be offered to the patients, not as a means of curing lymphedema but rather as an adjunct to control of the symptoms related to the increased swelling and size of the extremity.

SUGGESTED READING

Fox U, Montrsi M, Romagnoli G. Microsurgical treatment of lymphedema of the limbs. Int Surg 1981; 66:53–56.

Miller TA. Surgical management of lymphedema of the extremity. Plast Reconstr Surg 1975; 56:633–641.

Miller TA. Lymphedema. In: Grabb WC, Smith JW, eds. Plastic Surgery, Boston: Little, Brown, 1979; 826.

Miller TA. Charles procedure for lymphedema: a warning. Am J Surg 1980; 139:290–292.

O'Brien BM. Shafiroff BB. Microlymphatico venous and resectional surgery in obstructive lymphedema. World J Surg 1979; 3:3–15, 121–123.

Puckett CL, Jacobs GR, Hurvitz JS, Silver D. Evaluation of lymphovenous anastomosis in obstructive lymphedema. Plast Reconstr Surg 1980; 66:116–120.

Tang H, Zhu J, Yu G, et al. Experimental observations of transportation of vein graft to lymphatics. Ann Plast Surg 1985; 15:285–295.

Thompson N. The surgical treatment of chronic lymphoedema of the extremities. Surg Clin North Am 1967; 47:445–503.

INDEX